Handbook on Children's Speech

DEVELOPMENT, DISORDERS, AND VARIATIONS

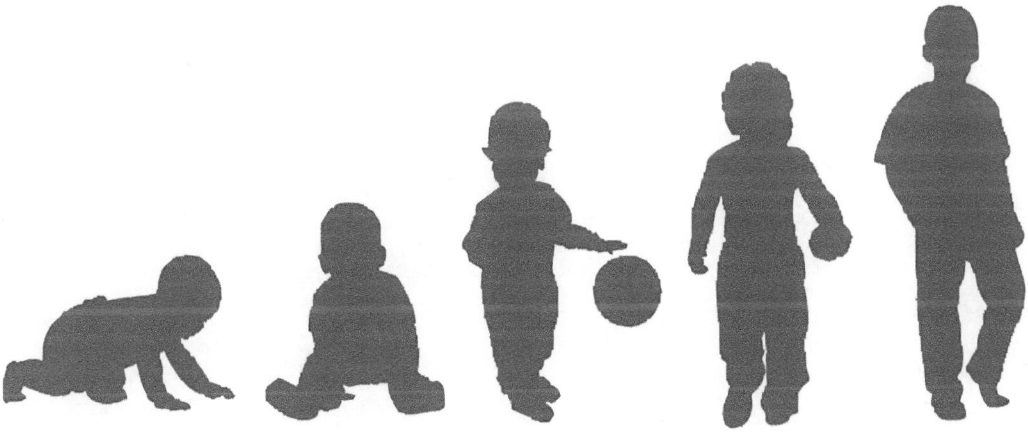

Handbook on Children's Speech

DEVELOPMENT, DISORDERS, AND VARIATIONS

Raymond D. Kent, PhD

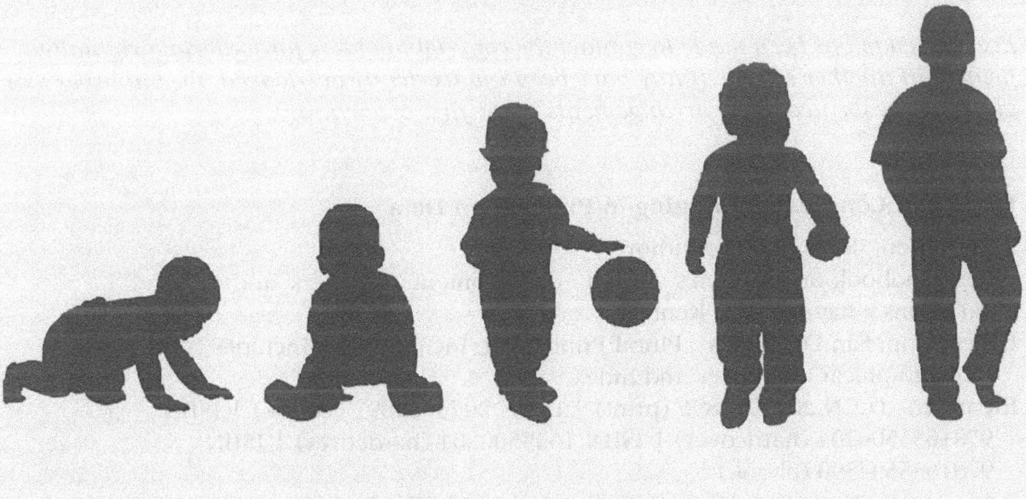

PLURAL PUBLISHING INC.

Plural Publishing Inc.

9177 Aero Drive, Suite B
San Diego, CA 92123

email: information@pluralpublishing.com
website: https://www.pluralpublishing.com

Typeset in 10.5/13 Garamond by Flanagan's Publishing Services, Inc.
Printed in the United States of America by Integrated Books International

Library of Congress Cataloging-in-Publication Data

Names: Kent, Raymond D., author.
Title: Handbook on children's speech : development, disorders, and variations / Raymond D. Kent.
Description: San Diego, CA : Plural Publishing, Inc., [2024] | Includes bibliographical references and index.
Identifiers: LCCN 2023024896 (print) | LCCN 2023024897 (ebook) | ISBN 9781635506204 (hardcover) | ISBN 1635506204 (hardcover) | ISBN 9781635504590 (ebook)
Subjects: MESH: Speech Disorders--diagnosis | Child | Speech Disorders--therapy | Speech Therapy--methods | Speech--physiology | Language Development
Classification: LCC RJ496.S7 (print) | LCC RJ496.S7 (ebook) | NLM WV 501 | DDC 618.92/855--dc23/eng/20230822
LC record available at https://lccn.loc.gov/2023024896
LC ebook record available at https://lccn.loc.gov/2023024897

CONTENTS

Preface *vii*
Acknowledgments *xi*

1 Introduction 1

2 Biological and Psychological Foundations of Speech Development 21

3 Systems and Processes in Spoken and Inner Language 57

4 Typical Speech Development 79

5 Assessment of Articulation and Sensorimotor Functions 117

6 Assessment of Voice and Prosody 159

7 Assessment of Phonology 191

8 Assessment of Intelligibility, Comprehensibility, and Other Global Features 217

9 Principles of Motor Development and Motor Learning of Speech 237

10 Bilingualism and Dialects 257

11 Clinical Populations and Conditions 279

12 Prevention, Treatment, and Clinical Decision Making 321

Appendix A. International Phonetic Alphabet (IPA) *353*
Appendix B. Variations of the Oral Mechanism Examination *355*
Appendix C. Cranial Nerve Summary *357*
References *359*
Index *455*

PREFACE

Speech is such a distinguishing feature of humans that Dennis Fry (1977) suggested we should be called *homo loquens* ("the talking animal"). For most people in the world, speech is the most used form of communication. It is estimated that on average we produce about 1000 words every waking hour, which makes speech one of our most highly practiced motor abilities. Development of speech in children is one of the most significant milestones observed by parents and specialists in child development. The word *infant* is derived from the Latin *infans*, meaning "unable to speak." There are many ways in which infants differ from adults, but the term given to this early phase of development pertains to only one—speech, or rather the lack of it. But, as discussed in this book, lack of speech in its adult form does not mean that children, at even the youngest ages, are not already on the path to spoken language. A great deal of research on infant vocalizations has produced what might be called "the book of babble," a collection of research articles that shows how cooing and babbling are foundations for speech development. Children produce their first words around their first birthday and then proceed on a course of rapid language development. Speech is a robust faculty that is acquired by most children despite large variations in language stimulation, socioeconomic level, and general health status. However, speech development can be disrupted or delayed in some children, with potentially profound consequences on quality of life. This book considers how speech develops in children, why speech disorders arise, and why variations such as dialect can occur in different populations. The book subtitle reflects this three-part goal: development, disorders, and variations.

The Facets of Speech

Speech in the general sense can be defined as the audible form of language expression. The systems of speech production convert an intended message to movements that generate an acoustic signal that is heard and decoded by listeners. Speech has several facets, as discussed in the following.

Language. The most obvious facet of speech is linguistic communication. Speech, along with gestures, is the earliest form of communication in childhood. It is also the primary means of human communication throughout the world. Speech offers several advantages as a means of communication. It is produced with our own body structures (therefore does not rely on tools or devices), can be transmitted by telephony, does not require visual cues, and contains different kinds of information in addition to the linguistic message (more on this below).

Gender and age. Speech provides cues as to a person's gender and age. When we receive a telephone call from an unknown person, we can quickly form opinions on whether the caller is male or female, young or old. Speech is highly sexually dimorphic, meaning that it is quite different between the sexes. Speech also changes with age, especially during childhood and adolescence.

Culture and language. Speech patterns are specific to individual languages. The imprint of a first language can influence learning another language, so that the additional language usually has a non-native accent. All speakers have a dialect that reflects geographic and social factors. The way we speak identifies us as part of a speech community that shares a language and a dialect.

Individual identity. We often can identify a familiar person just from the sound of his or her voice, as when the person says "hello" over a telephone. Speech is a personal identifier in which idiosyncratic features are combined with aspects of gender, age, and culture. Speech, like our faces, is individually distinctive. When we speak, we announce ourselves.

Emotion. Aside from facial expression, speech is the major way of expressing emotions. Children learn very early in life that vocalization can signal discomfort, pleasure, and other emotional states. Speech is nearly always imbued with emotion. Even the so-called neutral tone of voice is a type of emotion. This emotional component has both expressive and receptive domains. We learn how to express emotions in our own speech and to recognize them in others.

Health. Speech can be affected by state of health, as when a listener detects that a speaker is tired or has a cold. Speech can be disordered in various ways, as detailed in this book. Some speech disorders arise for unknown reasons, whereas others are associated with developmental conditions such as autism spectrum disorder or hearing loss.

Speech as Complexity

Even a simple utterance can combine these various facets. Speech also is a combination of skills related to audition, somatosensation, phonology, and motor control. It is one of the fastest and most precisely timed of human behaviors. Ordinary speech is extraordinary in many ways, and decades of research have been conducted to understand it. Although most six-year-old children are highly intelligible to strangers, the development of various aspects of speech continues into puberty and adolescence. But even in adulthood, speech undergoes continual refinement in an apparent effort to achieve optimal performance. The scientist Karl S. Lashley took speech as the prime example of serial ordering of behavior, and it is prowess in this domain that sets speech apart from other human skills and activities.

Contemporary understanding of speech in children is multidisciplinary, including the fields of developmental biology, developmental psychology, genetics, linguistics, medicine, neuroscience, and speech-language pathology. These and other fields are needed to create an account of how speech develops, how it can be disordered, and how it reflects cultural and individual experiences. A natural consequence of this synthesis is the emergence of new subdisciplines, such as the developmental neuroscience of speech disorders, which enfolds speech development, speech disorders, and neuroscience to portray new methods of diagnosis and treatment.

Because speech draws on many body systems and processes, it is not surprising that many different conditions can imperil speech development. Many, but surely not all, of these conditions are outlined in this book. But for many speech disorders, the cause simply is not known. In medical parlance, these are idiopathic disorders (idiopathic denotes a disease or condition that arises spontaneously or for which the cause is unknown). Many different therapies have been developed to improve speech production, and this book describes more than 30 such treatments along with summaries of evidence for their effectiveness.

Speech as we usually think of it is directed to others for the purpose of communicating thoughts, feelings, and experiences. But speech takes two other common forms. One is private speech, that is, speech directed to oneself and not to others. The other form is inner or covert speech, which is not really spoken but nonetheless shares many properties with spoken speech. Inner speech has important functions of monitoring, self-regulation, and reflection. Textbooks on speech development and disorders usually pay little attention to inner speech. To be sure, inner speech is not easily studied, but the scientific literature attests to its importance. Sometimes we speak not to be heard but rather to reflect and self-direct.

Risk Factors in Speech Disorders

Although many different factors can pose risks for speech disorders in children, research shows that the most prominent risk factors in different countries are male sex, family history, and birth difficulties. Speech disorders also occur in many different diseases and conditions, including anatomic anomalies, neurodevelopmental disorders, genetic syndromes, hearing impairment, and socioeconomic disadvantage.

Adultcentrism

This book suffers from a limitation that is all too common in discussions of child development—it has an adultcentric point of view. Adultcentrism is the tendency of adults to view children and their experiences from a biased, adult perspective (Goode, 1986). As Petr (1992) points out, this perspective is evident in the formulation of stage theories of child development that lead to the implicit presumptions that children are incomplete and essentially incompetent. Adults, being on the far end of maturity on any such stage model, become the standard of completion and competence. Children, by definition, fall short. Stage models are presented several times in this book because they are convenient and economical in portraying development. Unfortunately, they tend to carry the misconceptions and distortions of adultcentrism. A consequence of adultcentrism is underestimation of children's abilities. At one time, it was proposed that human infants were basically subcortical in their neural processes and largely unaware of the complexities of human speech. But it is now clear that infants are capable of statistical learning, defined as the ability to detect statistical regularities in their environment. This kind of learning potentially applies to virtually all levels of human language (Romberg & Saffran, 2010) and compels a new perspective on how even the youngest members of our species recognize structure in their environments and use this information to fuel the development of language and cognition. It has been shown that some language tracts in the brain are already formed at birth.

The author has no real remedy for adultcentrism in this book, but a remedy in practice is to try to see children at any point of development as being complete and competent within the circumstances of their lives. Words such as immature, undeveloped, unsophisticated, and simplistic should be used (if used at all) with due regard to the powerful phenomena that underlie lifelong development. Merrick and Roulstone (2011) wrote, "Children have the right to express their views and influence decisions in matters that affect them. Yet decisions regarding speech-language pathology are often made on their behalf, and research into the perspectives of children who receive speech-language pathology intervention is currently limited" (p. 281). Adult perspectives and opinions should be balanced by consideration of how children view themselves and their abilities. Children and their parents do not always share the same attitudes (McCormack, McLeod, & Crowe, 2019).

Intended Audience

This book may be of interest to anyone who seeks to understand speech development in children, but it is focused especially on disorders and variations. The challenge facing speech-language therapists and other professionals is illustrated by the example of a 6-year-old child who has a speech disorder accompanied by a mild hearing loss, a dental malocclusion, and a family history of communication disorder. As a further complication, this child is learning English as a second language that is not spoken at home.

References

Fry, D. (1977). *Homo loquens: Man as a talking animal.* Cambridge University Press.

Goode, D. (1986). Kids, cultures, and innocents. *Human Studies*, *9*, 85–106.

McCormack, J., McLeod, S., & Crowe, K. (2019, March). What do children with speech sound disorders think about their talking? *Seminars In Speech and Language*, *40*(02), 94–104.

Merrick, R., & Roulstone, S. (2011). Children's views of communication and speech-language pathology. *International Journal of Speech-Language Pathology*, *13*(4), 281–290. https://doi.org/10.3109/17549507.2011.577809

Petr, C. G. (1992). Adultcentrism in practice with children. *Families in Society*, *73*(7), 408–416.

Romberg, A. R., & Saffran, J. R. (2010). Statistical learning and language acquisition. *Wiley Interdisciplinary Reviews: Cognitive Science*, *1*(6), 906–914. https://doi:10.1002/wcs.78

ACKNOWLEDGMENTS

Many thanks to Plural Publishing for bringing this book to reality. Valerie Johns helped me to design the work plan and offered valuable advice throughout the process. Jessica Bristow and Lori Asbury handled production matters with grace and efficiency. It has been a pleasure to work with them. Angie Singh has ably directed the publishing company since the death of her husband, Dr. Sadanand Singh—a visionary, philosopher, and extraordinary friend. He was a vigorous champion of books and authors, and I am indebted to him for a rewarding personal relationship filled with thoughtful and inspiring conversations. He is fondly remembered.

Deep thanks to my wife Jane, who is steadfast in her encouragement and support. As my partner in life for more than 50 years, she has been patient, wise, and loving. For that and more, I am forever grateful.

Sixty years ago, I took a class called Introduction to Speech Pathology at the University of Montana. I was intrigued by a field of study that combined biology, psychology, and linguistics with a clinical focus (the mission and basic content of this book). I hold in great esteem Professors Charles D. Parker and Richard M. Boehmler, who shined a light on my academic path. I followed their example and pursued graduate studies at the University of Iowa, where I was deeply influenced by Professors James F. Curtis and Kenneth L. Moll, who modeled the practice of clinical and basic science. After obtaining my PhD, I took a postdoctoral fellowship at the Massachusetts Institute of Technology, where I had the great fortune to delve more deeply into speech acoustics and speech synthesis, with guidance from Professor Kenneth N. Stevens and Dr. Dennis H. Klatt. I acknowledge them all with admiration and gratitude.

My career was based at the University of Wisconsin-Madison and the Boys Town Institute for Communication Disorders in Children (Omaha, Nebraska). Along the way, I had the opportunity to interact with many scientists and clinicians, as well as a host of undergraduate and graduate students. They are part of a fulfilling life. The standard form of a curriculum vitae is a listing of positions, publications, and presentations, but it often fails to note the very important contributions of people who helped to shape interests, aspirations, and goals. This acknowledgment is a humble effort in that direction.

To SLPs and SLTs who help children on the path to spoken language.

1

INTRODUCTION

This book considers the various processes underlying speech development and speech disorders in children. Speech is defined as movements or movement plans that produce acoustic patterns that accord with the phonetic structure of a language. This definition implies that speech should be understood as a motor activity, an acoustic signal, an encoding of a linguistic message, and reception of that message in a listener's brain. But that is not all. Speech is a primary means of individual recognition and emotional expression. Even a simple utterance can carry information on the intended linguistic message, the speaker's identity and cultural background, and the speaker's emotional state. Speech is a motor act that is learned and maintained through sensory information, primarily but not exclusively from the auditory and somatosensory (kinesthetic and tactile) channels. The intimate connections between motor and sensory aspects compels use of the term *sensorimotor*.

A major part of learning to speak is learning the sensorimotor skills of what is very likely the most highly coordinated motor behavior that most humans possess. The task is complicated by the large number of muscles involved (100 or so different muscles in the oral, laryngeal, and respiratory organs), the precise control of spatial and temporal parameters, and the essential linkage to cognition and language. It should be emphasized that a focus on sensorimotor processes does not mean that this book pertains only to children's motor speech disorders as typically defined. Rather, the effort is to examine how sensorimotor and other processes factor into the general experience of learning to produce intelligible speech and how these processes are disrupted in children's speech disorders, of which there are several kinds.

It is well to note that speech is a distinctive feature of humans, so much so that it has been argued that our species may as well be called *homo loquens* ("talking animal") as *homo sapiens* ("wise man") (Fry, 1977; Pulgram, 1970). The uniqueness of speech to humans is relevant to this book because it implies specialties that underlie the development and use of speech as a tool of communication and cognition. Perhaps chief among these specialties are the neural connections between the cerebral cortex, cerebellum, and the vocal organs. Interestingly, the word *infant* is from the Latin for "unable to speak" or "speechless." There are many things that infants cannot do, but inability to speak is a common label for this stage of life and signals the importance attached to the faculty of speech.

> "Speech, as the preferred output modality for human language, is an unusual feature of our species that depends upon a complex but well-understood set of mechanisms, including vocal/motor, auditory/perceptual, and central neural mechanisms. The capacity for speech clearly differentiates humans from other primates . . . " (Fitch, 2018, p. 256)

Coverage of the book's topic includes two major interrelated domains: (1) speech development and (2) pediatric speech disorders focusing on the ages of birth to puberty. Because speech disorders in children occur against a complex developmental background, the understanding of these disorders requires knowledge about how speech develops and how it is affected in children with disorders. These topics are introduced in the following two sections.

Speech Development

Speech development can be defined as the continuous, age-related process of change in speech patterns over the lifespan. The process of change is influenced by both maturation and experience. Motor control is adapted to anatomic, physiologic, and cognitive changes that occur over the lifespan, even into advanced age. Understanding speech development requires consideration of developmental changes in the anatomy and physiology of the speech production system, the maturation of sensory and cognitive capabilities, the refinement of language skills and abilities, and the social experience of communication. This book concentrates on the early part of the process of speech development (when speech and language are largely developing) but many of the principles can be extended to later phases such as adolescence and adulthood. A child's journey to intelligible speech begins with infant vocalizations such as coos and babble. Most infants utter their first words at about one year of age, produce about 50 to 200 different words at two years of age, and learn about 21 words each day in early childhood.

> "That every child learns to talk is such a commonplace observation that we have to stop and think about it to appreciate what a miracle of development it really is. And once it is appreciated, it is almost impossible to suppress your curiosity. I find it one of the most challenging mysteries on the agenda of psychological science." (G. Miller [1977] *Spontaneous apprentices: Children and language* [pp. 19–20]. Seabury Press.)

Speech production is malleable to some degree in both children and adults, probably more so in the former, as discussed in Chapter 10, which deals with the issues of bilingualism and dialect. It is commonly believed that malleability is limited, especially in adults, which could explain the difficulty that adult speakers have in acquiring another language (L2) that is free from the influences of the first language (L1). It has been proposed that L2 learning is limited by maturational constraints. According to Lenneberg (1969, p. 639), " . . . the maturation of the brain marks the end of regulation and locks certain functions into place." Scovel (1988) suggested that a critical period for L2 speech learning closes at about 12 years owing to decreased brain plasticity that accompanies neural maturation. Patkowski (1980, 1990) concluded that a critical period for the learning of both L2 speech and morphosyntax closes at about 15 years of age. However, other authors assert that plasticity can be observed in both language and the brain. Even in adults, L1 is not rigid and permanent but rather dynamic and fluid. Research reviewed by Chang (2012) has shown restructuring of sound patterns in L1 through the influence of L2 (a phenomenon known as **phonetic drift**), and significant, sometimes rapid, adjustments to L1 speech in response to a variety of environmental factors. The concept of life-long plasticity is discussed in detail by de Leeuw and Celata (2019) and other articles in a special issue of the *Journal of Phonetics*. The topic of a critical period (or several critical periods) is examined more fully in Chapter 10.

Languages have their own phonetic systems, with different repertoires of vowels and consonants, different melodies, and different rhythms. It has been proposed that languages even have their own **phonetic settings**, that is, a tendency for the speech production system to return to a language-specific habitual configuration (Honikman, 1964). Mennen et al. (2010) wrote of this configuration as follows, "For example, languages may differ in their degree of lip-rounding, tension of the lips and tongue, jaw position, phonation types, pitch range and register" (p. 13). Perhaps speakers adopt phonetic settings to facilitate the demanding sensorimotor functions in speech production that are keyed to the phonetic and phonological features of a language. If so, learning a second language is not just a matter of learning its phonemes or other segments but a matter of learning the optimal settings of the speech production system.

Information relating to typical speech development (covered in Chapter 4) is essential to understanding speech itself and the nature of speech disorders. The process begins in utero, given that the fetal auditory system is capable of processing aspects of the speech signal, such as the mother's voice and the overall prosody. Newborns typically announce their arrival with a robust cry, which is evidence of a healthy respiratory system and the beginning of vocal behavior. Thereafter, vocal development proceeds from cooing and babbling vocalizations to first words and eventually to multisyllabic utterances with syntactic structure. Understanding typical patterns of development is essential to clinical assessment and treatment. Chapter 4 summarizes how speech takes form as the consequence of processes of maturation and experience. The developmental process draws on several capabilities and resources, including sensory function, motor control, and phonological acquisition.

Pediatric Speech Disorders and Variations

The second component of this book, pediatric speech disorders and other speech variations, pertains to aspects of impaired (or atypical) speech development and to speech development in bilingualism. These two broad categories are sometimes labeled disorders and differences. The disorders are not easily defined and are not well understood with respect to their prevalence and incidence. MedlinePlus (n.d.), an information source of the National Library of Medicine, defines **speech disorder** as "a condition in which a person has problems creating or forming the speech sounds needed to communicate with others. This can make the child's speech difficult to understand" (https://medlineplus.gov/ency/article/001430.htm#:~:text=A%20speech%20disorder%20is%20a,Articulation%20disorders). This source goes on to identify the common speech disorders to include articulation disorders, phonological disorders, disfluency, voice disorders, and resonance disorders. But this is only a partial list—one that is expanded in this book, especially in Chapter 11. A further complication is that a specific speech disorder may co-occur with other disorders, such as another type of speech disorder (e.g., articulation disorder accompanied by developmental stuttering), as well as language and hearing disorders. For present purposes, a **speech disorder** is defined as any impaired, habitual pattern of speech production that members of the speaker's sociolinguistic community regard as atypical or significantly inappropriate. A **speech difference**, for lack of a better term, is the effect of bilingual or multilingual experience on a child's speech development. This effect is not a disorder. but it can co-occur with a disorder, and that poses challenges to clinical assessment. Much more is said about this in Chapter 10.

Unfortunately, it is not always straightforward to differentiate speech disorders from language disorders, and this difficulty has complicated efforts to determine the incidence and prevalence of these disorders. Raghavan et al. (2018) concluded from a review of studies on this topic that, "existing data sources do not capture the condition [speech and language disorders] in a reliable, uniform, or systematically valid manner, which poses a barrier to population level ascertainment of the condition. Current survey data also do not sufficiently permit the separation of speech and language disorders into speech, language, and other communication disorders" (p. 11).

A further complication is that speech disorders often are comorbid with various health and socioeconomic factors (Keating et al., 2001), a point that recurs throughout this book. But whatever the exact percentage of affected children may be, a significant number of children have a speech disorder that affects their quality of life, and, in some individuals, the disorder can have lifelong consequences.

Clinical conditions can be described in terms of several aspects, as follows:

1. **Phenomenology** is the systematic description and classification of phenomena without efforts at explanation or interpretation. A phenomenological description pertains to the observed signs and symptoms of a disorder (e.g., a listing of misarticulations in a child's speech without interpretation as to cause). Such descriptions are useful in determining the presence and/or severity of a disorder.
2. **Etiology** is the cause or causes of a disease or abnormal condition (e.g., identifying hearing loss as contributing to a child's speech disorder). Speech disorders in children are linked to several different etiologies,

and a significant proportion are considered **idiopathic** (meaning "unknown cause"). Some disorders are thought to have a **multifactorial etiology** in which two or more factors play a role in causing or exacerbating the condition. Frequently occurring etiologies, either alone or in combination, include hearing impairment, structural anomaly such as cleft palate, motor disorder, genetic influences, and sociocultural factors.

3. **Epidemiology** is the study of the distribution and determinants of health-related states or events in specified populations. Epidemiologic studies tell us how often diseases, disorders, or other conditions occur in different groups of people and why (e.g., showing that speech disorders occur more frequently in boys than girls).
4. **Pathogenesis** is the course of an illness or condition, from its origin to manifestation and outbreak (e.g., showing that a speech disorder in early childhood may be linked to a later disorder of reading). A similar concept is the **natural history** of a disorder or condition (i.e., how it changes over time). Speech disorders often have a developmental profile that reflects general processes of maturation as well as a child's social interactions.
5. **Treatment** is intervention to normalize a disorder, provide compensations if normalization is not possible, or to prevent worsening (e.g., initiate therapy to correct misarticulations and improve speech intelligibility). Across clinical specialties, treatments are increasingly studied with the principles of evidence-based practice, in which outcomes are evaluated with standardized tools.
6. **Prevention** is any course of action that decreases the likelihood that a person will have a disease or other condition (e.g., identify and modify conditions that put a child at risk for a communication disorder). As explained in Chapter 12, prevention takes several different forms.

Many speech disorders can be associated with atypical motor patterns of speech production, and it is important to distinguish motor speech disorders from general motor processes in speech development. Discussions of **motor speech disorder (MSD)** in children usually identify three or four disorders: **childhood apraxia of speech (CAS)**, **dysarthria**, **motor speech delay (MSD)**, and perhaps a yet-to-be defined disorder (let's call it Disorder X, which may not be a single disorder at all but rather a group of disorders). CAS has attracted a great deal of clinical attention and substantial progress has been made in its diagnosis, treatment, and etiology, although differing views persist about its nature and treatment. Childhood dysarthria, unlike adult dysarthria, has no widely recognized classification of types, although some progress has been made in identifying the responsible neural lesions. It does not appear that classifications used in acquired dysarthria in adults align with the speech disorder in children (Morgan & Liégeois, 2010; Schölderle, Haas, & Ziegler, 2021). Motor speech delay was described by Shriberg et al. (2019) as a pediatric motor speech disorder distinct from childhood dysarthria and CAS, and it was proposed as an addition to the Speech Disorders Classification System (SDCS; Shriberg et al.,

1997). The 10 signs of speech motor delay found in more than 50% of the children who were positive on the sign included age-inappropriate precision and stability behaviors in speech, prosody, and voice domains, with the most frequently occurring signs involving speech production.

The hypothetical Disorder X mentioned earlier is not established as a clinical entity, but the reason for its mention is to recognize growing evidence that motor factors contribute to speech disorders that are not confidently categorized as CAS, dysarthria, or speech motor delay. Vermiglio (2014) wrote that a clinical entity is defined by the Sydenham-Guttentag criteria (Guttentag, 1949), namely that it must (1) have an unambiguous definition, (2) represent a homogenous group with a perceived limitation, and (3) facilitate a diagnosis and intervention. Defining a clinical entity is important for many reasons, including effective diagnosis, treatment, and reimbursement for clinical services. Naming a disorder is an important step because it distinguishes the disorder from others and leads to clinical descriptions relevant to assessment and treatment.

Aside from the commonly recognized MSDs, motor issues are important to understanding speech sound disorders in the general sense, including **articulatory/phonological disorder**, which is a general term for speech sound disorders of nonspecific origin. The terms **articulatory disorder** and **phonological disorder** are used in research and clinical practice, but the distinction between them is not clearly specified. For this reason, the term articulatory/phonological disorder (or phonological/articulatory disorder) is used to encompass a broad range of speech sound disorders. However, the more neutral term **speech sound disorder (SSD)** appears to be gaining favor, partly because it is not always clear how to distinguish articulatory from phonological components for an individual child. Namasivayam et al. (2020) wrote,

> The present definition describes SSD as a range of difficulties producing speech sounds in children that can be due to a variety of limitations related to perceptual, speech motor, or linguistic processes (or a combination) of known (e.g., Down syndrome, cleft lip and palate) and unknown origin. (p. 2)

The term **speech sound** is frequently used without definition. When a definition is offered, it may be something like *individual units of speech production* (which could be phonetic segments, phonemes, or perhaps some other element). Lindblom (1990) wrote, "What is a speech sound? Although phonetics is the study of speech sounds, textbooks do not normally present a standard definition" (p. 137). Lindblom goes on to note that definitions often have a circular nature, in that the term being defined becomes part of the definition. Defining a speech sound as a unit carries the risk of reducing speech production to a sequence of units, rather like keys on a keyboard. But, as discussed in Chapters 6 and 7, speech is more than a sequence of elements. Rather, speech is organized at several different levels that are integrated into a rhythmic and melodic pattern in which segments are very difficult to identify because speech movements are context-adaptive, overlapping with one another in their segmental affiliation, and subject to a variety of influences including speaking rate and speaking style.

The segmental assumption (i.e., speech sounds are units) runs through discussions of development (acquisition of speech sounds, which typically is a chronology of phoneme mastery in childhood) and disorder (speech sound errors, which usually focuses on phonemes). The American Speech-Language-Hearing Association (n.d.) defines speech sound disorders as "an umbrella term referring to any difficulty or combination of difficulties with perception, motor production, or phonological representation of speech sounds and speech segments—including phonotactic rules governing permissible speech sound sequences in a language" (first paragraph of https://www.asha.org/practice-portal/clinical-topics/articulation-and-phonology/). This definition mentions both speech sounds and speech segments but does not explain how these terms differ and why both should be recognized. The subsequent mention of *speech sound sequences* in the definition also lacks clarity. The definition of speech sound disorder conflates three critical terms: speech sounds, speech segments, and speech sound sequences (none of which is defined).

Given the ambiguity of the term *speech sound*, it is understandable why so many books, articles, and online sources on speech sound disorders simply do not define it. But it is necessary to define it to give an understanding of related terms such as *speech sound disorders* and *speech sound acquisition*. Simply put, the concept of speech sound is central to the study of speech, much as the concept of an element is central to chemistry. This book uses the following definition: a **speech sound** is a unit in the acoustic signal of speech, with the duration of the unit ranging from a phonetic segment to a larger prosodic unit, depending on the purpose of the analysis. By this definition, speech sounds include units such as phonetic segments, phonemes, syllables, and intonational patterns, whether produced by people or machines. Although this book is concerned primarily with speech produced by humans, machine speech has clinical relevance in systems such as a **voice output communication aid (VOCA)**, also known as a **speech generating device (SGD)**, which is any device producing intelligible speech that allows a person who is nonvocal (or who has great difficulty in producing speech) to communicate with another person or with some electromechanical system. A speech sound is an acoustic entity; however, this entity may be produced—by a human, a robot, or a computer using synthetic speech. Technological advances have taken speech from a purely human activity to one that is adapted to a world of artificial intelligence.

Accordingly, a speech sound disorder is an atypical production of a specified unit in the acoustic signal of speech. The units that are commonly recognized are phonetic segments or phonemes, but these are not the exclusive domain of the disorders, which can extend to larger units such as syllables, words, or intonational phrases. The rationale and implications of this definition are discussed more fully in Chapter 11. In comparing different systems for the classification of speech sound disorders, Waring and Knight (2013) concluded that there is general agreement on three major subgroups: an articulation-based subgroup, a motor planning subgroup, and a phonological subgroup. However, the means to identify the subgroups are not necessarily consistent across the major classification systems. Chapter 11 discusses the possibility that each of these subgroups can be understood in part through consideration of sensorimotor factors. The chapter also considers the possibility that " . . . children with SSDs do not typically fall neatly into a binary pattern of either having a particular impairment (e.g., phonologic vs. CAS) or not" (Strand et al., 2013, p. 516). This inquiry examines the possibility of sensorimotor factors in accounting at least in part for the difficulties of children labeled as having speech sound disorders. To this point, Namasivayam et al. (2013) concluded that, "the severity of speech motor planning and sequencing issues may potentially be a limiting factor in connected speech intelligibility and highlights the need to target these issues early and directly in treatment" (p. 246).

"Theoretical accounts and clinical management of pediatric speech sound disorders (SSD) are limited by previous research. Participants' speech difficulties have been inadequately described, reflecting the lack of clarity in existing diagnostic guidelines. Performance measures have primarily focused on the articulation of consonants in single words rather than phonological competence and the cognitive-linguistic abilities underlying speech development" (Dodd, 2014, p. 189).

Speech disorders are associated with a host of conditions. It is now evident that motor problems, sometimes subtle, accompany disorders such as specific language impairment (also called developmental language disorder), autism spectrum disorder, Fragile X syndrome, fetal alcohol syndrome, Down syndrome, developmental coordination disorders, and many others (as considered in Chapter 11). Therefore, there is a need for valid, reliable, and sensitive tools to assess speech motor function. Although not a disorder per se, problems with speech may appear in children and adults learning a second language. These problems are classified as differences rather than disorders, but speech-language pathologists often are called upon to offer services in accent modification (also called accent reduction), which is designed to alter patterns of regional or foreign dialects so that the client's speech conforms more closely to the speaking patterns of a target community, such as a new country of residence. This issue is of growing concern as the bilingual population increases and is discussed in detail in Chapter 10.

Theoretical and Methodological Approaches

Several different approaches have been proposed for the study of disorders of speech. Among the most prominent approaches are those listed in the following.

Medical and Health-Related Models

The traditional **medical model** assumes that a disease or disorder is fully accounted for by deviations from the norm of measurable biological variables. For example, it might be suspected that a speech disorder in a child is related to a hearing loss, which could be assessed with audiometry to determine the type and severity of the loss, and the likely effects of the loss on the discrimination of speech sounds. The medical model is basically atheoretical and is concerned with identifying a disease or disorder and treating it. A negative consequence of this model applied to speech development is that it can pathologize dialect differences rather than recognizing their cultural foundations. A newer version of the medical model, called the **biopsychosocial model** (Figure 1–1) seeks to address not only disease, but illness or disorder in its full character, thereby overcoming the mechanistic and reductionist features of the older model. In the biopsychological model, hearing loss, for example, is considered in the broader context of a child's life, to include factors such as temperament and family characteristics. This model is intended to understand the nature of a disorder within a specific framework of assumptions and constructs.

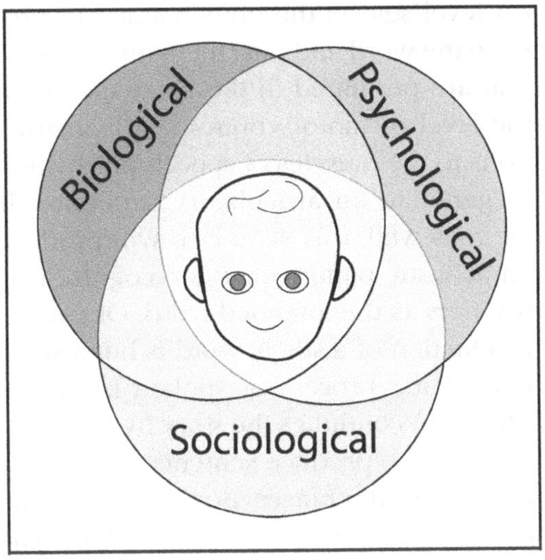

Figure 1–1. The biopsychosocial model depicted as a Venn diagram in which a child's status is an intersection of biological, psychological, and sociological factors.

The **International Classification of Functioning, Disability and Health: Children & Youth Version (ICF-CY;** WHO, 2007) seeks to understand a child's functioning, health, and well-being in a broad framework that includes (1) body functions and structures, (2) activities, and (3) participation, as all three of these relate to environmental and personal factors. The model is illustrated in Figure 1–2. The ICF-CY also includes a classification with a hierarchical structure having four levels of detail. This classification complements the model by identifying activities and participation. The ICF-CY is significant especially because of its worldwide usage and its recognition that well-being is not sufficiently understood by reference to body functions and structures (as

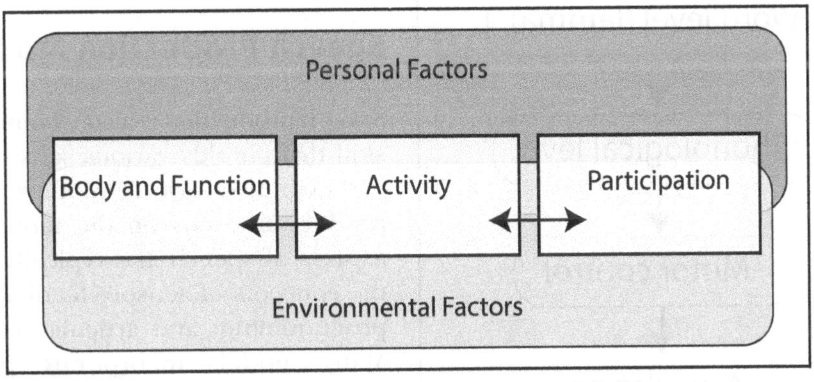

Figure 1–2. The ICF model. The components of body and function, activity, and participation are viewed in the context of personal and environmental factors.

in the traditional medical model). The ICF-CY offers important perspectives relevant to speech disorders in children, but, as discussed in Chapter 12, its implementation is not always straightforward.

Psycholinguistic Models

Psycholinguistic models describe and analyze the acquisition, use, and breakdowns of verbal behavior in terms of psychological or cognitive processing, usually addressing the three basic processes of reception or comprehension, storage or underlying representation, and speech production. Identification of a specific breakdown in one or more processes is key to diagnosis and treatment of a disorder. This model is often schematized as a box and arrows diagram, as shown in Figure 1–3, which illustrates processes involved in the production of a single word. The topmost box is the concept that is to be expressed. This phase is prelexical, meaning that it precedes selection of actual lexical items. The next phase is the word level in which a **lemma** is selected. In psycholinguistics, a lemma is the conceptualization of a word before it can be expressed as a sound pattern. That is, a lemma is an abstract form that precedes the production of the word as an articulatory and acoustic pattern. The phonological level selects the units needed to produce the word and puts them into patterns that are permitted in the language. Next, the level of motor control sends instructions to the muscles of speech production to generate an articulatory sequence. If all goes well, this sequence will produce an acoustic pattern that is recognized by listeners as the intended word. Of course, production of a single word is but a small part of the process of spoken language. Chapter 3 continues the story by considering how we produce sentences and other multi-word utterances. Box and arrow diagrams often are used in psycholinguistic models of spoken language (Baker et al., 2001), as discussed in later chapters. Individual boxes typically represent stages of processing and the arrows connecting them are information signals.

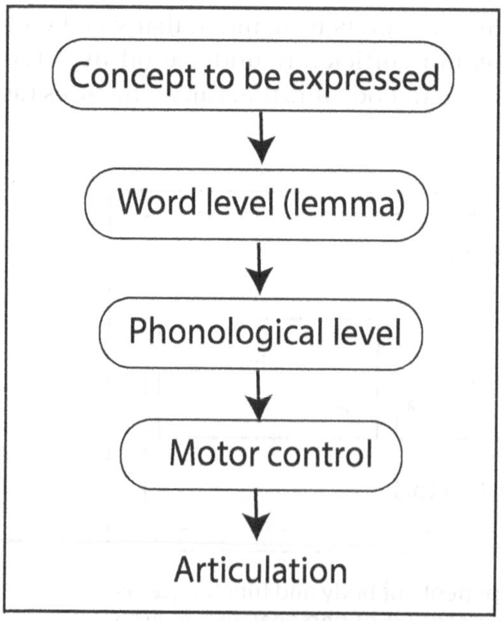

Figure 1–3. Box and arrows diagram of the basic processes in producing a word.

Speech Production Models

Speech production is a consummate motor skill that enfolds various sensory, motor, and cognitive aspects. Models of speech production focus on the motor control aspects of speech and typically embrace the concepts of sensory feedback, motor programming, and articulatory control. Many models incorporate principles of **system control theory**, defined as a strategy that controls the behavior of dynamical systems, often by incorporating a controller and feedback loops. Some basic examples are shown in Figure 1–4. Part A of the diagram shows a system of open-loop control in which instructions are sent to the muscles and muscle contractions produce the desired movements. This type of control works well if the controller knows exactly what instructions are needed for a desired result. As applied to speech, this kind of model supposes that the motor commands to produce a given sound such as /p/ are prepackaged and can be executed without reliance on sensory feedback. Part B of the diagram shows a simple closed-loop control in which auditory and somatosensory feedback is used to amend the instructions sent to the muscles. This kind of model recognizes that feedback plays an essential role in producing speech sounds by compensating for errors or unexpected conditions. Part C of the diagram shows a feedforward type of control in which a component in the controller predicts the sensory consequences of a movement and can use the predicted pattern with the actual pattern identified by feedback signals. As applied to motor control, this kind of system can predict and even suppress feedback if desired.

Several different approaches to speech motor control have been advanced, some of which are summarized below.

Dynamic Systems Theory (DST)

Dynamic systems theory (DST), in its general formulation, pertains to natural phenomena whose state or instantaneous

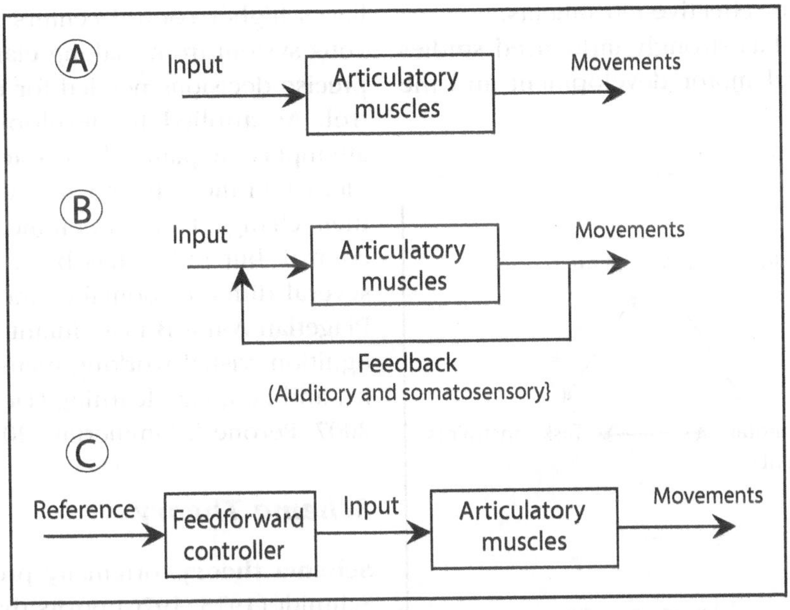

Figure 1–4. Models of motor control. Part A: open-loop control in which instructions are sent to the muscles and muscle contractions produce the desired movements. Part B: a simple closed-loop control system in which auditory and somatosensory feedback is used to amend the instructions sent to the muscles. Part C: a feedforward type of control in which a component in the controller predicts the sensory consequences of a movement and can use this prediction to make corrections.

description changes over time (therefore *dynamic*). DST is formalized as an application of mathematics, in which dynamic equations account for changes in complex systems over time. According to DST, each step in a developmental process is determined by the state of the system at a previous moment and succeeding steps can yield unpredictable, nonlinear developmental patterns. As applied to movements, DST proposes that a movement is the emergent product of the interaction of multiple subsystems within the individual, task, and environment (Figure 1–5). Each of these factors is associated with various constraints that operate to select movement features that accomplish a particular goal. This theory predicts that novel complex behaviors can emerge when intervention destabilizes the system and then stabilizes subcomponent skills needed for effective movements.

DST has strongly influenced studies of general motor development and the clinical practice of physical therapy. As it pertains to speech production, DST proposes that action responses in speech are based on task-determined synergies that operate with few degrees of freedom and well-defined control parameters (Kelso & Tuller, 1986; van Lieshout, 2004). The **problem of degrees of freedom** in motor behavior is especially critical for a multi articulate system such as speech production, and reduction of the degrees of freedom facilitates the control of the articulators and may benefit a child who is learning to speak. One way of limiting the internal degrees of freedom in high-dimensional systems like speech production is to constrain the elements to act together in functional groupings of muscles and joints that act synergistically. These synergies are called **coordinative structures**.

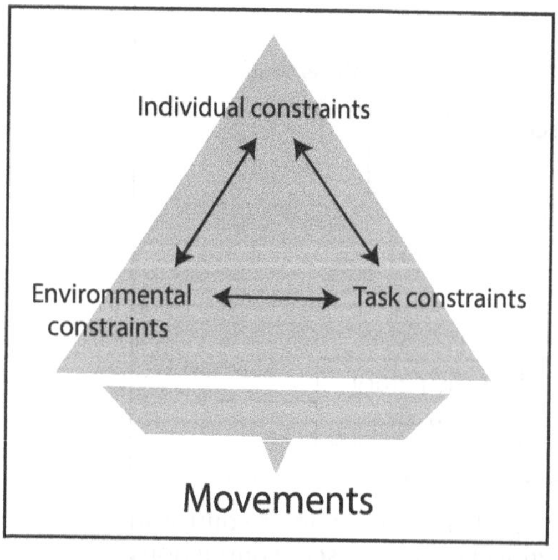

Figure 1–5. A diagram of the major components in DST, which asserts that a movement is the emergent product of the interaction of multiple subsystems within the individual, task, and environment.

A major appeal of DST is that it relieves higher control centers in the nervous system from making elaborate and precise decisions needed for motor control. As applied to development, DST attempts to explain when systems are stable, when they change, and what makes them change. DST is not limited to motor control, but rather has been applied to several different domains, including the Piagetian A-not-B task, infant visual recognition, visual working memory capacity, and language learning (De Bot et al., 2007; Perone & Simmering, 2017).

Schema Theory

Schema theory, originally proposed by Schmidt (1975, 1976) posits that a movement pattern is produced by means of a **generalized motor program (GMP)**, which is a set of motor commands prepared before the initiation of movement and is retrieved from memory and adapted as needed to the demands of a particular circumstance. The GMP is somewhat analogous to a computer program that specifies the operations to be performed. Flexibility of motor control depends on learning the relations between the initial conditions (e.g., the positions of the articulators), the generated motor commands, the sensory consequences of these motor commands (e.g., auditory and somatosensory signals in speech production), and the outcome of the movement. The theory relies on two types of schemata. A **recall schema** is built from experience and provides parameter values to the GMP. A **recognition schema**, also built from experience, yields the expected feeling of the movement. The main features of schema theory are shown in Figure 1–6. The GMP consists of invariant features (the basic signature of a movement) and parameters (specific features learned from experience). Information from the movement is stored in short-term memory to create the recall and recognition schema. The schema rules are updated as needed and used to modify the parameters in the GMP. Unlike DST, GMP asserts that mental representation is essential for the performance of skilled movement. Evidence that supports the concept of mental representation comes from studies showing that learning a movement can be facilitated by imagining the movement or by observing another individual perform the movement. These effects are not predicted by the standard version of DST. Imagery and observation point to the operation of a mental representation such as a motor program. These ideas are developed more fully in Chapter 9.

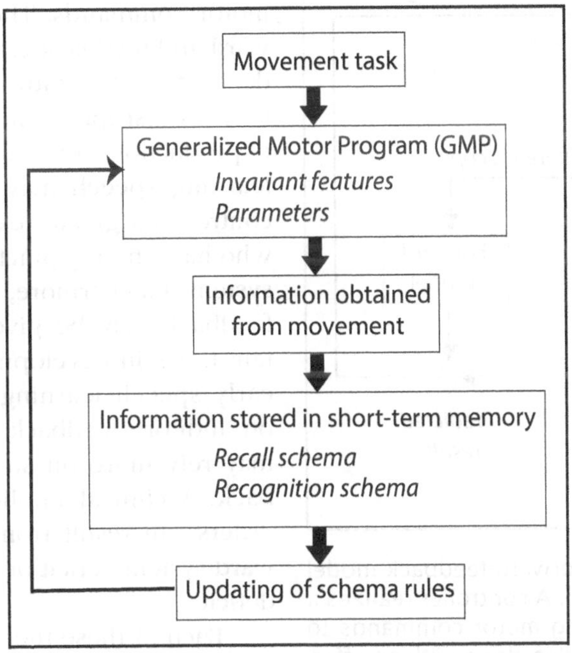

Figure 1–6. Diagram of the processes in a schema model of motor control. A core feature of this model is a generalized motor program that is updated through motor experience.

Computational Models

Several different computational models have been proposed to account for speech production (Parrell et al., 2019). One of these, the **Directions Into Velocities of Articulators (DIVA) model** (Guenther, 1994; Tourville & Guenther, 2011), considers the roles of internal models, feedback control, and feedforward control in learning and refining movements. These concepts are discussed in more detail in later chapters and brief definitions are introduced here. Basic components that are common to several versions of computational modeling are illustrated in Figure 1–7. An **internal model** is a neural system that mimics the actions of a sensorimotor system such as speech production, enabling the central nervous system to predict the consequences of motor commands and to determine the motor commands needed to perform specific tasks. Internal models are the basis for feedforward control in which internal action representations plan the initial motor output before sensory feedback is available. Feedback control enables the motor system to use sensory inputs to make corrective adjustments as needed. **Efference copy**, which is an internal duplicate of the motor signals sent to the muscles, is used to predict, and sometimes suppress, the sensory consequences of voluntary movements. That is, the controller issues two sets of instructions, the motor commands that are sent to activate muscles and an internal copy of these commands that is used to predict the results of the motor commands. The roles of feedforward and feedback control can vary with developmental status and other factors such as disruption of the normal means of production. For example, a young child learning speech may rely on feedback control to a greater extent than an adult who has a highly practiced speech motor system. Furthermore, different kinds of feedback may be given priority at certain times in development. For example, early speech learning may rely heavily on auditory feedback and later learning may rely more on somatosensory feedback. A clinical implication is that disorders can result from either a feedforward system deficit or a feedback system deficit.

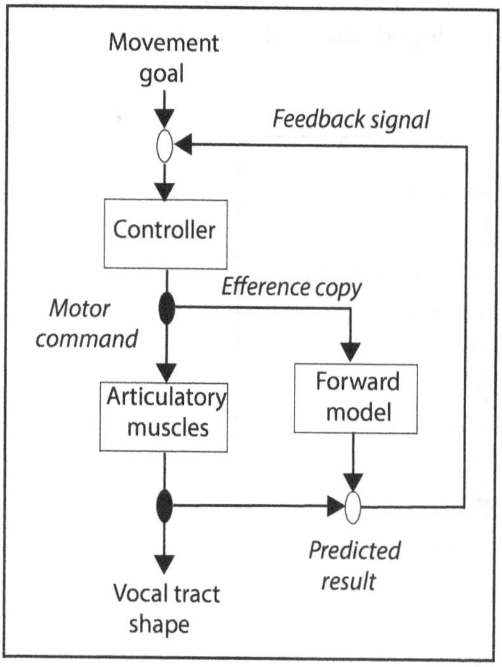

Figure 1–7. A feedforward-feedback model of speech production. A controller realizes a motor goal by issuing motor commands to the articulatory muscles along with an efference copy (an internal duplicate of the motor commands). The predicted result determined from the efference copy is compared with the actual result to generate a feedback signal.

Each of these theoretical alternatives has its advocates, strengths, and limitations. Setting aside the very important issue of clinical entity, there is another reason to consider motor factors in speech development, namely, that speech is a motor skill and aspects of this skill could be compromised even in children who are not given a confident diagnosis of MSD. That is, learning motor skills are part and parcel of speech development, and the interaction of motor skill learning with other aspects of spoken language is critical to understanding the developmental processes.

Artificial Intelligence and Expert Systems

Expertise in a specialty is based on accumulated knowledge and the ability to use this knowledge to make effective decisions. An expert in speech disorders is equipped with a broad base of knowledge and a set of clinical decision-making skills. A broad effort has been made to construct computer-based expert systems that use techniques of artificial intelligence, and these efforts are interesting here for two main reasons: (1) they can serve as models of human expertise, and (2) they are increasingly used in teaching and clinical applications. Expert systems were the foundation of current developments in artificial intelligence, deep learning, and machine learning systems. The essential core of an AI-based expert system has three components (Saibeneet et al., 2021):

1. It is knowledge-based, which typically means that it is associated with a database consisting of all the information needed to solve a particular problem.
2. It emulates the decision-making process of a human expert, which is accomplished mainly through an inference engine based on a rule set derived from the collected knowledge.
3. It is an application of AI that affords technical solutions for data collection and system behavior modeling.

On the surface, speech may seem to be a rather simple human behavior. But as this book reveals, speech is a highly complicated behavior that depends on multiple skills and types of knowledge, including the following domains:

a. hearing and other senses that provide information from outside sources (e.g., other speakers) and inside information (e.g., auditory and kinesthetic feedback of one's own speech production),
b. cognition (the process of acquiring and accessing knowledge),
c. language formulation, including word selection and the arrangement of words in a syntactic pattern,
d. phonology, or the patterning of sounds to form words,
e. sociocultural aspects of language use (e.g., pragmatics and emotion), and
f. motor control over the processes of respiration, phonation, articulation, and resonance.

Each domain is complicated on its own, but the interaction of these domains presents a substantial challenge to understanding how speech develops and how it can be disordered. Clinical expertise draws on each knowledge domain to determine diagnosis, prognosis, and treatment choices. The system relies on heuristics that emulate human decision making. Examples of progress in this area are the systems developed by Robles-Bykbaev et al. (2015) and Toki et al. (2012).

Chapter Summaries

Chapters are organized in a way that supports clinical knowledge and process, as shown in the chapter diagram of Figure 1–8. The first four chapters provide background information on spoken language and its development. The next four chapters cover issues in clinical assessment, followed by a chapter on motor development and motor learning, and then a chapter on bilingualism and dialect. The final two chapters address clinical populations in which speech disorders are likely and the prevention and treatment of speech disorders in children. Chapter summaries follow.

Chapter 2. Biological and Psychological Foundations of Speech Development. This chapter describes the developmental background of speech development and includes summaries of changes in the anatomy, physiology, and function of the speech production system, along with developments in psychological domains such as emotion. Lying at the heart of this discussion are two major principles: (1) children are not simply small adults but rather differ in very important ways from adults in the biological and psycho-

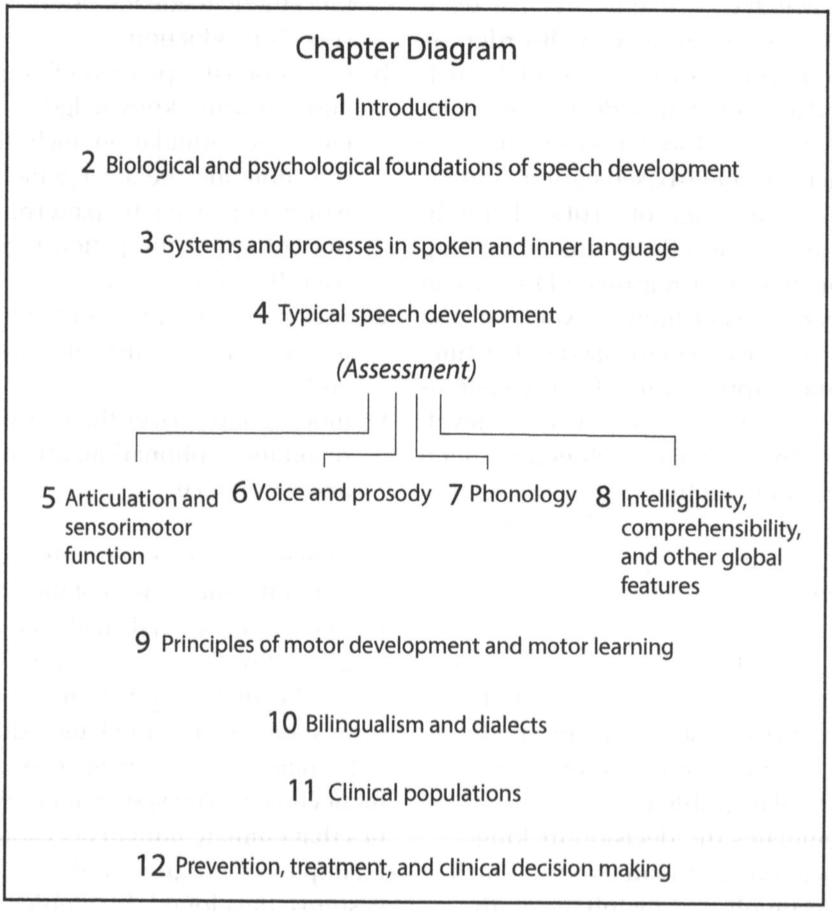

Figure 1–8. Diagram of the chapter content of this book.

logical foundations of speech production, and (2) the processes associated with speech development have a multilayered and protracted maturation that may extend to adolescence and sometimes even young adulthood. These principles are relevant to understanding how speech develops, as well as the assessment and treatment of speech disorders. Included in this chapter is a chronological profile of developmental and maturational changes relevant to speech.

Chapter 3. Systems and Processes in Spoken and Inner Language. Producing an utterance has been conceptualized as a multi-stage process that begins with an idea to be expressed and ends with articulatory movements that give rise to an acoustic signal of speech that can be perceived and decoded by listeners. Identifying the number and nature of the stages in this process has occupied the imagination and efforts of scientists in many different specialties. This chapter describes the commonly recognized stages and relates them to aspects of human cognition and emotion. Speech is a primary means of emotional expression, beginning in the early weeks of life and continuing through the lifespan. In the proposed model of spoken language, emotion and language are integrated into several components that generate speech as a signal for linguistic and emotional communication.

Chapter 4. Typical Speech Development. Speech development has been described in three major ways: the chronology of speech sound mastery, the presence or absence of phonological processes, and the development of speech motor control. Underlying these approaches is an understanding of speech development as a sensorimotor phenomenon, especially the formation and refinement of movements that are at the core of speech production. This chapter summarizes major milestones in speech production and relates them to other developmental domains.

Chapter 5. Assessment of Articulation and Sensorimotor Functions. Included in this chapter are the methods of assessment routinely used in the examination of children who may have a speech disorder. These assessments cover a range of nonspeech and speech tasks that provide insight into the possible mechanisms of disorder. Included in this chapter are the following methods of assessment: oral mechanism examination, maximum performance measures, articulation, phonological processes, perceptual rating scales, and tests of speech motor function.

Chapter 6. Assessment of Voice and Prosody. Speech development is more than speech sound acquisition, and speech is more than an inventory of phonemes or other segments. Speech includes the regulation of voice quality and prosody, which are closely related and involve some of the same underlying systems and mechanisms. Prosody is also known by the term suprasegmental, implying that the features of interest transcend the segmental (phonemic) building blocks of speech. The basic components are the melody and rhythm of speech, but it is not always easy to cleave speech production into the domains of segmental and suprasegmental because these domains interact to form the spoken message. This chapter summarizes the development of voice and several aspects of prosody and outlines tools for clinical assessment.

Chapter 7. Assessment of Phonology. This chapter briefly reviews phonological theories as they relate to speech development and disorders and discusses the topics of phonological memory, phonological access to lexical storage, phonological awareness, and phonological patterns in speech production. The role of auditory processing, which is typically neglected in formal theories of phonology, is emphasized as an important component in phonological development and disorders.

Chapter 8. Assessment of Intelligibility, Comprehensibility and Other Global Features. We speak to be understood. That statement seems simple enough but attempts to measure and analyze speech intelligibility and related aspects of communication have given rise to a substantial literature and a diversity of approaches. The primary goals of this chapter are to identify the underpinnings of intelligible speech and to describe methods for the clinical assessment of intelligibility, comprehensibility, accuracy, communicative efficiency, fluency, and accentedness. Strengths and weaknesses of various assessments are described as they relate to different clinical populations.

Chapter 9. Principles of Motor Development and Motor Learning. Like other motor skills, speech must be learned in a process that includes goal formulation, muscle activation, practice, and feedback. Motor learning is relevant to many different disciplines, and the principles discovered through extensive research efforts in several specialties are relevant to speech development and speech-language pathology. Principles of motor learning are discussed in a growing number of papers that reflect an increasingly sophisticated knowledge of the motoric and neurophysiological bases of speech production. As discussed in this and other chapters, these concepts are incorporated in some therapies for MDSs in children, as well as for second language acquisition. Some aspects of motor development and learning are mentioned in earlier chapters, but this chapter integrates and consolidates theory and data pertaining to these topics.

Chapter 10. Bilingualism and Dialects. An atypical pattern of speech production traditionally has been categorized as a delay, disorder, or difference. However, these categories can occur in combination in an individual child, especially when the child has a dialect. This issue is of growing concern as the number of bilingual speakers increases in the United States. This chapter discusses the clinical challenges of distinguishing delay, disorder, and difference.

Chapter 11. Clinical Populations. Speech disorders are associated with a large array of clinical entities or conditions. This chapter describes many of these and identifies characteristics of the speech disorder in each based on a review of the recent literature. It also examines the traditional classifications of speech disorders into functional and organic and explains that many disorders are multifactorial in origin, which forces a different perspective on etiology.

Chapter 12. Prevention and Treatment, and Clinical Decision Making. This chapter briefly considers prevention strategies but is concerned mainly with treatment methods. Treatment alternatives are summarized, including relevant theoretical background and available levels of evidence. Key references are identified as sources of detailed information on procedures of treatment. Treatments are considered for the broad range of speech disorders in children, not just speech sound disorders as commonly understood.

Recurrent Themes

Certain concepts recur often enough in this book to qualify as major themes in understanding children's speech development and disorders. These concepts are as follows.

1. Speech production and perception have a protracted development, with some aspects maturing into adolescence and adulthood. Although some sources suggest that children have intelligible speech by the age of 4 years, detailed studies of speech indicate a much longer maturational period, indicating adaptation of the speech perception and production systems to a variety of developmental factors. In addition, speech production appears to be malleable in some respects throughout life, as shown by studies of both native and later learned languages.
2. To some degree, speech can be understood by general principles from disciplines such as biology, linguistics, and psychology. However, speech is specialized in its sensory and motor implementation. For example, speech as a motor skill draws on a specialized craniofacial musculature that is deployed to meet exacting demands of temporal organization.
3. Speech development and speech disorders have a multifactorial background that combines cognition, language, speech motor control, sensory processing, and emotion, to mention a few. Several of the disorders considered in later chapters have a complex etiology, often involving genetic and environmental factors. Genetic factors often involve the interactions among several genes, and perhaps epigenetic influences in which environmental factors play a role.
4. Speech is spoken language, which means that speech is intimately tied to language structure and processes, and that the speech signal carries information at several levels, including segmental (i.e., phonemes), prosodic (i.e., rhythm and melody), emotional, and pragmatic.
5. One approach to understanding complex systems is to identify their modular composition, and this approach applies to speech and its development, including anatomic, motor, and cognitive elements. A **module** is defined as a set of interconnected elements that function as a semi-autonomous unit in a larger assembly of other elements. A simple example from anatomy is the human skull, which has two major modules, a craniofacial skeleton and the cranium, which grow at different rates during development.
6. An important concept that frequently arises in discussions of human development is that of **scaffolding**. In the construction industry, a scaffold is a temporary structure that supports a work crew and gives access to needed materials. In psychology and child

education, scaffolding provides temporary support in learning, taking account of current strengths and limitations and aligning with learning objectives. Scaffolding is mentioned frequently because it captures the active, goal-directed nature of many developmental processes as well as interventional methods.

7. Children learning to speak are emotional, cognitive agents who actively construct the motor patterns of speech production from their current physiological and psychological status. Research has shown that emotion and spoken language are intimately connected in cognitive development and that speech, from its earliest beginnings in the vocalizations of infants, is imbued with emotion.

Summary

1. Speech production draws on a variety of skills and knowledge. Speech is a motor act that is closely tied with cognition, language, and emotion. Aside from sign language, there is no behavior other than speech that is rooted in the most sophisticated dimensions of human life.
2. Aspects of speech perception and production have a protracted development and maturation, extending to at least the age of puberty.
3. Understanding, assessing, and treating disorders of speech in children requires knowledge about typical speech development and the various ways in which development can be delayed or disturbed. Recent models of both development and disorders embrace the complexity of speech by acknowledging the need to consider biological, psychological, sociological, and linguistic factors that underlie speech communication.
4. Speech can be analyzed into interacting sensory, motor, and linguistic components that have individual trajectories of development and maturation.

2

BIOLOGICAL AND PSYCHOLOGICAL FOUNDATIONS OF SPEECH DEVELOPMENT

Speech in children develops against a background of anatomic and physiologic changes in the respiratory, laryngeal, and supralaryngeal systems of speech production, including motor and sensory maturation. It also develops along with changes in sensory function, cognitive abilities, social interactions, and other motor behaviors such as locomotion and manual dexterity. This chapter reviews some of the major developmental changes associated with speech production in children and serves as a background for the succeeding chapters. It heeds the advice from Malik and Marwaha (2022) that "To apply knowledge regarding human growth and development, healthcare [or other] professionals need to be aware of 2 areas: (1) milestone competencies, for example, growth in the motor, cognitive, speech-language, and social-emotional domains and (2) the eco-biological model of development, specifically, the interaction of environment and biology and their influence on development."

Anatomic and Physiologic Development

Children are not simply small versions of adults, which is especially true of the speech production system. During development, the structures involved in speech production change in size, shape, relative position to other structures, and tissue properties of biomechanics, cytology, and histology. These changes are continuous and often interactive. The following sections summarize changes in the three major speech production systems—respiratory, laryngeal, and supralaryngeal—during the period between infancy and adolescence. These systems are complex in several respects. They are composed of a large array of muscles, and some muscles have properties that appear to be unique to the craniofacial apparatus and perhaps to speech production. The uniqueness is multidimensional, including genetic, embryologic, histologic, and functional aspects (Kent, 2004).

It is often said that speech is an overlaid function, meaning that it is produced with biological systems that serve other purposes vital to life (e.g., breathing, eating). But it also has been asserted that the requirements of speech may have shaped the organs that produce it. The evolution of speech is a topic of much uncertainty and controversy, but there are reasons to believe that it is a tractable problem and important progress has been made (De Boer, 2019; Fitch, 2018). This book is concerned more with ontogeny, the development of the individual organism, than with evolution. The primary goal is to summarize how the relevant anatomy and physiology of speech change with development and how these changes relate to speech production at different ages. The overarching theme of this chapter is that speech has a long maturational trajectory, extending from the fetus to adolescence, with many significant events along the way. The following sections summarize developmental patterns in the anatomy and physiology of the systems of speech production. Each system is complex, but a specific goal in understanding speech production is to determine how these systems are coordinated in a unitary motor act. Unfortunately, terminology is not entirely consistent in the relevant literature. Carey et al. (2009) suggest a standard terminology for the lips, mouth, and oral region, and it would be helpful to have a standard terminology for all systems of speech production.

Respiratory System

Speech is produced as a modulation of airflow from the lungs, and ordinary conversation is a sequence of breath groups, with each group composed of syllables and words. The **respiratory system** has two major divisions, the conducting zone and respiratory zone. The former consists of the airways of the mouth, nose, pharynx, larynx, trachea, bronchi, bronchioles, and terminal bronchioles. For ventilatory purposes, this zone is basically a conduit for airflow. The respiratory zone, where gas exchange occurs, consists of the lung parenchyma formed from the respiratory bronchioles, alveolar ducts, and alveolar sacs. The respiratory system also can be considered to have two main muscular systems, the rib cage and the diaphragm. The **rib cage** consists of the sternum (breastbone), costal cartilage (cartilaginous connections between the ribs and other bones), 12 pairs of ribs, and the bodies of the thoracic vertebrae. The ribs elevate for inspiration and depress for expiration. The **diaphragm** is a musculotendinous sheet that takes the form of two domes, situated at the inferior boundary of the rib cage. It has two main functions, to separate the thoracic and abdominal cavities and to assist in ventilation by changing the volume of the thoracic cavity and the lungs. The rib cage and diaphragm cooperate to produce the air pressures and flows needed to sustain life and to support functions such as speech.

The infant's respiratory system differs markedly from that in adults (Di Cicco et al., 2021; Hammer & Eber, 2005; Jones et al., 2000). The neonatal thorax has a pyramidal shape that contrasts with the barrel shape in adults, and an infant's ribs have a horizontal orientation in comparison to the oblique orientation in adults. The obliqueness of the adult ribs is a factor in explaining the "bucket handle" mechanical action observed in adult ventilation (i.e., the motion of the ribs causes a lateral expansion of the thoracic cavity). Developmental changes also occur in the shape and stiffness of the rib cage during early life. Growth of the respiratory system can be seen in lung volumes, capacities, and airflows, as well as in the cellular structure of the lungs. Lung volume doubles by about 6 months of life and triples by the first year, with growth continuing until adulthood. Between 6 and 13 years, vital capacity increases from about 1000 mL to about 2500 mL, with somewhat larger values in boys than girls (H. E. Jones, 1955). A stunning increase occurs in the number of alveoli, the basic functional unit of gas exchange. The neonate has about 17 to 71 million alveoli, compared with about 200 to 600 million in adults. Alveolar multiplication continues to the age of 2 or 3 years (Di Cicco et al., 2021; Jones et al., 2000; Joshi & Kotecha, 2007). Respiratory rate declines from birth to early adolescence, with the steepest fall in infants under 2 years of age. The rate at birth is about 44 breaths per minute, compared with 26 breaths per minute at 2 years of age, and about 16 breaths per minute in adulthood (Fleming et al., 2011).

These developmental achievements are relevant to speech production because the respiratory system provides the aerodynamic power of sound production. Lung volume is a limiting factor in the duration of phonation or other speech behaviors. As reviewed in Kent (2022), the durations of infant vocalizations are typically in the range of 1 to 4 s for cry and about 0.2 to 2 s for syllables. In comparison, the mean duration of a breath group in adults is about 4 s for passage reading and about 5 s for spontaneous speaking (Wang et al., 2010). However, as discussed in Chapter 6, adults can sustain vowel phonation for 20 s or longer. During infancy, breathing for vocalization acquires its own characteristic pattern that differs from breathing for ventilatory purposes. An infant in rest breathing has a tight coupling of the rib cage and abdomen, but this coupling becomes looser during vocal behaviors (Connaghan et al., 2004). In the second half of the first year of life, infants show a decreased compliance of the chest wall and a greater potential for neuromotor control (Reilly & Moore, 2009). Following the emergence of a pattern of speech breathing by about 18 months, refinement of the breathing pattern continues from about 3 to 10 years of age (Boliek et al., 2009; Hoit et al., 1990). The typical pattern is to initiate breath groups in the midrange of vital capacity and make stable and rapid inspirations to achieve these volumes. This gradual maturation of speech breathing fits with the developmental pattern in other subsystems of speech, as discussed later in this chapter and in Chapter 4.

Typically developing children usually do not have difficulty in meeting the respiratory demands of speech production. They can generate subglottal air pressures and air volumes that are well beyond those needed for ordinary speaking tasks such as conversation or oral reading. However, children with developmental conditions such as cerebral palsy may lack the needed respiratory abilities (Edgson et al., 2021). Implications for assessment are described in Chapter 5 and for treatment in Chapter 12.

Supralaryngeal System

The vocal tract of the newborn human neonates looks more like that of nonhuman primates than an adult human (P. Lieberman et al., 1972). Figure 2–1 compares the vocal tracts of a human neonate

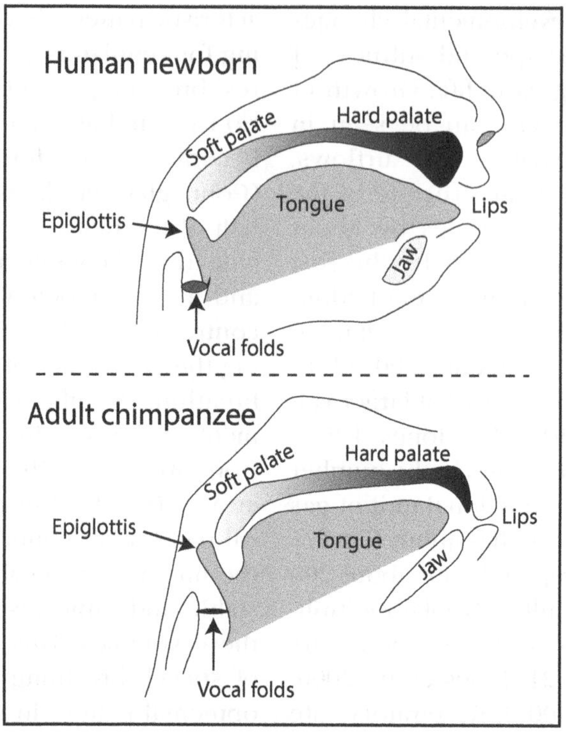

Figure 2–1. The vocal tracts of a human neonate (*top*) and an adult chimpanzee (*bottom*).

and an adult chimpanzee. Among the similarities are a compact arrangement of the soft palate and epiglottis (called velic-epiglottic engagement), a relatively short pharynx compared to the oral cavity, a high position of the larynx relative to other structures of the craniofacial complex, and a gradual angle between the oral and pharyngeal cavities. The vocal tract of the human infant is shown in Figure 2–2 as a shaded region surrounded by the oral structures that contain it. The diagram at the bottom of the figure represents the three major cavities: oral, nasal, and pharyngeal. These cavities define the overall geometry of the vocal tract. Figure 2–3 shows the vocal tracts of a 1-year-old child and an 18-year-old woman. The adult female has a marked separation of the soft palate and epiglottis, a lengthened pharyngeal cavity, and a right-angle configuration of the oral and pharyngeal cavities. During the first few months of life, the vocal tract is remodeled to take a more distinctively human shape. Along with lengthening of the pharynx, there is a substantial decrease in the size of the tongue relative to the size of the supralaryngeal cavity. These anatomical changes are likely to enhance articulatory movements of the tongue and therefore facilitate speech production (Denny & McGowan, 2012a, 2012b).

Growth of the vocal tract and its constituent structures is nonlinear, and the structures of the vocal tract do not follow the same growth trajectory (Barbier et al., 2015; Kent & Vorperian, 1995;

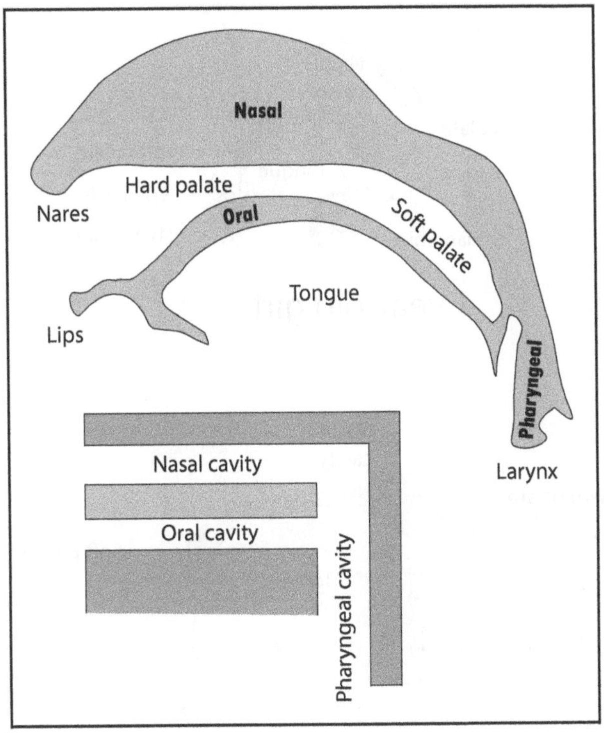

Figure 2–2. *Top:* The vocal tract of the human infant shown as a shaded region surrounded by the oral structures that contain it. *Bottom:* The three major cavities comprising the vocal tract: oral, nasal, and pharyngeal.

Vorperian et al., 2009; Wang et al., 2016). De Boer and Fitch (2010) concluded that the supralaryngeal vocal tract does not achieve an adult-like configuration until the age of about 6 to 8 years. This conclusion is based on data from Fitch and Giedd (1999), D. E. Lieberman and McCarthy (1999), and Vorperian et al., (2005). Between 3 and 10 years, the vocal tract and related structures have a relatively gradual growth but are affected by changes in dentition (emergence and shedding of primary dentition, emergence of secondary dentition), hypertrophy of pharyngeal tonsils (adenoid) with maximum thickness reached at 7 to 10 years (Vogler et al., 2000), and a decreasing ratio of size of the tongue to the size of the supralaryngeal cavity (Denny & McGowan, 2012b). In older childhood and adolescence (11 to 18 years), the vocal tract has a pubertal growth spurt, especially in males, for whom there is a marked increase in size of the length of the pharynx. Sexual dimorphism is strongly evident at this period and is reflected in acoustic measures such as vocal fundamental frequency and formant frequencies (Kent & Vorperian, 2018; Vorperian & Kent, 2007).

Now we take a closer look at individual structures of the vocal tract, with the goal of defining their essential properties and patterns of development.

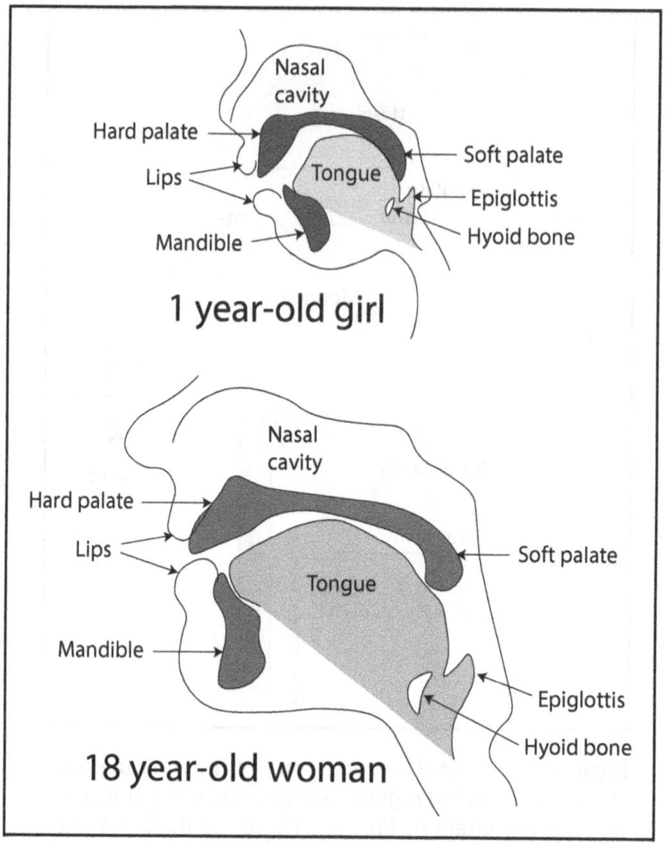

Figure 2–3. The vocal tracts of a 1-year-old girl and an 18-year-old woman. Major structures are labeled.

The Tongue

The tongue has both extrinsic and intrinsic muscles, as shown schematically in Figure 2–4. The extrinsic muscles attach the tongue to surrounding structures such as the palate, styloid process of the temporal bone, hyoid bone, and jaw. The intrinsic muscles have their origins and insertions within the tongue. The tongue is a **muscular hydrostat**—a biological structure that is composed largely of muscle and lacks skeletal support in the form of bone or cartilage (Kier & Smith, 1985). The musculature itself serves to provide both skeletal support and movement. The supporting function is possible because muscles are like fluids that are incompressible at physiological pressures, so that volume is preserved even as the shape of the structure is changed. A water-filled balloon is a useful analogy. The balloon can be squeezed in one dimension but a compensatory expansion in another direction preserves its volume. The tongue is capable of such adjustments because it consists of a 3-dimensional array of muscle fibers, as shown in Figure 2–4. Movements are performed relative to the internal mechanism of support. A child learning to speak must master the control of the tongue to achieve

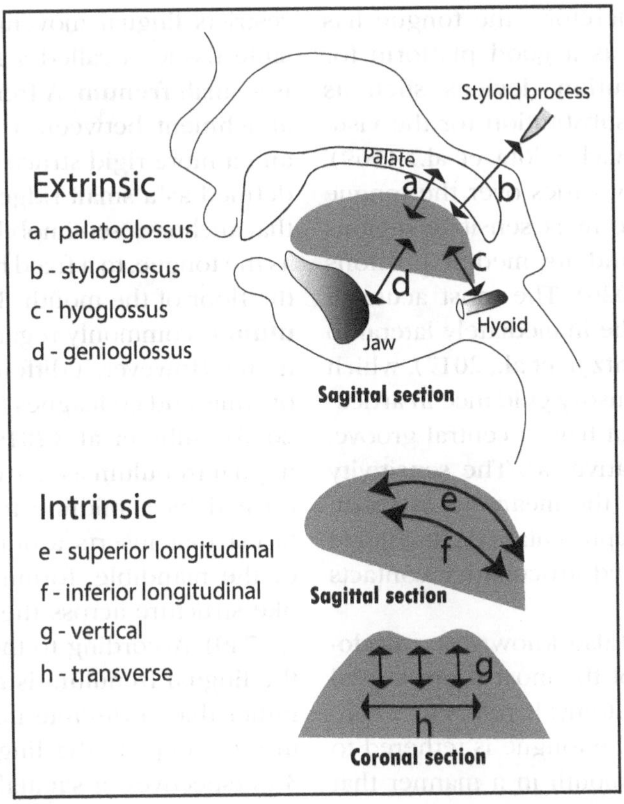

Figure 2–4. The extrinsic and intrinsic muscles of the tongue. Note the 3-dimensional array of intrinsic muscle fibers in the tongue.

the overall position in the vocal tract, the muscle activation needed for support, and the muscle activation needed for local deformations (i.e., articulations such as raising the tongue tip). In early infancy, the tongue functions rather like a piston in a cylinder, which is well suited to sucking and swallowing. But with the changes in the vocal tract described earlier in this chapter, the tongue gains greater mobility within the vocal tract. Also contributing to this mobility is a child's ability to deploy the extrinsic and intrinsic muscles of the tongue to achieve changes in position and shape. At the level of microanatomy, the tongue has a variable distribution of muscle fiber types (Sanders et al., 2013). The posterior tongue has predominantly slow-twitch Type I fibers that are suited to perform tonic contractions and postural support with fatigue resistance. The anterior tongue has predominantly fast-twitch Type II fibers that are capable of rapid phasic movements. The heterogeneity of muscle fiber types in the tongue endows it with a range of motoric capabilities.

The tongue is well endowed with sensory receptors that help to fulfill its role in ingesting and tasting foods, mastication, swallowing, and speech. The tongue has greater sensitivity and spatial resolution compared to other body parts (Miles et al., 2018; Pamir et al., 2020), except perhaps the upper lip (Grossman et al., 1965). Therefore, the tongue has been proposed as a good platform for sensory substitution devices such as visual-to-tactile substitution for the visually impaired (Bach-y-Rita et al., 1969). Tactile sensitivity varies over the tongue surface, with the most sensitive regions being the tip and its medial portions (Pamir et al., 2020). The most acute of all regions may lie immediately lateral to the midline (Moritz Jr. et al., 2017), which could provide sensory guidance in articulating sounds that have a central groove, such as the fricative /s/. The sensitivity of the tongue is the means to establish somatosensory representations that guide and affirm desired articulatory contacts during speech.

Tongue-tie (also known as **ankyloglossia**) is one of the most controversial topics in oral anatomy. It refers to a condition in which the tongue is tethered to the floor of the mouth in a manner that restricts lingual movement. The responsible tissue is called a **frenulum**, which is a small **frenum**. A frenum is a mucosal attachment between a mobile structure and a more rigid structure. A frenulum is defined as a small ridge or fold of tissue that anchors a semimobile body part, such as the tongue, to a fixed body part, such as the floor of the mouth. The **lingual frenulum** is commonly regarded as a band of tissue. However, a different view is given by Mills and colleagues (Mills et al., 2019, 2020). Mills et al. (2019) described the lingual frenulum as "a dynamic structure, formed by a midline fold in a layer of fascia that inserts around the inner arc of the mandible, forming a diaphragm-like structure across the floor of mouth" (p. 749). According to their observations, the lingual frenulum is a sheet of fascia, rather than a discrete midline band. Figure 2–5 depicts the lingual frenulum in 3 perspectives: a sagittal section, a fron-

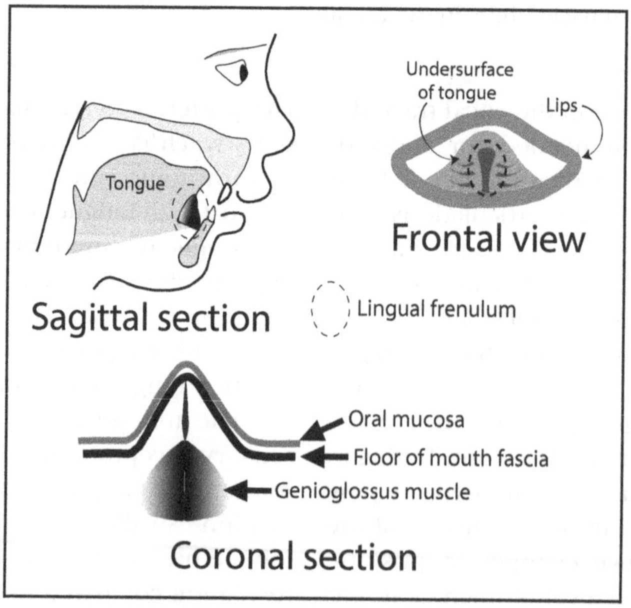

Figure 2–5. The lingual frenulum in three perspectives: a sagittal section, a frontal view, and a coronal section.

tal view, and a coronal section. Note that the frenulum is a fold of tissue in which the oral mucosa overlies the fascial of the mouth floor. A frenulum that is too short or too tight could possibly restrict mobility and interfere with functions such as speech and swallowing. Estimates of the prevalence of anterior ankyloglossia (restriction of the tongue tip) range between 4% and 10% (Segal et al., 2007). Among the notable consequences of tongue-tie are difficulties with breastfeeding, including poor latch, maternal nipple pain, mastitis, poor weight gain and early unnecessary weaning. Accordingly, ankyloglossia has been of particular interest to physicians and lactation consultants. Katz et al. (2020) conducted a Delphi study to formulate a definition of ankyloglossia. The result recognizes two separate pathways for identifying a newborn with this condition. One pathway is based on a single pathognomonic anatomic feature, whereas the other specifies a single functional deficit that is accompanied by at least 2 of 12 other diagnostic items (functional, anatomic, or behavioral). A surgical remedy for ankyloglossia is tongue-tie division or frenotomy. The effects of ankyloglossia on speech production are discussed in Chapter 11.

The Velopharynx

This structure is critical to intelligible speech and feeding. Its function is adapted during development to the changing anatomy of the soft palate and adjacent structures. Early vowel-like vocalizations in infants tend to be nasalized and are likely to be classified as quasi-resonant vowels, that is, vowels that lack the fully resonant structure of oral vowels (Oller, 2000). The capability for reliable velopharyngeal closure during vocalization is acquired during the first year of life, with a rapid increase between 6 and 9 months, which corresponds to the emergence of canonical babbling, as discussed in Chapter 4. By the age of 12 months, nearly all stop consonants and vowels in syllables are produced with continuous velopharyngeal closure, which is an important threshold for the development of intelligible speech. This closure is accomplished in different ways (Croft et al., 1981), and the four major forms are illustrated in Figure 2–6. Differences in velopharyngeal anatomy likely account for these different patterns. One such factor is the **adenoid (pharyngeal tonsil)**, which grows rapidly during infancy, so that nearly all infants have adenoids by the age of 5 months (Jaw et al., 1999). The adenoid is part of a circular arrangement of lymphatic tissue called **Waldeyer's Ring** (Figure 2–7). Between the ages of about 3 to 5 years, the soft tissues of the velopharynx grow more rapidly than does the nasopharynx, resulting in a reduction of the airway.

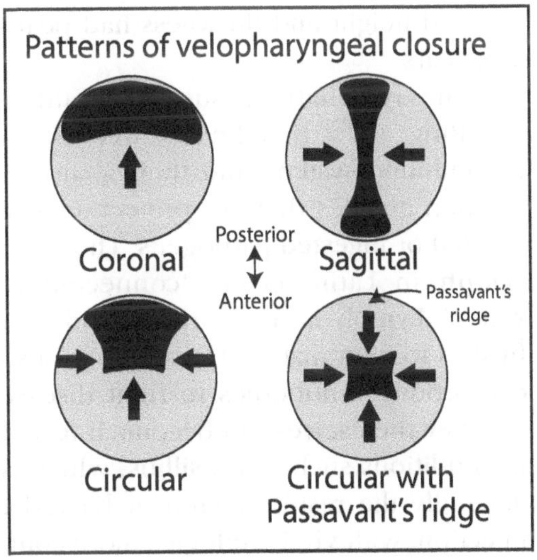

Figure 2–6. The major forms of velopharyngeal closure, as viewed from above the velopharyngeal sphincter.

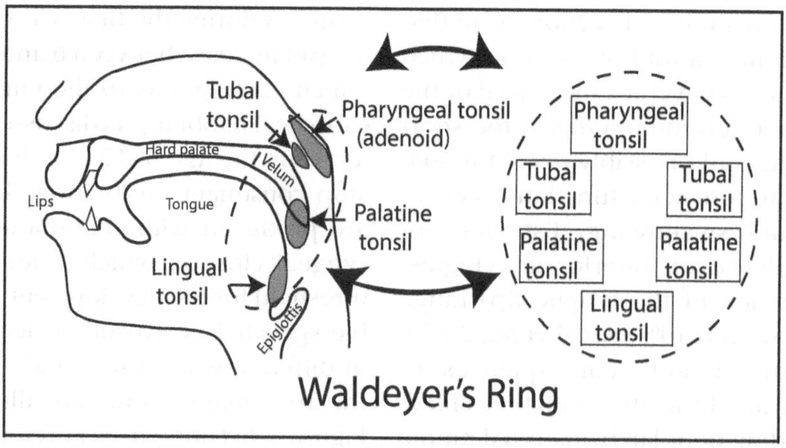

Figure 2–7. The circle of lymphatic tissue is called Waldeyer's Ring. *Left:* sagittal view. *Right:* diagram of the ring.

A child at this age may adopt a different pattern of velopharyngeal closure to accommodate the change in anatomy. After this period, the nasopharynx grows faster than the soft tissue, so that the size of the airway increases (Jeans et al., 1981). The different dimensions of the adenoid appear to have different growth patterns. Perry et al. (2022) reported that adenoid depth had peak growth at 4 years, but adenoid height and thickness had peaks at 8 years.

The lymphatic tissues of Waldeyer's Ring are a first line of defense in the immune system, and their anatomic location enables them to protect against inhaled or ingested pathogens. The word **lymph** in Latin means "connected to water." Lymph is a colorless fluid that flushes foreign matter. These tissues also can produce antibodies to fight disease but they themselves can become infected in conditions such as tonsillitis, which is generally the result of viral or bacterial infection, with viral etiologies more common. Tonsillitis is typically an inflammation of the palatine tonsil, which can be seen adjacent to the pharyngeal arches. On their surface, tonsils have specialized antigen-capture cells known as M cells that capture antigens generated by microorganisms. When the M cells recognize an antigen, they activate other tonsillar cells called T and B cells to trigger an immune response.

Age-related (physiological) **adenoid hypertrophy** (growth of the adenoid) is a frequent issue in specialties such as otolaryngology, pediatrics, and speech-language pathology. The incidence of functional disorders of the oropharynx in children is second only to disorders of the musculoskeletal system (Volkov et al., 2020). A condition of growing concern is **obstructive sleep apnea syndrome (OSAS)**, which in children is related mainly to upper airway obstruction in the regions of the nasopharynx and oropharynx. Untreated OSAS in children has been linked to failure to thrive, enuresis, attention-deficit disorder, behavior problems, poor academic performance, and cardiopulmonary disease (Chan et al., 2004; Thomas et al., 2022). Another airway problem of increasing clinical interest is **mouth breathing**, that is, breathing through the mouth rather than the nose. Achmad and Ansar (2021) categorized mouth breathing into three etiologic types (obstructive, habitual, and anatomical) and identified risk factors as nasal obstruction, adenoids, and children who are not exclusively breastfed. Although the etiology and incidence of mouth breathing have not been securely established, the condition warrants professional attention as it has been related to a host of consequences, including learning difficulties, speech and language problems, asthma morbidity, upper respiratory tract infections, and periodontal disease. It has been recommended that speech-language pathologists be involved in identifying and treating habitual mouth breathing and sleep-disordered breathing (Bonuck et al., 2021; Mohammed et al., 2021). Mouth breathing is considered in more detail later in this chapter and in Chapter 11.

The Lips

The lips are the central feature of the lower face and have a complex musculature consisting of the orbicularis oris muscle (OOM) and several facial muscles arranged in a fan-like fashion with the lips at the center (Figure 2–8). The OOM is like the intrinsic muscles of the tongue in not having a bony or tendinous origin. Accordingly, it may be regarded as a muscular hydrostat. Peeters et al. (2019) point out that the OOM consists of two major parts, deep and superficial. The deep part is older in evolution and has a sphincteric action for purposes such as food ingestion. The superficial part consists of eight radiating facial muscles and serves the precise muscular actions needed for speech, facial expressions, and playing wind instruments. D'Andrea and Barbaix (2006) similarly classified the facial muscles into two functional units, with the inner ring of the OOM being part of the deep unit and the outer ring of the OOM being part of the superficial unit. The lips, like the tongue, have a mechanical linkage with the mandible, so that both labial movements are predicated on mandibular position and movement.

A feature of clinical interest is **incompetent lip seal (ILS)**, in which children

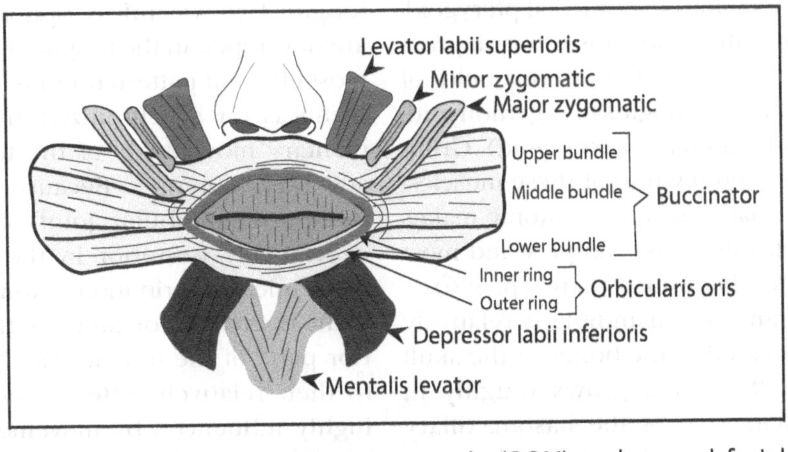

Figure 2–8. The orbicularis oris muscle (OOM) and several facial muscles arranged in a fan-like fashion with the lips at the center.

tend to maintain an open mouth and appear to close their lips with some difficulty (Drevenšek et al., 2005; Inada et al., 2021). Children with ILS use higher levels of activity in the OOM to make labial closure (Yoshizawa et al., 2018). ILS frequently co-occurs with mouth breathing (discussed earlier), a behavior that is of increasing concern in fields such as dentistry, otolaryngology, pediatrics, and speech-language pathology. It is estimated that the prevalence of ILS in Japanese children is at least 30% and increases with age (Nogami et al., 2021). Comparable prevalence data do not appear to be available for children in the U.S.

The Mandible

The development of the mandible or jaw is a basis for understanding normal occlusion of the teeth (discussed in the following section), the generation of the forces needed in mastication, and the production of speech. The mandibular musculature is versatile. It can generate powerful forces for biting and chewing but also permits finely graded adjustments in degree of opening. The muscles can be grouped into two sets, those that elevate or close the mandible (masseter, medial pterygoid, and temporalis) and those that depress or open the mandible (anterior belly of the digastric, genioglossus, geniohyoid, mylohyoid, and lateral pterygoid). Grünheid et al. (2009) wrote of these muscles, "Their special functional anatomy makes jaw muscles the most complex and most powerful in the human body" (p. 596).

In infants, the mandible is relatively small compared to the bones of the skull (Figure 2–9), and it grows roughly in parallel with that of the nasomaxillary complex, tongue, and dentition. The newborn's mandible is largely occupied by the tooth buds that eventually will give rise to the primary dentition. Smartt Jr. et al. (2005) remarked that, "while the presence of a particular mandibular subunit and its surrounding tissues is genetically determined, the development of that subunit, and its subsequent maintenance, is a function of the local mechanical strains to which it is subjected" (p. 15e). The mandible is a skeletal support for the tongue and lips in the behaviors of sucking, swallowing, chewing, and speech. In a study of individuals from birth to 19 years of age, Kelly et al. (2017) concluded that the growth of the mandible is nonlinear, with rapid growth during the first five years of life in both sexes and a pronounced growth spurt in males during puberty. Growth patterns are not uniform across the different regions of the mandible. Structures in the horizontal plane have a predominantly neural growth, whereas structures in the vertical plane have a somatic growth.

Major aspects of mandibular participation in oral behaviors are discussed in the following.

Tongue movements can be analyzed into jaw-dependent and jaw-independent components. When the jaw moves, the tongue follows unless opposing forces are developed in the tongue muscles. The most efficient pattern for most oral movements is for synchronized and complementary movements of the tongue and jaw (i.e., synergy). Because the hinge (temporomandibular joint) of the jaw is relatively posterior in the head, the mechanical contribution to tongue movement is greater for anterior than posterior parts of the tongue. The lips, owing to their relatively anterior location, are highly influenced by movements of the jaw. Tongue-jaw and lip-jaw coordination is a basic requirement of speech produc-

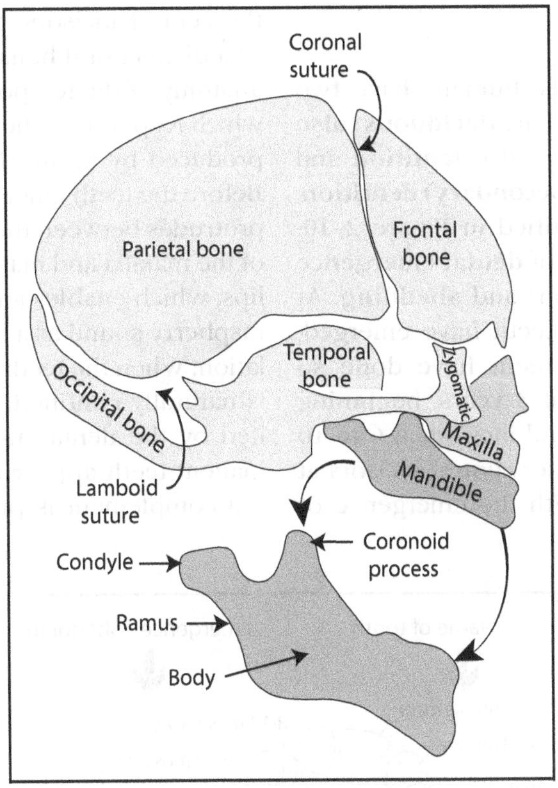

Figure 2–9. The infant skull, showing the relative proportions of the bony components.

tion. As discussed in later chapters, a jaw block can be used to stabilize the jaw during speech production as a means of isolating the muscular actions of the tongue and lips.

Jaw movement has been linked with the emergence of babbling, on the assumption that rhythmic movements of the jaw are a motor platform for repetitive babbling (as proposed in frame/content theory; MacNeilage, 1998). It also has been proposed that oscillatory patterns of jaw movement for purposes such as chewing are the precursors of speech. More is said about this in Chapter 4. Stability of position and movement of the jaw is important in behaviors such as speech and swallowing. Deviations from midline can compromise the accuracy and efficiency of movement of the jaw and the structures it supports, as discussed in Chapter 9.

Motor control of the jaw matures before that of the lips. Jaw movements in 1- and 2-year-old children are more adult-like than movements of the upper and lower lips, which are more variable (Green et al., 2002). An implication of this result is that the earliest stages of speech motor development reflect nonuniform maturation of articulatory control. It is advantageous for jaw movement to mature before movements of the lips and tongue, given that the jaw is skeletal platform for the performance of labial and lingual movements.

The Teeth

Like most mammals, humans have two generations of teeth: the **deciduous (also called primary or milk) dentition** and the **permanent (or secondary) dentition**. The teeth are identified in Figure 2–10, along with the ages of **dental emergence** (also called eruption) and **shedding**. At birth, none of the teeth have emerged, but all deciduous teeth have done so by the age of about 3 years, beginning with the lower central incisors at 6 to 10 months and the upper central incisors at 8 to 12 months. With the emergence of the central incisors, biting now appears as a distinct oral behavior and affects the anatomy of the temporomandibular joint, which responds to the mechanical loading produced by biting (Nickel et al., 2018). Before the teeth emerge, the tongue often protrudes between the alveolar processes of the maxilla and mandible to contact the lips, which enables an infant to make the raspberry sound as a lingual-labial articulation. When the teeth emerge, the tongue is naturally confined to the space delimited by the dental arches. The first permanent teeth appear by 6 years, and the full complement is present at or around

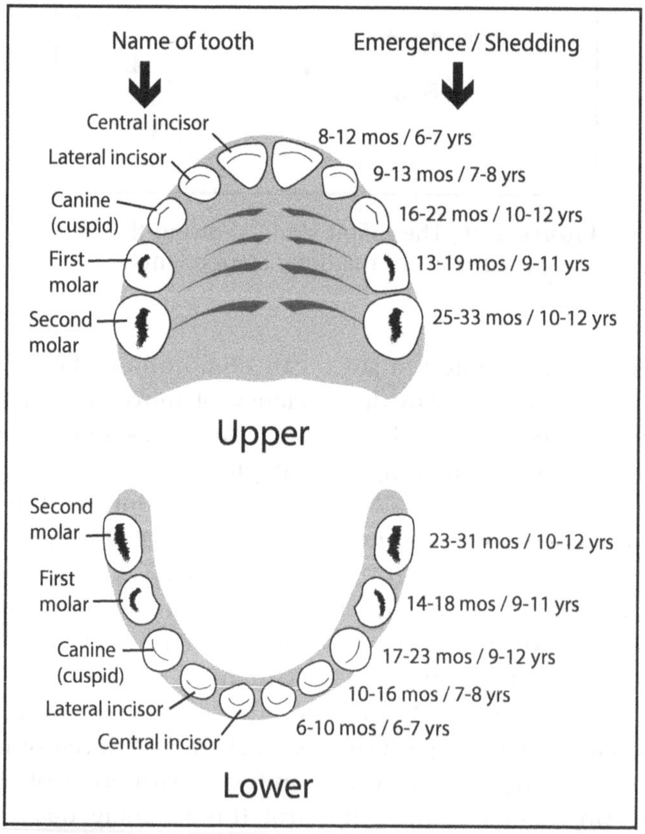

Figure 2–10. The primary or deciduous dentition, showing the tooth names and their approximate ages of emergence (also called eruption) and shedding.

the age of 18 years, with the emergence of the third molars, the so-called wisdom teeth. The permanent dentition is shown in Figure 2–11.

Dental occlusion is the pattern of surface contact between a tooth in a dental arch and its opposing tooth in the other arch when the jaws are closed. **Malocclusion** is an abnormal contact pattern that can result in inefficient or idiosyncratic biting patterns, and as discussed in Chapter 11, the possibility of speech sound disorder. Malocclusions are defined in three dimensions or planes—sagittal, vertical, and transverse, as shown in Figure 2–12. Three commonly reported classes of occlusion are known as Angle's classes, illustrated in Figure 2–13. In Class 1 (normal) occlusion, teeth are aligned in cusp fossa relationship with their antagonist teeth. In Class 2 (overjet) occlusion, the anterior maxillary teeth protrude horizontally or extend beyond the mandibular teeth. The tips of the buccal cusp tips are positioned anteriorly relative to the class 1 position. In Class 3 occlusion, the anterior maxillary dentition is positioned posteriorly to the mandibular anterior teeth. This condition is also known as a reverse overjet.

It is estimated that the worldwide prevalence of malocclusion in different stages of dentition is 56%, and the proportion of children estimated to have a definite need for orthodontic treatment is about 17%, and borderline need is about

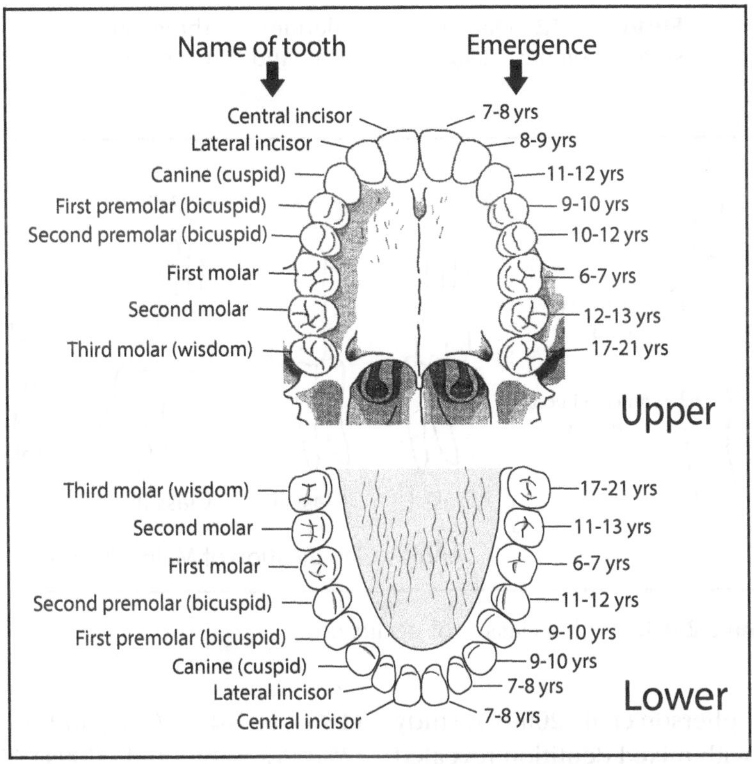

Figure 2–11. The adult or permanent dentition, showing the tooth names and the approximate ages of emergence.

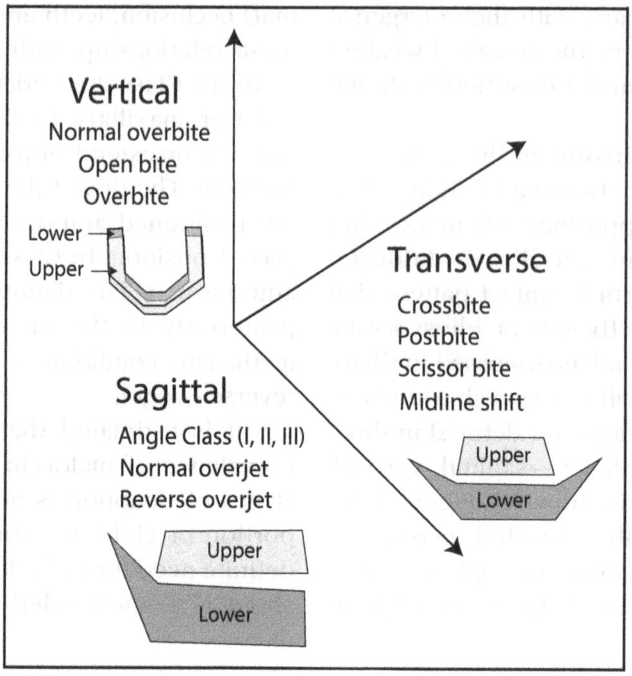

Figure 2–12. Malocclusions defined in three dimensions or planes—sagittal, vertical, and transverse.

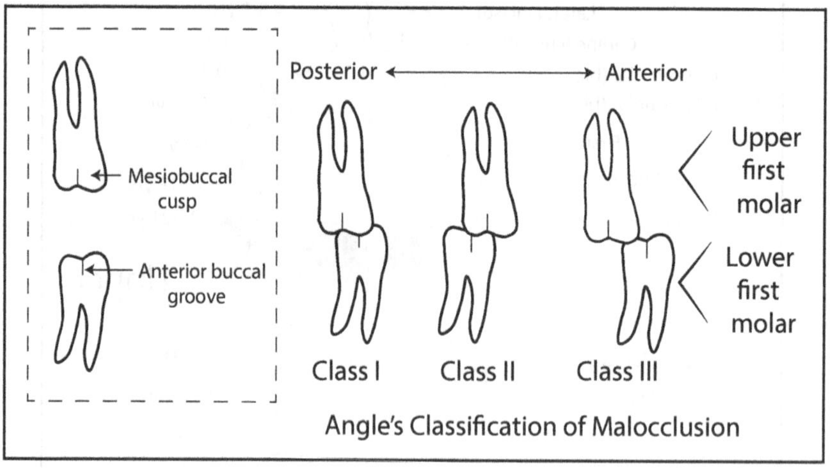

Figure 2–13. Angle's classes of occlusion.

34% (Christopherson et al., 2009). A study of children with mixed dentition revealed that the malocclusions were, in order of highest to lowest frequency: deep overbite (46%), overjet (38%), anterior open bite (18%), crossbite (8%), and reverse overjet (3%) (Tausche et al., 2004). The etiology of different malocclusions is complex and variable, including both hereditary and environmental factors, and self-correction

Malocclusion Terminology

Crossbite—the upper teeth bite inside the lower teeth

Crowding—inadequate spacing required for the teeth to be in correct alignment

Diastema—a space between two teeth, often affecting the central incisors

Midline shift (also called midline deviation or asymmetry)—a misalignment of the line between the lower teeth and the line between the upper teeth

Open bite—lack of vertical overlap of the maxillary and mandibular anterior teeth, or no contact between the maxillary and mandibular posterior teeth

Overbite (also called a deep bite)—the amount of overlap of the mandibular anterior teeth by the maxillary anterior teeth measured perpendicular to the occlusal plane

Overjet—the upper teeth extend past the lower teeth horizontally

Postbite—a lack of posterior occlusal contact

Reverse overjet (also called a Class III malocclusion)—the lower teeth are further forward than the upper teeth

is most likely for anterior open bite, sagittal malocclusions, and posterior crossbite (Dimberg et al., 2015).

The Laryngeal System

In the first few months of life, the larynx descends relative to the cervical vertebrae (of which there are seven, numbered C1 to C7). The thyroid cartilage in the newborn is attached to the hyoid bone, which is situated approximately opposite to the junction between C2 and C3. The high position of the larynx facilitates the suck-swallow-breathe pattern typical of neonates. The hyoid bone and larynx begin to descend by the age of 6 months. The descent continues to a location of C2 to C5 at 2 years, C5 at 5 years, and C7 at adulthood. A newborn has a larynx that is about one third the size of the adult larynx (Monnier, 2011). The neonate's vocal folds are approximately 7 mm long, compared to 12 to 17 mm in adult females and 17 to 23 mm in adult males.

The adult vocal folds have a laminated structure called the **lamina propria** (Figure 2–14) that is fundamental to modern theories of phonation, such as the **cover-body theory** (Hirano, 1974). The lamination is a developmental or emergent phenomenon in that the vocal folds of the newborn have a relatively uniform histology that lacks the layered structure

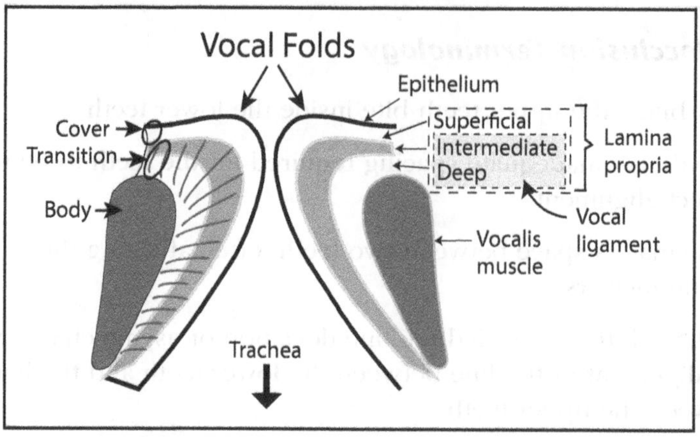

Figure 2–14. The structure of the vocal folds in adults. Each fold can be described in terms of layers. Shown at the left are the cover, transition, and body. Shown at the right are the epithelium, lamina propria, and vocal muscle.

seen in adults. The maturational pattern proceeds from a monolayer of cells in the neonate to a bilaminar structure by about two months, to a more fully constituted bilaminar structure by five months, to a trilayer by the age of seven years, and to adult-like composition by 12 years. (Boseley & Hartnick, 2006; Hartnick et al., 2005; Hirano et al., 1983; Rosenberg & Schweinfurth, 2009). It appears that mechanical stimulation of the vocal folds is required for the full development of the lamina propria, as shown in a study of three young adults with severe cerebral palsy who had never vocalized (Sato et al., 2008). Because of an intractable health problem, all three had a laryngectomy, which permitted examination of the vocal folds. The study revealed that the mucosae were hypoplastic and rudimentary, lacking a vocal ligament, Reinke's space, and the layered structure seen in healthy adults. The uniform structure of the lamina propria resembled the state described in infants. However, the detailed developmental sequence is not entirely clear. Nita et al. (2009), using light and electron microscopy to examine the larynges of human fetuses aged 7 to 9 months, found a nonuniform distribution of both collagenous and elastic system fibers in the lamina propria, indicating that vocal ligament is present before birth. The essential point is that development of the laminated structure of the vocal folds continues to the age of about 12 years. Further laryngeal development continues to the age of about 18 years, especially in males, as the laryngeal tissues undergo considerable growth in size.

The Orofacial Reflexes

Infant reflexes (also known as primitive, newborn, or neonatal reflexes) are involuntary motor responses that originate in the brainstem and are assumed to have survival value for purposes such as protection or nourishment. These reflexes are seen in typically developing infants, but many of them disappear or are integrated in voluntary motor behavior in the first year of life. It is commonly believed that these reflexes are suppressed during development of the frontal lobes of the brain. Orofacial reflexes can be observed prenatally or postnatally and are part of oral motor behavior in the first year of life and beyond (Kondraciuk et al., 2014). Table 2–1 lists the primary orofacial reflexes along with their effective stimulation, behavioral appearance, age of appearance, and age of integration or disappearance. These orofacial reflexes co-occur with early vocal behaviors and could have either facilitative or interfering effects on voluntary movements for vocalization. In addition, these reflexes are clinically important as a gauge of neurologic maturity or integrity in the developing infant. For example, persistence of a reflex beyond its usual timeframe can be an indication of neurological disorder. Kondraciuk et al. (2014) review the implications of the orofacial reflexes for the development of speech and other oral activities. They concluded that abnormalities of the orofacial reflexes can contribute to delayed speech development and articulation disorders.

Table 2–1. The Primary Orofacial Reflexes in Infants, Showing the Name of Reflex, Effective Stimulation, Behavioral Appearance, Age of Appearance, and Age of Integration or Disappearance

Infant Reflex	Stimulus	Appearance	Age of Appearance	Age of Integration or Disappearance
Rooting	Touching corner of mouth	Head turns toward stimulus, mouth opens with tongue thrusting	28 weeks GA	3 to 6 months
Sucking/ swallowing	Touching roof of mouth	Tongue protrudes to contact lips, followed by peristaltic tongue movements	14 weeks GA	6 to12 months
Tongue thrust or extrusion	Touching or depressing tongue	Tongue thrusts forward	Present at birth	4 to 6 months
Bite	Pressure applied to gums	Jaw opens and closes	Present at birth	9 to 12 months
Transverse tongue	Touching, food contact, or taste to lateral part of tongue	Tongue moves toward side of stimulation	28 to 29 weeks GA	9 to 24 months
Gag or pharyngeal reflex	Stimulation of posterior pharyngeal wall, tonsillar area, or base of tongue	Contraction of muscles in posterior pharynx	Present at birth	Diminishes by about 6 months but persists through life

"Several studies have shown persistence of primitive reflexes in children with cerebral palsy, attention-deficit/hyperactivity disorder, and autism spectrum disorder. Persistence of primitive reflexes varies in relation to the type and severity of symptoms in cases of cerebral palsy and attention-deficit/hyperactivity disorder and with the presence of comorbid intellectual disability in children with autism spectrum disorder. Primitive reflexes have also been shown to persist in adults with Down syndrome." (Sigafoos et al., 2021)

Modular Growth of the Head and Skull

A popular approach to the study of complex biological structures is to consider them as being composed of **modules**, or semi-autonomous units that interact in the overall system. An example is the identification of modules in the growth of the human skull and craniofacial system (Esteve-Altava et al., 2015). This approach is well-suited to the study of the speech production system, given that structures of the head and neck grow at different rates, as shown in Figure 2–15. There are two super-modules, the **neurocranium** (the brain case), consisting of 8 bones, and the **viscerocranium** (the facial skeleton), consisting of 14 bones that do not contact the intracranial space. The neurocranium follows a growth trajectory that Scammon (1930) called **neural growth**, which has an early growth and reaches nearly adult size at about 6 years of age. In contrast, structures of the viscerocranium follow a growth trajectory called **general or somatic growth**, in which adult size is reached much later, usually in late adolescence. These two growth trajectories are evident in Figure 2–15. The structures that are involved in speech and voice production are slow to reach adult size, which is further evidence of the general conclusion that speech development is a protracted process. Figure 2–15 also shows selected milestones in the developmental anatomy of the systems that underlie speech. At any given age in childhood, the system is in flux, so that a child must adapt motor control to changes in the size, shape, relative configuration, and tissue composition of the component structures.

The Auditory System

The ear usually is considered to have three anatomic divisions, the **external ear** comprised of the ear canal, the **middle ear** consisting of the tympanic membrane (eardrum) and the ossicular chain, and the **inner ear** consisting primarily of the cochlea and vestibular apparatus. The sense of hearing is accomplished by a series of mechanical and electrophysiological events reaching from the tympanic membrane to the higher centers of the cerebral cortex. A much-simplified version of the pathway of the auditory nervous system is shown in Figure 2–16. Some important features of this pathway are (1) the stimuli received in one ear are sent primarily to the opposite side of the brain by virtue of contralateral connections, (2) there are several opportunities for collateral interaction, and (3) different stages of processing are present. It should be emphasized that the pathways

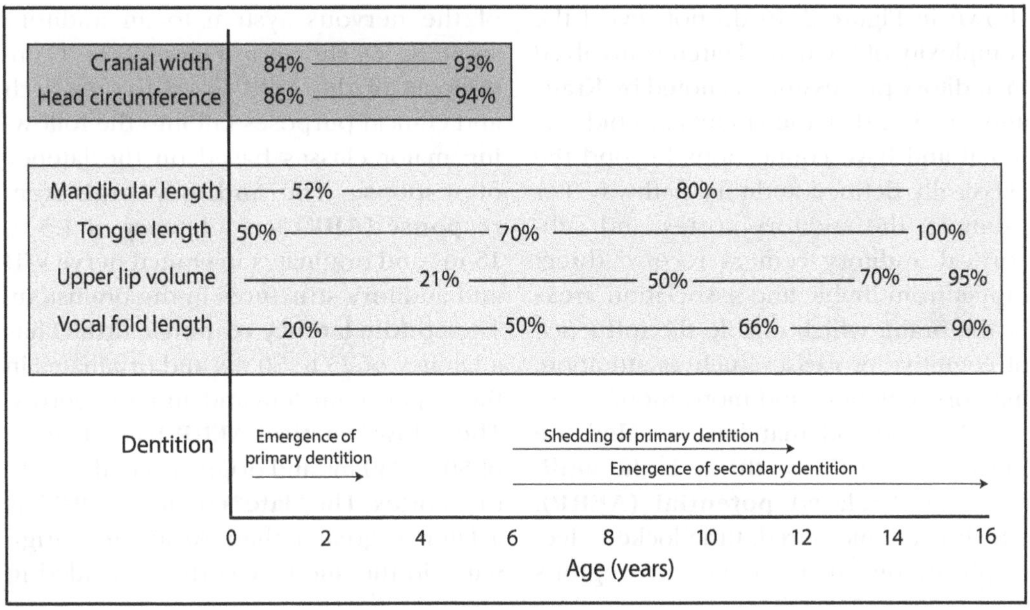

Figure 2–15. Growth trajectories of selected craniofacial structures, shown as percentages of adult size reached at various ages. The box with darker shading contains structures of the neurocranium, and the box with lighter shading contains structures of the viscerocranium and larynx. Also shown is the development of the dentition.

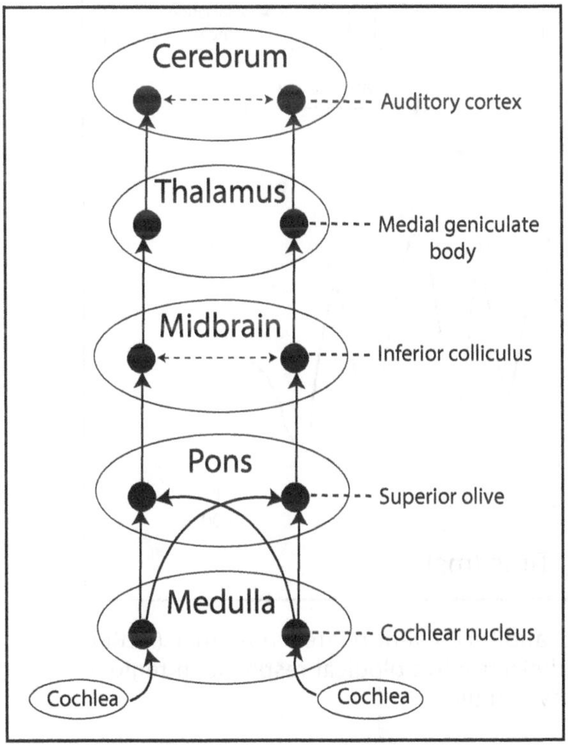

Figure 2–16. Diagram of a simplified version of the pathway of the auditory nervous system extending from the cochleae to the auditory cortex in the cerebrum. The dotted lines with double arrowheads indicate contralateral connections.

shown in Figure 2–16 do not reveal the complexity of the neural circuits involved in auditory processing. As noted by Kraus and Nicol (2014), the circuits are bidirectional and have connections beyond the classically defined auditory pathway. For example, the auditory cortex and subcortical auditory centers receive direct inputs from limbic and association areas of the brain, which enable the influence of cognitive processes such as attention, memory, emotion, and motivation.

One method that has revealed the functioning of this pathway is the **auditory event-related potential (AERP)**, which is the measured, time-locked electrophysiological response in regions of the nervous system to an auditory stimulus, as shown in Figure 2–17. Components of the AERP used for research and clinical purposes fall into the following major classes based on the latency of response. The **auditory brainstem response (ABR)** has a latency of 1.5 to 15 ms and originates in cranial nerve VIII and auditory structures in the brainstem. The **middle latency response (MLR)** has a latency of 25 to 50 ms and originates in the upper brainstem and auditory cortex. The **"slow" cortical AERP** has a latency of 50 to 250 ms and originates in the auditory cortex. The **"late" cortical AERP** has a latency greater than 80 ms and originates in the auditory cortex. Included in

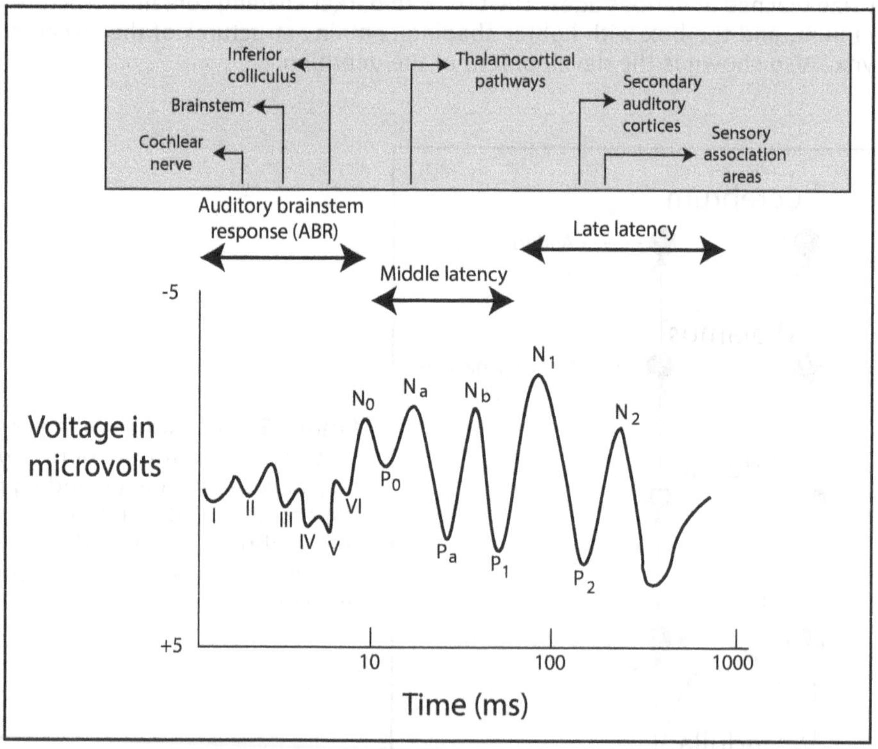

Figure 2–17. Components of the auditory event-related potential (AERP), which is the measured, time-locked electrophysiological response in regions of the nervous system to an auditory stimulus.

this late response is the mismatch negativity (MMN), which is a response to a change in the stimulus.

Spoken language processing is a term used for the complex system that supports the ability to understand and retain the acoustic signal of speech (Medwetsky, 2011). It has been suggested that spoken language processing can be divided into two major components, a low level of speech perception and a high level of listening comprehension (Schiller et al., 2020). During speech perception, acoustic cues are mapped onto phonetic or linguistic representations such as phonemes, syllables, or words. These representations are accessed by the level of listening comprehension, which integrates semantic, syntactic, and pragmatic information to determine the meaning of the spoken message. Spoken language processing provides a general framework for understanding the development of the auditory perception of language, as considered next.

The following discussion is based on summaries of the development of the auditory system in Eggermont and Moore (2012), Fior (1972), Jensen and Neff (1993), Litovsky (2015), Moore and Linthicum, Jr. (2007), and Werner (2007). A major part the of auditory pathway, including the inner ear, brainstem pathway, and cortex, is formed in the human embryo. Following a period of rapid growth and development during the second trimester of fetal development, the cochlea in the final trimester has an adult-like configuration. A study of the relationship between the duration of intrauterine development and the neural discrimination of speech identified a critical threshold of auditory cortex development around 32 weeks of gestational age, indicating that babies born before this age are vulnerable to early speech discrimination deficits that may lead to delays in language development (Alexopoulos et al., 2021). From full-term birth to about 6 months of age, maturation is observed in the middle ear and the brainstem auditory pathways. Brainstem activity is associated with behavioral responses to sound, phonetic discrimination, and evoked brainstem and early middle latency responses (aspects of speech perception in the SLP model). In the first few days and weeks of life, infants readily attend to speech and prefer speech over non-speech sounds (Vouloumanos & Werker, 2007). During the first 6 months, infants perform as **universal language receptors**, meaning that they can differentiate among all phonemic categories, including those that are not in their native language (Werker & Tees, 2005). This universal discrimination ability changes by the first year of life, when infants retain the ability to discriminate phonemes in the languages to which they are frequently exposed but lose the ability to discriminate phonemes in other languages (Werker & Yeung, 2005). This process has been called **perceptual attunement** and reflects a perceptual reorganization in which infants become highly adept at discriminating sounds in their native language at the expense of a more general discriminative ability. The benefit of such attunement is that it permits efficient and reliable discrimination of the most salient sounds. Native language perceptual categories are formed between 4 and 6 months of age for vowels, and between the 10 and 12 months, for consonants (Kuhl et al., 1992; Tsuji & Cristia, 2014; Werker & Tees, 1984). Infants in the first year of life are capable of statistical learning of sound patterns, specifically, the detection of consistent sound patterns in syllables. Syllables contained in the same word tend to occur in a predictable order, but syllables that cross word boundaries do not. Infants can detect and use the statistical properties of syllable co-occurrence to segment novel words. Not only do they detect the frequency of occurrence of syllable pairs, but they also learn the probabilities with which one syllable predicts another. Word boundaries are most likely to occur for syllable pairs that have low transitional probabilities. Infants as young as 8 months demonstrate this phenomenon with as little as 2 minutes of exposure to the sound stimuli.

Research on speech perception has led to important theoretical developments, two of which are considered here. The **native language magnet/neural commitment theory** (Kuhl et al., 2008) accounts for how infants' ability to discriminate speech sounds is progressively adapted to their native language. The theory proposes that early auditory experience with a language induces a neural commitment to the phonetic units of that language to result in prototypical representations of the phonemic inventory. This developmental process enhances the auditory processing of sounds in the native language but can interfere with detection of the sounds in non-native languages. This initial neural commitment can be altered by later auditory experiences, as in learning another language. The magnet metaphor implies that the perceptual spaces near the centers of phoneme categories are warped so that category goodness (prototype) affects the discriminability of sounds in the native language. Figure 2–18 illustrates this phenomenon in a hypothetical perceptual space in which the prototypes of the phonemes are labeled 1, 2, and 3, and various sounds are identified with alphabet letters.

Another theory, the **processing rich information from multidimensional interactive representations (PRIMIR)** (Werker & Curtin, 2005) proposes that the speech signal is processed by three dynamic filters: initial biases, developmental level of the child, and requirements of the specific language task at hand. This theory was developed to address two fundamental issues in infant speech perception: (1) that speech perception is both categorical and gradient, and (2) that perception is influenced by both ontogenetic development and online processing. The first issue is addressed by multidimensional planes, and the second, by assuming that performance is continually changing and flexible as a function of age and task so that processing and representations are interwoven.

The stages of auditory processing shown in Figures 2–16 and 2–17 apply in general to the development of audition, but with an important exception. Goodrich and Kanold (2020) discovered that an additional specialization of neurons, called subplate neurons, are found in the auditory cortex before the thalamic connections to the cortex are formed. Kanold (2022) explains that these subplate neurons participate in relay circuits connecting the thalamus with the input layer of the auditory cortex and thereby "form a specialized development structure that provides a functional scaffold for the permanent wiring of the cortex" (p. 34). From the age of 6 months to the age of 5 years, progressive maturation is observed in the thalamic projections to the cortex and of the longer latency Pa and P1 evoked potentials. Sophisticated auditory processing is accomplished by higher centers in the cortex. Yathiraj and

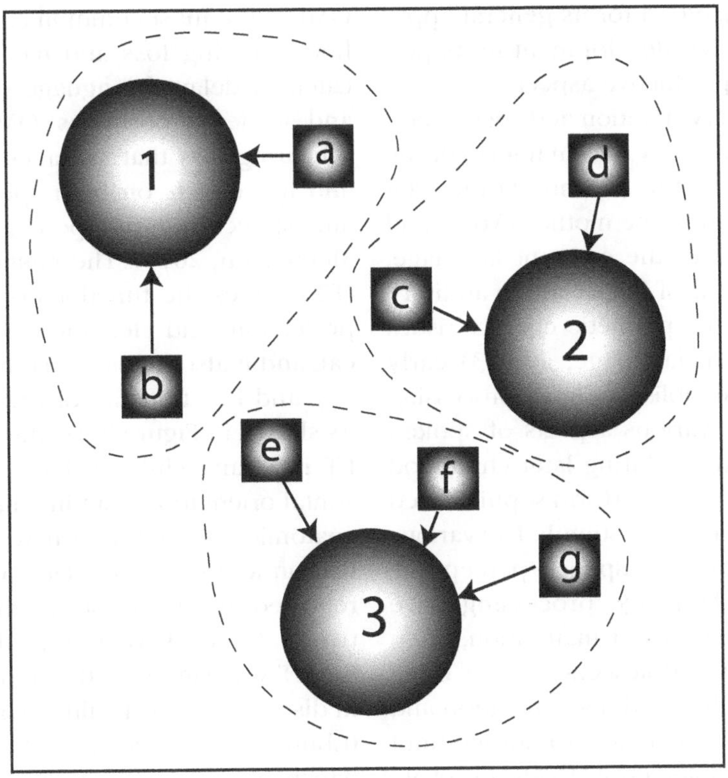

Figure 2–18. Illustration of the perceptual magnetic effect in which hypothetical perceptual space contains the prototypes of 3 phonemes (labeled 1, 2, and 3) and various sounds (labeled with alphabet letters) that are attracted to the prototypes.

Vanaja (2015) concluded that different auditory processes have different rates of development and that these differential gradients of maturation indicate regional variation in the maturation of the auditory nervous system. From 6 to 12 years, maturation occurs in the superficial cortical layers and their intracortical connections, which is related to the appearance of the N1 potential and improved linguistic discrimination. Among the late-maturing auditory abilities is the ability to distinguish rapidly presented auditory stimuli, which improves until early adolescence, as evidenced by performance on various psychophysical tasks (A. M. Fox et al., 2012). This slowly maturing feature of auditory perceptual processing may be related to language development. The **rate-constraint processing theory** of language and literacy development maintains that a child's ability to parse rapidly presented auditory material is related to the development of oral language skills (Tallal, 2000). Such parsing requires a fine degree of temporal resolution to identify phonetic segments that play a role in learning to read. The temporal resolution is on the order of tens of milliseconds.

The development of speech perception may result from cascading and multisensory influences, as suggested by Choi et al. (2018). This concept is explored further in Chapter 4 for its general application to speech development in its perceptual and productive aspects.

In summary, audition and speech perception have an early start in human development, functioning during (1) the fetal stage to recognize the mother's voice and some features of the ambient language, (2) the first year of life to attune auditory processes to the phonetic characteristics of the ambient language, and (3) early childhood to establish auditory processing that supports various aspects of spoken language, and (4) during later childhood and adolescence to perform sophisticated judgments of auditory stimuli. The various aspects of audition, speech perception, and spoken language processing have different trajectories of maturation, often extending into adolescence. Even basic skills of speech sound discrimination and categorization continue to improve until puberty and adolescence (McMurray et al., 2018; Stollman et al., 2004).

Anatomic development of the middle ear and related structures may be related to disease conditions such as **otitis media with effusion (OME)**, a collection of noninfected fluid in the middle ear space. OME is the most common cause of childhood hearing loss and has been implicated in delayed language development and academic problems. OME results in a hearing loss that averages 18 to 35 dB and has effects on both speech-in-quiet and speech-in-noise perception (Cai & McPherson, 2017). The **eustachian tube (ET)** serves the functions of ventilation, protection, and clearance of the middle ear, and it also helps to maintain physiology and functionality of the middle ear. As shown in Figure 2–19, the angle of the ET in young children has a more horizontal orientation than in adults, and this anatomic configuration may hinder ventilation and clearance. Dinç et al. (2015) reported in a study of patients aged between 8 and 79 years that the angle of the ET was significantly more horizontal in diseased versus healthy ears. Also contributing to OME is adenoid hypertrophy, which, together with other anatomic variations, can cause obstructive hypertrophy of the upper airway (Aslıer et al., 2022). (See discussion of adenotonsillar hypertrophy in Chapter 11).

Disorders of hearing are discussed in Chapter 11. The Centers for Disease

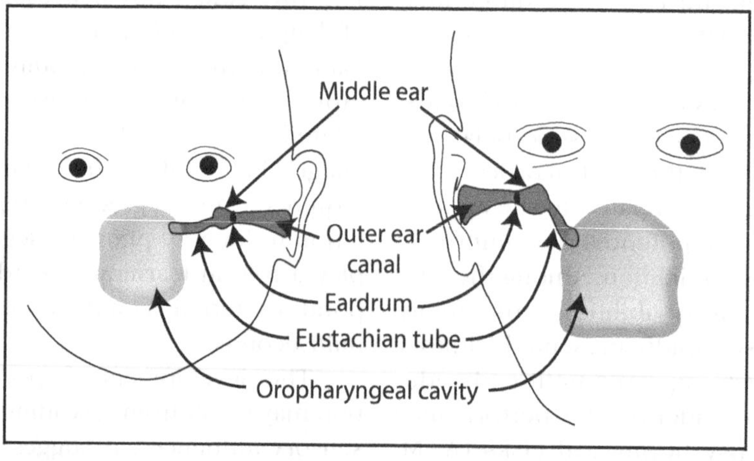

Figure 2–19. The orientation of the Eustachian tube in young children (*left*) and adults (*right*).

Control (CDC, 2020) reports that "hearing loss affects between 1 and 2 per 1,000 infants in the United States and, when left undetected, can delay a child's speech and language, social, and emotional development." Early Hearing Detection and Intervention (EHDI) programs have been established in many states and territories. The goals of these programs are to screen infants for hearing loss, ideally before 1 month of age; provide diagnostic audiologic evaluation for infants who do not pass the screening, ideally before 3 months of age; and enroll infants in early intervention if they have been identified as having permanent hearing loss, ideally before 6 months of age.

Genetics and Epigenetics

It has been estimated that about two-thirds of human genes contribute to the development of the craniofacial system (Doshi & Patil, 2012). This system is vulnerable to an "unusual number of developmental abnormalities or teratologies" (Gans, 1988, p. 3), which may reflect its formation by multiple cranial and facial elements that have differential growth patterns. According to Chai and Maxson (2006), craniofacial malformations are involved in about 75% of all congenital birth anomalies in humans. The rich genetic investment in the craniofacial system is fundamental to an understanding of typical and atypical growth and function. Genetics determines the **genotype,** the heredity material (DNA) within genes that is passed from one generation to the next. The **phenotype** is the combination of physical and behavioral traits of the organism (e.g., size and shape, metabolic activities, and patterns of movement). Genetic studies have profoundly affected the understanding of communication disorders. It is estimated that about 50% of prelingual hearing loss can be attributed to hereditary factors (Mchugh & Friedman, 2006), and genetics is implicated in several speech and language disorders, including stuttering, speech sound disorders, specific language impairment, and childhood apraxia of speech (Benchek et al., 2021; Newbury & Monaco, 2010). But in many of these disorders, etiology is multifactorial, often involving genetics with environmental and other conditions.

The **chromosome** is a threadlike body that carries genetic information in the form of genes (Figure 2–20). Of the total 46 chromosomes, 23 are inherited from the mother and 23 from the father. There are two sex chromosomes that are specialized to transmit sexual status. All cells contain at least one X chromosome, received from the mother, but female offspring have two X chromosomes (XX), whereas males have one, along with a Y chromosome received from the father (XY). The remaining 44 chromosomes are called **autosomes**. A **pedigree** (or **pedigree chart**), such as that shown in Figure 2–21, is used to analyze the pattern of inheritance of a particular trait, variant, or disease throughout family members. The pedigree also shows the vital status (living or dead) of the family members.

Sex and Gender

Sex is a primary factor in the prevalence of communication disorders. Nearly all developmental disorders that affect communication, speech, and language skills are more frequent in boys (Adani & Cepanec, 2019; Chapter 4), and sex must be considered in the diagnosis and treatment of a wide array of health and educational

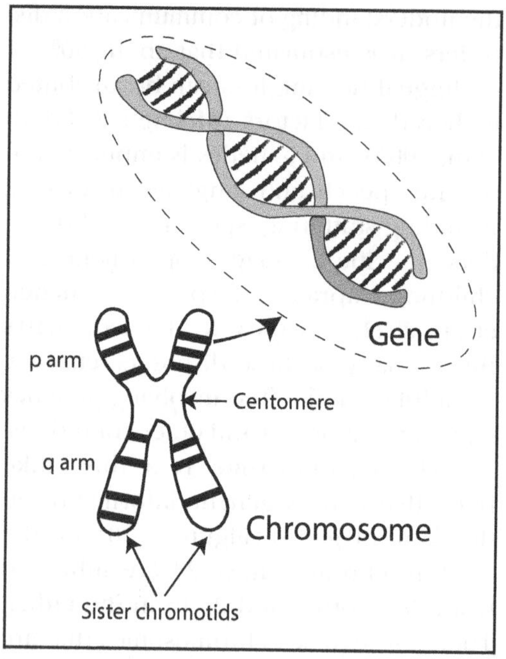

Figure 2–20. The chromosome and gene. The p arm is also called the short arm, and the q arm is also called the long arm.

problems (Zanon et al., 2019). Sex and gender differences are mentioned frequently in this book, so it is important to define these terms. The World Health Organization (WHO) discusses the difference between sex and gender. According to the WHO, **sex** relates to "the different biological and physiological characteristics of males and females, such as reproductive organs, chromosomes, hormones, etc." In contrast, **gender** refers to "the socially constructed characteristics of women and men—such as norms, roles and relationships of and between groups of women and men. It varies from society to society and can be changed. The concept of gender includes five important elements: relational, hierarchical, historical, contextual and institutional." Spoken language is strongly affected by sex or gender. Voices usually can be classified as either male or female based primarily on

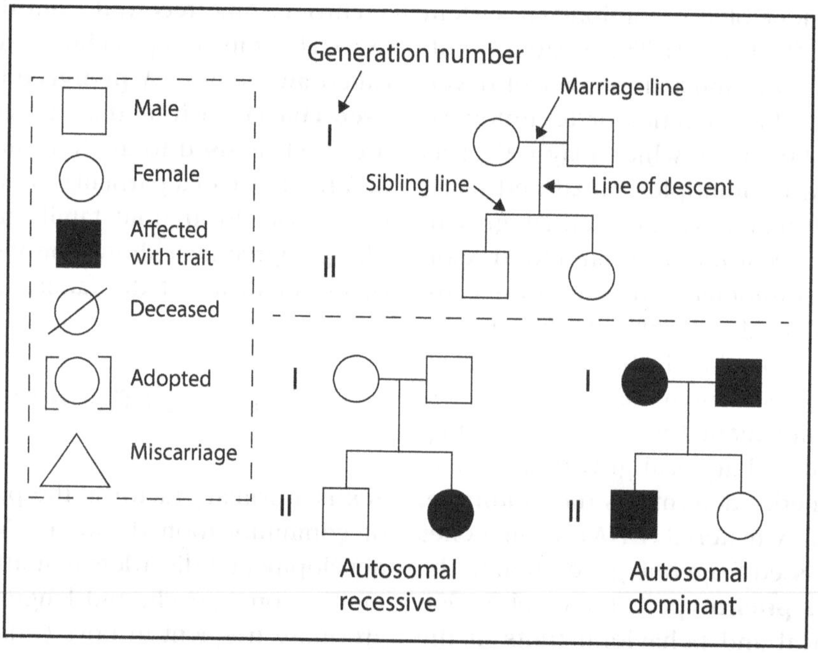

Figure 2–21. Symbols and patterns commonly used in a pedigree chart that shows the genetic history of a family over generations.

vocal pitch (as discussed in Chapter 6). In addition, there are sex or gender differences in various patterns of communication, as considered in Chapters 3, 4, and 5. In this book, the term *sex* is used to refer to biological and physiological differences between male and females, and the term *gender* is used to refer to differences in the overall patterns of social and communicative behaviors.

Patterns of Inheritance

The primary patterns of inheritance are described in terms of if and how family members are affected (i.e., carrying a trait, variant, or disease). The patterns are as follows.

Autosomal Dominant Patterns

- If both parents are affected and an offspring is not, then the trait must be dominant (the parents are both heterozygous).
- All affected individuals must have at least one parent who is affected.
- If both parents are unaffected, then all offspring must be unaffected (homozygous recessive).
- Huntington's disease is an example of an autosomal dominant genetic disorder.

Autosomal Recessive Patterns

- If both parents are unaffected and an offspring is affected, then the trait must be recessive (parents are heterozygous carriers).
- If both parents show a trait, all offspring must also show the trait (homozygous recessive).
- Cystic fibrosis, sickle cell anemia, and Tay-Sachs disease are examples of autosomal recessive disorder.

X-Linked Inheritance

- Pedigree charts are not sufficient to show X-linked inheritance because autosomal traits could possibly generate the same results.
- Certain patterns or trends can confirm that a trait is not X-linked dominant or recessive.

X-Linked Dominant Inheritance

- If a male shows a trait, then all daughters and his mother show it as well.
- An unaffected mother cannot have affected sons (or an affected father)
- X-linked dominant traits tend to be more common in females because they have two X chromosomes.
- Fragile X syndrome (FXS), also called Martin-Bell syndrome, is an X-linked dominant genetic condition. It is the most prevalent inherited cause of mild to severe intellectual disability and accounts for about half of the cases of X-linked mental retardation and is the most common cause of mental impairment after trisomy 21 (Down syndrome). Both Fragile X syndrome and Down syndrome are discussed in more detail in Chapter 10.

X-Linked Recessive Inheritance

- If a female shows a trait, then all sons and her father must show it as well.
- An unaffected mother can have affected sons if she is a carrier (heterozygous).
- X-linked recessive traits tend to be more common in males because they have only one X chromosome.
- Duchenne muscular dystrophy, some types of colorblindness, and hemophilia are examples of X-linked recessive disorders.

Genetic and Epigenetics of Speech Anatomy

The shape of the face is determined mainly by the geometry of underlying skeletal elements, adipose tissue, and muscles (Murillo-Rincón & Kaucka, 2020). Well before puberty, sex differences can be seen in the forehead, buccal region, and chin (Matthews et al., 2018). Knowing variations in typically developing anatomy is a necessary foundation for the identification of clinical conditions, some of which can be subtle. Weinberg et al. (2016) stated in their rationale for a craniofacial repository that, "Thus, all descriptions of dysmorphology are inherently comparative by nature . . . an understanding of what constitutes the range of normal variation for craniofacial features is essential." (pp. e185–e186). In the same vein, Tubbs et al. (2016) remarked that, "the line between an anatomic variation that is pathologic or predisposes one to pathology and one that is just a trait that is outside of what is considered normal is very gray" (p. xvii).

The most common orofacial anomaly is **clefting** (a fissure or longitudinal opening), which has a worldwide incidence of 1 in 700 births. Clefting can be **nonsyndromic** (isolated) or **syndromic** (occurring as part of a constellation of features, as in velocardiofacial syndrome). It can also occur in **sequences** (in which malformations occur in a temporal pattern, as in Pierre Robin sequence). Cleft lip is associated with 171 syndromes, but only about 15% of individuals with cleft lip-cleft palate are syndromic (Eppley et al., 2005). Craniofacial anomalies have been described in many different syndromes or sequences, including Apert, Carpenter, Cri du chat, Crouzon, Down, Fetal Alcohol Spectrum (Fetal Alcohol Syndrome and Fetal Alcohol Effect), Fragile-X, Long-face, Noonan, Pfeiffer, Pierre Robin, Roberts, Saethre-Chotzen, Treacher Collins, Velocardiofacial, and Williams.

More subtle craniofacial anomalies have been reported for attention deficit hyperactivity disorder (ADHD; Andersson & Sonnesen, 2018), autism (Manouilenko et al., 2014), and cerebral palsy (Alaçam et al, 2020; Edvinsson & Lundqvist, 2016). These less obvious anomalies, which may be considered as part of the general category of **minor physical anomalies (MPAs)**, are of particular interest in understanding relationships in cerebro-craniofacial development. The brain and craniofacial tissues develop in concert and under mutual influence with some common genetic signaling pathways (Francis-West et al., 2003). MPAs may provide important insights into neurodevelopmental models of disorders such as autism (Boutrus et al., 2017; C. Cheung et al., 2011; Ozgen et al., 2010) and schizophrenia (Compton & Walker, 2008). Compton and Walker (2008) explain that "both genetic and environmental factors contribute to structural and functional brain changes in the intrauterine and perinatal periods that predispose one to developing schizophrenia" (p. 425). As noted by Ozgen et al. (2010), research shows a rapidly increasing number of genes in the regulation of cerebro-craniofacial development.

Historically, the two main methods of following the growth and reconfiguration of craniofacial structures were superimposition of images (such as lateral cephalograms) or structural measurements. Superimposition has been a mainstay in fields such as orthodontia in which successive images for an individual patient can be obtained over the course of treatment. Superimposition can be done with a best-fit method for the overall cephalogram, or the identification of landmarks, either metallic implants or relatively stable structures of the maxilla or mandible. Superimposition in 2-dimensional studies often is referenced to the cranial base, which changes little after neural growth is completed. With the introduction of 3-dimensional cone-beam computed tomography, the typical approaches for superimposition are registration points or mathematical algorithms. The alternative to superimposition is to make linear or angular measurements of structures and structural relationships. This approach has a long history in cephalography, originally based on x-ray cephalograms but now also including images obtained through CT or MRI. Some of the commonly performed measurements depend on the identification of landmarks, such as reference planes, lines, or points (Figure 2–22).

The development of speech is influenced by both genetic and epigenetic factors. The word **epigenetics** has been

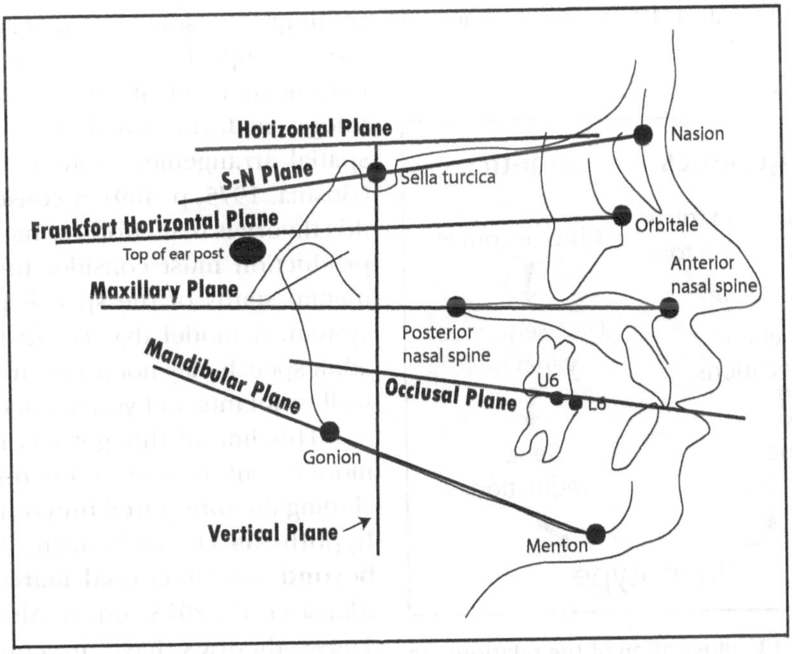

Figure 2–22. Reference points, lines, and planes used in craniofacial measurements.

variously defined since it was introduced by Waddington (1942). For present purposes, epigenetics is defined as the different phases or processes extending from genotype to phenotype, including intrinsic factors (e.g., hormonal effect on cells; Buschang & Hinton, 2005) to extrinsic factors (e.g., biomechanical and/or environmental stimuli that affect gene expression; Carlson, 2005). Roosenboom et al. (2016, p. 1) summarized the matter as follows, "The craniofacial complex is the billboard of sorts containing information about sex, health, ancestry, kinship, genes, and environment." Figure 2–23 illustrates how genetic and epigenetic influences mutually determine the phenotype. Neither genetics nor epigenetics operates in isolation in determining the developmental path of an organism.

The concept that the anatomy of the craniofacial system is partly determined by its functions has a long history, but the present account takes up this history in the 1960s and 1970s. In a series of articles, Moss (1962, 1963, 1968; 1997a, 1997b, 1997c, 1997d) proposed and refined his **functional matrix hypothesis**. A functional matrix is an inclusive term that integrates soft tissues (e.g., muscles, glands, nerves), the teeth, and functioning spaces (e.g., the cavities of the vocal tract). Moss proposed that the functional matrix is primary in development and that any associated skeletal unit is secondary, which means that the functional matrix drives changes in the size, shape, and spatial position of the skeletal components. The growth of the skeletal framework that supports a function (e.g., speech) is influenced by both the growth and the operational activity of the related functional matrixes. Bosma (1975) independently developed a similar theory that he called performance anatomy, in which the functions performed by a system contribute to the developing anatomy of that system. He wrote as follows concerning speech development, "The gestures of prelinguistic sounds and early speech are accomplished by structures at their current moment of development in histology, in form and dimension, and in spatial arrangement within this region" (Bosma, 1975, p. 469). A consequence of this theory is that efforts to model speech production must consider the developmental status of the speech production system. A model that is satisfactory for adult speech may not necessarily apply as well to infants and young children.

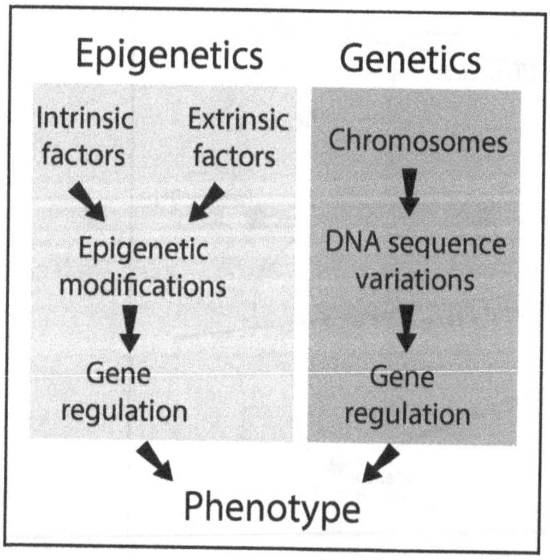

Figure 2–23. Illustration of the relationship between epigenetics and genetics in giving expression to the phenotype.

This line of thought has resulted in more recent theories and hypotheses, including the **integrated functional matrix hypothesis** (D. Lieberman, 2011), and **beyond the functional matrix** (Esteve-Altava et al., 2015; Esteve-Altava, 2020). These theories have in common the principle that craniofacial structures are shaped by experience and function, that is, epigenetic factors. Lieberman (2011) emphasized an epigenetic perspective, which he describes as the "vast set of processes by which alternative, variable phenotypes—cellular, anatomical, physiological, even behavioral—derive from a given genotype" (p. 271). This principle is important in specialties such as orthodontia and airway dentistry, but it is relevant as well to speech-language pathology. A clinical example is considered in Chapter 10 on a condition called **long-face syndrome**, which may be the result of the behavior of mouth breathing.

Socio-Emotional Development

"Emotions are a 'grammar of social living' that situate the self within a social and moral order; they structure interactions, like scripts in pieces of fiction, in relationships that matter" (Keltner et al., 2019, p. 3). This "grammar of social living" is played out in different ways—facial expressions, body postures or movements, vocalizations, touching, or emoticons (emotional icons) that are added to text messages. Emotion and vocal behavior are closely linked because (1) emotions are expressed through vocalizations through the lifespan, (2) language is a vehicle for recognizing and classifying different emotional states, and (3) speech production is affected by an individual's emotional state. Emotion is often neglected in accounts of speech and language development even though spoken language is almost always accompanied by emotional expression of some kind. Even a so-called neutral emotion is an emotional state. Both speaker and listener make use of emotional information for communicative purposes, and speech and emotion develop mutually and interactively as children relate with others and with the environment. The two major domains of research on emotional expression are the face and the voice, as discussed in the following.

Facial Expression of Emotions

Facial expressions are accomplished by the facial muscles, also called the **mimetic muscles** (the word *mimetic* means imitation or mimicry). Studies of facial expressions of emotions have been highly influential in defining emotion and determining the number of emotions that can be expressed. A difficulty is that the science of emotion lacks a common definition of its subject. Izard (2010) interviewed 34 emotion researchers to get their definitions of emotion. From the varied responses, he distilled the following:

> Emotion consists of neural circuits (that are at least partially dedicated), response systems, and a feeling state/process that motivates and organizes cognition and action. Emotion also provides information to the person experiencing it and may include antecedent cognitive appraisals and ongoing cognition including an interpretation of its feeling state, expressions or social-communicative signals, and may motivate approach or avoidant behavior, exercise control/regulation of responses, and be social or relational in nature. (p. 367)

This definition may not be satisfying, and Izard himself comments that it says more about what emotion does than what it is. Definitional problems aside, efforts have been made to determine how many emotions humans (and animals) have. In the *Expressions of the Emotions in Man and Animals*, Charles Darwin wrote that there are about 34 emotions. Paul Ekman (1993) concluded that there are six basic emotions, including sadness, happiness, fear, anger, surprise, and disgust. Plutchik (1980), in his Wheel of Emotion, grouped eight basic emotions in pairs of opposites: joy-sadness, anger-fear, trust-distrust, and surprise-anticipation. Jack et al. (2014) identified only four basic emotions: happiness, sadness, fear/surprise, and anger/disgust. Cowen and Keltner (2017) concluded from a study of reactions to emotionally evocative short videos that the emotional experiences reported by participants took the form of 27 different categories. The discordant results are due in part to differences in methods and in theories. Malik and Marwaha (2022) commented that the distinct emotions present from birth are anger, joy, and fear, as revealed by universal facial expressions. The typical approach used in the study of emotional expression in children is to determine the ages at which specific emotions are acquired, so that development is a matter of adding emotions, rather than changing their quality. But it is not certain that an emotion such as fear in early childhood is the same as in adults. Children also differ from adults in having a greater tendency to make decisions based on emotions rather than logic and reason (Grisso, 2000). Emotional development is potentially multidimensional and not just a matter of adding discrete items to an emotional palette.

The two most widely accepted theories are the basic emotion theory and dimensional theory. Basic emotion theory holds that emotions are discrete entities or categories, whereas dimensional theory regards emotions as independent dimensions (Cowen & Keltner, 2017). The neural circuits of emotion are extensive within the central nervous system. Grandjean (2021) proposed an integrated model of the functional and brain levels of emotional processing that encompassed five main systems of cortical and subcortical neural networks that account for perception and sound organization, related action tendencies, and associated values that integrate complex social contexts and ambiguous situations. Although it is often assumed that emotions are basically the same across cultures, Mesquita (2022) argues to the contrary, citing evidence that emotions are not innate but culturally determined as to type and expression. For example, anger is not the same across cultures and situations, and some cultures discourage the expression of emotions. If Mesquita is correct, then the experience of emotions in Western, Educated, Industrialized, Rich, and Democratic (WEIRD) cultures should not be generalized worldwide.

Vocal Expression of Emotions

The vocal expression of emotion (emotional prosody) has been studied in two major ways: emotional prosody of connected speech (e.g., conversation or reading a text) and vocal bursts (brief, nonword utterances such as laughs, shrieks, growls, sighs, oohs, and ahhs). Juslin and Laukka (2003) concluded that listeners can judge emotional prosody with an accuracy of about 70% for the five emotions of anger, fear, happiness, sadness, and tenderness. In a study that included individuals from ten different nations, Cordaro et al. (2016) found that listeners could identify vocal bursts of six positive emotions (amusement, awe, contentment, desire, interest, relief, and triumph) and six negative emotions (anger, contempt, disgust, embarrassment, fear, pain, and sadness).

It has been shown that infants can discriminate emotional expressions in non-verbal vocalizations (Soderstrom et al., 2017) and prosodic cues (Flom & Bahrick, 2007). Infants in the second half of the first year have a vocal repertoire that contributes to regulating cooperative interaction with their mothers, which is thought to be important in language acquisition (Papaeliou et al., 2002). However, perception and production of emotional prosody has a long developmental trajectory. Aguert et al. (2013) summarized the matter by noting that the ability to use emotional prosody to attribute an emotional state is present early in life, but this ability develops over a considerable period before attaining the level observed in adults.

Developmental Interactions of Emotion, Language, and Socialization

Emotion and language interact so that emotions can be labeled by children as they experience them during development. Hoemann et al. (2019) proposed that emotional development is the process of developing emotion concepts, and that emotion words are critical to this process. They suggested that infants and children learn emotion categories much as they learn other abstract conceptual categories, namely, by observing others who use emotion words to label events that are themselves highly variable. Lindquist et al. (2015) also draw attention to the language-emotion interaction in their Conceptual Act Theory, which proposes that an instance of emotion occurs when information from one's body or another body is given meaning in the present situation by concept knowledge about emotion. Language is a primary means to support conceptual knowledge that interprets the meaning of sensations from the body and world in different situations.

Atypical recognition of emotions has been observed in several developmental conditions, including autism spectrum disorder, developmental stuttering, Down syndrome, attention deficit hyperactivity disorder, and a variety of child psychopathologies and neuropathologies (as considered in more detail in Chapters 7 and 10). Moreover, it has been reported that the recognition of vocal emotions is positively related to socio-emotional adjustments in typically developing 4-to-8-year-old children (Neves et al., 2021). It is important to recognize the interaction of emotion with the act of speaking. A study of psychosocial stress testing revealed that a large portion of the physiological response that typically would have been attributed to emotion was due to vocalization alone. Speaking, especially public speaking, induces physiological responses, such as increased blood pressure (Grimley et al., 2018). Although these responses have been studied largely in people who stutter, it is possible that similar responses occur in many individuals and a variety of circumstances, including children with other types of speech disorders.

Verbal and Nonverbal Communication

Speech communication consists of both verbal and nonverbal components. Verbal communication is the linguistic message, and nonverbal communication is the behavior of the face, body, or voice with the linguistic content removed. However, communication usually involves an interaction of verbal and nonverbal cues, and it is not easy to separate them (Hall, Horgan, & Murphy, 2019). For example, emotions often are expressed by a combination of verbal and nonverbal cues. An often-cited statistic is that 93% of communication is nonverbal. This statistic comes from studies by Merhabian and Ferris (1967) and Merhabian and Wiener (1967) in which the participants judged words as positive, neutral, or negative when presented by a speaker with or without facial cues. Analysis of the data showed that the listeners' perceived attitudes were a combination of three cues in the following proportion: 7% verbal, 38% vocal (tone), and 55% facial expression. But generalizing these results to everyday communication is risky because we usually communicate not with single words but with multiword utterances in more complicated social circumstances. Nonverbal cues certainly are important in communication, but their contribution may not be as great as suggested in these studies. Children learn to use nonverbal communication in the form of gestures (emblems such as waving goodbye), vocal emotional cues, facial expressions, and body movements. The relative use of verbal and nonverbal cues depends on the communicative setting and the personal characteristics of the interactants.

Conclusions

The biological and psychological foundations of speech have developmental trajectories that are relevant to the acquisition of skilled behaviors needed for speech. The main conclusions of this chapter are as follows.

1. In many respects, the growth and maturation of the biological and psychological systems relevant to speech extend to late adolescence and even young adulthood. This protracted maturation is important background for understanding the processes of speech development and their vulnerability to delay or disorder, as well as their plasticity as a factor in intervention for speech disorders.
2. Heterochrony (different rates of development and maturation) is evident in the overall biological system relevant to speech as well as in its component subsystems. Therefore, growth and development should be understood in terms of differential rates for the various components and processes underlying speech and other oral behaviors.
3. The system is highly complex, consisting of a large array of muscles that vary in their histologic properties and their functional specializations. Furthermore, some tissues involved in speech production are highly specialized and are not found in other parts of the body. Speech is special in many ways.
4. Mounting evidence points to the principle that the functions of the craniofacial system determine aspects of its developmental anatomy (i.e., function helps to shape structure).
5. The two main ways of expressing emotion are facial expressions and vocal behaviors. Human vocalization is an interaction of linguistic and affective communication, and this interaction is a lifelong process.

3

SYSTEMS AND PROCESSES IN SPOKEN AND INNER LANGUAGE

For all its ordinariness in everyday life, speaking is a remarkable behavior. It is the most common means of learning and expressing language. It is a motor activity that has few rivals in terms of its demands on the precise timing of movements. It is the product of dozens of muscles in the respiratory, laryngeal, and supralaryngeal systems. Models of spoken language reveal the multiple processes involved in producing an utterance. One such influential model is presented by Dutch psycholinguist Willem J. M. Levelt in his book *Speaking: From Intention to Articulation* (1993). Many of the ideas described in the book resonate in contemporary writings on speech production, and they serve as core concepts in this chapter.

Speech can be overt or covert. Overt speech is speech that is spoken aloud, whether to others or oneself. Covert speech, also known as inner speech, is known only to the person who formulates it. Speech is important not only because it is a primary means for communicating with others (overt speech), but also because it helps us to regulate our own behaviors, make decisions, monitor our actions, and reflect on our experiences (covert speech). This chapter considers efforts to model the production of overt speech by breaking it into component stages of processing. But it also examines the understanding of inner speech and how this knowledge relates to the overall phenomenon of language and to our own sense of self. Language learning includes the two domains of overt and inner speech. Understanding the development of speech in children should consider both domains.

Spoken language usually is conceptualized as a multilevel or multistage process that begins with an idea or mental message to be communicated and ends with articulatory movements that generate an acoustic signal (Levelt's, 1993, intention to articulation). This output signal is received by a listener who decodes the acoustic signal and uses language processes to derive the intended message. The nature and number of stages vary considerably across different models and theories, and only selected examples are considered here. In their classic book *The Speech Chain*, Denes and Pinson (1963) included a diagram of the process of speech communication that has been reproduced hundreds of times. Figure 3–1 follows Denes and Pinson in showing the components of speaker, medium, and listener at the left side of the figure, along with the basic levels of processing in the central panel (i.e., the linguistic and physiological levels in the speaker, the acoustic level, and physiological and linguistic levels in the listener). Research has elaborated and refined the processes of spoken language, as shown in the elements to the right side of Figure 3–1. The goal of this chapter is to discuss the processing of spoken language with reference to speech development and disorders. The discussion begins with an unpacking of the elements in Figure 3–1, with special reference to speech and language development in children.

The Linguistic Level

Levelt (1993) summarized a line of investigation into language processing that has deeply influenced the contemporary understanding of how we communicate with speech, especially how words are retrieved from long-term memory and produced as articulatory patterns. Several aspects of Levelt's theory of language production are shown in the upper right section of Figure 3–1 and in a more elabo-

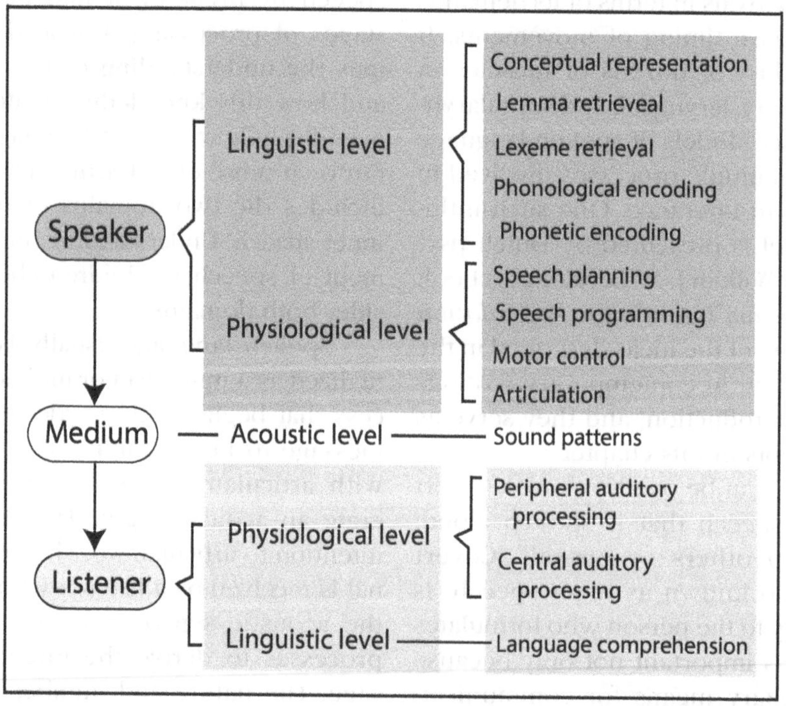

Figure 3–1. The "speech chain" in relation to associated components in an elaborated model of spoken language.

rated diagram of Figure 3–2. The following discussion is keyed to the levels in Figure 3–2, which serves as a graphic outline of what follows.

Conceptual Representation

This level in Figure 3–2 is one of mental representation of a message to be conveyed. It is not yet tied to specific choices of words or syntax but rather guides the overall process of spoken language to ensure that the intended message (concept or idea) is produced. The early stages of the communicative process are the intention to communicate and the formulation of a thought to be expressed. These operations are prelinguistic in the sense that they precede language formulation

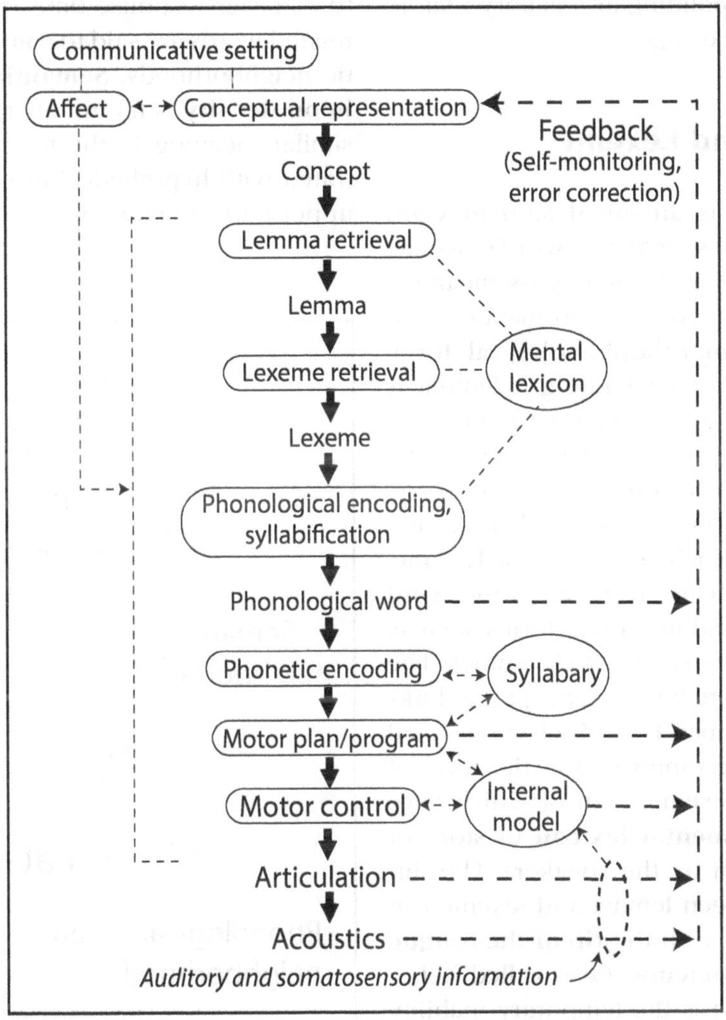

Figure 3–2. A model of the production of spoken language modified from Levelt (1993).

per se. The nature of the conceptual representation depends on the speaking task. For example, repetition of a modeled utterance ("Say the word *elephant*") differs from picture naming ("What is the name of this animal?") and from remembering a trip to the zoo ("What were the largest animals that you saw?"). The present discussion presumes that the speaker is formulating a message to be communicated and needs to select words, a suitable syntactic arrangement of the words, and a corresponding articulatory plan to convey the message.

Lemma and Lexeme

The **lemma** is an initial step in word retrieval that specifies a word's syntactic properties and possibly its meaning. A second step retrieves information about the word's morphophonological form. One way of understanding a lemma is to look in a dictionary for the entry of a particular word. The main entry is the lemma. But the dictionary may group several other forms of the word under the same entry; each of these is a **lexeme**. A frequently cited example is the word *go* (lemma) and its variant forms such as *goes, going, gone, went* (lexemes). The lemma is a core lexical concept that links different lexemes. Lexical selection (word finding) is accomplished at the level of lemma and lexeme, both of which have access to a **mental lexicon** (a store of words known by the speaker). The difference between lemma and lexeme can be illustrated with the **tip-of-the-tongue (TOT) phenomenon** (also called lethologica), which is the temporary inability of a speaker to recall a well-known word. Very often, the speaker can recall partial information about the hard-to-recall word, such as its initial sound, number of syllables, or meaning. The speaker knows that the word is present in the lexicon (indicating awareness of the lemma) but cannot retrieve the word itself (the lexeme). The mental lexicon is characterized in part by **semantic neighborhoods**. Research on word recognition has shown that a speaker activates semantically related words along with a target word. This activation is demonstrated experimentally as advantages in word recognition (e.g., faster response time). Semantically related words are said to compose semantic neighborhoods. **Semantic neighborhood density** is the number of words of similar meaning in the lexicon, as illustrated with hypothetical examples in the upper part of Figure 3–3.

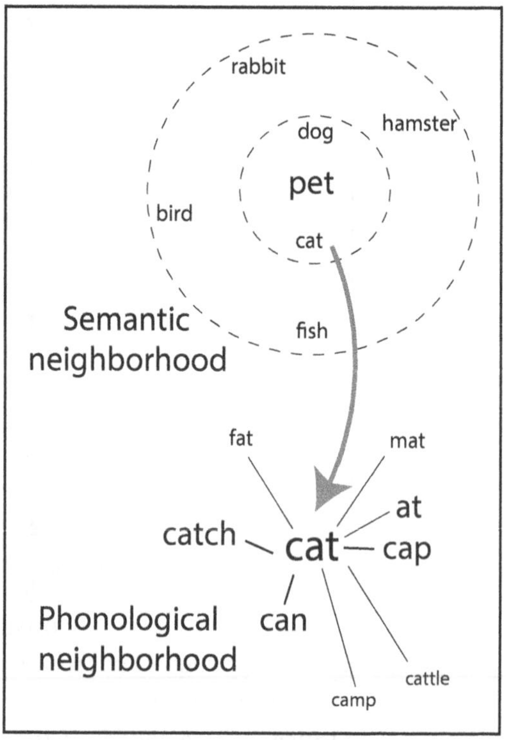

Figure 3–3. Hypothetical semantic and phonological neighborhoods.

Phonological Encoding

Phonology deals with the ways in which sounds are systematically organized to form words in a language or dialect (a topic that is discussed in Chapter 7). Phonological encoding translates a lexeme into sound patterns that conform to the rules of the language. This level has access to the mental lexicon. A **phonological representation (PR)** for a word is the underlying sound structure stored in long-term memory. This representation has roles in word learning, speech production, and literacy. There are two different perspectives on children's PRs. The first, called the **accessibility account**, holds that PRs are adult-like from infancy (Liberman et al., 1989; Rozin & Gleitman, 1977) The second, called the **emergent account**, proposes that PRs become gradually restructured with development (Metsala & Walley, 1998; Ventura et al., 2007; Ziegler & Goswami, 2005). Walley et al. (2003) proposed that children's PRs, compared to adults', are more holistic and underspecified, which can result in reduced discrimination among vocabulary items. If a child stores words as detailed acoustic codes, a storage challenge arises as new words are learned. This challenge forces the child to restructure the storage to a more economical one based on segments such as phonemes rather than acoustic patterns. The process continues to develop until the age of about 8 years. As a child's lexicon grows, there are corresponding changes in semantic neighborhood density.

Clinical implications are discussed in Chapter 7 with reference to PRs in disorders of speech, language, and reading. Sutherland and Gillon (2005) stated that the precision and accessibility of underlying PRs of spoken words may contribute to problems in phonological awareness and subsequent reading development for young children with speech/language impairment. They recommended the use of receptive-based assessments that examine underlying PRs to provide clinically relevant information for children with communication impairment. An example of such an assessment is the **Quality of Phonological Representations (QPR)** task (Claessen et al., 2009), in which children judge correct or incorrect productions of words shown on a computer screen. Using this method, Claessen and Leitão (2012) found that children with specific language impairment had lower quality phonological representations than children with typical language development.

Phonological theories are briefly reviewed in Chapter 7. The goal of this book is not to consider such theories in depth but rather to give an overview of how these theories relate to children's speech production and to identify central concepts in speech development and disorders. One of the more controversial issues in phonology is the status of the syllable. Kohler (1966) attacked the concept of the syllable as being unnecessary, impossible, or harmful, or some combination of these. His criticisms dealt mainly with the difficulty of segmenting syllables in a spoken message. In defending the utility of the syllable, Anderson (1969, p.196) admitted, "The syllable is a traditional, if often ill- or undefined, notion in phonological studies, though it is often mentioned only to be neglected." The position taken in this book is that the syllable is a fundamental unit of language structure and processing. The syllable finds numerous applications, including analyzing the early vocalizations in infancy, specifying phonological processes in children's speech development, describing patterns of misarticulation, characterizing the auditory encoding of the acoustic signal of speech, and understanding the organization of articulatory movements in typical and atypical speech production. The syllable is indispensable as it lends conceptual unity to a variety of phenomena mentioned in almost every chapter of this book. As shown in Figure 3–3, syllabification is part of phonological encoding, and a **syllabary** (a catalog of syllables that can be accessed in perceiving and producing speech) is associated with phonetic encoding. The relationship between words, syllables, segments, and phonetic features is shown in Figure 3–4, a depiction of phonological representation.

As mentioned earlier, words have semantic neighborhoods. They also have a phonological neighborhood, as depicted in the lower part of Figure 3–3. A **phonological neighborhood** is defined as the number of phonologically similar words in the lexicon, and usually is determined as the number of words that are created by adding, deleting, or substituting a single sound in a target word. **Phonological neighborhood density** is a measure of neighborhood size based on the number of words that can be generated by replacing a phoneme in a target word with another phoneme in the same position. The semantic neighborhood density increases with age and language experience, and the same is true of phonological neighborhood density. In addition, density holds implications for language processing. It has been shown in studies with adults that words with more phonologically similar neighbors are recognized with less efficiency than words with fewer neighbors. Apparently, greater neighborhood density increases lexical competition. The same principle applies to children. Donnelly and Kidd (2021) found that the lexicons of 30-month-olds showed lexical-level competition that increased with vocabulary size. Dollaghan (1994) calculated sizes of phonological similarity neighborhoods for expressive lexicons for two vocabulary lists representative of children aged 1;3 to 3;0. She reported that more than 80% of the words in the lexicons had at least one phonological neighbor and almost 20% had six or more phonological neighbors. Stokes (2014) suggested that words with high neighborhood density in adult language could facilitate word learning in children because they are less demanding of working memory than words of lower neighborhood density. A related question is: What are the units that children are most likely to store in the process of word learning? Grimm et al. (2019) concluded from a study of the rate of word learning in children that short utterances, rather than frequently occur-

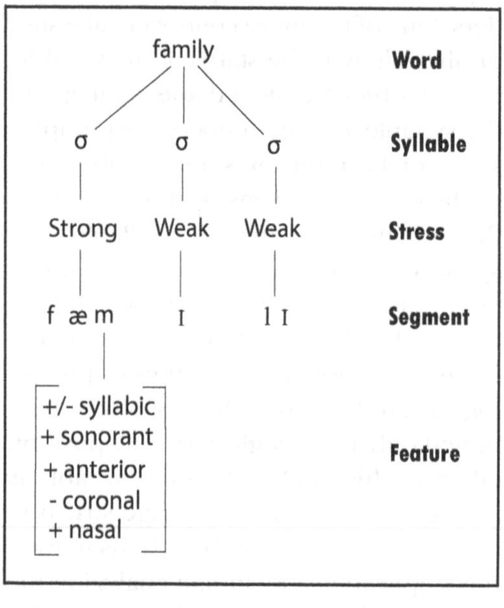

Figure 3–4. Levels of phonological representation of a word.

ring or predictable chunks, predict the acquisition of words. They also noted that short utterances are likely to correspond to words—a feature that may facilitate word learning.

Phonetic Encoding

Phonological encoding deals with relatively abstract elements. Phonetic encoding translates these abstract elements into a more concrete level of phonetic segments, essentially a narrow phonetic transcription of the intended utterance. This level includes specification of allophones and other features that are finer than those of the level of phonological encoding. Phonetic encoding is responsible for language-specific information that is adequate for the formulation of motor commands to the speech production systems. The syllabary is an attractive concept in phonetics because there are fewer syllables than words, and syllables are economical packages for phonetic and motoric information. As children gain expertise with a language, they learn to use phonetic principles and regularities that are specific to the language at hand. Children learning two or more languages face the challenge of learning the phonetic features of the separate languages, as discussed in Chapter 10.

Physiological Level of Speech Production

The phonetic sequence generated at the level of phonetic encoding is not yet sufficiently detailed to produce the required patterns of muscle activation. The physiological level is responsible for converting phonetic segments into motor commands that achieve the desired articulatory results. For example, the bilabial stop /b/ can be produced with different combinations of lip and jaw movement, depending on phonetic context and other factors. If the muscles of the lip are relatively inactive, lip movements are still possible because the lower lip is carried by the jaw. Decisions regarding the timing and degree of activation of the speech muscles are made at the physiological level, or the speech production level in Figure 3–2.

Speech Planning and Programming

The terms motor planning and motor programming are used differently by different authors, and it should not be assumed that a single definition of these terms is universally accepted. The *APA Dictionary of Psychology* (VandenBos, 2007) defines a **motor program** as "a stored representation, resulting from motor planning and refined through practice, which is used to produce a coordinated movement. Motor programs store the accumulated experience underlying skill at a task." This definition implies that **motor planning** is an activity that precedes motor programming. As applied to speech, motor planning is the selection and assembly of a basic articulatory plan, such as a sequence of phonetic units. Motor programming is a more detailed, subsequent process in which movements are specified in terms of the sequence of muscle activations. Planning and programming are followed by the actual execution of speech movements.

A similar view was expressed by Van Der Merwe (2021), who proposed a four-level model of speech production that includes two pre-execution phases (motor planner and motor program generator) and an execution phase. The four levels are as follows. Level 1 is linguistic-symbolic planning, which is a necessary first step in the process of speech production. Level 2 is a motor planner and incorporates an inverse model, an efference copy, and a forward model specific to each sound or highly practiced utterance. Also included is a forward predictive planner with the capability of planning several sounds as well as their coarticulation. Level 3 is a motor program generator and predictive controller that is characterized by an integral forward model architecture. Level 4 is the final execution phase that is presumed to act under closed loop control. This model holds implications for both the development and disorders of spoken language. Regarding development, the model suggests that a child's progress in spoken language involves maturation of separate but related processes of planning, programming, and execution. Regarding disorders, the model identifies potential points of breakdown or fragility in the overall process of speech production. This issue is discussed in later chapters, especially Chapter 5.

> "Indeed, speech, alongside the gestures used in sign language, is the only level of language which has at its foundation motor control." (p. 90) [deLeeuw, D. E., & Celata, C. (2019). Plasticity of native phonetic and phonological domains in the context of bilingualism. *Journal of Phonetics*, *75*, 88–93. https://doi.org/10.1016/j.wocn.2019.05.003]

Speech Motor Control

A broad definition of **speech motor control** is that it includes the planning, programming, and execution components of speech production (Kent, 2000). The motor plan is a relatively abstract prescription of the movement goals for the overall speech production system (including the respiratory, laryngeal, and supralaryngeal structures, although many studies and models focus only on the last of these). The goals for the vocal tract structures could be in the form of gestures (e.g., open the velopharyngeal port) or articulatory targets (e.g., contact of the tongue tip with the alveolar ridge), or acoustic targets (e.g., a specific spectral pattern of noise energy). The motor program is more detailed in determining which muscles are activated to achieve the goals in the motor plan, considering the current state of the system including the positions of the articulators. A stage of movement specification completes the process by determining the patterns of muscle activation including duration and strength of contraction, in accord with the motor program. Movement specification embraces general and speech-specific principles of movement control. An example of a general principle is Fitts' Law, which states that the amount of time required for a movement to reach a target area is a function of the distance to the target divided by the size of the target, so that the greater the distance and the smaller the size of the target, the longer it takes to reach the target. This law appears to apply to speech movements, at least for fast ones (Kuberski & Gafos, 2021). Chapter 9 considers in detail motor learning and motor control relevant to speech production.

Articulation

Articulation is the pattern of speech movements observable by imaging methods such as x-ray, MRI, or ultrasound (discussed in Chapters 4 and 5). Discussions of articulation typically focus on the supralaryngeal structures (jaw, tongue, lips, and soft palate), but the movements of these structures are coordinated with actions at the respiratory and laryngeal levels. Therefore, a complete model of speech production should include the respiratory, laryngeal, and supralaryngeal subsystems. To some degree, articulation can be inferred from acoustic analyses. The description and analysis of articulatory movements is complicated because multiple movements often co-occur in rapid sequence, sometimes simultaneously and sometimes overlapping. Articulatory data are the raw material from which inferences are drawn on the nature of speech motor control. A major focus of research on speech production at the supralaryngeal level has been the phenomenon of **coarticulation**, which is a change in the production of a speech segment due to the influence of neighboring sounds, especially the flanking segments. Coarticulation is manifest as a shingling of articulatory features across segments, such that a given feature can extend across two or more segments. Coarticulatory effects are commonly labeled as forward or backward. **Forward coarticulation** (also known as anticipatory, regressive, or right-to-left coarticulation) is the presence of an articulatory feature in advance of the phonetic segment to which it belongs. For example, as shown in Figure 3–5, nasalization of the vowel /u/ in the word *spoon* occurs in anticipation of the nasal feature of the following consonant /n/. For the same word, rounding occurs in the fricative /s/ in anticipation of the rounding feature of the vowel /u/. **Backward coarticulation** (also known as progressive, retentive, or left-to-right coarticulation) is the presence of an articulatory feature after the production of its parent segment. For example, nasalization of the vowel /i/ in the word *knee* is retention of the nasal feature of the preceding consonant /n/. The vowel /i/, like all vowels in American English, generally is produced only with oral resonance, but it is nasalized when preceded or followed by a nasal consonant. Coarticulation arises in part because of articulatory inertia (i.e., the articulators cannot move instantaneously) and because of strategies in motor control (primarily efforts to achieve efficiency and economy in speech production). The extent of the contextual influence varies but can reach across several consecutive segments, as in the case of anticipatory lip rounding in words such as *construe*, for

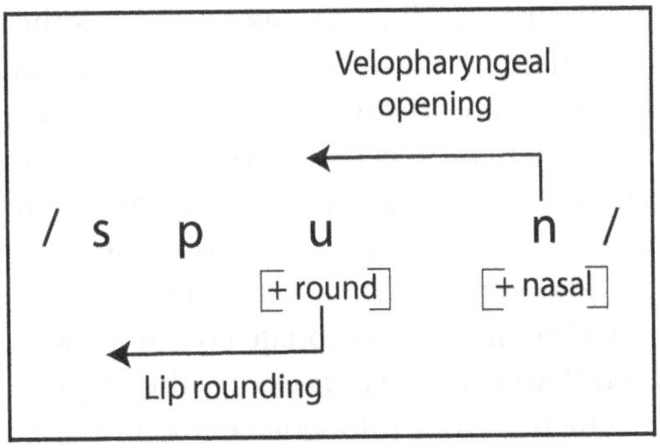

Figure 3–5. Illustration of examples of forward coarticulation in production of the word *spoon*. Velopharyngeal opening in anticipation of the nasal feature for consonant /n/ is evident during the vowel /u/, and lip rounding in anticipation of the rounded feature for vowel /u/ is evident during the production of the initial consonant /s/.

which lip rounding begins as early as the consonant /n/, four segments away from the rounded vowel. The mere presence of coarticulation is not surprising, but the patterns of coarticulation have intrigued those who study speech production.

Phonetic segments differ in the degree to which they accommodate coarticulation. **Coarticulation resistance** is the degree to which a given phonetic segment resists accommodation to neighboring phonetic segments. A segment with high coarticulation resistance has an articulation that varies little with changes in phonetic context. For example, the palatal fricative /ʃ/ is resistant to context effects, whereas the bilabial stop /p/ can accommodate a variety of co-occurring tongue shapes. **Coarticulatory aggressiveness** is the degree to which a phonetic segment exerts a strong coarticulatory influence on neighboring segments and exhibits little effect of contextual variation on its own production.

Coarticulation has been studied in typically developing children and in children with speech and language disorders, often with the goal of using coarticulation as a window into the processes by which speech movements are organized and coordinated. A basic question is whether children differ from adults in the presence or spread of coarticulation. Research on typical development has led to contradictory conclusions, with some studies showing less extensive coarticulation in children and other studies showing more extensive coarticulation. The contrary results are reconciled in large part by recognizing gradients of coarticulation degree within a continuum from a syllabic to a segmental type of organization As Noiray et al. (2018) explained,

> Taken together, previous research and present findings suggest that a crucial step in becoming mature speakers may not be for children to globally increase or decrease coarticulation but to achieve flexible patterns of coarticulation depending on the combination of segments. (p. 1363)

This conclusion is highly relevant to the study of coarticulation in speech and language disorders.

Coarticulation has been studied in speech disorders to gain insight into the nature of speech disturbances. In the case of children's speech disorders, it is imperative to consider age-level developmental patterns of coarticulation in typically developing children to identify deviations. Atypical coarticulation has been reported for subtypes of speech sound disorders (Maas & Mailend, 2017); CAS (Nijland et al., 2002) and hearing disorders (Waldstein & Baum, 1991). As discussed in Chapter 11, CAS is a disorder in which atypical coarticulation has emerged as an apparently characteristic feature.

Contemporary theories often emphasize internal models as the means to achieving adaptive and accurate motor control of speech production. As explained in Chapter 1, internal models achieve motor control through interactions of the articulatory system and the neural controller (which includes the internal model). Through the operations of the controller, the articulatory system receives information from the central nervous system (CNS), feedback signals, and the efference copy. The four major advantages that internal models offer in motor control were summarized by Wolpert et al. (1995) as follows. (1) Feedback control is limited because the delays in sensorimotor loops are too long to be effective as a control strategy, but internal models offer a faster means of control. (2) Internal models can use motor outflow (efference copy) in the nervous system to anticipate and cancel the sensory consequences of movements. (3) By comparing the desired and actual sensory consequences of a movement, the internal model generates signals to support motor learning. A similar strategy can be used in mental practice (imaging a movement without performing it). (4) The forward component of an internal model can perform state estimation, a process that combines efferent copies of motor commands with afferent sensory signals to create a representation of the current status of the peripheral motor system. An implication is that children achieve speech motor control in part by constructing internal models that are revised and updated during the developmental process. There is very little research on this topic, but the continuous development of the cerebellum in childhood may be an important neural basis for establishing internal models (Ego et al., 2016). This topic is taken up in Chapter 12. The cerebellum also appears to play important roles in monitoring and error detection, topics that are discussed in the following section.

Monitoring and Feedback in Speech Production

Models of language processing often assume an architecture that is hierarchical and unidirectional (i.e., with information preceding only from top to bottom without provision for interactions across levels). This assumption does not have universal acceptance, because research has been interpreted to show such interactions (Dell, 1985; Harley, 1984). One way of accounting for such interaction is to incorporate feedback, as shown in Figure 3–2. Feedback signals allow for processing at one stage to influence operations at another higher stage. The role of feedback is considered more fully in the next section. Another solution to potential interaction across levels is the concept of **spreading activation**, that is, activation in one component may inhibit or facilitate activation in another component (even at a higher level). Such spreading activation is a prominent feature in some connectionist models of language comprehension and production (Dell, 1985). We take a closer look at monitoring after a discussion of speech errors in the following section.

Errors in Speech Production

Speech production is hardly an error-free process, no matter how highly practiced speakers may be. Slips of the tongue are a universal human experience, and efforts have been made to collect examples and analyze their properties. Research on speech errors has helped to shape understanding of (1) points of vulnerability or breakdown in the planning and execution of speech, (2) mechanisms of self-monitoring and error detection, and (3) disordered speech, especially in individuals with neurologic disorders such as aphasia or apraxia of speech. A **speech sequencing error** is an error in speech production in which units such as phonemes, syllables, morphemes, or words are transposed, repeated, added, or deleted. Errors of this kind sometimes are called **spoonerisms**, after the Oxford don and ordained minister William Archibald Spooner (1844–1930), who was famous for committing such errors with remarkable frequency. An example of a transposition is "a mice nan" produced instead of "a nice man." An example of repetition is "one one-way" instead of "one runway." Sequencing errors committed by neurotypical adults and adults with neurological disorders have been studied in detail to understand the planning and execution processes of speech production, usually on the assumption that these slips reflect points of fracture or vulnerability in these processes, analogous to a fault line causing earthquakes. A general conclusion is that these errors do not occur randomly but rather follow general rules or regularities involving properties such as syllable position and stress.

In an article entitled "The Non-Anomalous Nature of Anomalous Utterances," Fromkin (1971) concluded that speech errors demonstrated the reality of phonological units such as features, phonemes, and syllables because manipulation of these units appeared to explain most of these errors. Meyer (1992) estimated that around 60% to 90% of all errors are misorderings of single segments, and that 10% to 30% are sequences of adjacent segments (two consonants or a consonant and a flanking vowel). Although such an analysis may indeed point to the primacy of phoneme-sized units as the vulnerable component in speech planning and execution, there is a risk that the method of analysis (i.e., presumed linguistic elements such as phonemes) determines the results. That is, the grain of the analysis assumes that the perceptually identified units involved in the errors are intact and faithful versions of the same units produced in error-free productions. This may not be true. Studies using acoustic or kinematic methods show variability in the articulatory or motoric levels of speech production (Cler et al., 2017; McMillan & Corley, 2010; Mowrey & MacKay, 1990; Pouplier & Hardcastle, 2005). These results raise the possibility that the planning and execution of speech production contends with several types of variability and vulnerability, some of which may not be perceived. Even speech that is judged by perceptual standards to be error-free may be associated with variability in its articulatory patterns.

A significant proportion of published error data based on phonetic transcriptions can be described as movement of a segment to an incorrect position within a prosodic "frame" (Dell, 1986; Shattuck-Hufnagel, 1983). Shattuck-Hufnagel (1983) observed that most phonological errors resulted from transposing, anticipating, or perseverating the syllable components of onsets, nuclei, and codas (these components are shown in Figure 3–6). She further noted that the speech errors usually involved single segments or clusters. To explain these results, she proposed a model in which a structurally tagged corpus of candidate segments is stored in a memory buffer during phonological encoding. A serial order

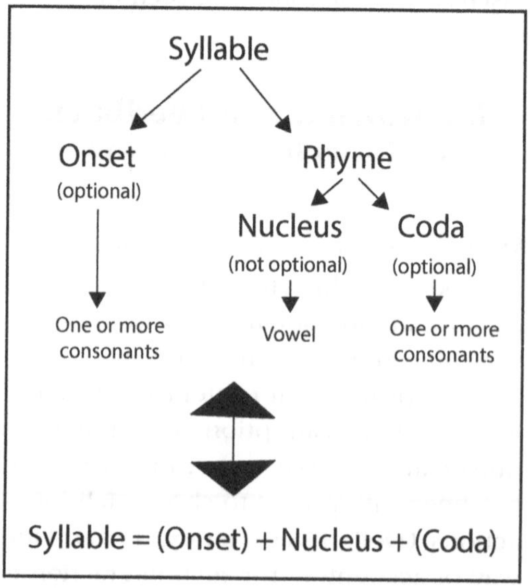

Figure 3–6. Phonological structure of a syllable.

processor then scans the items and copies them into stressed and unstressed syllabic frames. Aspects of this hypothesis have been incorporated in models of speech production that account for speech errors in terms of the distributed representation and gradient activation of linguistic elements during speech planning (Alderete et al., 2021; Goldrick & Chu, 2014).

Speech sequencing errors in children have been studied less often than errors in adults, but there are notable research contributions to affirm that children do commit such errors. Stemberger (1989) collected 576 such errors in diary studies of his two children. Children's errors were very much like those of adults, but some differences were noted, including a slower decay in the activation of accessed elements and less interdependence between different phonological elements in a word or segment. Jaeger (1992, 2004) conducted an analysis of 907 slips from 32 children, ages 1;4 to 6;0, collected in naturalistic settings. The results showed a general similarity to the types and proportions of slips in data for adults, with phonological errors outnumbering errors at the lexical and phrasal levels. In phonological errors, the rank order of frequency of error was as follows: anticipations, perseverations, and exchanges. Jaeger also reported that children produce more completed anticipations and exchanges than adults, which she attributed to less maturity in self-monitoring. Like adults, children make more substitutions than additions or omissions. For a fuller account of this research see Jaeger (2004).

Self-initiated speech repairs have been reported in children as early as the single-word stage of 1;6 to 2;0 (Clark, 1982; Forrester, 2008; Laakso, 2006). The frequency of self-initiated speech repairs increases during childhood, with 5-year-old children making fewer repairs than older school-aged children (Evans, 1985; Rogers, 1978). Redford (2019) concluded that children do not demonstrate an adult-like capability in self-monitoring until the age of about 4 years, at which age they begin to use external feedback to update and revise representations and processes of speech production. Terband, Van Brenk, and van Doornik-van der Zee (2014) summarized research on this topic as follows: "The increased ability to successfully use auditory feedback for compensation and adaption suggests that crucial steps are made in the development of auditory–motor integration around the age of 4" (p. 66). If this is correct, then this age is a watershed event in the development of speech production, with implications for the treatment of speech disorders, especially aspects of treatment that require tasks of monitoring.

These studies of children's speech errors are relevant to the clinical issue of self-monitoring in speech disorders. Much of the work on this topic pertains to the relationship between self-monitoring and generalization (Koegel et al., 1986, 1988; Shriberg & Kwiatkowski, 1990). Self-monitoring promotes generalization of correct productions, especially outside the clinical setting (Koegel et al., 1988). A complication is that children's speech errors can arise from two different conditions, one being a sequencing error such as those in the classical speech error literature, and the other being an articulatory/phonological error. Children's speech errors are more likely to occur in multiword utterances (McCauley et al., 2021) and inconsistency of word production also increases in multisyllabic utterances with complex syllable structure (Holm et al., 2022). Multiword utterances appear to challenge children's ability to formulate and produce spoken language.

Mechanisms of self-monitoring and error detection are considered next.

Self-Monitoring and Error Detection

A general definition of **self-monitoring** is the ability of speakers to inspect their own speech for errors or other undesired properties. Some writers distinguish internal monitoring (e.g., speech planning) from external monitoring (articulation and acoustics). It is often asserted that monitoring can occur at different linguistic levels. Self-monitoring is a necessary step in error detection. But error detection is of limited value unless it is accompanied by error correction, which is the revision of detected deviations from the intended target. Figure 3–2 shows possible feedback loops that might support self-monitoring and error correction. This diagram is intended to be inclusive of the various proposals for feedback and to allow for the possibility that children may use different types of feedback during different phases of speech development. It also allows for the possibility of impairments in auditory self-monitoring, as may be case for children with complex speech sound disorders (Terband & van Brenk, 2023). Auditory feedback may play a more critical role in early speech development than it does in mature speech. Verbal self-monitoring is needed both to detect errors and to assess vocal attributes such as loudness, rate, voice quality, and emotion.

Monitoring can be accomplished with both external and internal feedback channels (Postma, 2000). The external channels include air- and bone-conducted feedback sent to the auditory nervous system, somatosensory feedback relating to the speech production system, and psychosocial effects of a speaker's utterances on listeners. The internal channels give feedback on the ongoing processes that precede speech output per se. Trewartha and Phillips (2013) presented evoked response data to show that speech errors can be detected during early stages of speech formulation processes, before actual articulation. Runnqvist et al. (2021) concluded that the cerebellum is involved in both internal and external monitoring, which was interpreted as evidence of forward modeling across the planning and articulation of speech. The external and internal channels pertain to several different stages or levels in the overall process, as shown in Figure 3–2.

Theories relating to self-monitoring and error correction are based largely on data from adults performing various language tasks. Less is known about how these processes develop in children. Postma (2000) summarized three major types of theories of self-monitoring. (1) The perception-based theory proposes that speakers monitor their speech using basically the same operations that are used to understand other speakers. An advantage of this approach is its parsimony and economy. Roelofs' (1997, 2000) comprehension-based model WEAVER++ (Word Encoding by Activation and VERification) states that internal monitoring forwards the phonological word to the central monitor, which compares it with selected production representations. It also has been suggested that a central monitor inspects the ongoing processes of speech production with three loops (conceptual, inner, and auditory) to verify the preverbal (propositional) message, the phonetic plan, and the auditory pattern. (2) The production-based theory relies on multiple local, autonomous monitoring operations to examine steps in the formulation of the spoken message. (3) Node structure theory explains error detection as a natural consequence of the activation patterns in the node system for speech production. Errors cause prolonged activation of uncommitted nodes, which can signal error. The approaches differ on the points of consciousness, volition and control, the number of monitoring channels, and their speed, flexibility, and capacity, and whether they can account for concurrent language comprehension disorders. (Lind & Hartsuiker, 2020).

Producing Words and Nonwords

Figure 3–2 depicts the overall process of producing a linguistic utterance (i.e., a word or sequence of words). We now look at how a child learns to perceive and produce single words or nonwords, as might be required in a task in which a child is asked to repeat a verbal stimulus. Some therapies for speech disorders involve the production of nonwords to avoid a child's reliance on learned patterns for real words. The use of words and nonwords can be informative because somewhat different processes are involved. For example, real words are represented in the child's lexicon, but nonwords are not. Children generally can produce phonetic patterns that are outside their vocabularies, so the question is: How do they do it? Figure 3–7 is a diagram of the processes involved, beginning with perception of an acoustic signal, and ending with an articulation that effectively reproduces that signal.

Perception has two components: a stage of initial auditory processing of a sound pattern and, if the signal is recognized as speech, a stage of speech perception. A signal that is perceived as speech

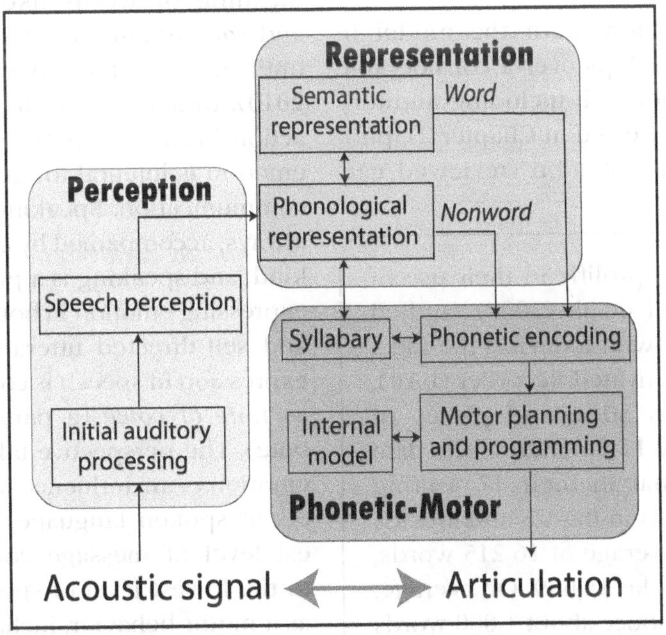

Figure 3–7. Diagram of the processes involved in perceiving and producing a phonetic pattern that is either a real word or a nonword.

is then processed as a phonological representation. (Chapters 2 and 7 discuss auditory processing in more detail.) In the case of a real word, the phonological representation matches a word in the lexicon (a semantic representation), so that learned linguistic information about that word is available for further processing. If the word is familiar and frequently used, these features may facilitate production in the following stages of phonetic encoding and motor control. Phonetic encoding may access a syllabary that stores information about individual syllables. Finally, motor control achieved through operations of planning and programming generates motor instructions that result in articulatory actions. In the case of a nonword, no matching item can be found in the lexicon, so that semantic information is not available. Therefore, the phonological representation bypasses the lexicon to feed directly into the stage of phonetic encoding and then to the stage of motor control.

Each component of the model in Figure 3–7 develops over a considerable period in childhood, including auditory perception (reviewed in Chapter 2), phonological representation (reviewed earlier in this chapter and discussed in more detail in Chapter 7), and speech motor control (reviewed in this chapter and in Chapters 2, 5, and 9). Adult-like performance may not be reached until puberty or even later. There are several points of vulnerability in the processes of Figure 3–6, and these points relate to clinical assessment, as discussed in Chapter 5.

> Humans are prolific in their use of words. Mehl et al. (2007) studied word usage with a device, the Electronically Activated Recorder (EAR), that records 30-second pieces of sound every 12.5 minutes. The data indicated that in their 17 waking hours women in the US and Mexico uttered an average of 16,215 words, and men spoke 15,669. On average, then, we produce about 1,000 words per waking hour.

Affect

Figure 3–3 departs from the typical model of processes in spoken language by recognizing affect as a component. As discussed in Chapter 2, emotion and language are closely linked, and evidence favors the psychological constructionist hypothesis that language supports the acquisition of emotion knowledge (Hoemann et al., 2019; Shablack & Lindquist, 2019). It has been reported that emotion word knowledge (e.g., knowing the meaning of words like *angry*, *happy*, and *sad*) roughly doubles every 2 years until the age of 11 (Baron-Cohen et al., 2010). In addition to the powerful interaction between emotions and language, emotion is integral to the process of oral communication. Speaking is often, if not always, accompanied by emotion of some kind, and speaking is a primary means of expressing emotion in both other-directed and self-directed utterances. Emotional expression in speech is commonly known as *tone of voice* (a paralinguistic attribute). The perspective taken here is that emotions can influence virtually all levels of spoken language, from the highest level of message conceptualization to the lowest level of speech production as a motor behavior, including aspects of articulation (Kim et al., 2015). A review of acoustic studies showed that emotion was expressed in speech through prosody, voice quality, and spectral features that often are specific to an individual speaker (Gangamohan et al., 2016).

The discussion of emotion in Chapter 2 emphasizes the challenge of studying emotional states, as well as progress in the development of emotion in childhood. Language is a means to emotional development as well as a primary means of emotional expression. Therefore, language and emotion are linked throughout development. Research on the neural correlates of emotion has emphasized prefrontal cortical networks that appear to operate in a top-down fashion to regulate attention, inhibition/cognitive control, motivation, and emotion by means of pathways connecting with posterior cortical regions and subcortical structures (Arnsten & Rubia, 2012). Neurodevelopmental processes associated with maturation of emotional regulation include a transition from broad to focal activation in the dorsolateral and ventrolateral prefrontal cortex, a shift from predominantly subcortical processing to predominantly cortical processing (especially the frontal cortex), and an increasing interaction between subcortical and cortical structures (Monk, 2008).

Emotion can enhance communication because it supplements and extends the linguistic aspects of a message. But emotion also can be disruptive. An extreme and well-known example is **stage fright**, the fear of public speaking or performance. Emotions and emotional disorders also have been associated with a variety of clinical conditions, including stuttering in children (Johnson et al., 2010), autism spectrum disorder (Grossman et al., 2013), and a range of speech and language impairments (Lee et al., 2020). The emotional components of spoken language probably deserve greater recognition in assessing and treating children with communication disorders.

Private Speech and Inner Speech

The discussion so far pertains to overt speech, that is, speech in the form of articulatory actions culminating in an acoustic signal. However, both children and adults are capable of other varieties of speech, including private speech and inner speech, which appear to serve functions of problem-solving, deliberation, self-awareness, and self-regulation. Talking to oneself, whether silently or aloud, can be beneficial and reflects the intimate connection between thought and language. **Private speech** is spoken speech that is addressed to oneself (also called **self-directed speech** or **self-talk**), whereas **inner speech** is unspoken and therefore inaudible. Inner speech has been defined as the "subjective experience of language in the absence of overt and audible articulation (Alderson-Day & Fernyhough, 2015, p. 931). Inner speech is also called covert speech, silent speech, verbal thinking, verbal mediation, inner monologue, inner dialogue, inner voice, articulatory imagery, voice imagery, speech imagery, and auditory verbal imagery. It has been proposed that there are two forms of inner speech (Fernyhough, 1996, 2004, 2008, 2013). **Expanded inner speech** is an internal dialogue that has many of the phonological properties and turn-taking aspects present in external dialogue (i.e., talking to others). Therefore, this kind of silent speech may have conversation-like properties in which thoughts are expressed in relatively complete linguistic form, like full sentences. Data from fMRI studies indicate that expanded inner speech activates processes of speech production to the level of articulatory planning to produce a predicted signal, the inner voice, with auditory qualities (Grandchamp et al., 2019). **Condensed inner speech** lacks many of these phonological details and assumes the form of simultaneous multiple perspectives. In Fernyhough's (2004, 2013) model, the default setting for inner speech is condensed, and the transition to expanded inner speech is likely to occur under situations of stress and cognitive challenge, as in trying to solve a difficult problem. Adults often use inner speech and private speech interchangeably and can switch from one to the other, depending on situation and objective. Heavy and Hurlburt (2008) found that inner speech occurred with an average frequency of 26% of all thoughts. However, individual variation was large, from 0% to 75% of the time across participants. Morin and Racy (2022) reported multiple functions of inner speech in university students, with the most frequent being problem solving.

> "Speech is external thought, and thought internal speech." (Antoine Rivarol, 1753–1801, French publicist, journalist, and epigrammatist)

The study of inner speech presents methodological challenges and is clouded by interpretive controversies. However, substantial strides have been made in several aspects of inner speech that are relevant to this book, including the following: development of inner speech in children, the possible role of inner speech in developmental disorders such as autism spectrum disorder, and the neural underpinnings of inner speech. These are reviewed in Chapter 4. It has been suggested that inner speech is a mental draft of covert speech production (Sekścińska, 2021). Inner speech appears to generate an efference copy, an internal duplicate of neural commands for movement (Whitford et al., 2017).

Vygotsky (1986) proposed that self-directed speech in children was important especially in self-regulation of cognition and behavior. He believed that private or inner speech was the intersection of the psychological processes of thought and language. Subsequent theorizing has suggested additional roles, including expression and regulation of emotions, planning for communicative interaction, theory of mind, fantasy, creativity, and autobiographical memory (Fossa, 2022; Geva & Fernyhough, 2019; Mulvihill et al., 2020). Private speech begins early in development, by the age of two years (Furrow, 1984) and has a developmental pattern during the preschool years (Winsler et al., 2000). Typical development of private and inner speech in children is summarized in Chapter 4.

Neural Networks of Spoken Language

Historical precedents in understanding the neural pathways of language were introduced by Prussian-born German psychiatrist and neurologist, Carl (or Karl) Wernicke (1848–1905) and German physician Ludwig Lichtheim (1845–1928). They proposed a dual-pathway model that linked "auditory word images" in Wernicke's area to "motor word images" in Broca's area. This theory is diagrammed in Lichtheim's house, which is shaped like an outline of a house and depicts processing centers and their connections (Figure 3–8). Wernicke's area was originally defined as the gyri forming the lower posterior left sylvian fissure (Brodmann's area 22) and was thought to support language comprehension. Broca's area is a cortical region in the left inferior frontal gyrus (the opercular and triangular parts of the inferior frontal gyrus, Brodmann's areas 44 and 45), an area that was considered critical to the production of speech. It is named after the French physician, anatomist, and anthropologist Paul Broca (1824–1880). Lichtheim's house is an early example of a centers and pathways model of the neural representation of language, based largely on data from individuals with aphasia.

Although Broca's and Wernicke's areas continue to be recognized in neural models of spoken language, current theories ascribe somewhat different roles to them. Mesulam proposed a neural network model in which information is processed in a hierarchy of networks according to levels of complexity involved in the task (e.g., simple repetition of an utterance as opposed to formulating a novel utterance). An important feature of the model is that brain regions involved in language are not fixed but rather take on different functions depending on the task. Important sites for integrating information are (1) the temporal pole of the paralimbic system which gives access to the long-term memory system and the emotional system, and (2) the posterior terminal portion of the superior temporal sulcus, which gives access to meaning. Semantic processing also is performed in the triangular and orbital portions of the inferior frontal gyrus. Mesulam's theory is like some other theories in proposing convergence or integration regions such as the inferior parietal lobule, which includes the angular gyrus and the supramarginal gyrus. The left inferior parietal lobule receives information from the right hemisphere as well as emotional information from the amygdala and cingulate gyrus.

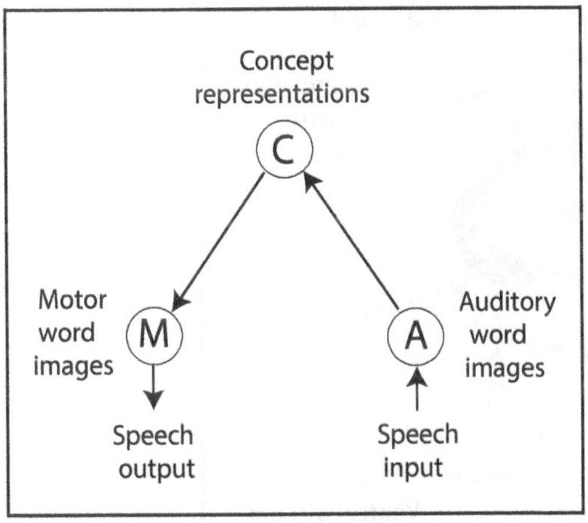

Figure 3–8. Diagram of Lichtheim's house, an early example of a centers and pathways model of the neural representation of language, based largely on data from individuals with aphasia.

Discovery of the neural pathways of language reception and production has been greatly advanced by neuroimaging methods. Of the various methods now available, the ones most suited to studies of children, including infants, are electroencephalography (EEG), magnetoencephalography (MEG), functional near-infrared spectroscopy (fNIRS), and functional magnetic resonance imaging (fMRI). Some important developments are reviewed next.

The Dorsal and Ventral Pathways of Language

Each hemisphere of the brain can be divided into two streams or systems of language processing: an upper dorsal and a lower ventral (Hickok & Poeppel, 2007), as shown in Figure 3–9. Each stream has distinct cortical regions connected by long association tracts running between the frontal lobe and posterior brain. The dorsal stream maps sound to articulation, and the ventral stream maps sound to meaning (i.e., structural analysis and semantics in different domains). These divisions relate to earlier descriptions of the dorsal (*where*)/ventral (*what*) division of the visual (Ungerleider & Haxby, 1994).) and auditory (Rauschecker & Tian, 2000) systems in the brain. The dorsal pathway described by Hickok and Poeppel (2007) consists of the arcuate and superior longitudinal fasciculi, and the posterior superior temporal lobe (including an area at the temporoparietal junction in the Sylvian fissure) terminating in the inferior frontal gyrus and premotor cortex (Saur et al., 2008). The ventral pathway consists of the middle and inferior longitudinal fasciculi, the uncinate fasciculus (Fridriksson et al., 2016), inferior fronto-occipital fasciculus (Martino et al., 2010), and the superior temporal gyrus ending near anterior portions of the inferior frontal gyrus (Saur et al., 2008). The dorsal pathway is linked to sensorimotor mapping of sound to articulation (Saur et al., 2008), and auditory feedback control in speech production (Hickok, 2012), making it important for supporting repetition (Ueno et al., 2011). By contrast, the ventral stream has been associated with the ability to map auditory input onto conceptual and semantic representations, as well as syntactic processing (Hickok & Poeppel, 2004; Ueno et al., 2011).

Brauer et al. (2013) studied the development of the dorsal and ventral pathways, finding that connections present at birth were the ventral pathway between the temporal areas to the inferior frontal gyrus and the dorsal pathway from the temporal cortex to the premotor cortex.

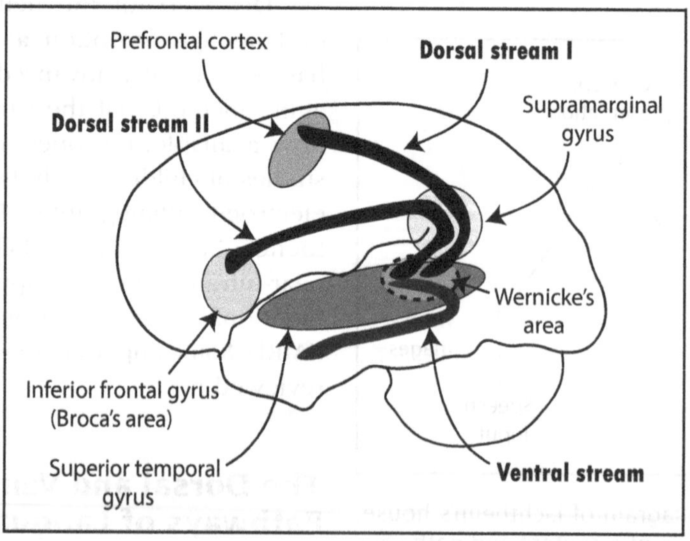

Figure 3–9. The two streams or systems of language processing: an upper dorsal stream that maps sound to articulation and a lower ventral stream that maps sound to meaning.

A subsequent maturation was observed for the dorsal pathway from the temporal cortex to the inferior frontal gyrus, which was thought to serve more complex language functions. Disruption to the dorsal pathway has been implicated in speech and language disorders including an inherited speech disorder (Liégeois et al., 2019), developmental stuttering (Kronfeld-Duenias et al., 2016), and various neurogenic communication disorders in adults (Fridriksson et al., 2016).

Cerebellum

The cerebellum is increasingly recognized as a critical structure in speech and language (Mariën, & Borgatti, 2018; Pleger & Timmann, 2018). Accumulating evidence also points to roles of the cerebellum in a variety of human behaviors such as balance, motor coordination, cognitive operations, and emotional functions. The cerebellum's protracted development in children, its sexual dimorphism, and its vulnerably to environmental influences (Tiemeier et al., 2010) help to explain why it is implicated in childhood onset disorders such as autism (Fatemi et al., 2012), ADHD (Goetz et al., 2014), and developmental stuttering (S. E. Chang et al., 2019). The cerebellum and the cerebrum are connected by two major pathways (Jobson et al., 2022). The cortico-ponto-cerebellar pathway projects from each cerebral hemisphere with decussation at the pons to terminate in the contralateral cerebellar cortex. The cerebello-thalamo-cortical pathway originates in the cerebellum, then crosses over to synapse on the contralateral thalamus, and continues to different regions of the cerebral cortex. A remarkable feature of cerebellar damage is that the effects of injury sometimes can resolve quickly with little or no residuals (see discussion of cerebellar mutism in Chapter 11). This feature is consistent with the hypothesis that a primary role of the cerebellum is to construct internal models of behavioral functions. Because internal models are continuously updated to ensure accuracy and stability of performance, the cerebellum is equipped to make rapid compensations for damage, except in the most serious instances. Furthermore, the different trajectories of maturation for different compartments of the cerebellum help to ensure a lifelong neuroplasticity to meet the demands of changing circumstances and needs (Romero et al., 2021).

Developmental Neuroscience of Speech

The preceding discussion is one step in advancing a developmental neuroscience of speech, that is, the specification of neural systems that support the development of speech in children. This topic is addressed in several chapters, especially Chapter 6 (which summarizes research on the neural correlates of prosody), and Chapters 9 and 11 (which provide information on processes and neuropathologies associated with speech development and its disorders). The information presented in this chapter is a basic introduction to the neural networks of speech production, including some aspects that are sometimes neglected, such as the processing of emotions involved in speech production. Speech production and perception involve widely distributed neural systems. The maturational gradients of these systems are being investigated with the tools of modern neuroscience. Maturation does not necessarily mean that fixed neural regions come to serve specific functions, but rather that networks continually adapt to capabilities and task demands.

Conclusions

1. Spoken language has often been modeled as a multistage process that proceeds from thought to articulation. The multiple stages are an index of the complexities involved in producing even a single word, let alone a multiword sentence, with a syntactic structure. Current theories of spoken language typically recognize several stages, with each stage responsible for processing certain types of information. An implication for the study of speech development is that children need to acquire the information needed at each stage and then integrate the various stages to produce the intended utterances.
2. Speech production is vulnerable to error, as shown most clearly in speech sequencing errors, in which units are deleted, added, or exchanged. Self-monitoring and error detection of speech involve both internal and external mechanisms.
3. Speech is often, if not almost always, accompanied by emotion. Speech and language are a primary means to emotional expression and fundamental to a child's learning about emotion words.
4. Overt speech is only one form of spoken language. We also engage in private speech and inner speech. Inner speech is used for problem-solving, deliberation, self-awareness, and self-regulation. Inner speech takes different forms that serve different functions. Overt speech and inner speech share certain properties and neural networks.
5. The neural systems of speech production are widely distributed, and the especially important components are the ventral and dorsal streams of the cerebral hemispheres, the cortico-ponto-cerebellar pathway, and the cerebello-thalamo-cortical pathway. Later chapters consider the role of laterality of the central nervous system.

4

TYPICAL SPEECH DEVELOPMENT

The development of speech has been described in three major ways: acquisition of speech sounds (typically the phonemes in a language), phonological processes, and learning motor patterns of speech. These approaches are reviewed in this chapter, along with related topics in the study of typical speech development, including acoustic and physiological correlates, gestural communication, and private and inner speech. Because speech development begins in infancy (and some aspects of speech perception begin even earlier—in the fetus), we begin this chapter with a look at the earliest vocalizations that put children on the path to spoken language.

Vocalizations in the First Year of Life

William Wordsworth wrote in his 1882 poem "My Heart Leaps Up" that, "The child is the father of the man." We might paraphrase this expression to say that the child's utterances are the progenitor of the adults' spoken language. It is now widely accepted that speech has its origins in vocalizations produced during infancy, and that sounds produced in the first year of life are continuous with subsequent speech and language development. Vocalizations, and not gestures, are the predominant mode of communication in the first year of life (Burkhardt-Reed et al., 2021) and are produced in remarkable quantity (Oller et al., 2019). Vocal behavior in infancy predicts later speech and language development (Werwach et al., 2021) and can help to identify children at risk for communication and developmental disorders (Lang et al., 2019). Therefore, it is important to establish procedures that enable valid conclusions to be drawn about patterns of vocal development in preverbal children, with the goals of identifying infants at risk and monitoring the effects of intervention. Vocalizations are grist for the clinical mill because they are usually highly abundant, progress though relatively predictable stages, and are continuous with later developments of speech and language.

Stage Models of Infant Vocalizations

Stage models have a long history in characterizing vocalizations in the first year of life. In the usual formulation, a **stage model** assumes that development is a discontinuous process in which qualitative differences in behavior emerge in an orderly and consistent fashion across individuals. Stages are identified by a discontinuity (a newly emerging form of behavior) followed by an interval of relative equilibrium. Some of the most recent (post 1980) stage models of early vocal development are shown in Figure 4–1. These models differ in the timing and naming of stages, but there is an overall similarity in the progression of certain vocal behaviors (Kent, 2022). Stage models are useful in that they are snapshots of relatively discrete points in an otherwise continuous pattern of development. Clinicians are not always able to make finely graded sequential or longitudinal observations of a child's development. Economic and other forces constrain clinical practice to make episodic or periodic observations of a child's development so that weeks or months may intervene between clinical appointments. Stages are a way of placing a given infant in a developmental progression, and parents or other caregivers can provide useful information on a child's development by reporting on stage-like behaviors.

A limitation in stage models is that they are generally descriptive and not explanatory. The stages describe behav-

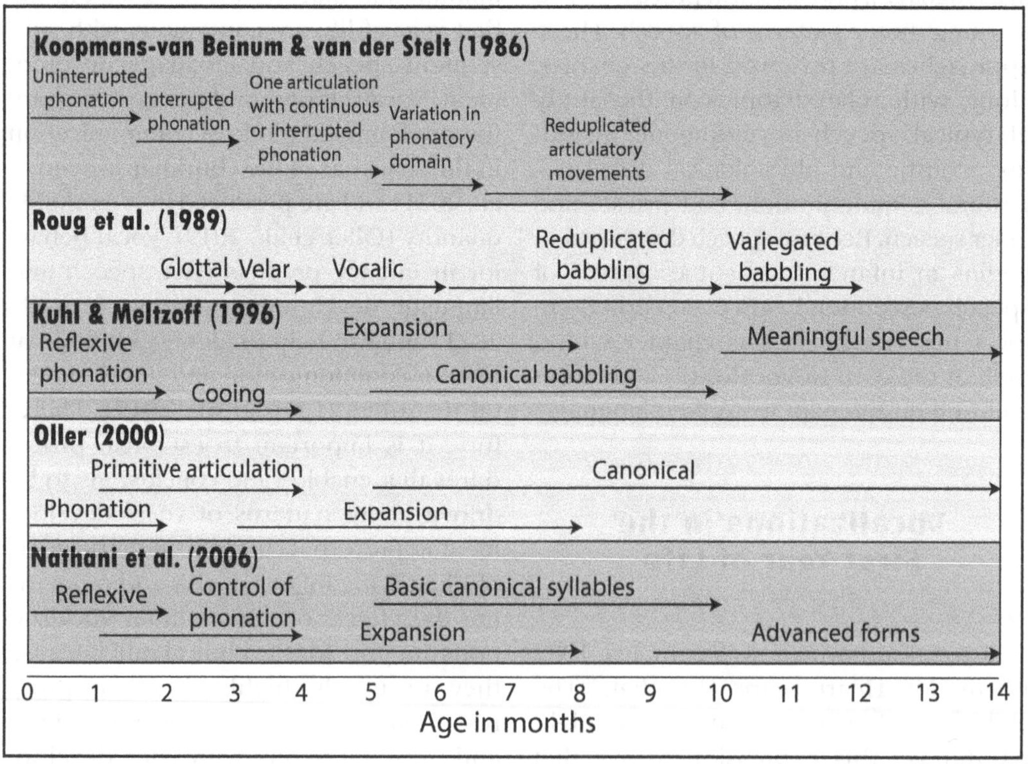

Figure 4–1. Selected stage models of vocalizations in early infancy. The lines with arrowheads indicate the approximate timing and duration of the individual stages.

iors but do not explain why these behaviors come about, for example, why one stage follows another, or even why there are stages at all. Commonly recognized stages are roughly as follows: simple phonation accompanied by little or no supralaryngeal articulation (e.g., cooing or vowel-like sounds), phonation accompanied by a simple oral articulation (e.g., the syllable /bɑ/), repetitive or canonical babble (e.g., the syllable sequence /bɑbɑbɑ/), and more advanced forms that may feature prosodic variation as well as more complex oral articulation (e.g., the syllable sequence /bɑbidɑ/). The latter stages may overlap with the production of first words. Stages usually are identified by noting the appearance or disappearance of certain kinds of vocalizations. One of the most important of these is the canonical syllable, discussed next.

A **canonical syllable** is defined as a syllable consisting of a consonant (excluding glottal consonants such as /h/ or /ʔ/) and a fully resonant vowel, with a rapid transition between them and normal phonation and pitch range. This combination of features describes a vocalization that has well-controlled phonation, predominantly oral resonance, and an oral constriction that is rapidly released into a following vowel. **Canonical babbling (CB)** generally is recognized as a repetition of a canonical syllable, which may or may not be identical across the repeated pattern. CB is recognized as a major advance in vocal behavior and is important for several reasons, including the following.

1. It is apparently a universal developmental phenomenon, as it has been reported in many languages (de Boysson-Bardies, 1999).
2. It typically has an onset between 6 to 9 months of age (Eilers et al., 1993; Morgan & Wren, 2018), even in the presence of environmental factors such as low socioeconomic status and multilingualism in the home (Oller et al., 1999). (However, the age of onset may reach as late as 15 months, according to data from McGillion et al., 2016).
3. It predicts subsequent development of speech and language (Werwach et al., 2021).
4. Because it is easily and reliably recognized by parents, it can be used in parent reports of development (Moeller et al., 2019; Oller et al., 1999).
5. Delay in its onset and other features may identify infants at risk for developmental disorders (Lang et al., 2019).

The **canonical babbling ratio (CBR)** is a measure of syllable usage calculated as the number of canonical syllables divided by the total number of syllables of any kind. Several different versions of CBR have been introduced (Molemans et al., 2012; Nyman et al., 2021). Some examples are as follows:

CBR^{TOT} = (number of canonical syllables)/(total number of syllables)

CBR^{utt} = (number of canonical syllables)/(total number of utterances)

CBR^{UTTER} = (number of canonical syllables)/(total number of utterances)

CBR^{syl} = (number of canonical syllables)/(total number of utterances)

CBR^{utt} = (number of true canonical syllables)/ (total number of utterances)

The proportion of vocalizations meeting the criterion of a canonical syllable is rather small, on the order of 15%, so that the typical calculation of CBR yields a value of 0.15 (Nyman et al., 2021).

Babbling and other infant vocalizations provide both sensory and motor experience that fosters later speech development. These early vocal behaviors give rise to multimodal representations in which motor processes are linked with auditory and somatosensory information (Fairs et al., 2021; Majorano et al., 2019; Werker & Tees, 1992). As mentioned in the introductory chapter of this book, vocal behavior is a refined sensorimotor accomplishment that adapts to biological maturation and communication needs and opportunities. CB may be a threshold behavior insofar as it represents a significant advance that prefigures a syllable-based organization of motor control. This behavior is notable both for its rhythmic structure and the coordination of articulatory movements within the component syllables of the sequence.

The age of about one year is a developmental milestone for several reasons. At about this age (with considerable variation), children produce their first words, respond to simple requests, can stand at least briefly without support, begin to walk, show increased use of communicative gestures, and can eat some foods independently. Some of these accomplishments are interrelated. Walking is associated with increased use of gestures but not vocalization (Iverson, 2021; West & Iverson, 2021). Bipedal (two-legged) locomotion frees the arms and hands, which promotes the use of gestures. It also encourages exploration of the environment, giving children greater opportunities to interact with their surround—people, animals, and objects. Bipedalism supports speech because walking on two legs yields the respiratory plasticity needed for speaking. Quadrupedal (four-legged) locomotion is achieved by synchronizing limb movements with respiratory cycles at a ratio of one stride to one breath. Quadrupedal animals that attempt to alter this ratio run the risk of falling flat because their limbs cannot find purchase in a rigid air chamber. Bipedal locomotion allows greater flexibility between limb movements and respiration. This advantage is not always evident in a one-year-old infant (Iverson, 2021) because vocalizations at this age are mostly brief and vital capacity is quite small (as discussed in Chapters 2 and 6). But eventually vocalizations become longer and vital capacity increases. Not only can humans walk and talk, but they can talk largely independently of their locomotion except when running.

To some degree, an infant's first words have articulatory properties continuous with those in babbling (Oller et al.,1976; Vihman et al., 1985). This developmental continuity reinforces the belief that prelexical vocalizations are relevant and informative regarding the overall process of speech development. It also points to the clinical value of assessing early vocalizations, which is addressed later in this chapter.

Capabilities or Processes

Another approach is to identify capabilities or processes in infant vocalizations. The objective is to establish the appearance of behaviors that are hallmarks of vocal development. Some examples are **functional flexibility, volubility, protophones**, and **repetitive babble**. These emergent behaviors may signal important advances in vocal development that prefigure intelligible speech.

Functional flexibility is observed when prelinguistic vocalizations express emotional valence (positive, neutral, and negative). Oller et al. (2013) concluded that at least three types of infant vocalizations (squeals, vowel-like sounds, and growls) express these emotions by 3 to 4 months of age. The linkage of vocalization to emotions is a powerful accomplishment that gives infants the capability to express their emotional status to caregivers. Throughout life, emotion is linked to vocal behavior, so much so that it is a common experience for a listener to reach conclusions about a speaker's emotional state even on brief utterances. This point is developed more fully in Chapters 3 and 7. Both the limbic vocal control and cortical vocal control pathways activate the musculature through the vagus nerve (cranial nerve X), the most complex and longest of the cranial nerves and serves multiple functions including somatosensory, special sensory, motor, and parasympathetic. **Polyvagal theory** (Porges, 2001, 2009; Porges & Lewis, 2010) proposes that the vagus nerve serves functions related to (a) social communication (e.g., facial expression, vocalization, listening), (b) mobilization (e.g., fight or flight behaviors), and (c) immobilization (e.g., freeze-or-faint response, vasovagal syncope, and behavioral shutdown. Vagal activity increases with positive parent-infant interactions and with positive vocalizations such as cooing and babbling (Field & Diego, 2008). Therefore, the vagus nerve is a neural connection for emotion, vocalizing, and listening.

Volubility is the quantity of vocalizations that are produced in early life (Long et al., 2020). Compared to nonhuman primates, human infants are remarkably prolific in their early vocalizations (Oller et al., 2019). Other motor systems exhibit the same phenomenon. Latash (2012) explained that the abundance of movements in infants is advantageous to motor development. Seemingly random movements are the raw material of motor skill development. In a study of walking, Adolph et al. (2012) concluded from observations of 12- to 19-month-old infants during free play that they averaged 2368 steps and fell 17 times/hour. Neither walking nor talking comes without ample practice! The sheer quantity of movements, whether vocal or otherwise, is a potentially important feature of development because it allows infants to explore movement possibilities, discover synergies, and recognize flexibility in movement patterns. Paucity of movement in infants is a clinical concern and may be a red flag for developmental disorders.

Protophones are defined by Buder et al. (2013, p. 105), as "those primitive categories of sounds that are thought to be speech-related, or precursors to mature speech . . . protophones can generally be divided into two categories: those related to phonation and those related to syllabification and/or articulation" (p. 105). Included in the former are quasivowels and full vowels, squeals and growls, whispers and yells, and various sounds produced on ingressive (in flowing) rather than egressive (out flowing) airflow. The categories of syllabification and articulation include raspberries, clicks, goos, glottal stop sequences, marginal and canonical babble. These sounds are characterized by a valving or articulation typically made at the supralaryngeal level accompanied by laryngeal activity of some kind. This dual character may be an early step in speech development, as it foreshadows the coordination of speech movements in syllables and words.

Repetitive babble is a striking feature of vocal development that is nearly universal and appears to be a bridge between earlier vocalizations and the emergence of early words. The usual form of repetitive babble is a sequence of CV syllables produced in a quasi-periodic rhythm. The babbling may be either **reiterated** (repetition of the same syllable) or **variegated** (composed of two or more different syllables), and there is not total agreement that one form necessarily precedes the other in development (Kent, 2022). Repetitive babbling (also called canonical babbling, CB) appears at about the same time as rhythmic movements in other body parts, including the limbs, fingers, and trunk (Ejiri, 1998; Piek & Carman, 1994; Thelen, 1979). These movements have been called rhythmic stereotypies in recognition of their rhythmic performance of a fixed movement. However, it has been shown that the movements may not be fixed but rather take variable forms across the repetition series, especially in early infancy (Adolph & Franchak, 2017).

Developmental Functional Modules

The concept of modules has been proposed for complex systems that can be decomposed into semi-autonomous units. A biological system is said to be modular if it can be divided into interacting components that are relatively autonomous with respect to each other. Bolker (2000) described three major properties of modules in evolutionary and developmental biology: (1) a module is a biological entity that has greater internal than external integration. (2) A module is an individualized element that can be distinguished from its surroundings or context, and whose function is based on integration with other modules and not simply their arithmetical sum (the whole being more than a sum of its parts). (3) A module is distinct from other entities with which it interacts in some way.

Developmental Functional Modules (DFMs) related to infant vocalizations are based on biological principles in genetics, embryology, muscle physiology, developmental anatomy, and principles of motor control (Kent, 2021, 2022). DFMs are developmental, functional, and modular. They are developmental in having an ontogenetic pattern of growth and remodeling that is semiautonomous in pattern formation or differentiation. They are functional in being discrete entities that perform actions distinct from other modules although they may cooperate and even overlap with other modules in global actions. They are modular in consisting of a set of spatially defined, interconnected elements. Briefly, a DFM is an assembly of vocal tract structures that function together to accomplish articulatory actions in speech. The modular concept recognizes that articulators do not act alone in producing vocal behaviors. Rather, they act in synergetic assemblies that reflect genetic, embryologic, and functional origins.

The DFMs defined in Kent (2021, 2022) are as follows:

1. Respiratory DFM consists primarily of the chest wall, diaphragm, and the upper airways (the last of these ensures patency during ventilation).
2. Laryngeal DFM consists primarily of the larynx and hyoid bone.

3. Mandibular DFM consists primarily of the mandible and hyoid bone. Because the mandible provides skeletal support for the tongue and lips and is, therefore, included within the the Labial Complex and Lingual Complex DFMs, described later.
4. Pharyngo-laryngeal DFM consists primarily of the larynx, hyoid bone, velopharynx, and posterior tongue. This DFM dissolves during the first few months of life as the larynx descends relative to the cervical vertebral column.
5. Velopharyngeal DFM consists primarily of the soft palate (velum) and the pharyngeal constrictors.This DFM matures after the Pharyngo-laryngeal DFM dissolves.
6. Labial Complex DFM consists primarily of the lips, facial muscles, and mandible. This DFM has 2 submodules: deep (which provides forceful movements for sucking) and superficial (which provides for finer movements in speech and other oral functions).
7. Lingual Complex DFM consists primarily of the tongue and mandible (which provides support and movement assistance). The tongue itself consists of 4 submodules: tongue body, coronal raising, dorsal raising, and pharyngeal.

Figure 4–2 illustrates 3 submodules of the Lingual Complex DFM. The tongue body submodule is the mass of the tongue and is involved in the overall carriage of the tongue as well as the production of vowels and vowel-like sounds. The coronal raising submodule elevates and lowers the tip and blade of the tongue, as appropriate for alveolar or dental consonants. The dorsal raising submodule elevates and lowers the dorsum of the tongue, as appropriate for velar consonants. The actions of these submodules together with the superficial submodule of the

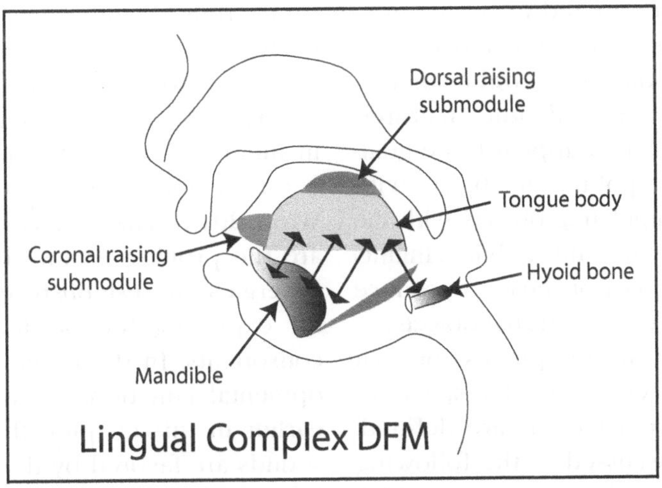

Figure 4–2. Illustration of the Lingual Complex DFM, showing the connections between the tongue, mandible, and hyoid bone, as well as the coronal raising and velar raising submodules.

Labial Complex DFM account for the predominance of coronal, velar, and bilabial sounds in early vocal development.

Goal Babbling in Vocal Development

A general question in the development of motor skills in infancy is: How can infants develop stable sensorimotor skills when their bodies are growing rapidly and undergoing non-linear changes in morphology (shape), along with changes in tissue composition? This question is germane to all motor skills including vocal development leading to speech. A possible solution is that infants do not simply perform random movements but rather perform goal-directed movements that support "learning by doing." Rolf et al. (2010) proposed a strategy of **Goal Babbling** in which an infant tries to achieve different goals and in doing so bootstraps sensorimotor coordination. This process helps infants to discover synergies in motor performance (e.g., tongue-jaw and lip-jaw synergy) and to refine internal models that can guide movements even as their bodies grow and change in relative dimensions and other features. Early movements that appear to be goal-directed include poking at objects with the fingers, manipulating objects with the hands, hand banging, and babbling. Infants can perform the last of these to produce sounds without using external objects.

A basic step in this process of goal babbling is to establish the space in which the internal models are defined. This space is discussed in the following for vowels first and consonants second. For both sound classes, the objective is to construct an articulatory space that accommodates early motor skills while allowing for expansion and refinement of motor skills as speech develops.

The typical pattern of vowel development was summarized by Kent and Rountrey (2020). At about 10 to 16 months, when early word production overlaps with babbling, the corner vowels /i u ɑ/ are often produced, and these are among the first vowels noted in developmental studies (Selby et al., 2000; Templin, 1957) and among the most frequently occurring vowels in natural languages (Maddieson, 1984). Because these vowels frame the extremes of vowel articulation, they are stable referents for articulation (Kent, 1992), acoustics (Kent & Rountrey, 2020), and auditory perception (Polka & Bohn, 2011). The relationships among articulation, acoustics and perception for this vowel triad are shown in Figure 4–3. These vowels represent the extremes in each domain of vowel description. Polka and Bohn (2011) proposed that these peripheral vowels are anchors within the **natural reference vowel framework**, which is potentially universal in vowel development. Further development of vowel production is influenced by the ambient language as the child hears vowels that fit into the vowel triangle of /i u ɑ/.

The consonants that predominate in infant babbling include the bilabials, coronals, dorsals, and glottals (Morgan & Wren, 2018). These places of articulation are the proving ground for articulatory synergies and establish reference points for exploring the production of other consonants. In the framework of Developmental Functional Modules discussed earlier in this chapter, these consonant sounds are favored by the structural and functional properties of the developing vocal tract. A general conclusion of studies on early vocal development is that a small set of consonants (/b d g m n/)

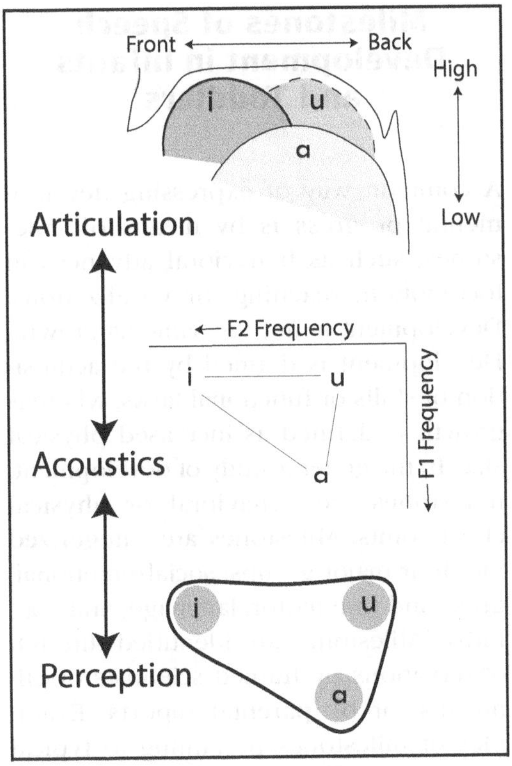

Figure 4–3. The point vowels /i u ɑ/, shown as articulatory configurations, acoustic patterns, and perceptual spaces. Articulatory description has the dimensions of tongue advancement (front vs back) and tongue height (low vs high). The acoustic representation is in the F1-F2 formant plane. The perceptual representation is a hypothetical space for vowels.

occur with notably high frequency (Morgan & Wren, 2018). These sounds achieve goal babbling in several respects: coordination of voicing with an oral articulation, three main types of oral constriction, control of velopharyngeal function (open or closed), and ballistic movements that underlie CV syllables in isolation or repetitive babbling. Prelexical vocalizations like babbling are initial steps in learning the voluntary movements needed for speech, and it is no accident that the sounds occurring with high frequency in babbling are often carried over to the production of first words (de Boysson-Bardies & Vihman,1991; Garmann et al., 2019; Oller et al., 1976; Vihman et al., 1985). Babbling is continuous with later speech development because prelexical vocalizations are goal-directed voluntary movements that build internal models that are robust to changes in vocal tract anatomy (Callan et al., 2000).

Metrics of Phonetic Development in Infants

Efforts have been made to develop quantitative indices of infant babbling. The CBR, discussed earlier, is frequently reported in studies of infant vocal development. Another metric is the **mean level of babbling (MLB)**, a scoring system developed by Stoel-Gammon (1987, 1991) that assigns levels of phonetic complexity to infant babbling. The three levels are determined as follows. Level 1 is assigned to vowel, syllabic consonant, consonant–vowel, or vowel–consonant combination in which the manner of consonant articulation is a glide or glottal. Level 2 is assigned to a consonant–vowel or vowel–consonant combination containing a true consonant (not a glide or glottal; the vocalization can contain repetitive sequences of sounds, but the place and/or manner of the consonant cannot change, except in voicing). Level 3 is assigned to consonant–vowel or vowel–consonant combinations in which the consonants are true consonants and the place and/or manner of articulation change at least once within the breath group.

Similar measures have been proposed for infants' first words. Paul and Jennings (1992) defined a measure of **syllable structure level (SSL)** with the following values.

1. Utterances composed of a voice vowel, voiced syllabic consonant, or CV syllable in which the consonant is a glottal stop or a glide.
2. Utterances composed of a VC or CVC syllable with a single consonant type, or a CV syllable that does not fit the criteria for Level 1. Voicing differences are ignored.
3. Utterances composed of syllables with two or more different consonant types, ignoring voicing differences.

For further discussion and examples of MBL and SSL, see Morris (2010).

> Jakobson (1941) argued that babbling was distinct from, and discontinuous with, speech development in children. Evidence now supports the contrary view that babbling shares characteristics with subsequent spoken language and is continuous with it in several important respects. The study of babbling has progressed through rigorous research using perceptual and acoustic methods. Babbling in infancy should be understood as an infant's deliberate effort to learn skills that lead to speech. It is quite different from another definition of babbling—that it is talking rapidly in a foolish, excited, or incomprehensible way.

Milestones of Speech Development in Infants and Toddlers

A common way of expressing developmental progress is by means of milestones, such as behavioral advances in locomotion, reaching, or vocalizations. Development is not the same as growth. Development is defined by the acquisition of skills or functional tasks, whereas growth is defined as increased physical size. In the general study of development, milestones are behavioral or physical checkpoints. Milestones are categorized into four major groups: social/emotional, gross and fine motor, language, and cognitive. Milestones are identified through observations by trained scientists or clinicians, or by parental reports. Examples of milestones pertaining to typical speech and language development in infants (birth to 24 months of age) are listed in Table 4–1. Milestones serve two important purposes. First, they point to orderly changes in a child's development of spoken communication. Some, but not necessarily all, of these changes are universal in the sense that they are observed across languages and cultures. Second, they can be used to formulate red flags that identify children at risk for communicative disorders or for developmental disorders in general. Red flags for communicative disorders are discussed in Chapter 5.

Table 4–1. Milestones in the Typical Development of Spoken Language in Infants, as Reported in Six Sources

Age (mos)	Feldman (2019)	Gerber et al. (2010)	Prath (2016)	Oberklaid & Drever (2011)	Visser-Bochane et al. (2020)	Prelock et al. (2008)
1		Throaty noises	Crying, vegetative sounds			
2		Coos, social smile, vowel-like noises		Social smile		
3	Differentiates cry, coos	Chuckles, vocalizes when talked to		Cooing		Cooing
4		Laughs out loud, vocalizes when alone		Turns to voice		
5		Says "Ah-goo," razzes, squeals, Expresses anger with sounds other than crying	Marginal babbling			
6		Reduplicative babble with consonants, listens, then vocalizes when adult stops, smiles/vocalizes to mirror		Babbling		Babbling
7		Increasing variety of syllables	Reduplicated babbling			
8		Says "Dada" (nonspecific), echolalia (8 to 30 months), shakes head for "no"				

continues

Table 4–1. *continued*

Age (mos)	Feldman (2019)	Gerber et al. (2010)	Prath (2016)	Oberklaid & Drever (2011)	Visser-Bochane et al. (2020)	Prelock et al. (2008)
9		Says"Mama" (nonspecific), nonreduplicative babble, imitates sounds	Phonetically consistent forms and jargon	Babbling		Intentional communication
10		Says "Dada" (specific), waves "bye-bye"				
11		Says first word, vocalizes to songs				
12	Says first words	Points to get desired object, uses several gestures with vocalizing (e.g., waving, reaching)		Says single words	Joint attention	Says first words
13		Uses 3 words, immature jargoning, inflection without real words				
14		Names one object, points at object to express interest				
15	Participates in conversation	Uses 3 to 5 words, immature jargoning with real words			Says words, 3-word sentence comprehension	
16		Uses 5 to 10 words				

Age (mos)	Feldman (2019)	Gerber et al. (2010)	Prath (2016)	Oberklaid & Drever (2011)	Visser-Bochane et al. (2020)	Prelock et al. (2008)
17						
18	Vocabulary of at least 50 words; Uses 2-word phrases; Learns new words easily	Uses 10 to 25 words, uses giant words (all gone, stop that), imitates environmental sounds, names one picture on demand				Vocabulary explosion; 2- to 3-word utterances (telegraphic language)
19						
20		Holophrases ("Mommy?" and points to keys, meaning: "These are Mommy's keys."), 2-word combinations, answers requests with "no"				

Speech Sound Acquisition in Children 3 Years and Older

By the age of 2 years, most children have a productive vocabulary of about 200 words and have begun to show reliable production of some phonemes. By the age of 3 years, progress in speech development is sufficient to warrant analysis in terms of the **mastery of phoneme production**. Speech sound acquisition often is expressed as the percentage of correct productions of a given sound. For example, a criterion of 50% mastery means that a sound is produced correctly 50% of the time when attempted. Figure 4–4 shows (a) a profile of speech sound mastery for the consonants of American English (based on an analysis of published studies by Crowe & McLeod, 2020), (b) the developmental classes of early 8, middle 8,

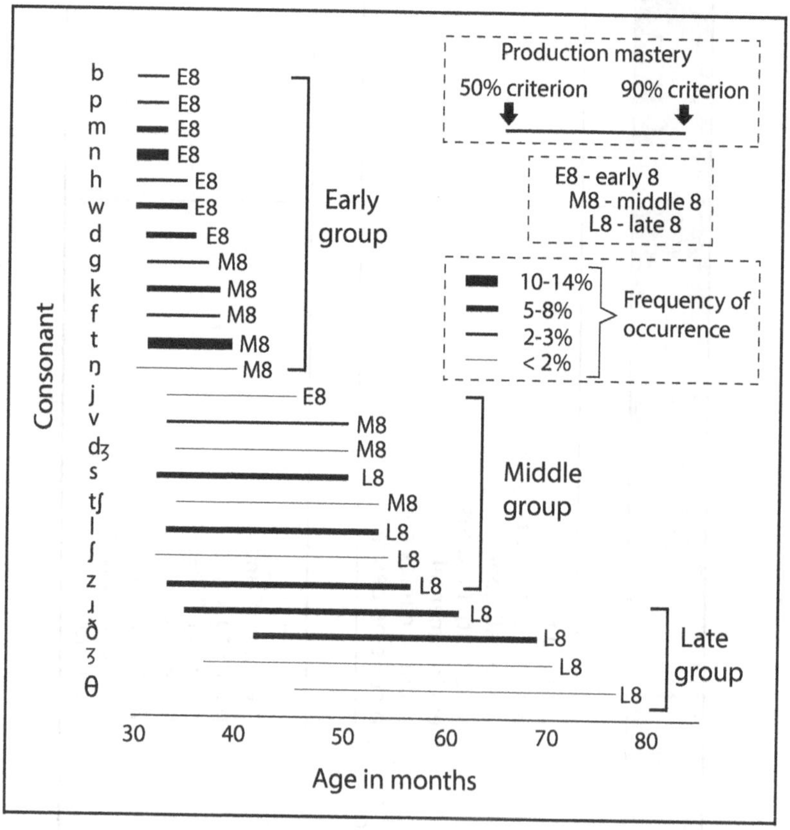

Figure 4–4. Profile of speech sound mastery and frequency of occurrence for the consonants of American English. Shown for each consonant phoneme is a line that connects two points, the 50% criterion of mastery and the 90% criterion of mastery (Crowe & McLeod, 2020). The consonants are grouped in 3 developmental sets: early, middle, and late mastery. The labels E8, M8, and L8 are the developmental groups identified by Shriberg (1993). Thickness of the lines for each consonant represents frequency of occurrence in American English (Shriberg et al., 2019).

and late 8 (Shriberg, 1993), and (c) estimates of the frequency of occurrence of the consonants in American English (Shriberg et al., 2019). Shown for each consonant phoneme of American English is a line that connects two points, the 50% criterion of mastery and the 90% criterion of mastery from the data in Crowe and McLeod (2020). The staggered profile of mastery across sounds makes it clear that acquisition is protracted over several years of childhood and that certain classes of sounds are mastered much earlier than others. As shown in the figure, the sounds might be classified into three major groups related to age of mastery, the early 12, the middle 8 and the late 4. This grouping differs somewhat from that proposed by Shriberg (1993), who identified 3 classes of 8 phonemes each in a study of children with speech sound disorders: the early eight (/m b j n w d p h/) are typically acquired by the age of 3 years, the middle eight (/t ŋ k g f v tʃ dʒ/) between the ages of 3 years and 6;6 years, and the late eight (/ʃ ʒ s z θ ð l ɹ /) between the ages of 6 and 8 years. The early eight, consisting largely of voiced stops, nasals, and glides, resemble sounds that predominate in infant vocalizations. The middle eight are characterized by the addition of voiceless stops, velar place of articulation, labiodental fricatives, and the palatal affricates. These additions reflect improved control of voicing and the relatively blunt places of articulation for labiodentals, velars, and palatals. The late eight are fricatives and the liquids /l/ and /r/. These sounds require finer articulatory adjustments for sustained frication and the formation of labial and rhotic articulations. Sounds with high frequencies of occurrence in American English are as follows: early group (/n t m w d k/), middle group (/s z l/), and late group (/ð ɹ/).

> "Consonants are muscles of the speech; they are the power, the frame, and the contour to the sound; they are the banks holding in the fluid essence of vowels" (S. Volkonsky [1913]. *An expressive word: A study and guide in speech mechanics, psychology, philosophy, and aesthetics in life and on the stage* [Russian]. St. Petersburg. Quoted by V. V. Nalimov [1974]. *In the labyrinths of language* [p. 189]. iSi Press.)

Vowel sounds are sometimes neglected in descriptions of speech sound mastery, apparently in the belief that they generally are acquired early and are seldom subject to production errors. But studies indicate that aspects of vowel production may have a mastery as late as 8 years (James et al., 2001) and that some children with speech sound disorders have vowel errors (Roepke & Brosseau-Lapré, 2021). Unfortunately, articulation tests are rarely designed to assess vowel production in any detail. Pollock (1991) concluded that of the articulation tests she evaluated, none provided an adequate sample to analyze vowel errors. Similarly, Eisenberg and Hitchcock (2010) observed that six of 11 standardized tests of speech articulation tested for vowels and that of the six, only two (Fisher–Logemann Test of Articulation [Fisher & Logemann, 1971] and Templin–Darley Tests of Articulation, [Templin & Darley, 1968]) had a phonetically controlled word for all 15 vowels of American English. Vowels are not acquired all at once. Rather, some vowels, like /i/ and /u/ are acquired early in life, by the age of 3 or 4 years, whereas others (especially the rhotic or r-colored vowels) may not be mastered by some children until much later. The general pattern of typical vowel development can be described in terms of three major sets: monophthongs (1 to 3 years), diphthongs (3 to 4 years), and rhotics (4 to 5 years), but there is substantial individual variation (Kent & Rountrey, 2020).

Phonological Processes

A **phonological process** is a difference (error) in speech sound production that is considered to reflect the operation of a simplification rule that is phonological in origin. The assumption is that children use simplifications when they are not capable of producing the phonological patterns of adult speech. For example, if children find it difficult to produce the fricative /s/, they may substitute it with the stop /t/ (for example, /sup/ is produced as /tup/, in a process known as stopping). The pattern of simplification eventually is suppressed as a child gains phonological ability (discussed more fully in Chapter 8). Among the frequently recognized processes are the following: **syllable structure processes (cluster reduction, final consonant deletion, syllable reduction)**; **substitution processes (deaffrication, fronting, gliding, stopping, vocalization)**, and **assimilation processes (prevocalic prevoicing, postvocalic devoicing)**. The ages of suppression (disappearance) of some of the commonly reported phonological processes are shown in Figure 4–5. A major appeal of phonological process analysis is that it reveals sound class patterns in children's speech production. For example, the process of final consonant deletion applies to all consonants occurring in a syllable-final position. The presence of a particular process is determined by examining how sounds are grouped together to account for error patterns (McReynolds & Elbert, 1981). It is usually assumed that phonological processes are the consequence of immaturity in the motor or physiological aspects of speech production (Chapter 7 considers this topic in more detail). The concept that phonological processes disappear or are suppressed with development is a rather destructive way of viewing development because it implies that something goes away to explain developmental advance. An alternative, more constructive view is that phonological processes reflect ongoing sensorimotor achievement in a child's development, that is, a child's capability to produce sound patterns is determined in large part by maturational processes, as discussed later in this chapter.

It has been concluded that children acquire an adult-like phonological system by the age of 5 to 6 years (Grunwell, 1987; Vance et al., 2005). Also, by this age, most typically developing children have speech that is highly intelligible to both familiar and unfamiliar listeners (see Chapter 8). However, as discussed later, the sensory and motor skills of speech continue to be refined for several more years.

Consistency and Variability of Speech Production

It is not surprising that children may show inconsistencies and variability in their speech production, even for sounds that are close to being mastered according to the usual clinical standards. It can be challenging to distinguish variability that is associated with typical development from inconsistencies that rise to the level of clinical concern. Holm et al. (2007) provide the following definitions:

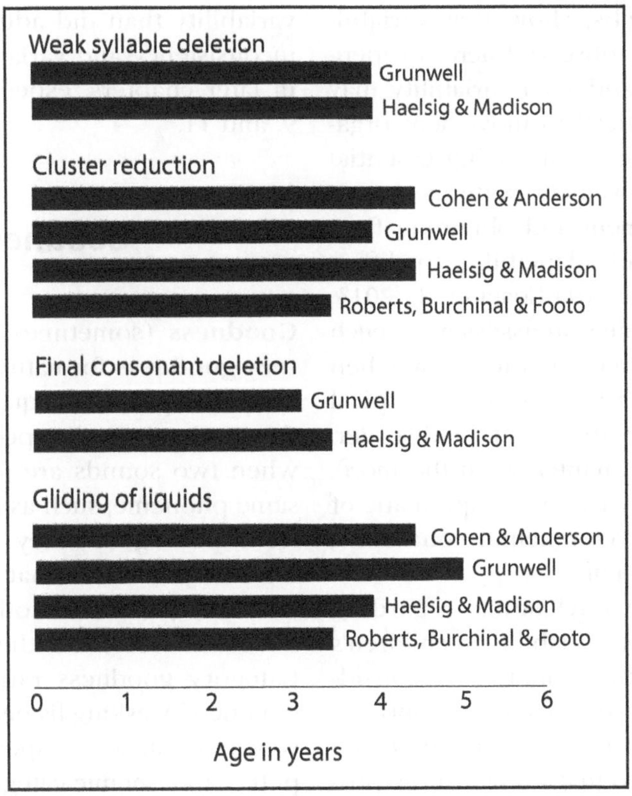

Figure 4–5. The ages of suppression (disappearance) of some of the commonly reported phonological processes. The data sources are Cohen and Anderson (2011), Grunwell (1985), Haelsig and Madison (1986), and Roberts et al. (1990).

> Variability is defined as productions that differ, but can be attributed to factors described in normal acquisition and use of speech. Inconsistency is speech characterized by a high proportion of differing repeated productions with multiple error types, both segmental (phoneme) and structural errors (consonant–vowel sequence within a syllable). (p. 467)

Holm et al. assessed variability and inconsistency by making phonemic transcriptions of a child's production of target words in three trials. Production of a word was considered as consistent if all three productions of a word were identical phonemically, even if the word was not produced accurately. Production of the word was considered variable when any differences were detected across the three trials.

Inconsistency and variability can be described at different levels, including the level of phonemes, the level of phonetic elements and features, and the level of movements. Segmental errors and variability are revealed by phonemic (broad) and phonetic (narrow) transcriptions. Movement error and variability are revealed by acoustic or kinematic methods. Studies of body movements, such as the limbs, show that variability is frequently observed across repetitions of a task and such variability may in fact be beneficial to movement organization and execution, "being essential for selecting movement patterns during motor development and obtaining flexible patterns and adaptability to different task demands" (da Costa et al., 2013, p. 2811). A problem in assessing speech production in children is to know when variability is an aspect of healthy typical development or an aspect of disorder, as discussed in Chapter 9. Furthermore, lack of variability can be symptomatic of certain neurodevelopmental conditions, such as cerebral palsy.

Therefore, conclusions regarding inconsistency and variability in children's speech should be tempered by consideration of the levels of analysis and the nature of the observed behaviors. Holm et al. (2022) noted that studies of the proportion of words produced consistently by typically developing preschool children vary from 17% to 87%, which is a range difficult to use as a clinical benchmark. Holm et al. determined the quantitative (consistency count) and qualitative (e.g., phonemic analysis) characteristics of word consistency in a large group of children aged 36 to 60 months. In a task of naming 15 pictures twice the mean consistency of production was 82%. McCauley et al. (2021) reported in a study of multiword units produce in spontaneous production that children aged 36 to 60 months were accurate and consistent 57% of the time or with two productions of a word having the same error 25% of the time. Goffman et al. (2007) found that both typically developing children and children with speech sound disorder had more segmental error and segmental variability and more movement trajectory variability than did adults. The issue of inconsistency and variability is taken up in later chapters, especially Chapters 5, 9, and 11.

Goodness

Goodness (sometimes called **articulatory goodness** for natural as opposed to synthetic speech) is a qualitative aspect of the production of a speech sound. Even when two sounds are judged to be the same phoneme, such as /d/, they can differ in how "good" they are in representing that phoneme. That is, one sound is a "better" /d/ than another even though both are heard as the phoneme /d/. Category goodness ratings are usually obtained by asking listeners to judge how well an instance of a speech sound exemplifies a phonemic category by assigning values from a numerical scale. Data from ratings of category goodness consistently show that phonological categories have an internal structure so that certain sounds are judged to be better than others as instances of that category (Drouin et al., 2016; Miller, 1994). A similar idea was described in Chapter 2 with respect to Kuhl's theory of perceptual magnets in speech perception. These findings have led to the formulation of models that view speech perception as a problem of statistical inference in which properties of the acoustic signal cue phonological category membership with varying levels of certainty (Kronrod et al., 2016). Goodness appears to be an aspect of speech that can be judged independently of other factors, such as intelligibility or phoneme identity (Sakash et al., 2023; Strömbergsson et al., 2015), and it, therefore, may be a useful index of speech production ability.

Motor Learning of Speech

If speech is in large part a motor achievement, then it should be possible to identify the motor substrates of speech development. The implication is that speech development can be described in terms of motor processes that underlie phoneme acquisition or phonological processes. A difficulty arises in that it is not a simple matter to differentiate motor aspects from other influences, such as phonological contrasts. It is reasonable, even necessary, to assume that motor skills of speech production develop simultaneously with phonological capabilities. The interaction between these two is an unavoidable circumstance of speech development. Later chapters, especially Chapter 9, have much more to say about motor learning, but for now it is sufficient to state some basic principles.

1. Speech is associated with spatiotemporal goals. That is, speech sounds are defined by positional targets (e.g., complete alveolar constriction) and temporal properties (e.g., a rapid movement away from the constriction). Phonemes are distinguished by these goals, so that learning to speak is in large part a matter of knowing how to achieve spatiotemporal goals. Speech makes exacting demands on both spatial positioning and the timing of movements. The motor skills of speech are learned through effort.
2. The learning of any motor skill takes practice and must account for the present status of the motor effectors (bones, muscles, and other tissues). As the vocal tract structures change in shape and size, adjustments must be made in motor control. Therefore, speech motor control is adapted and refined as its biological substrate changes, and additional demands are placed on the complexity of the linguistic message.
3. Acquisition of a motor skill establishes stable yet flexible representations in the central nervous system. These ostensibly conflicting requirements are satisfied by establishing motor patterns that are reliable but plastic enough to meet changing demands.
4. Speech motor control does not have a steady pattern of growth but rather one that is characterized by different phases. For example, early speech motor control has been described as having three phases: a period of little or no change, a rapid increase followed by a decrease at 18 months co-occurring with the vocabulary burst, and a steady increase from 21 to 60 months (Iuzzini-Seigel et al., 2015).
5. Auditory feedback is thought to be critical to speech motor learning, as it is the means to establish sensory-motor maps that guide speech production. But different aspects of auditory feedback may be used during early development. Scheerer et al. (2020) concluded that toddlers are more sensitive to changes to postural properties such as fundamental frequency, compared to phonemic properties such as formant frequencies.

Although the concept of movements underlying speech production is by no means novel or new, there are few systematic proposals of speech development based on movements or motoric variables. Preference has been given to more abstract concepts such as phonemes or phonological processes, even if these ultimately are sometimes described and defined in motor terms. An influential theory based on a movement-based approach is **Articulatory Phonology** (Browman & Goldstein, 1992; discussed in more detail in Chapter 7). This theory proposes that an articulatory gesture is a goal that can be achieved through a variable combination of articulatory movements. For example, in producing the bilabial /b/, a goal is to bring the lips tightly together to make a complete closure. But this goal can be achieved through different combinations of lip and jaw movement, varying from no jaw participation at all to a high level of jaw movement and relatively little lip movement apart from the jaw. In articulatory phonology, the phonological representation is in terms of articulatory gestures, rather than features or segments. In the formal development of articulatory phonology, articulatory gestures have been defined as tract variables, that is, parameters that pertain to adjustments of the vocal tract. The seminal work on this theory was done by linguist Catherine P. Browman (1945–2008) and by linguist and cognitive scientist Louis Goldstein. Figure 4–6 gives an example of articulatory gestures in the production of the word *pan*.

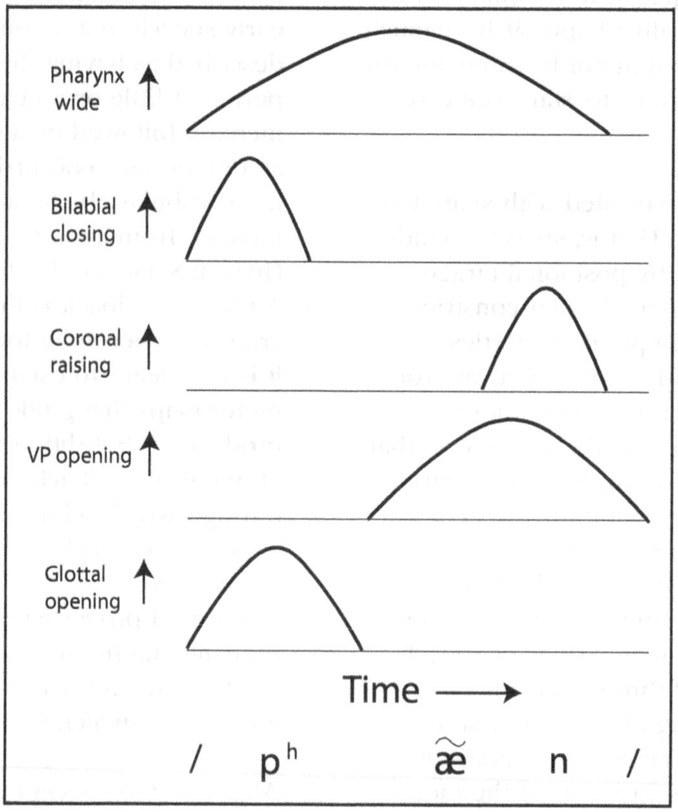

Figure 4–6. Diagram showing the gestural score for production of the word *pan* based on the articulatory gestures of pharyngeal widening, bilabial closing, coronal raising, velopharyngeal (VP) opening, and glottal opening.

Articulatory phonology is not the only means of representing speech in terms of movement variables, but it is one of the most systematic efforts to do so. Chapter 7 discusses several phonological theories.

Tongue Bracing

The classic depictions of lingual function in speech are based on classifications of place and manner of articulation for consonants, and vowel height and advancement for vowels (the International Phonetic Alphabet is reproduced in Appendix 1). These descriptions impute that the essential articulation is discrete and adequately described by concepts such as a single point of contact in most cases. But this view is changing, as recent studies indicate that during speech production the tongue has nearly continuous contact with other oral structures, such as the upper molars (Gick et al., 2017). This phenomenon, called **lateral bracing,** illustrated in Figure 4–7, and is accomplished through muscle activation and may be an essential biomechanical property of speech production. This bracing affords not only a biomechanical advantage to tongue movements but may also provide sensory feedback on the placement of the tongue. (Note: this type of bracing should be distinguished from lingual bracing, an appliance used in orthodontics.) It is likely that the role of lateral bracing is adapted to the current state of the dentition in children (discussed in Chapter 2).

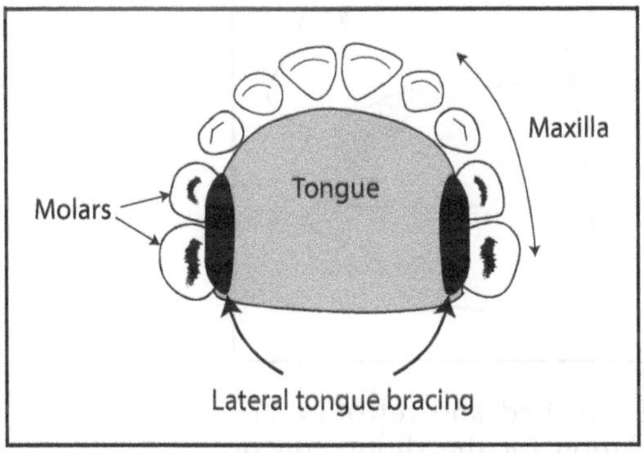

Figure 4–7. Lateral tongue bracing in which the tongue is stabilized by contact with the upper molars.

Late Acquired Sounds

This section addresses the late four sounds (see Figure 4–4) and sounds that are most likely to be in error in children judged to have residual speech sound disorder (R-SSD). Children with R-SSDs are likely to misarticulate liquids, sibilants, or both. Errors on liquids usually involve /ɹ, ɝ, ɚ/ and sometimes /l/. Sibilant errors typically occur with /s, z/ and sometimes /ʃ, ʒ, tʃ, dʒ/.

The story of /ɹ/

The liquids /ɹ/ and /l/ are produced with coordinated actions of the tongue tip and tongue body to form anterior and posterior constrictions, respectively (Boyce, 2015; Gick, 1999; Gick et al., 2002; Proctor, 2011; Sproat & Fujimura, 1993). The movements that form these constrictions are made with different timing, which poses another complication in producing the liquids. The rhotic consonant /ɹ/ is a sound that is acquired relatively late in typical speech sound acquisition (see Figure 4–4) and is often identified as an error sound in children with speech disorders. Historically, the articulation of /ɹ/ has been described as taking one of two major forms, **retroflex** (made with a backward turning of the tongue tip) and **bunched** (made with a bulging of the tongue in the palatal or velar region) with each form often associated with a constriction in the pharynx (Howson & Monahan, 2019). These articulations are illustrated in Figure 4–8. The pharyngeal constriction may be a secondary articulation (Boyce et al., 2016), which makes the rhotic consonant a challenge in speech development. Westbury et al. (1998) concluded from a study of 53 young adults that tongue shapes for /ɹ/ vary widely across speakers within a given phonetic context, and more continuously rather than categorically. Some commonalities emerged from the data, including the observation that tongue shapes vary by context in ways that are similar for most speakers. Kabakoff et al. (2021) and Preston et al. (2019) decided against classifying tongue shapes as either retroflex or bunched because perceptually acceptable rhotics often are produced with tongue shapes that do not match either of these categories. These results point to the possibilities that articulation of /ɹ/ is adapted to its phonetic environment and that speakers differ in their articulatory patterns for this sound. Dediu and Moisik (2019) deduced that the two common articulatory strategies of retroflex and bunched may be attractors on a multi-dimensional continuum, and that the selection of one strategy over the other is influenced by individual anatomic characteristics in the anterior region of the vocal tract. They also drew attention to the importance of pharyngeal bracing for both variants of /ɹ/. As children pursue articulatory precision, they may discover the advantages of biomechanical stability and feedback provided by various forms of bracing for lingual articulation. These observations suggest that considerations of anatomy and potential for bracing should be part of the treatment for disordered production of /ɹ/.

Howson and Monahan (2019) presented evidence that rhotics are a natural class and that they often are paired with a lateral in the phonetic inventories of

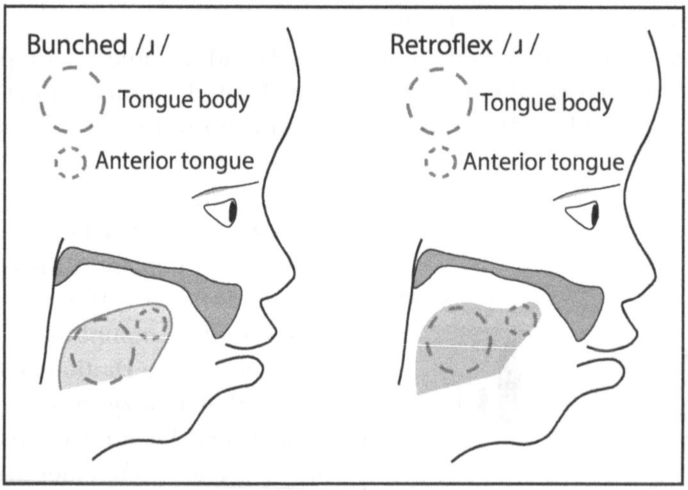

Figure 4–8. Production of the bunched and retroflex /ɹ/, the two major classes of articulation for the rhotic consonant according to classic phonetic description. Participation is shown for the tongue body and anterior tongue.

languages. This observation strengthens the grouping of rhotics and laterals as liquids and helps to explain the co-occurrence of these sounds. The word **liquid** is a cover term for the lateral and rhotic consonants, which have a greater degree of articulatory constriction than that for vowels but a lesser degree than that for the obstruents (stops, fricatives, and affricates). A difficulty for children learning to produce /ɹ/ is that there is no single well-defined articulation for this sound, and individual solutions may be needed (Byun et al., 2014). Howson and Redford (2021) interpreted their acoustic data on /ɹ/ to mean that children adopt an articulation strategy of tongue–body-first (i.e., tongue body articulation precedes articulation of the anterior tongue). This developmental sequence is consistent with the concept of the tongue behaving as a muscular hydrostat: the posture or support is established before local deformations are made to accomplish refined articulatory actions. Howson and Redford also observed a stronger anticipatory effect of vowel context on children's coarticulatory patterns compared to adults. This effect was interpreted to mean that anticipatory posturing (coarticulation) for tongue–body targets is given priority over posturing for tongue blade targets. These results pertain to children who were judged to have perceptually acceptable /ɹ/ production, which indicates that perceptual data do not necessarily tell the whole story of motor maturation in speech production.

Rhotics, more than most consonants, can take on double duty, as both consonant and vowel. In American English, the rhotic consonant /ɹ/ has the vowel counterparts /ɝ/ and /ɚ/, with the former being stressed and the latter unstressed. These rhotic forms share some acoustic properties, such as a relatively low frequency of the third formant (F3) or a close positioning of the second formant (F2) and F3 so that the two formants merge in auditory perception as a single band of energy, called the *rhotic formant* (Kent & Rountrey, 2020).

The Story of /l/

The lateral consonant /l/ can present difficulties for young children and for some persons learning English as a second language. Like /ɹ/, the lateral /l/ is formed with two constrictions, one made with the tongue tip and the other with the tongue body. The tongue tip makes a midline closure with the alveolar ridge of the hard palate, but the sides of the tongue allow a lateral opening on either side of the midline closure, as shown in Figure 4–9. As with the /ɹ/ sound, the articulation of /l/ requires positioning of both the tongue body and the anterior tongue. The associated movements may pose difficulty for children because they are opposite in direction, with the tongue body being retracted, rather like the position for vowel /o/, and the tongue blade and tip extended forward to contact the alveolar ridge. The /o/-like position of the tongue body may explain why children sometimes produce the /l/ with a vowel /o/ (e.g., saying the word *wheel* as /wio/.

The Story of /ð/ and /θ/

The interdental fricatives are among the last sounds to be mastered in typically developing children and among the sounds frequently in error in children with speech sound disorders. They appear to be more difficult than the fricatives /s/ and /ʃ/. Why should this be the case? A likely

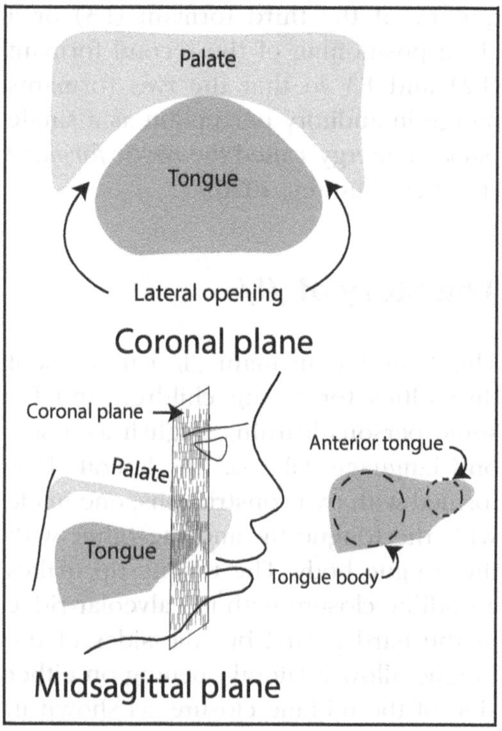

Figure 4–9. Production of the lateral consonant /l/, shown in the coronal and midsagittal planes. The articulation involves midline closure and lateral opening.

reason is that interdentals are very weak, having the lowest intensity of almost any speech sound, which makes them difficult to hear, for both children learning speech and for clinicians who are conducting articulation tests. These sounds are difficult to identify even at 60 dB sensation level by normal-hearing young adults (Kent et al., 1979). The voiceless /θ/ was correctly identified only about half the time at 60 dB, a level that ensured nearly 100% correct identification for all other sounds except /ð/. Because these sounds are weak, clinicians may have limited ability to discriminate error productions and should therefore be cautious in reaching decisions about production accuracy. With respect to production, the interdental fricatives are made by forming a narrow constriction between the tongue tip and the upper central incisors, as illustrated in Figure 4–10, which shows the articulatory configuration, a corresponding acoustic tube model, and the spectral shape of the fricative noise. The essential components of the vocal tract configuration are a back cavity, a constriction, and a front cavity that is very short and therefore has little effect on shaping the noise energy in the audible frequencies, which results in a diffuse spectrum of low intensity. Fortunately, the weak energy of these sounds is somewhat compensated for by the visibility of their interdental articulation. In respect to frequency of occurrence in American English fricative /ð/ has a relatively high frequency and occurs in frequently used words such as *this, that, then, than, they*, and *the* (Shriberg et al., 2019). In contrast, /θ/ is one of most infrequently occurring sounds in American English.

The Story of /s/ and /z/

These sounds are called stridents or sibilants in recognition of their strong frication energy, stronger than any other fricative in American English. Production requires formation of a narrow constriction, typically near the alveolar ridge but sometimes closer to the upper incisors. This constriction is needed to generate turbulence noise, and the placement of this constriction provides the resonance effects of a small cavity that lies between the constriction and the lip opening. This cavity is just long enough to shape the fricative energy to have a high-frequency dominance that contributes to the perceptual salience of these sounds. The articulation is illustrated in Figure 4–11 as a vocal tract configuration, an acoustic tube model, and a spectrum of the fricative

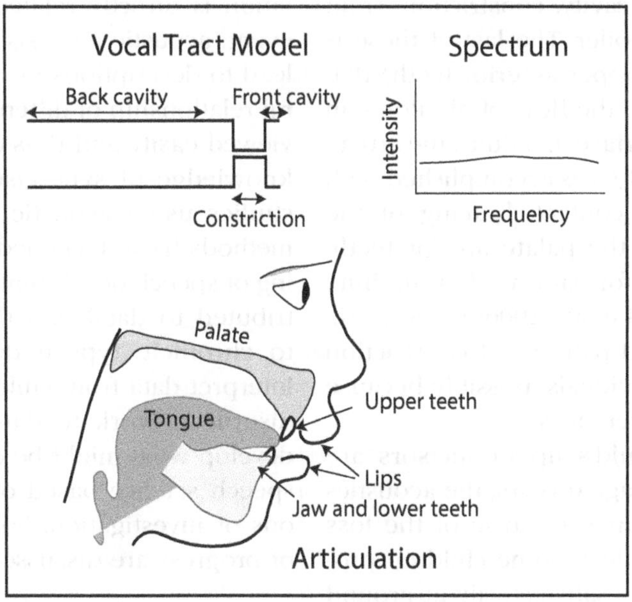

Figure 4–10. Production of the interdental fricatives /ð/ and /θ/, shown as a vocal tract model, acoustic spectrum, and articulatory configuration.

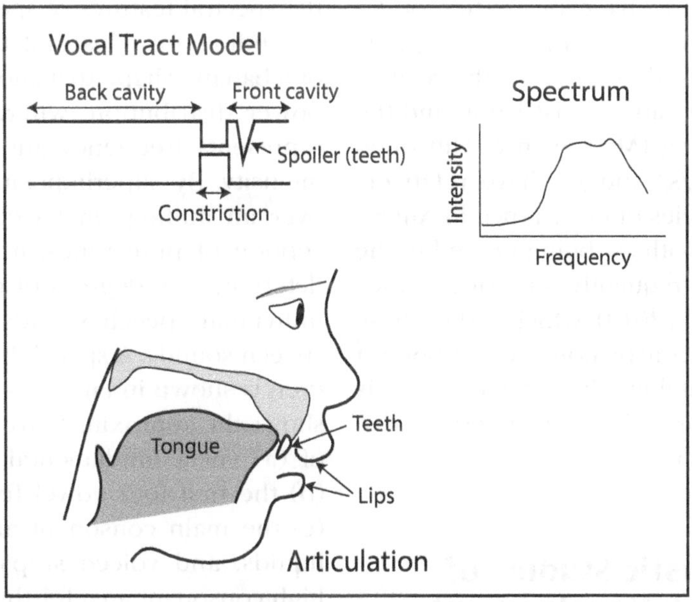

Figure 4–11. Production of the alveolar fricatives /z/ and /s/, shown as a vocal tract model, acoustic spectrum, and articulatory configuration.

noise. The vocal tract configuration consists of a back cavity, constriction, front cavity, and a spoiler. The last of these is an object (the upper anterior teeth) that acts to break up the flow of air along an aerodynamic surface. In adults, the articulation of /s/ and /z/ is accomplished with lingua-alveolar contact, bracing of the tongue against the palate and/or teeth, and (usually) formation of a midline groove (McLeod et al., 2006; Stone et al., 1992). The exact patterns of constriction vary across individuals, possibly because of anatomic differences.

When a child's upper incisors are shed at around age 6 years, the acoustics of /s/ often change because of the loss of the spoiler effect. Some children produce /s/ and /z/ satisfactorily at around age 4 years but later are judged to have a distorted production of these sounds (Dodd et al., 2018). Changes in dentition (Chapter 2) could be a contributing factor in this apparent reversal of speech sound mastery. The acoustic properties of /s/ differ between children and adults, possibly related to differences in the relative sizes of the fricative constriction and the glottal opening (McGowan & Nittrouer, 1988). Both /s/ and /z/ have relatively high frequencies of occurrence in American English, with /s/ being ranked in the top five most frequently occurring sounds (Shriberg et al., 2019), which makes these sounds both conspicuous and important for speech intelligibility. Malocclusion is another factor to be considered, as discussed in Chapter 11.

Acoustic Studies of Speech Development

Lenneberg (1964, p. 115) wrote optimistically on the potential of acoustic studies of speech: "Since every acoustic modulation is directly related to some motor event, acoustic analysis is quite likely to lead to descriptions in which the temporal relationship of different events can be viewed easily and thus contribute to our knowledge of synergism." Instrumental studies using acoustic and physiologic methods have deepened the understanding of speech development and have contributed to databases that can be used to chronicle typical development and interpret data from children with speech disorders. Work to date has helped to develop what might be called a pediatric speech science based on modern methods of investigation. Some major points of progress are discussed next.

The Speech Banana for Children

Fant (1995) described a plot that relates the spectral features of speech sounds to an audiogram. This plot takes the form of a banana-shape that shows the speech power distribution, where the abscissa represents frequency and the ordinate, intensity. By superimposing this banana over an audiogram based on the perception of pure tones, it is possible to determine the degrees of gain or loss of individual speech sounds or classes of speech sounds. A speech banana for children is shown in Figure 4–12. This figure shows the approximate frequency ranges of (a) vocal fundamental frequency, f_0, (b) the first four vowel formants F1-F4, (c) the main consonant area for glides, liquids, and voiced stops, and (d) the high consonant area for the sibilant fricatives /ʃ ʒ s z/ and the affricates /tʃ dʒ/. Because children have shorter vocal tracts than adults, the frequencies of vocal tract resonances in children are conspicuously

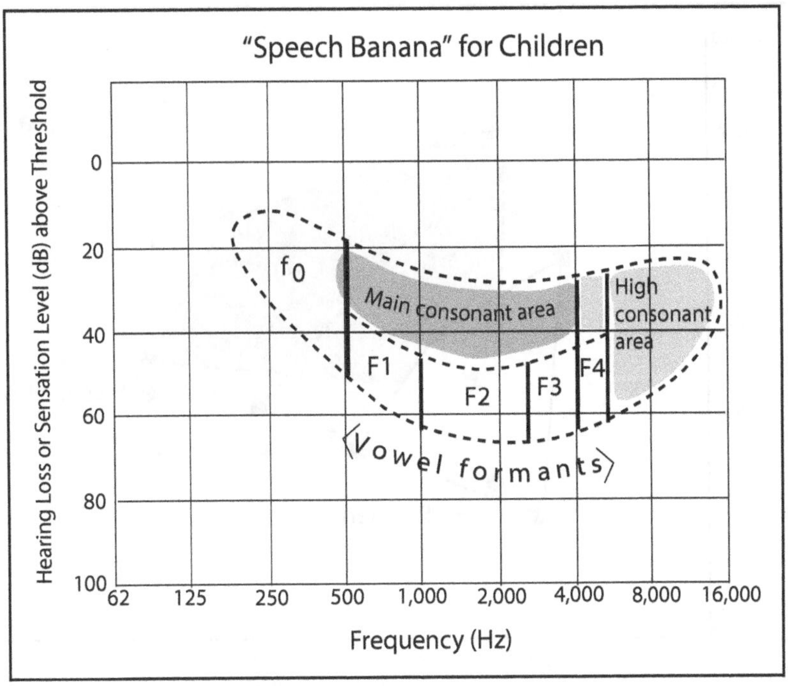

Figure 4–12. The speech banana for children, depicting the major frequency regions of sound energy for fundamental frequency, vowel formants (F1-F4), main consonant area, and high consonant area.

higher than those in adults. The energy for children's sibilants can extend to nearly 16 kHz. This acoustic property has implications for the effects of hearing loss on speech development, the acoustic display of speech features in treatment programs such as acoustic biofeedback, the selection of recording devices for speech studies, the transmission of children's speech, and the perception of children's speech by adults with hearing loss. It is little wonder that children's speech can be difficult to understand over telephones that have a restricted bandwidth, such as analogue telephones that have a bandwidth of about 3 kHz (passing energy from about 300 to 3400 Hz). Things do not get much better with 2G digital mobile networks, but 3G and 4G networks have a bandwidth of about 7 kHz and 5G networks offer additional advantages.

Vowel Formant Frequencies

As classically demonstrated by G. E. Peterson and Barney (1952), vowel formant frequencies vary with the age and sex of speakers. Subsequent research has led to a more detailed picture of how formant frequencies vary with age and sex (Kent & Vorperian, 2018; Vorperian et al., 2019). Figure 4–13 shows for 3 groups of speakers the vowel quadrilaterals defined by the corner vowels /i/ (high front), /æ/ (low front), /u/ (high back), and /ɑ/ (low back). This variation in formant frequencies with age and sex forces the conclusion that these factors must be considered in using acoustic data to study speech development or its disorders. The area contained within the vowel quadrilateral is commonly called the vowel space area (VSA) and has been correlated with

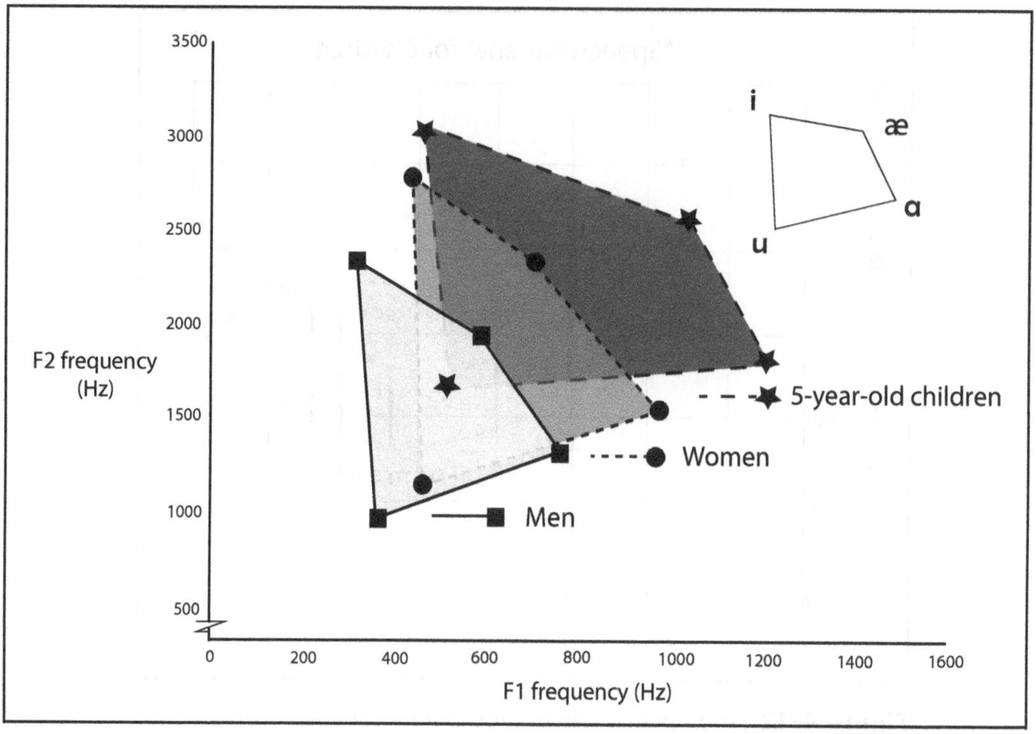

Figure 4–13. The vowel quadrilaterals for three groups of speakers: men, women, and 5-year-old children. The quadrilaterals are derived from the F1 and F2 values of the corner vowels.

speech intelligibility in both healthy and disordered speech (as reviewed in Kent & Vorperian, 2018). Graphs of VSA values for children aged 5 years and older are available in Flipsen and Lee (2012) and Kent and Rountrey (2020).

Voice

See Chapter 7 for discussion of voice and prosody in typical and atypical speech development. It also describes methods of clinical assessment suitable for children.

Spectral Moments

An approach to the acoustic analysis of fricatives is calculation of spectral moments (Jongman et al., 2000; Maniwa et al., 2009; Nissen & Fox, 2005). An advantage of spectral moment analysis is that the first four spectral moments, M1, M2, M3, and M4, offer a concise and quantitative description of fricative spectra. M1, also called centroid or center of gravity, is the weighted mean frequency of the energy distribution. M2, or standard deviation, is the spread of the energy distribution and is calculated as the averaged squared distance from the centroid. The higher moments M3 and M4 are useful to describe other features of the energy distribution. M3, or skewness, is an index of asymmetry in the energy distribution and is calculated as the difference between the energy above and below the centroid. M4, or kurtosis, is calculated as the average distance from the centroid raised to the fourth power, divided by the squared variance of the distribution. It has been described as a measure of either the "peakedness" of the spectrum or the "thickness" of the tails of the distribution, compared to the normal distribution of the same variance. Spectral moments have been used to characterize fricatives in the speech of typically developing children (Flipsen et al., 1999; Nittrouer, 1995; Nissen & Fox, 2005) and children with speech disorders (Karlsson et al., 2002; Maas & Mailend, 2017; Shriberg et al., 2003). For both children and adults, the fricative /ʃ/ has a lower M1 than fricative /s/, presumably because of the longer front cavity for /ʃ/ and perhaps also because of the presence of a sublingual space created when the tongue approximates the palate (Perkell et al., 1979; Perkell, et al., 2004).

Temporal Patterns

In motor skills generally, children's performance is slower and more variable than that of adults. Speaking rate in children usually is slower than that in adults and is reflected in longer durations of segments such as vowels. But a slower rate does not imply greater accuracy of production. A gauge of the accuracy of motor control is to determine the variability of temporal or spatiotemporal patterns in repeated tokens of a speech sequence. Research with acoustic, aerodynamic, electropalatographic and kinematic measures shows that children typically have greater variability than adults (Koenig et al., 2008). Furthermore, this greater variability in children is not simply a consequence of their typically slower speaking rate, as the same result pertains to a relative measure, the coefficient of variation (the standard deviation divided by the mean). Such variability also has been reported for the **spatiotemporal index (STI)**, a measure of variability in displacement records, which is obtained by summing the standard deviations calculated across amplitude and time-normalized records, usually 10 or more (A. Smith et al., 1995). This procedure usually is based on records of lip movements, but it can be generalized to other articulators. Variability is of interest for several reasons, including its possible use as an index of maturity of speech motor control, application to the study of speech disorders in children, and understanding why children's speech is less intelligible than that of adults. Regarding the latter, if speech perception depends in part on the expectation of regular or predictable timing patterns, then deviations from those patterns may contribute to reduced intelligibility. The rhythm of speech may aid listeners in effective direction of auditory attention (Wöstmann et al., 2016).

One of the most heavily researched aspects of timing is **voice onset time (VOT)**, the relative timing of the articulatory release of a stop consonant and the onset of voicing for the syllable in which the consonant occurs. In early vocalizations, the most frequently occurring consonants are /b d g/, that is, consonants perceived as voiced stops. In sound mastery, voiced stops are mastered somewhat earlier than their voiceless cognates (see Figure 4–4). Apparently, voiced stops are easier for children to produce, if only because they follow the principle of "everything moves at once" (i.e., there is no need to establish patterns of relative timing of movements). The acoustics of voiceless stop production are illustrated in Figure 4–14, which shows the following properties: release burst, aspiration,

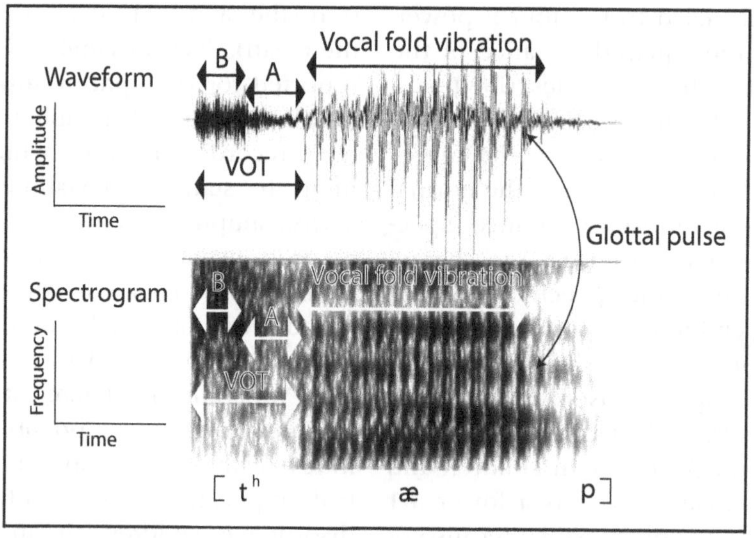

Figure 4–14. Voice onset (VOT) shown as a waveform at the top and spectrogram (bottom). VOT is the difference in time between the articulatory release of a stop consonant and the onset of voicing. The pattern is for the word tap. B is the interval of frication for the burst, and A is the interval of aspiration,

and onset of voicing. In American English, voiceless stops in syllable initial position are produced as aspirated stops. But some other languages have a category of unaspirated voiceless stops (i.e., they have a release burst followed by short lag of voicing onset). Different timing patterns of articulatory release and onset of voicing are shown in Figure 4–15. The patterns include simultaneity of release and voicing onset, a short delay of voicing relative to the release, and a long delay of voicing relative to the release.

Instrumental Methods

The main appeal of instrumental methods, such as those just described and those discussed in Chapter 5, lies in their potential to yield objective, quantitative data on speech production, thereby overcoming some of the limitations of a purely auditory-perceptual approach. But this appeal is offset to some degree by the cost of the devices and the need for training in their use. Acoustic methods are within the reach of clinicians in a variety of settings and the costs are very low, provided that a computer of adequate speed and memory is available (which is becoming less and less an obstacle given the rapid progress in digital technologies). Advances in automatic acoustic analyses should facilitate the use of acoustic methods in the clinic for the analysis of speech articulation, voice, and prosody. Discussed next is an example of how instrumental methods can add to our understanding of speech development.

Covert Contrasts

Before children produce a contrast between two given phonemes such as /p/ and /b/, they may pass through an intervening stage in which they produce a

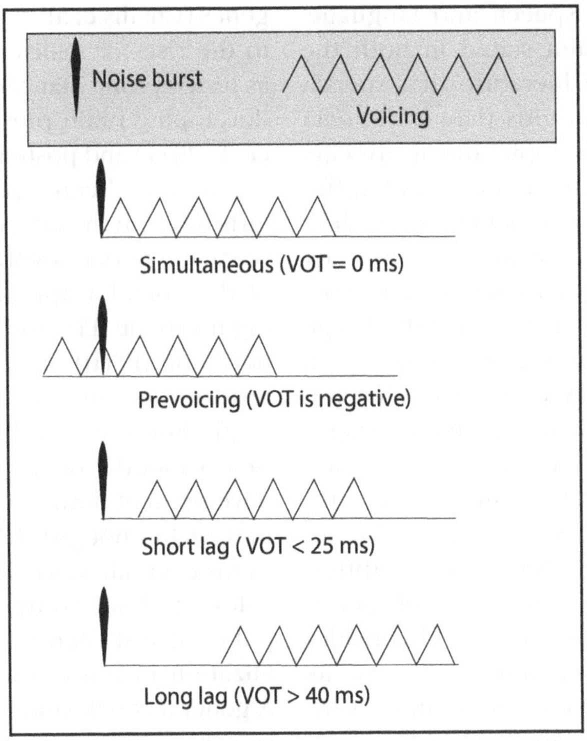

Figure 4–15. Illustration of four major categories of VOT based on the timing of voice onset relative to articulatory release: simultaneous voice onset, prevoicing (negative VOT), short lag voice onset, and long lag voice onset.

covert contrast, which is defined as a subphonemic difference in the production of the sound. These contrasts can be difficult or perhaps even impossible to detect by perceptual methods such as phonetic transcription. Covert contrasts can occur in both typical and atypical speech development, and they have been identified almost exclusively through acoustic and physiological methods (Gibbon & Lee, 2017a; Glaspey & MacLeod, 2010; Macken & Barton, 1980; McAllister et al., 2016; Scobbie et al., 2000; see also the special issue of *Clinical Linguistics & Phonetics*, Gibbon & Lee, 2017b). Gibbon and Lee (2017a) commented that, " . . . recent studies have provided convincing new evidence that covert contrasts are likely to be widespread in child speech" (p. 4). The implication is that commonly used methods of perceptual analysis may be insensitive to aspects of progress in speech development. A similar conclusion was reached by Munson et al. (2010), who suggested that covert contrasts are ubiquitous and may be a common feature of speech development but is poorly documented because of the insensitivity of auditory-perceptual judgments.

Sex and Gender Differences

Much has been written about sex and gender differences in the development and disorders of speech and language. Although it is often stated in both the scientific and lay literature that speech develops earlier in girls than boys, data are mixed on this topic and it appears that differences are modest and influenced by a variety of other factors, including socioeconomic status, age and sex of siblings, and environmental stressors (Etchell et al., 2018; Feldman, 2019; Lange et al., 2016; Wallentin, 2009). Etchell et al. concluded that sex differences that are prominent at certain developmental stages may be negligible in other stages, owing to the influence of different rates of maturation between the sexes. Statistical comparisons should go beyond mean differences in the age of achievement of speech and language skills and should consider variability and longitudinal patterns as well. It appears that boys are more variable than girls in group statistics (i.e., there are more boys at both ends of the distribution).

It is well established that boys are more vulnerable to communication disorders than girls, and this generalization pertains to a variety of conditions including developmental language disorder, stuttering, autism spectrum disorder, and speech sound disorders (May et al., 2019; Wallace et al., 2015). Why is this so? The explanation may lie at least partly in prenatal factors, beginning with the **trophoblast**, the layer of tissue on the outside of the blastula that supplies the embryo with nourishment and subsequently forms a substantial part of the placenta. Studies indicate that the trophoblast in the presence of a male fetus may generate a more pro-inflammatory environment, and that there are sex differences in the maturation of the hypothalamic–pituitary–adrenal axis and the expression of placental genes (Challis et al., 2013). Further adding to the risk for males are hormones such as testosterone that can strongly affect the developing brain prenatally (Durdiakova et al., 2011) and postnatally (Nguyen et al., 2013). It has been reported that boys and girls differ in the effects of minipuberty, a postnatal period involving a transient rise of the gonadotropic hormones (luteinising hormone [LH] and follicle-stimulating hormone [FSH]) and of the sex steroids testosterone and estradiol. The gonadotropic hormones and sex steroids in the first 5 months of life influence physical development during the following 6 years in boys but not girls (Becker et al., 2015). Beking et al. (2018) determined from a longitudinal study that prenatal and pubertal testosterone affect brain lateralization in boys in a task-specific way. A general conclusion is that hormones act in sex-specific ways throughout human development and not only in puberty. Hormonal activity appears to be a major factor in explaining sex differences in the vulnerability to communication disorders. There are indications of sex differences in the cortical circuitry associated with speech perception and production (de Lima et al., 2019).

Speech differences between boys and girls also may result from learning the sex-specific features of speech (Meditch, 1975; Sachs et al., 1973). Evidence for a learning or sociocultural basis of boy-girl differences comes from research on voice gender (Cartei et al., 2014; Cartei, Cowles, & Reby, 2012; Cartei & Reby, 2013). When speakers, both adults and children, are asked to make their speech sound more feminine or masculine, the acoustic changes in formant pattern are in the direction expected from studies of sex differences. Cartei et al. (2012) suggested that speakers can spontaneously adopt a "gender code" to vary the expression of gender and related (e.g., masculinity/femininity) characteristics. Pisanski et al. (2016) concluded that both men and women can imitate (a) larger body size by increasing vocal tract length and decreasing vocal fundamental frequency, and (b) smaller body size by reducing vocal tract length and increasing vocal fundamental frequency.

Speech conveys attributes related to both sex and gender. Biological and sociocultural factors interact to give speakers characteristics that go beyond a simple dichotomy of male and female. Speech is a mirror of several interacting processes in human development, and individual children can assume different speech patterns that are adapted to their social interactions.

Sex as a risk factor for developmental communication disorders is taken up in Chapter 11, which goes into more detail on how male sex interacts with other factors to pose risk for disordered speech and language.

Typical Development of Communicative Gestures

A **gesture** is defined as a movement of the hands, arms, head, or other body part to express an idea, feeling, or need. Gestural communication depends on joint attention that usually emerges by 12 months of age and is manifest as gestures that signal pragmatic language functions such as requests, affirmations, or protests. At about 9 to 10 months of age, infants begin to produce proximal triadic gestures such as holding out an object, giving an object, or reaching (Bates et al., 1975). Pointing emerges about the same time or shortly after, around 9 to 12 months of age (Carpenter et al., 1998). Gestures predict subsequent communication abilities in children (Goldin-Meadow 2015), and use of gestures in infants co-occurs with early stages of verbal development and may contribute to acquisition of spoken vocabulary (Özçalışkan et al. 2017). Mishra et al. (2021) classified gestures into three subtypes: (1) deictic gestures are joint attention-based movements indicating objects, locations, and people; (2) ideative gestures are culturally recognized facial and body movements; and (3) nominal gestures are play-based movements with the referent-object in hand. Another type of gesture, representational gesture, emerges before the onset of the 25-word milestone of spoken language and has been called by several other names including symbolic, iconic, empty-handed, or referential (Capone & McGregor, 2004). Representational gestures are not instrumental, meaning that the referent is not being manipulated as is the case with play-based nominal gestures. Deictic gestures, first produced between 9 to 12 months of age, are used to express needs and to engage in communicative exchanges and predict the emergence of first words (Colonnesi et al. 2010). Ideative, nominal, and representational gestures appear between 12 and 18 months of age and make further contributions to the development of verbal language (Özçalışkan et al. 2016). Crais et al. (2004) categorized the communicative functions of gestures seen in typically developing children aged 9 to 24 months as behavior regulation, social interaction, and joint attention. Underlying all of these is intentionality.

The Typical Development of Private Speech and Inner Speech in Children

Children produce not only speech directed to others, but also private (self-directed) speech and inner (covert) speech, both of which may help to shape a child's cognitive, communicative, and social abilities. Talking to oneself is a way of building oneself. Private and inner speech were introduced in Chapter 3, with information pertaining mostly to adults. Both Piaget and Vygotsky theorized about private and inner speech in children. Piaget (1926) concluded from his studies of children talking to themselves in classrooms that self-talk, which he called **egocentric speech**, reflected an immature cognition and would later develop into mature speech. Vygotsky took a more constructivist point of view in characterizing egocentric speech as integral to the normal development of communication, self-guidance, self-regulation of behavior, planning, pacing, and monitoring skills. He believed that private speech is rooted in a toddler's social interactions and peaks during preschool or kindergarten when children tend to talk to themselves. Vygotsky's (1986) influential model of the developmental significance of self-directed speech emphasized the roles of self-regulating cognition and behavior.

However, it has been suggested that private speech has multiple roles, including emotional expression and regulation, planning for communicative interaction, theory of mind, self-discrimination, fantasy, creativity, and the mediation of children's autobiographical memory. A review of the literature revealed that the most general functions of private speech in children in naturalistic classroom settings was to regulate task engagement and cope with social challenges (R. M. Flanagan & Symonds, 2022). The use and functions of private speech appear to change in early childhood. Winsler et al. (2000) found that private speech in 3-year-old children did not vary as a function of the child's immediate activity, but that private speech in 4-year-old children was more likely to occur during activity that was sustained and goal-directed as opposed to activity that was rapidly changing and not goal-directed. Bono and Bizri (2014) concluded from a study of language skills, private speech, and self-regulation in 3- to 5-year-old children that the frequency of private speech mediated the association between language ability and self-regulation. Children with better language skills used private speech less often and had better self-regulation.

Vissers et al. (2020) proposed four stages in the development of private and inner speech. Stage I, which occurs during early language acquisition, is the period in which a child masters the fundamentals of an external dialogue, which involves communication and regulation of one another's behavior. Stage II, which occurs at about 3 to 4 years, is marked by increasing linguistic experience and the onset of self-directed talk or private speech. One interpretation of this behavior is that children act as though an adult is talking to them, which assists in regulating or guiding behavior. Compared to external dialog, private speech is simplified in its compositional and syntactic features. External dialog and private speech are both overt speech that typically focuses on the current, planned, or sometimes recalled events. Private speech appears to be universal, occurring in all languages. Stage III, beginning at about the age of 6 to 7 years, exhibits increased flexibility in covert speech, as children achieve more complete internalization of their thoughts during various cognitive tasks such as remembering, reading, and writing. This stage has been characterized as expanded inner speech, which is like private speech in that both are task-driven and conscious, focusing on current or planned activity, and involving top–down processes. Both also involve the use of utterances that are linguistically well-formed (hence expanded). Stage IV, condensed inner speech, is the final stage of speech internalization, which incorporates both top-down and bottom-up processes. Utterances often take the form of single grammatical structures, which explains why this stage is called condensed. The developmental progression is illustrated in Figure 4–16, which includes early vocal behaviors (cooing, babbling, first words, external dialog), private speech, and two stages of inner speech corresponding to the expanded and condensed types.

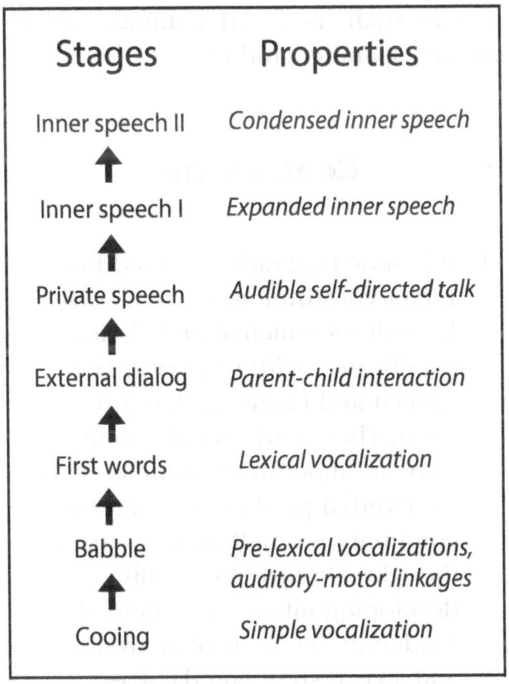

Figure 4–16. Stages in the typical development of overt, private, and inner speech.

Investigations of the neural correlates of inner speech give insights into its nature and function. Geva and Fernyhough (2019) reviewed evidence pointing to an association between inner speech and the maturation of the dorsal language stream, especially its fronto-temporal and fronto-parietal segments. (See Chapter 2 for discussion of the dorsal stream and its relationship with spoken language.) Whitford et al. (2017) demonstrated that inner speech is associated with an efference copy that has detailed auditory properties. In a study using both electroencephalography (EEG) and functional near-infrared spectroscopy (fNIRS), Stephan et al. (2020) concluded that when linguistic aspects are involved, as in the speech execution phase, children do not have adult-like processes of phonological encoding or complex auditory feedback mechanisms. These findings show the feasibility of neurophysiological studies of inner and private speech and should contribute to a model of speech production that integrates overt and covert speech over the lifespan.

Cascades and Systems Views of Speech Development

Bornstein et al. (2013) identified two major themes in developmental science. One theme emphasizes the developmental trajectory of domain-related age-appropriate constructs leading to the mature phenotype within the domain. Examples in the study of speech development are the trajectories in the domains of audition (discussed in Chapter 2), articulation (discussed earlier in this chapter), and phonology (discussed in this chapter and in Chapter 7). Each of these domains can be assigned a development trajectory that leads to adult-like capability. The second theme focuses on the relative contributions of multiple determinants from different domains to the expression of a mature phenotype. For example, in speech development, this approach might consider jointly the contributions of audition, motor control, and phonology to result in patterns of speech that converge on the adult form. Bornstein et al. point out that the first theme is concerned with the discovery of different forms of developmental stability, whereas the second theme is concerned with developmental systems. The two themes are not mutually exclusive, and Bornstein et al. tied them together in their account of children's academic achievement.

In developmental psychology, the term *cascade* usually means a process or processes "by which function at one level or in one domain of behavior affects function at higher levels or the organization of competency in later developing domains of general adaptation" (Cox et al., 2010, p. 497). This construct has broad application, including the development of spoken language. Iverson (2021) noted that there has been increasing interest in "studying links between motor and language development in infancy and in exploring the downstream, cascading effects of motor achievements on infants' developing language skills" (p. 228). Choi et al. (2018) proposed that the development of speech perception can be explained by cascading multisensory influences in a critical period framework, in which critical periods are considered as epochs of maximal receptivity to different aspects of language.

Figure 4–17 gives an example of cascading effects across multiple domains, specifically speech perception, general motor, and speech production The categories for speech perception from Choi et al. (2018) are used as a general framework of developmental progression. The shaded boxes show the linkage across speech perception, general motor, and speech production at each stage of development. Linkages within and between domains can have facilitating effects of development. For example, relationships have been shown between sitting and language development (Libertus & Violi, 2016), between walking and use of gestures (Iverson, 2001), and between babbling and early speech perception (Fagan, 2015; Vilain et al., 2019). Figure 4–17 greatly simplifies the developmental paradigm. A fuller account would include factors such as social communication, emotions, and cognition.

Conclusions

1. It is now generally accepted that infant vocalizations such as babbling have developmental and clinical significance with respect to later speech and language development. These early vocalizations have an important continuity with later verbal productions, and this continuity is a hallmark of current thought. Studies of typically developing infants have helped to identify methods of analysis and a corresponding database that can be used as a reference

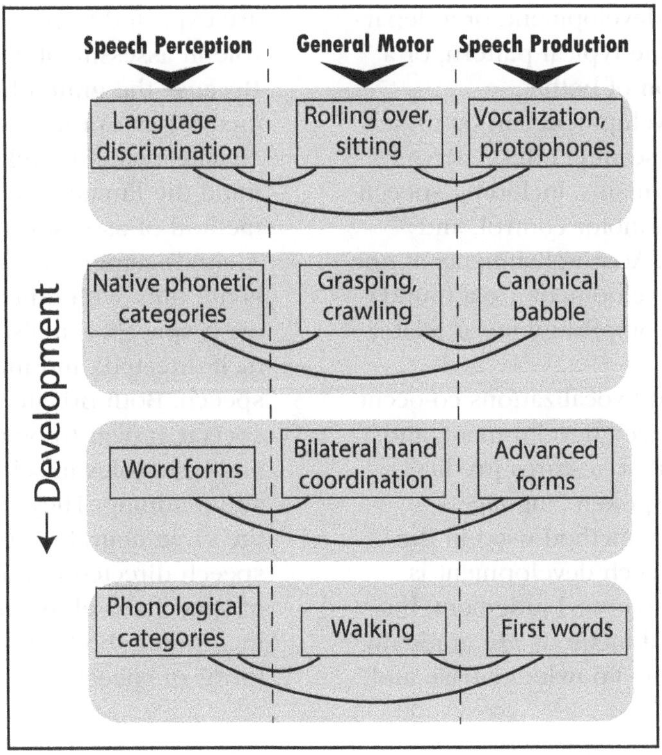

Figure 4–17. Cascading effect across the domains of speech perception, general motor, and speech production during infancy. The connecting lines between boxes represent linkages that can facilitate development across domains.

in clinical assessments, which are predominantly conducted with the examiner's eyes and ears.

2. Speech development extends over several years and does not reach maturity in its more refined sensorimotor aspects until adolescence or later. Basic aspects of development that are most often reported occur before the age of eight years when mastery of sound production is essentially accomplished, phonological patterns are adult-like, and speech is highly intelligible even to unfamiliar listeners. However, even this mature form of speech is malleable to some degree, allowing for the learning of a second language.
3. Speech development depends on several maturational processes including anatomic development, refinement of speech motor control, auditory analysis, and learning of phonological patterns. Information on typical development is a foundation for the assessment and treatment of speech disorders, as considered in later chapters. For example, a common question is whether a given disorder represents a delay of an otherwise typical

pattern of development, or a departure from the typical pattern, or a combination of both.

4. Speech development can be understood as cascading effects across multiple domains, including speech perception, motor control, and phonology. Accomplishments at one point in development are a foundation for accomplishments at a later point.
5. Gestures and vocalizations co-occur in early speech development, and it appears that gestures predict aspects of spoken language.
6. The primary method used in the study of speech development is auditory-perceptual judgment, but instrumental methods are gradually adding to the knowledge base and are expected to play an increasing role in assessment and treatment. Because the grain of observation or analysis can profoundly influence conclusions, it is well to bear in mind the limitations of any specific method of assessment.
7. A child's experience with speech is not only with other-directed overt speech, but also with private (self-directed) and inner (covert) speech. Both private and inner speech appear to be used frequently and have roles in self-regulation and planning. They use some of the same neural systems as overt speech directed to others. A theory of speech development should incorporate both overt and covert forms of speech.

5

ASSESSMENT OF ARTICULATION AND SENSORIMOTOR FUNCTIONS

This chapter focuses on the assessment of speech in children 3 years of age or older. Children of this age usually can participate in activities such as conversation and naming, which provide the substance for assessment of speech skills. Chapter 4 includes information on measures that have been used with younger children, and this chapter discusses clinical implications of these and other measures for infants and toddlers.

Speech production can be assessed with a variety of methods, including perceptual, acoustic, aerodynamic, and kinematic. Each method has advantages and limitations. Methods also are selected in accord with the characteristics of the child being examined—characteristics such as age, cognitive ability, and presence of comorbid conditions (e.g., hearing loss, visual impairment, and general motor impairment). Perceptual methods are the mainstay of speech-language pathology and are often the only means of assessment used in routine clinical services. Even when other methods are used, they often are interpreted against or with findings from perceptual assessments. For some purposes, perceptual methods are the only practicable tool, as they can be used in a variety of settings and with a spectrum of abilities and limitations in individual children. The primary methods of assessment are discussed in this chapter as they pertain to children with suspected speech disorder of any type or severity. The goal is to provide a general survey of assessments that are in common use or could have future application. Subsequent chapters offer detailed discussions of the assessment of voice and prosody (Chapter 6), phonology (Chapter 7), and intelligibility and other global properties of speech (Chapter 8).

International Classification of Functioning, Disability and Health (ICF)

The **International Classification of Functioning, Disability and Health (ICF)** is a framework for describing and organizing information on functioning and disability. A major advantage of the ICF is that it provides a standard language and conceptual basis for the definition and measurement of health and disability throughout the world. It was approved for use by the World Health Assembly in 2001, based on an extensive testing program conducted across the world and including people with disabilities and a range of relevant disciplines. A companion classification for children and youth **(ICF-CY)** was published in 2007. The ICF integrates the major models of disability by recognizing the role of environmental factors in creating disability, along with the relevance of associated health conditions and their effects. A diagram showing the interactions among the components of the ICF is shown in Figure 5–1.

The application of the ICF-CY to communication disorders is discussed in several articles (Barnes & Bloch, 2019; Cunningham et al., 2017; McCormack et al., 2010; McLeod & Bleile, 2004; McLeod & McCormack, 2007). These papers explain how various assessments relate to the categories of the ICF-CY. However, there is not total agreement on some categorizations (Barnes & Bloch, 2019), and it would be helpful to have consensus to ensure consistent use across clinicians.

Efforts have been made to develop comprehensive speech-language pathology outcome measures for preschool children to meet the need for detecting changes in life-participation. These measures include the American Speech-Language-Hearing Association (ASHA) **Pre-Kindergarten National Outcome Measure System (Pre-K NOMS)**, **Therapy Outcome Measures (TOM**; Enderby, 1997), and **Focus on the Outcomes of Communication Under Six** (FOCUS, Thomas-Stonell et al., 2010). For further discussion of outcome measurement, see Chapter 12.

Oral Mechanism Examination

This examination, also known as the **oral peripheral examination** or **speech mech-**

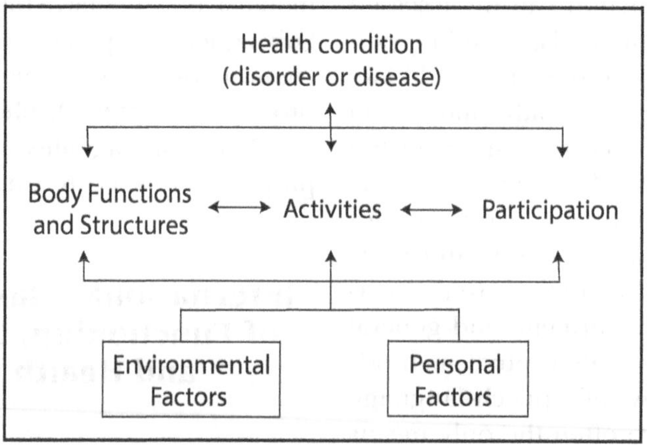

Figure 5–1. Diagram of the major components of the International Classification of Functioning, Disability and Health (ICF).

anism examination, is part and parcel of the clinical assessment of children with a speech disorder (Fox, 2018; Farquharson & Tambyraja, 2019). Despite its common, if not universal, use in clinical assessments in speech-language pathology and other specialties, there does not appear to be a widely adopted, standardized cross-disciplinary and international procedure. Lack of standardization hinders the effort to establish well-defined and reliable descriptions of anatomic variants to be shared across clinicians and clinical sites. Several different checklists and data forms are available online or in published print versions, and many clinics or subspecialties have developed their own procedures and recording forms. Commercially available instruments are described by Ruscello (2000). Apparently, the only standardized and valid instrument recognized for use in clinical trials is the **Frenchay Dysarthria Assessment-2nd edition** (FDA-2; Enderby & Palmer, 2008), which was developed to assess dysarthria in individuals aged 12 years to adulthood (Cardoso et al., 2017).

Standardized definitions and methods of observation are essential starting points for descriptions and classifications of dysmorphology. A key reference for the mouth, lips, and oral cavity is Carey et al. (2009), which reflects an effort to standardize terminology by an international group of clinicians and scientists working in the field of dysmorphology. Methods of observation also need to be standardized to ensure that the results of an examination are comprehensive, valid, and reliable. For example, it is important to specify the postures and movements of the structures under study (Fox, 2015).

Table 5–1 lists assessments that are suitable for general use with children. These assessments vary widely in their construction, with some concentrating on function, others on both structure and function. Structural observations are often limited to features such as size and symmetry. Functional assessment typically addresses motor integrity of the major articulators and larynx (tongue, jaw, lips, velopharynx, and vocal folds). Only rarely do published assessments provide guidance on the evaluation of sensory integrity of the orofacial region. This topic is considered later in this chapter.

A frequently cited clinical protocol was developed by Robbins and Klee (1987) to assess the oral and speech motor abilities of children. The authors administered an 86-item test to 90 typically developing children aged 2:6 to 6:11. Because only 10 children served in each age group, the resulting data are not truly normative in the statistical sense. Structure was scored as a binary judgment (normal or abnormal) and function was rated on a 3-point scale (2 = adult-like function, 1 = emerging adult-like precision, and 0 = absent function). Developmental changes were not observed in the structural integrity of the vocal tract but were seen in oral and speech motor functioning. Structural observations vary from basic categories (e.g., symmetry and size for the maxilla) to more elaborated descriptions (e.g., structure of the tongue at rest was assessed in terms of carriage, fasciculations, furrowing, atrophy, and hypertrophy). It is presumed that clinicians scoring the test possess internal standards for the evaluation of the protocol's components. Robbins and Klee did not identify structural abnormalities in any of the children in their study, but the dichotomous nature of their scale may not have been sensitive to anatomic variations (e.g., malocclusion). A study of children with SSD persisting after the

Table 5–1. Structures and Functions Considered in Different Systems of the Orofacial Examination

Structure or Function	1	2	3	4	5	6	7
Breathing	x		x	x	x	X	
Phonation (voice)				x	x		x
Jaw structure				x	x	x	x
Jaw function	x	x		x	x	x	
Lip structure	x		x	x	x	x	x
Lip function		x		x	x	x	x
Tongue structure	x		x	x	x	x	x
Tongue function	x	x		x	x	x	x
Velum/velopharynx structure			x	x	x	x	x
Velum/velopharynx function	x	x		x	x	x	
Hard palate structure		x		x	x	x	x
Pharynx structure			x	x		x	x
Pharynx function				x		x	
Dentition		x	x	x	x	x	
Nares structure			x				
Nares function				x			
Face at rest	x	x		x			x
Facial expressions	x			x			
Diadochokinesis	x			x	x	x	
Speech motor function	x	x		x	x		
Orofacial sensation							
Swallowing			x	x			

Sources: 1. Bakke, M., Bergendal, B., McAllister, A., Sjogreen, L., & Asten, P. (2007). 2. Dworkin, J. P., & Culatta, R. A. (1980). 3. Grandi, D. (2012). 4. Johnson-Root, B. A. (2015). [Note: clinical observations are grouped in the two major categories of routine and discretionary.] 5. Robbins, J., & Klee, T. (1987). 6. St. Louis, K. O., & Ruscello, D. (2000). 7. Vitale (1986).

age of 6 years revealed that the most affected orofacial domains were chewing and swallowing (41%), masticatory muscles and jaw function (38%), and sensory function (38%) (Mogren et al., 2020). The same domains often are affected in other speech disorders, such as those associated with dysarthria.

Oral mechanism examinations that are intended to serve a screening function are necessarily less detailed than examinations designed for more comprehensive evaluations. A screening type of examination has the advantage of clinical efficiency but may not draw the examiner's attention to relevant but sometimes subtle clinical features. Other variations of the oral mechanism examination have been developed for specific purposes or clinical populations, as listed in Appendix B. Included in some oral mechanism examinations are tests of maximal performance, a topic considered in a later section of this chapter.

Assessing Sensory Function in the Orofacial System

Although sensory functions of the orofacial system are generally regarded as highly important in speech and feeding, there is little agreement on how these functions should be assessed in children (or adults for that matter). General discussions of this topic are available in Bahr and Hillis (2001), Gironda et al. (2011), and Kent et al. (1990). The primary test methods, as summarized by Jacobs et al. (1998); Lee et al. (2022); and Sivapathasundharam and Biswas (2020), are as follows.

1. **Two-point discrimination tests** apply adjacent stimuli to a cutaneous surface and participants are asked to indicate when they are aware of two points of stimulation. However, this method is not a true measure of spatial acuity and has poor test–retest reliability.
2. The method of **von Frey fibers** applies synthetic microfibers to the surface and participants are asked to state the presence or absence of stimuli. This method activates slow adapting mechanoreceptors (Merkel's disks and Ruffini endings) and is, therefore, not a satisfactory index of mechanoreceptors in general. Test kits are commercially available.
3. **Oral stereognosis** is the ability to identify the shape and form of a three-dimensional object with tactile manipulation of that object without access to visual and auditory stimuli. Various objects have been designed to test oral stereognosis and some are available commercially. Kumin et al. (1984) assessed oral stereognosis in children and found that performance improved with age and that girls performed better than boys. A variant is the alphabet letter recognition test that uses as stimuli alphabet-letter shapes of varying sizes that are placed on the surface, and participants are asked to identify the letters. This method activates both fast and slow adapting mechanoreceptors, and it can measure both oral stereognosis and spatial acuity. However, alphabet letters are not uniformly identifiable because they differ from one another in number of edges and other geometric features (e.g., compare the letter *W* with the letters *O* and *I*). It also requires cognitive abilities that relate somatosensory impressions to letter recognition, which is learned through the visual modality. The task may pose difficulties for younger children and individuals with cognitive impairments. Another problem that often

affects tests of oral stereognosis is that they generally involve manipulation of the test objects, which makes the tests sensory and motor rather than purely sensory.

4. The **grating orientation test** uses custom stimuli with varying groove dimensions. The grates are applied to the tongue either horizontally or vertically in a random order, and participants are asked to discriminate the orientation of the grooves. This method seems to be gaining favor but reports of its use in children are limited.
5. A test developed specifically for individuals with fluency disorders is the **Movement, Articulation, Mandibular and Sensory awareness (MAMS) assessment** (Cook et al., 2011). This test, perhaps in modified form, may have general value in assessing sensory functions of the orofacial system.

There is sparse evidence for the value of these procedures in relation to speech development and disorders, which is unfortunate given the sensitivity of the orofacial structures and the likely importance of sensory information in speech and feeding. The most sensitive tissues in the orofacial region are the tongue, lips, and hard palate. The last mentioned of these has been rather neglected in studies of sensation, but it appears to rival the fingertips in its capacity for pressure sensing and spatial localization of mechanical stimuli (Moayedi et al., 2021). Taken together, these oral tissues provide a rich supply of somatosensory information that can be used in speech and feeding.

Little wonder, then, that sensory assessment is often neglected. But the difficulty of assessment should not stand in the way of future developments. Useful information may be obtained from even simple tasks such as: touching a tongue depressor to different orofacial regions and asking a child to point to the region that was touched on a doll or facial image (a test of punctate sensitivity), moving the instrument from the midline to one side or the other of a structure and asking a child to point in the direction of movement (a test of kinetic sensitivity). Testing of oral sensation is a much-needed area of research. The oral structures are among the most sensitive tissues in the human body, and there is little question that sensory information contributes in important ways to the development of speech and feeding.

> ASHA's Practice Portal regarding Speech Sound Disorder describes an oral mechanism examination as a key component of a comprehensive speech evaluation. A range of knowledge and experience is needed to ensure valid and reliable observations.

Maximum Performance Tasks and Measures

Maximum performance tasks pertain to maximal efforts in aspects of voice or speech production, such as prolonging a sound for as long as possible on a single breath or repeating a syllable as fast as possible on a single breath. These tasks assess the envelope of motor functions related to aspects of speech production, even if the tasks themselves are not necessarily regarded as speech per se. The term *envelope* is apropos because the measures derived from these tasks define the upper limits or ranges of the target variables. Conversational speech in healthy adults is performed well within these limits, except perhaps for the rate of syllable repetition (Kent et al., 1987). But for adults with compromised health and for very young children, even conversational speech may approach some of these limits. The clinical utility of maximum performance measures for general-purpose speech assessment has been questioned, especially because of concerns related to poor reliability, lack of standardized procedure, and uncertainties as to clinical interpretation. An overall review of these problems along with possible solutions is available in Kent et al. (1987) and Kent, Kim, and Chen (2022). It is not clear if all concerns have been, or can be, addressed to general satisfaction. But, as discussed in this chapter, maximum performance tasks and measures can be of clinical value for certain populations and purposes. The commonly used tasks are described in this chapter, with comments on rationale for use, task protocol, derived measures, and reference data. (Normative data in the strict sense of the term are not always available for these tasks, but sources of reference data are identified for children younger than 12 years).

Maximum Phonation Time (MPT) or Maximum Prolongation Time (MPT)

Maximum Phonation Time (MPT), also known as **Maximum Phonation Duration (MPD)**, is a task in which speakers are asked to inhale deeply and produce a sound for as long as they can. MPT often is taken as a proxy for lung volume, on the assumption that duration of sound prolongation is a first-order reflection of the amount of air available to support sound production. K. Lewis et al. (1982) concluded that there is a "significant and dominant relationship between vital capacity and the length of sustained phonation of /a/" (p. 47). **Vital capacity** is the maximum amount of air that can be expelled from the lungs after a maximum inhalation (see Chapter 2 for deeper discussion). However, because MPT reflects both lung volume and type of phonation (Solomon et al., 2000), caution should be observed in clinical interpretation. MPT for vowel production should be regarded as a phonation task that reflects both respiratory and laryngeal functioning. For example, if a child produces a vowel phonation with a severely breathy voice quality, MPT may be reduced compared to reference values because air is wasted during the breathy phonation and not necessarily because of respiratory insufficiency. The sound to be produced is usually a vowel, such as /ɑ/, but continuant consonants such as /s/ or /z/ also are used, depending on the purposes of the examination. The protocol that follows is based primarily on the task of vowel production as described by Rvachew et al. (2005).

1. The clinician produces a prolonged /ɑ/ for approximately 2 s on one breath with steady and normal pitch and a comfortable level of effort. The child is then asked to imitate the model. This step can be repeated if needed to obtain a satisfactory production.
2. Same as #1 above except the clinician models a sustained vowel for 4 to 5 s and then asks the child to imitate the model.
3. The clinician asks the child to say /ɑ/ for as long as possible on one

breath (no model provided). The instruction can be repeated two more times to enable the child with several opportunities to prolong the vowel.

4. If the child produces only a very brief vowel phonation, the clinician can use a visual aid to encourage a longer production. One way of doing this is for the clinician to hold a finger or toy in the air as a visual cue for sound prolongation.

The measurement typically used is simply the duration of phonation, as determined with a stopwatch or computer display of the waveform. Several sources of reference data are available. Figure 5–2 displays data from several sources for children. MPT increases at about 0.5 to 1.0 s per year, beginning with a value of 4 s at 2 to 3 years of age. It has been shown that MPT values are affected by the number of trials and feedback given to the child. Although it is common to use 3 trials, this number may not be sufficient to obtain the greatest value of MPT. K. Lewis et al. (1982) found that MPT in children increased over at least 10 trials. However, it is questionable if such a large number is justified in respect to either clinical efficiency or possible health risks

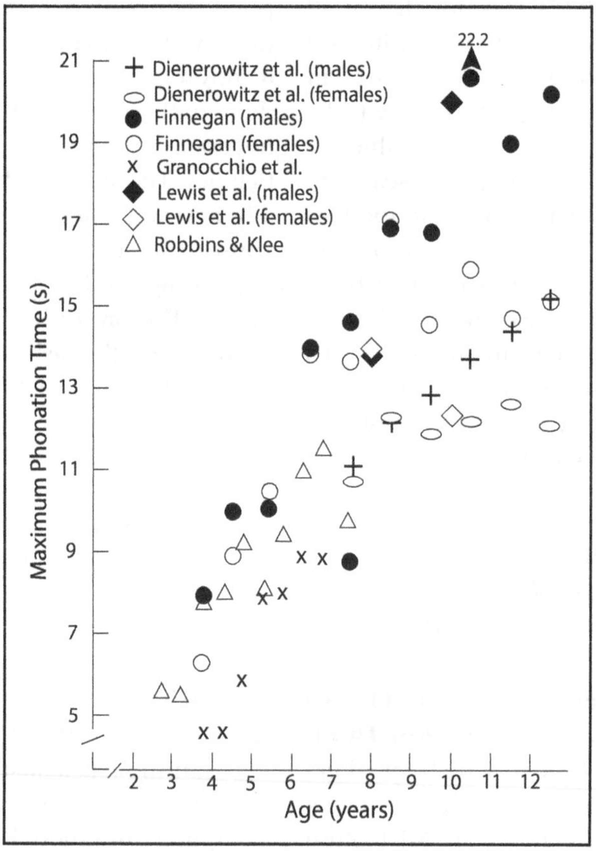

Figure 5–2. Mean values of maximum phonation time (MPT) from several studies of typically developing children.

(Kent et al., 1987). It may be sufficient for most clinical purposes to determine if a child is capable of a value of MPT that is adequate for ordinary speech production. A useful criterion in this respect is the **"five-for-five rule"** (the ability to maintain an air pressure of 5 cm H_2O for 5 s) recommended by Netsell and Hixon (1978). With this guideline, a child could be judged to have adequate respiratory support for speech if he or she can produce a phonation with steady pitch and loudness for at least 5 s. If it is judged important to inquire further into respiratory capability, then the clinician could ask the child to blow into a straw that has one end immersed in a container of water (Hixon et al., 1982). If bubbles appear when the straw is immersed to a depth of 5 cm and the bubbles can be maintained for 5 s, then the child has satisfied the criterion of "five-for-five." Whatever the number of trials, it is preferable to report the maximum number rather than a mean or other measure of central tendency. The reason is the same as that for a track-and-field event, in which a competitor is given credit for the maximum performance (e.g., the fastest time for a 100 m race). A mean value is almost always an underestimate of maximum performance. In general clinical practice, a reasonably accurate measure of maximum performance is the best of three trials. In the case of children with severe motor disorders such as cerebral palsy, consideration should be given to body position and respiratory capacity, as these factors may limit sound prolongation.

Reference values vary considerably across studies, no matter what statistic is used to express the results. MPT values considerably below those in Figure 5–2 were reported by Cielo and Cappellari (2008), Cielo et al. (2016), and Tavares et al. (2012). The discrepant results are perhaps explained largely by procedural variation. The main point is that reference values vary widely across sources and may differ by a factor of two or more for a given age and sex. MPT values for healthy adults range from about 15 to 35 s, with longer times for men than women (Kent et al., 1987). These values are in proportion to vital capacity and may have some bearing on spoken language. Boucher and Lalonde (2015), finding that vital capacity correlates strongly with mean length of utterance (MLU) in speakers aged 5 to 27 years, proposed that increased vital capacity could support increasingly long utterances that, in turn, might influence lexical diversity. Alternatively, it is possible that production of longer utterances stimulates increased vital capacity. The MPT tasks are relatively simple, but it not always easily or reliably performed by children younger than 3 years of age, which places a lower limit on age-based reference values. For comparison purposes, the durations of infant vocalizations generally are in the range of 1 to 4 s for cry and about 0.2 to 2 s for syllables (Kent, 2022).

The protocol for maximum prolongation duration of the fricatives /s/ and /z/ (or any other sound judged to be of clinical interest) is essentially the same as that described previously for vowel prolongation. Strictly speaking, maximum duration of production for the fricative /s/ is not a phonation task because /s/ is a voiceless sound. Determining the maximum duration of production for /s/ and /z/ has been of particular interest in assessing voice function through the s/z ratio, which is the ratio of /s/ duration to /z/ duration (Eckel & Boone, 1981). Both the MPT for vowel phonation and the s/z ratio were selected as components in a minimal protocol for the pediatric voice clinic (Cohen et al., 2012). Reference data for /s/ and /z/ durations and the s/z ratio are available in Tavares et al. (2012). The guideline is that individuals with normal voices have approximately equal prolongation times for /s/ and /z/ so that the s/z ratio is about 1.0. Individuals with vocal pathologies tend to have shorter durations for /z/ than for /s/ so that the s/z ratio is larger than 1.0.

Diadochokinesis (DDK), Alternating Motion Rate (AMR), and Sequential Motion Rate (SMR)

The word **diadochokinesis (DDK)** is derived from the Greek *diadochos* (succeeding) + *kinesis* (movement). Diadochokinesis or diadochokinesia is the ability to perform a rapid succession of antagonistic movements such as flexion and extension of the arm, pronation and supination of the hand, or tapping with a finger. In speech-language pathology, DDK refers to rapid repetitions of individual syllables or a combination of syllables. The syllables typically used (and for which reference values are most available) are the monosyllables /pʌ/, /tʌ/, /kʌ/ (often called **alternating motion rate, AMR**) and the trisyllable /pʌtʌkʌ/ (often called **sequential motion rate, SMR**). The vowel /ʌ/ is used in this description, but different vowel sounds appear in the literature on DDK. Another DDK task is **laryngeal diadochokinesis (LDDK)** which involves alternating adjustments of the vocal folds, as in repeated production of the syllable /hi/. The protocol that follows is based primarily on Rvachew et al. (2005), with modifications from Kent et al. (2022).

1. Ask the child to say /pʌ/, and then /pʌpʌpʌ/, and then /pʌpʌpʌpʌpʌ/.
2. Model the repetition of approximately 12 /pʌ/ syllables on a single breath at a rate of about four syllables per second and ask the child to imitate the model.
3. Ask the child to repeat step 2 but this time as fast as possible. The task can be stopped when the child has produced 12 or more syllables. The child might be given two additional opportunities to maximize the repetition rate, especially if the production is uneven or lacks precision of articulation.
4. If the child has difficulty producing a syllable train that is rapid and regular, the clinician can use a visual aid, such as tapping on a desk surface. Saying a sound as fast as possible can be a difficult concept for some children to grasp, and it may help to use another motor system, such as hand tapping, to convey the concept of rapid alternating movement.

If desired, the task can be repeated for other monosyllables, a disyllable such as /pʌtʌ/ or a trisyllable such as /pʌtʌkʌ/. Some children (and even some adults) may have difficulty producing a trisyllable, such as /pʌtʌkʌ/, but can do quite well with real words such *buttercup*, *pattycake* or *pat-a-cake*. If a client stumbles while attempting to say /pʌtʌkʌ/, the clinician may suggest rapid repetition of the word *buttercup* as an alternative.

The basic measure is the number of syllables produced in 1 s. This rate measure can be obtained in either of two ways: (1) counting the number of syllables produced in a certain interval of time (count-by-time method), or (2) determining the amount of time used to produce a given number of syllables (time-by-count method; S. G. Fletcher, 1972). The time-by-count method is preferred by some clinicians because it is simple and easy to use (Williams & Stackhouse, 2000). It is preferable to make syllable counts from an acoustic display of waveform and/or spectrogram to ensure an accurate value (Kent et al., 2022). Figure 5–3 shows mean DDK rates from several sources for AMR and SMR tasks. The general pattern is one of increasing rate from 2 to 12 years of age. Mean DDK rates for adults in these tasks are about 6 syllable/s (Kent et al., 2022). Diepeveen et al. (2019) concluded that a sequence of at least 5 syllables is sufficient, with the mean rate based on measuring the duration of at least 3 syllables, disregarding the first and last syllables in the sequence. However, such a small number is not sufficient to assess irregularities in timing or intensity across syllables (Kent et al., 2022).

In addition to determining a simple rate measure, analyses of accuracy of production can be made. One approach is to determine inventories of types of phonetic errors such as voicing change, manner change, exchange, regressive assimilation, progressive assimilation, addition of segment, and deletion of segment (Preston & Edwards, 2009; Yaruss & Logan, 2002). Raters should be phonetically trained and ideally would have substantial experience with speech sound disorders. Icht and Ben-David (2021) introduced a scale to rate the accuracy of DDK production. The scale has 5 points: (0) all productions in a sample were inaccurate and non-consistent, or unable to compete the task; (1) poor accuracy and consistency, with articulation errors ≥7; (2) medium accuracy and consistency, with articulation errors ≤4 and ≤6;

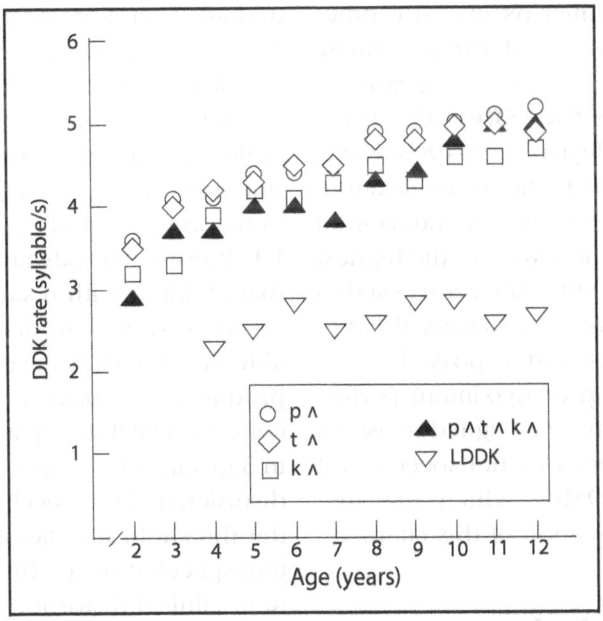

Figure 5–3. Mean diadochokinetic (DDK) rates reported for typically developing children. The data are for the monosyllables /pʌ/, /tʌ/, /kʌ/, the trisyllable /pʌtʌkʌ/, and laryngeal diadochokinesis (LDDK).

(3) good accuracy and consistency, with articulation errors ≤3; and (4) accurate and consistent productions of all targets, with flawless performance.

Aside from measures of rate and accuracy of production, several other measures have been proposed to quantify the regularity of syllable production. These measures typically focus on either the temporal or intensity variability within a syllable train, as determined from a computer display of the speech waveform. For discussion of alternative measures and their application in different speech disorders see Kent et al. (2022). There is little standardization of these measures for children's productions.

Other Maximum Performance Tasks

Especially when it is desired to assess vocal function, clinicians may use other tasks, such as the **vocal range profile (VRP)**, also called a **phonetogram**, or **speech range profile (SRP)** (D'Alatri & Marchese, 2014; Heylen et al., 1998; Wuyts et al., 2002). For VRP, clients are asked to sustain the vowel /ɑ/ as soft and as loud as possible from the lowest to the highest vocal pitches. For SRP, clients are asked to read or repeat a list of sentences aloud in a soft voice and as loud as possible.

Another group of maximum performance tasks are those designed to assess the range and speed of nonspeech oral movements (NSOMs), which are discussed in a later section of this chapter.

Notes on Clinical Applications

A basic clinical motivation in using maximum performance tasks is that they can give information on a child's ability to generate adequate forces for speech production and to achieve gross coordination of the speech production systems. Both maximum sound prolongation and DDK tasks require participation of the respiratory, laryngeal, and supralaryngeal subsystems of speech production. Deviations from smooth and steady performance of these tasks can indicate the need for deeper assessment. Maximum phonation time requires respiratory drive, suitable adjustment of the vocal folds to achieve phonation, and a stable vocal tract configuration. Maximum sound prolongation for the fricatives /s/ and /z/ makes similar demands but also requires a precise and sustained articulatory configuration to generate turbulence. The DDK tasks of AMR and SMR make further demands of varying place of articulation either across or within trials. Different tasks isolate different components of speech production and are, therefore, useful to assess motor performance that is relatively immune to linguistic factors.

DDK is not uniformly atypical in children with speech sound disorders, but slow rate and irregularity have been noted in some studies (Kent et al., 2022). J. L. Preston and Edwards (2008) reported that children with residual speech sound errors were less accurate and more variable than typically developing children in production of /pataka/. Wren et al. (2012) compared DDK for /pətəkə/ and /bədəgə/ in 3 groups of children: persistent speech disorder (PSD), speech errors but below the threshold for classification as persistent speech disorder (non-PSD), and common clinical distortions only (CCD). The CCD and PSD groups were judged to have a weakness in oromotor skill as revealed in DDK performance. Tafiadis et al. (2021) reported that children with phonological disorders performed significantly slower than typically developing children in all speech DDK tasks, but not in nonspeech oral-motor tasks.

Thoonen et al. (1996) developed a procedure for the differential diagnosis of dysarthria and dyspraxia, based on maximum performance data collected from children aged 6 through 10 years. The process begins with the assignment of a dysarthria score of 0, 1, or 2, where 0 indicates that the child is not dysarthric and a 2 indicates that the child is primarily dysarthric. AMR is the primary diagnostic marker for dysarthria, but MPD is considered. Scores are assigned as follows: a score of 0 if AMR is greater than 3.5 syllable/s, a score of 1 if AMR is between 3.0 and 3.5 syllable/s and MPD is more than 7.5 s, a score of 2 if AMR is less than 3.0 syllable/s or if AMR is between 3.0 and 3.5 syllable/sec and MPD is less than 7.5 s. Next, a dyspraxia score of 0, 1, or 2 is assigned as follows: a score of 0 if SMA is produced correctly at a rate of at least 4.4 syllable/s without requiring more than two additional attempts; a score of 1 is assigned if the SMA is between 3.4 and 4.4 syllables/s if the MFD is greater than 11 s without requiring more than two additional attempts to achieve a correct sequence; a score of 2 is assigned if either SMA is between 3.4 and 4.4 syllable/s and more than two additional attempts were required for a correct sequence or if MFD is less than 11 s.

Atypical DDK is a common feature of both CAS, childhood dysarthria, and perhaps subtypes of speech sound disorder. Slow, inaccurate, and disrupted DDK is commonly observed in CAS (see review by Kent et al., 2022). Murray et al. (2015) concluded that "polysyllabic production accuracy and an oral motor examination that includes DDK may be sufficient to reliably identify CAS and rule out structural abnormality or dysarthria" (p. 43). Studies of children with dysarthria related to cerebral palsy have shown slow DDK rate (Nam et al., 2006; Nip, 2013; Ozawa et al., 2001) and articulatory inaccuracies (Nam et al., 2006). Also in cerebral palsy, atypical performance has been observed in double nonspeech movements such as a blow–smile sequence, which often were performed with asymmetry, imprecision, reduced smoothness, and reduced lip excursion (Mei et al., 2020). Diepeveen et al. (2022) concluded from a cluster analysis of a large set of measures that DDK performance is important to the diagnosis of speech sound disorders because it was a primary factor in distinguishing between two of the subtypes and, together with phonological components, distinguished between two other subtypes. They wrote, "The current study confirms that MRR performance has a distinctive contribution to the diagnosis of SSD" (p. 18).

General conclusions are as follows.

1. Maximum performance tasks have a long history in speech-language pathology. Progress has been made in standardizing procedures and developing reference databases. However, published reference data vary widely, especially for measures of sound prolongation such as MPT.
2. Routine use of these tasks does not necessarily seek to establish the actual limits of performance, but rather to determine if the motor systems have sufficient capability to meet the basic demands of speech production in respect to respiratory drive, laryngeal function, and supralaryngeal articulation.
3. Children aged 4 years and older should be capable of a MPT of at least 5 s and an AMR of at least

3.5 syllable/s. Children who do not meet these criteria may need to be assessed in more detail, especially to determine if they are affected by respiratory limitations.

4. DDK (AMR and/or SMR) may be affected in children with speech sound disorders, dysarthria, or CAS. DDK has been recommended as part of the assessment procedure for CAS.

Consideration should be given to obtaining at least two measures: DDK rate (syllables/s) as an index of movement limitations and DDK regularity (e.g., standard deviation in the time difference between two consecutive syllables), as an index of the ability to maintain a uniform temporal pattern. More detailed analyses can be used to describe the quality and accuracy of the DDK task.

Nonspeech Oral Movements (NSOMs)

The use of **nonspeech oral movements (NSOMs)** is a subject of considerable controversy in speech-language pathology. One difficulty in reaching a confident conclusion is that NSOMs often are not clearly defined or standardized, so it is difficult to distinguish among tasks that might be classified as speech or nonspeech (or somewhere between). A definition proposed by Kent (2015, p. 765) is that "NSOMs are motor acts performed by various parts of the speech musculature to accomplish specified movement or postural goals that are not sufficient in themselves to have phonetic identity." Examples of NSOMs are jaw opening/closing, protrusion and lateral movements of the tongue, and lip opening/closing. Such tasks resemble range of motion (ROM) maneuvers in neurology and physical therapy. There has been substantial debate over the role and value of nonspeech oral movements in relation to speech production, but nonspeech oral movements can provide useful information for certain purposes, including conduct of a cranial nerve examination (Appendix 3 lists the cranial nerves and their functions), assessing movement control in severely involved children (e.g., those with dysarthria associated with cerebral palsy), and children with orofacial dysmorphology (e.g., cleft palate). The clinician may make observations of the range and symmetry of motion, along with other features. As discussed in subsequent chapters, the performance of nonspeech movements is not necessarily related to the performance of speech movements, which hinders clinical interpretation of the results. The role of NSOMs in the assessment of motor speech disorders in children is discussed later in this chapter in a section on *Praxis and Speech Motor Control.*

Perceptual Methods

This section considers conventional articulation tests, phonemic and phonetic transcription, rating scales, phonetic inventories, and other perceptual methods.

Articulation Tests

An **articulation test** is a standardized or nonstandardized examination of a child's ability to produce speech sounds in a particular language. These tests are generally relational in nature because a child's performance is judged relative to standards for age-related peers. Several different forms of these tests have been developed, most using pictures or photos of items or actions to elicit words containing the target sounds. These tests rely largely or exclusively on the production of single words, with performance judged by the clinician who administers the test. Standardized tests usually provide normative data of articulation performance for different chronological ages of children. The tests typically use judgments of speech sound errors such as substitutions, omissions, distortions, and additions (abbreviated **SODA**). Norm-referenced articulation or phonological tests commonly used in the United States and United Kingdom are the following:

Arizona Articulation Proficiency Scale, 3rd ed. (AAPS–3; Fudala, 2000).

Bankson–Bernthal Test of Phonology (BBTOP; Bankson & Bernthal, 1990).

Clinical Assessment of Articulation and Phonology (CAAP; Secord & Donohoe, 2002).

Diagnostic Evaluation of Articulation and Phonology: Articulation Assessment (DEAP; Dodd et al., 2006).

Fisher–Logemann Test of Articulation (FLTA; Fisher & Logemann, 1971).

Goldman–Fristoe Test of Articulation, 2nd ed. (GFTA–2; Goldman & Fristoe, 2000).

Khan–Lewis Phonological Analysis, 2nd ed. (KLPA–2; Khan & Lewis, 2002).

Hodson Assessment of Phonological Patterns, 3rd ed. (HAPP–3; Hodson, 2004).

Photo-Articulation Test, 3rd ed. (PAT–3; Lippke et al., 1997).

Smit–Hand Articulation and Phonology Evaluation (SHAPE; Smit & Hand, 1992).

Structured Photographic Articulation Test, 2nd ed. (SPAT–II; Dawson & Tattersall, 2001).

Templin–Darley Tests of Articulation (TDTA; Templin & Darley, 1968).

An advantage of using a standardized test is that "this gives parents a clearer understanding of how their child is performing in comparison to his/her same-age peers" (Tyler & Tolbert, 2002, p. 217). However, standardized tests do not ensure complete coverage of articulatory or phonological ability, and they may be misleading when used with children who are bilingual or do not have a mainstream dialect (Chapter 10). In a review of articulation tests for the objective of determining a child's phonetic inventory, Eisenberg and Hitchcock (2010) concluded that, "Although useful for identifying children with SSD, currently available standardized tests do not provide the requisite number of opportunities in the right types of words for generating a complete phonetic inventory of either the consonants or the vowels of English. The test words must, therefore, be supplemented with probes of phonetically controlled words to establish the sounds that are and are not in a child's phonetic inventory." Morrison and Shriberg (1992), in a comparison of articulation tests with conversational speech sampling, found that the articulation accuracy profiles from these two methods differed at all linguistic levels examined, including overall accuracy, phonological processes, individual phonemes, manner features, error-type, word position, and allophones.

They concluded that "In comparison to the validity of conversational speech samples for integrated speech, language, and prosodic analyses, articulation tests appear to yield neither typical nor optimal measures of speech performance" (p. 259). Masterson et al. (2005, p. 229) offer a more positive view, commenting that, "the results of this study suggest that a single-word task tailored to some extent to the client's phonological system gives sufficient and representative information for phonological evaluation." They also note that a brief conversational sample is useful to assess prosody, intelligibility, and other aspects of language, and to confirm the representativeness of the single-word sample.

Transcription Methods

A **transcription** is a written record of sound patterns. A **phonemic or broad transcription** is used in the general study of spoken language to record the nature and distribution of phonemes used in the words and other linguistic units in a particular sociolinguistic community. Attention is given to the broad phonemic class, so that allophones of a given phoneme are transcribed with the same phoneme symbol, regardless of their structural and environmental context. For example, the initial and final sounds in the word *tot* are transcribed with the same phoneme symbol even if the initial /t/ is released as a plosive and the final /t/ may be unreleased. Similarly, in speech-language pathology, phonemic transcription has the goal of representing the phonemes produced in a speech sample. By convention, phoneme symbols are enclosed within virgules or slashes, for example, /s/. The internationally standard set of such symbols is the alphabet of the International Phonetic Association (IPA) included in Appendix A.

Phonetic or narrow transcription is used when it is desired to provide a more detailed transcription, including allophonic variations. The symbols for these transcriptions are enclosed in square brackets, for example, [t]. Modifications of a phoneme are represented with **diacritic marks** that are placed in positions around the parent (phoneme) symbol. Diacritic marks for general application have been developed as part of the IPA. But for clinical purposes, other systems of diacritics are available, including the system used in *Clinical Phonetics* by Shriberg et al. (2019). An advantage of this system is that the diacritic marks are placed in systematic positions related to the type of modification. For example, modifications of the sound source are indicated by diacritic marks positioned below the parent symbol. Narrow transcription can be time consuming, which limits its application in the routine assessment of speech disorders. In addition, skills in transcription can be difficult to learn and maintain (Knight et al., 2018). However, its clinical value has been reported in several studies (Ball et al., 2009; Knight et al., 2018; Shriberg et al., 2019).

Transcription provides the raw material for several different analyses, including accuracy in producing speech sounds, phonological processes or other sound class errors, intelligibility at the syllable or word levels, prosody, language features, and compensatory articulations. Accurate transcription requires training and experience on the part of the transcriber, as well as careful attention to the task. Because it can be time-consuming, clinicians may use it selectively rather than routinely in clinical assessments (Knight et al., 2018). Analysis procedures related to transcription data are considered next.

Speech accuracy is the correspondence between a speech target (usually a phoneme or a word) and the production of that target by a client. Examples of accuracy measures are **percent consonants correct (PCC)** and **percent vowels correct (PVC)**, or a rating on a scale of accuracy. These measures sometimes are considered as proxies of speech intelligibility, but some speakers can have notable inaccuracies without sacrificing intelligibility. In clinical usage, accuracy often pertains to whether a production is considered correct according to the standards of a given language, dialect, or speech community. The term accuracy also has been used in relation to variability of production, as in the case of repeated productions of a target. With this definition, an accurate production is one that is highly repeatable.

Percentage of consonants correct (PCC) is a quantitative measure of severity of speech sound disorders introduced by Shriberg and Kwiatkowski (1982). It is based solely on the judged production of consonants, which are classified as correct or incorrect based on sampling rules. The clinician determines the percentage of correctly articulated consonant sounds out of all consonant sounds attempted during a 3- to 4-minute conversational speech sample. According to Shriberg and Kwiatkowski (1982), PCC correlates to a corresponding severity level of the SSD as follows: PCC > 85% is mild, 65% < PCC < 85% is mild-moderate, 50% < PCC < 64% is moderate-severe, 50% < PCC is severe. A modified version of the PCC is called **Percent Consonants Correct-Revised (PCC-R)**, which bases the calculation on substitution and omission errors but not distortion errors, which are excluded from analysis. That is, PCC-R is the percentage of correctly articulated consonants (disregarding distortion errors) in a speech sample out of all opportunities for consonant production in that sample. Despite research indicating the value of PCC as an index of severity of disorder and a proxy for speech intelligibility, its adoption in wide-scale clinical use may be limited. A survey of SLPs revealed that PCC was rarely used, and respondents often reported limited academic and clinical exposure to the metric, inconsistent knowledge of PCC rules, and a lack of confidence using the measure (Dale et al., 2020). It was also noted that an obstacle to its use is that PCC requires transcription skills and can be time consuming. Although the number of respondents in the survey was not large (62 out of 900 invited participants), the results are nonetheless concerning.

Transcribing conversational samples from children with severe speech problems can be difficult. A particularly vexing problem is how to represent words or other utterances that are unintelligible. These are of high interest because they can serve as an index of severity and may give insight into a speech disorder. Barnes et al. (2009) marked with an "X" each unintelligible word or syllable in language sampling transcripts. An advantage to this method is that it permits calculation of MLUw, mean number of syllables per word, or mean number of syllables per utterance (Flipsen, 2006). However, it does not convey information on why the item was unintelligible. Alves et al. (2020) proposed the **Percentage of Intelligible Correct Syllables (PICS)**, which is calculated on all speech material, based on the following equation:

Number of accurate syllables /
(number of accurate syllables +
number of inaccurate syllables +
number of unintelligible syllables)

They also calculated **Percentage of Intelligible Syllables (PINTS)** by counting vowels as well as the number of unintelligible syllables. This was done automatically, via a Perl script. An intelligibility score was calculated as the number of transcribed syllables divided by the total number of syllables in the transcript, multiplied by 100.

Phonological Mean Length of Utterance (pMLU) is the length of a child's word productions (in segments) plus the number of correct consonants in each production divided by the total number of word tokens (Ingram, 2002). This measure, therefore, reflects both the length of words and the number of consonants correctly produced.

Babatsouli and Sotiropoulos (2018) proposed the **Measure for Cluster Proximity (MCP)** as a quantitative index of consonant cluster production in children's speech. Specifically, this measure addresses the issue of quantitatively differentiating stages in cluster production: reduction; vowel epenthesis; and two-members, substituted or correct. In comparing MCP with PCC, Babatsouli (2021) reported that there can be large differences between the two measures in individual clusters within and between children, but there is a strong and statistically significant correlation when averaged over all clusters per child, or over all children per cluster class based on manner of articulation.

Other approaches to clinical assessment focus on whole words or conversational speech. Jing and Grigos (2022) determined the interrater reliability of clinician ratings of the accuracy of whole words rather than individual sounds. Results indicated a substantial interrater reliability to a consensus judgment using a 3-point rating scale, with higher levels of reliability for correct productions and productions with extensive errors as opposed to minor errors. Vowel distortions were particularly challenging to rate. Phonetic transcription of conversational speech is challenging in terms of the mental effort and time investment needed to obtain accurate data. The **Connected Speech Transcription Protocol (CoST-P)** (Barrett et al., 2020) was designed for the transcription of connected speech produced by children with speech disorders. This tool offers guidelines for analysis that may promote both efficiency and accuracy of transcription.

A basic question in the analysis of connected speech is: How large a sample is needed for adequate and valid analysis? Wren et al. (2021) provide an answer based on data for a range of measures obtained from 776 5-year-olds who participated in a story retell task. Measures included: a range of profiles of percentage consonant correct; frequency of substitutions, omissions, distortions, and additions (SODA); percentage of syllable and stress pattern matches; and a measure of whole word complexity (Phonological Mean Length of Utterance, pMLU). Statistical analyses that compared these measures at different sample sizes show that sizes of 75- word tokens or greater have minimal differences in most measures, although 100-word tokens were needed for pMLU and measures of substitutions and distortions.

Phonetic Inventories

A **phonetic inventory** is a repertoire of speech sounds. Bates et al. (2021) stated that,

> A phonetic inventory in its simplest form lists the speech sounds that a child can physically articulate irrespective of how he/she uses them in words. Thus, it will include speech sounds that are used both accurately and inaccurately when targeted by the child. (p. 3)

Inventories are accomplished in two different ways. An **independent analysis** counts the number of native-language consonant or vowel types and the syllable shapes, without reference to the adult system. A **relational analysis** assesses the accuracy of the produced consonant or vowel forms relative to the adult system, so that the inventory contains only correctly produced sounds. Independent analyses are more appropriate for prelexical sounds such as babbling, and to the production of words and word approximations.

A common criterion for inclusion of a sound in a phonetic inventory is that the child must produce the sound at least twice in a sample of spontaneous speech (Stoel-Gammon, 1985). The source of data can be transcriptions of conversation or more structured tests such as articulation tests. However, as noted earlier in this chapter, Eisenberg and Hitchcock (2010) concluded that the currently available standardized tests cannot provide a complete phonetic inventory of either the consonants or the vowels of English. Table 5–2 shows the syllable-initial consonant inventories of young children between 8 and 39 months of age.

Table 5–2. Initial-Position Consonant Inventories in Young Children of Different Ages, as Reported in Three Studies

Age (mos.)	Robb & Bleile (1994)	Stoel-Gammon (1985)	Dyson (1988)
8	/d t k m h/		
9	/d m n h w/		
10	/b d t m n h/		
11	/d m n h/		
12	/b d g m h/		
14	/b d g t k m n h w l/		
15	/b d h/	/b d h/	
18	/b d m n h w/	/b d m n h w/	
21	/b d g t k m n h w/	/b d t m n h/	
24	/b d p t k m n h s w/	/b d t g k m n h w f s/	/b p d t g k f s h m n w j l/
29			/b p d t g k f s h m n w j l/
39			/b p d t g k f s h m n w j l r/

The sounds present in most inventories across age beginning with the first year of life are /b d m n h w/. McCune and Vihman (1987) proposed that early articulatory skills could be characterized as the learning of **vocal motor schemes (VMS)**, defined as generalized action patterns that yield consistent phonetic forms. In a study of children aged 9 to 16 months, McCune and Vihman (2001) reported that the most common VMS consonants were: /t d p b k g s m n l/, a set of sounds very similar to those listed in Table 5–2. From the point of view of articulatory phonetics, the sounds produced in infancy are produced with (1) bilabial, coronal, dorsal, and glottal places of articulation; (2) stop or nasal manner of production (distinguished by velopharyngeal function), and (3) a gradual appearance of the voicing contrast. Stops and nasals have in common a closure at some point in the vocal tract and may share some dynamic properties of the oral articulation such as the release of the oral closure.

Rating Scales

Rating scales are used in speech-language pathology to obtain information on listener judgements of aspects of speech such as intelligibility, quality, or naturalness. A **rating scale** is a method of registering a perceptual judgment on a graphic of some kind. A commonly used rating scale is the **Equal Appearing Interval Scale (EAIS)**, also known as the Thurstone technique of attitude measurement after its primary author, L. L. Thurstone (1928). This scale is an interval (or category, or partition) scale of measurement designed for rating psychological attributes such as attitudes, but it is frequently used in speech-language pathology to rate judgments of attributes such as voice quality, speech intelligibility, fluency, and swallowing. It is usually assumed that intervals on the scale are equidistant and equally distributed, so that the distance between any single value, such as 3, and its flanking value, such as 4, is the same

The *APA Dictionary of Psychology* (VandenBos, 2007) defines developmental delay as a delay in the age at which developmental milestones are achieved by a child or delay in the development of communication, social, and daily living skills. It is usually assumed that the milestones and skills eventually will be achieved. Speech delay can be similarly defined as a delay in reaching the developmental milestones of speech or delay in the development of the skills of speech communication. Criteria for diagnosing speech delay are not uniform, but an often-used criterion is that the child's conversational speech is characterized by age-inappropriate speech sound omission errors and/or substitution errors (that may occur along with distortion errors). Speech delay may be accompanied by a language delay. A late talker is a child who has expressive and/or receptive language that lags normative milestones. The word delay can be disturbing to a parent or other caregiver, and it is important for clinicians to be aware of this possibility and to provide assurance that delay does not mean lifelong difficulty or a general cognitive disability.

as the distance between any other pair of values, such as 1 and 2. This assumption has analytic significance because it means that rating data can be analyzed with parametric statistics to yield means, standard deviations, and other summarizing values. For example, speech intelligibility in a child might be judged on a scale of 7 equal intervals, from a value of 1 (representing extremely unintelligible speech) to a value of 7 (representing a high degree of intelligibility). The EAIS has had numerous applications in many specialties, including psychology, medicine, rehabilitation, and marketing. EAIS resembles the popular Likert (pronounced /l ɪ k ɚ t/ and named after Rensis Likert [1903–1981]) rating scale, in which respondents note their degree of agreement on a bipolar scale with something like "Do not agree at all" at one end and "Agree completely" at the other.

In his classic studies of psychometric scaling, Stevens (1946) distinguished prothetic and metathetic attributes. **Prothetic** attributes are additive in nature and are sometimes called quantitative. An example is sound intensity. **Metathetic** attributes are substitutive in nature and are sometimes called qualitative. An example is pitch. With respect to the attributes of speech, it has been concluded that prothetic attributes include speaking rate (Cartwright & Lass, 1975), intelligibility (Schiavetti, Metz, & Sitler, 1981; Schiavetti, 1992), severity of stuttering (Schiavetti et al., 1983), nasality (Whitehill et al., 2002; Zraick & Liss, 2000), and severity of disorder (Eadie & Doyle, 2002). Metathetic attributes include naturalness (Eadie & Doyle, 2002), degree of foreign accent (Southwood & Flege, 1999), and activity and participation (Ma & Yiu, 2007).

Why does it matter if an attribute is prothetic or metathetic? The reason is that different psychometric scaling methods are preferable for the two types of attributes. Prothetic dimensions are more appropriately scaled with **Direct Magnitude Estimation (DME)** than with EAIS. In DME, the magnitude of a subjective experience such as speech intelligibility is expressed by assigning a number to it. For example, a judge may assign the value of 100 to a particular sample of speech and a value of 200 to a sample that is judged to be twice as intelligible. Some of the most important attributes of speech (e.g., speaking rate, intelligibility, severity) are better assessed with DME than EAIS. But EAIS is far more frequently used in clinical settings across specialties. The preference for EAIS is based primarily on convenience and economy. DME is more difficult to implement than EAIS. EAIS applications abound in the literature and clinical reports in the field of speech-language pathology (and many other specialties as well). There may be little point in resisting the tide of popular choice. The perfect should not be the enemy of the good, and perhaps the best investment of time and energy is to make EAIS as valid and reliable as possible.

A basic decision in using interval scales is selecting the number of scale values. In his classic article, G. A. Miller (1956) concluded that people tend toward 7 points of gradation in short-term memory and categorization (hence, the "magic number seven, plus or minus two"). But even if the value of 7 represents a limiting value in decision-making, it is necessary to use a scale of more than 7 points to achieve that level of performance, which is why scales of 10 or more points sometimes are used. But in contemporary usage, scales of 3, 4, or 5 points appear to be increasingly common in specialties such as speech-language pathology, neurology, rehabilitation medicine, and physical therapy. Studies of the optimal number of response categories in rating scales have yielded discrepant results, as discussed in Ludlow et al. (2019). Wu and Leung (2017) concluded from a simulation study that using a larger number of Likert scale values gives a closer approach to the underlying statistical distribution, and hence normality and interval scales. They recommended that social work practitioners use 11-point Likert scales from 0 to 10, which is a natural and easily comprehensible range. The current shift to 5 scale points notwithstanding, it may ultimately be the optimal solution to adopt 11-point scales for perceptual judgments. For now, clinicians should feel free to adopt the number of scale values that they prefer.

A hybrid rating scale, the dichotomous-ordinal scale, is an ordinal scale that has two aspects: (a) a category denoting absence of a particular attribute (e.g., nasality), and (b) two or more levels of ordered presence (i.e., severity) of the phenomenon. An advantage of this scale is that severity ratings are done only when an attribute is present, so that scoring and recordkeeping are simplified (Ludlow et al., 2019).

An alternative method of scaling that is attracting considerable interest is the **Visual Analog Scale (VAS)** that commonly takes the form of a horizontal (HVAS) or vertical (VVAS) line, usually 10 cm in length, anchored by two verbal descriptors at the ends of the line. Other versions include meter-shaped scales (curvilinear analogue scales) and box scales (rectangles containing circles equidistant from each other). These are illustrated in Figure 5–4. Perceptual judgments are made by marking a tick on the scale at the point that corresponds to a judgment

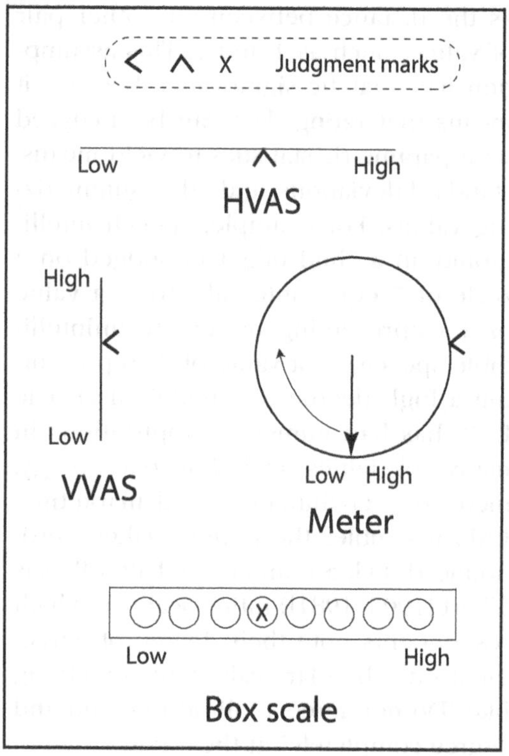

Figure 5–4. Different versions of the visual analog scale (VAS): horizontal VAS (HVAS), vertical VAS (VVAS), meter, and box scale.

of magnitude, and the data are derived by simple linear measurement with a ruler or by computer. Advantages of this approach include a potentially fine degree of registering judgments with a relatively simple task. VAS has been used across a wide range of perceptual attributes, including speech sound learning (Munson, 2012), intelligibility (Abur et al., 2019), hypernasality and audible nasal emission (Baylis et al., 2015), and swallowing efficiency and safety (Curtis et al., 2022).

Given its ease of use and accumulating reports of satisfaction with its reliability, VAS is likely to be increasingly adopted in clinical applications. Some limitations should be noted. Torrance et al. (2001) noted two biases that can affect the results. The first, **context bias**, relates to the fact that a VAS score for an item depends on the number of presented items that are better and worse than that item. If an item to be judged is presented with many items that are more positive (e.g., less severe speech involvement), then its value is likely to be depressed. Conversely, if a given item is presented together with many items that are more negative (e.g., more severe involvement, then its value is enhanced. The second bias, **end aversion**, is the tendency to avoid using the extreme categories of a category scale or to avoid the portion of the scale near the ends of a continuous scale. Torrance et al. (2001) cautioned that in the assessment of health states, VAS always should be accompanied by other types of assessment. Similarly, Franchignoni et al. (2012) recommended that, "investigators, particularly in fields such Physical and Rehabilitation Medicine (PRM), should think twice before selecting a VAS as an outcome measure for clinical use (particularly when used as a standalone tool)" (p. 44). These warnings deserve notice, but research on the use of VAS in speech and voice assessment generally supports the use of this tool. In short, VAS may be a good choice given the need to balance ease of use against possible limitations as a metric.

The foregoing discussion attempted to identify the advantages and disadvantages of perceptual rating scales, and readers may very well be frustrated that there is no clear best solution. Experts may not be in complete agreement about rating scales, but these scales are used across many specialties and the number of such scales seems to be ever increasing. Perhaps the best advice is to proceed with due caution, recognizing that any perceptual rating scale is imperfect but can nonetheless have clinical value. For certain aspects of speech, rating scales may be the only, or the most practicable, method of measurement. For example, goodness of articulation, discussed in Chapter 4, is usually assessed by asking listeners to judge the extent to which a particular instance of a sound is representative of the phoneme (Dugan et al., 2019; Strömbergsson et al., 2015).

Praxis and Speech Motor Control

This section considers two general issues in assessing speech motor disorders in children: praxis and differential diagnosis. **Praxis** is a general term for action or exercise, typically referring to a motor skill of some kind. **Orofacial praxis** is the ability to perform volitional skilled movements of speech and other orofacial functions following verbal command or demonstration (Kools & Tweedie, 1975). Imitation, discussed earlier in this chapter, often is used to assess praxis. Whether praxis is assessed with demonstration (modeling) or verbal command, the behavior to be assessed is an integrated sensorimotor skill that builds on experience as well as the integrity of the sensory and motor systems. For example, Guilleminault et al. (2019) assessed what they termed "lingual gnosis" (defined as the ability to recognize an object with the tongue) and "lingual praxis" (motor planning or programming of coordinated tongue movements). They conceived of the development of lingual motor coordination as proceeding from lingual gnosis (which begins in utero) to lingual praxis (gained through experience with specific movement patterns). This idea can be generalized to the other components of the oral mechanism. Bearzotti et al. (2007) reported on the ability of typically developing children aged 4 to 8 years to perform 6 gestures, 24 single and 12 complex, elicited through verbal and imitative request. The results showed a progressive development of the orofacial praxis, with imitation being more effective than verbal request, especially for younger children, and with mastery of sequences of gestures and oroverbal movements by the age of 6 years.

The three main diagnostic categories of pediatric motor speech disorder are CAS, dysarthria, and speech motor delay. As explained in Chapter 1, these categories may be revised or expanded in the future, but for present purposes these three categories are the focus of discussion and present in themselves significant clinical challenge. Murray et al. (2021) reviewed studies on the speech features that differentiate CAS from other speech sound disorders and concluded that there were no studies of the highest diagnostic quality although 15 studies had potential to identify features for differential diagnosis (see Chapter 11 for further discussion). Iuzzini-Seigel, Allison, and Stoeckel (2022) conducted a web-based survey of 359 pediatric speech-language pathologists to determine clinical confidence levels in diagnosing childhood apraxia of speech and dysarthria. The majority (60%) of respondents reported low or no confidence in diagnosing dysarthria in children, and 40% reported that they consequently tend not to make this diagnosis. Uncertainty also surrounds the diagnosis of CAS. Chenausky and Tager-Flusberg (2022) commented that many of the characteristics of different dysarthrias resemble the core impairments in CAS. They note a further complication in that dysarthria may co-occur with CAS, which makes diagnosis even more difficult.

Several factors contribute to this diagnostic challenge. As noted in Chapter 1, childhood dysarthria lacks a widely accepted classification system, and it is doubtful that the classifications used in adult acquired dysarthrias are suitable for use with children (Morgan & Liégeois, 2010; Ruessink et al., 2021; Schölderle, Haas, & Ziegler, 2021; van Mourik et al., 1997). Acquired dysarthria in adults is quite different from childhood dysarthria in that affected adults have established premorbid sensorimotor linkages that can serve as a reference for relearning. But many children with dysarthria have not established the sensorimotor patterns needed for highly intelligible speech. Motor programs are experience-dependent insofar as performance and practice are needed for their development and refinement. Neilson and O'Dwyer (1981) address this issue by stating that, "Dysarthria in cerebral palsy might result, therefore, from the distortion of motor commands by transmission through damaged descending pathways or because appropriate motor commands are not correctly formulated in the first place" (p. 1018). They agreed with Kent and Netsell (1978) that the speech disorder can be viewed as a motor learning deficit. It follows, then, that both childhood dysarthria and CAS involve deficits in motor learning, and it is not surprising that they may share some features of atypical speech production.

The distinction between apraxia of speech and dysarthria in adults is sometimes explained by designating the former as a programming disorder and the latter as a disorder of execution. This concept, popular as it may be, has been questioned for use in adults (Lowit et al., 2022) and may come under even more intense questioning for children. Dysarthria in adults is a group of neurogenic speech disorders characterized by abnormalities in the strength, speed, range, steadiness, tone, or accuracy of movements needed for respiratory, phonatory, resonatory, articulatory, or prosodic components of speech production (Duffy, 2019). Description of the movement irregularities is difficult in adults and even more so in children. In common clinical practice, the movement disturbances are inferred from auditory-perceptual judgments and the speech mechanism examination. More is said on this topic later in the chapter, following a review of contemporary assessment tools that were designed to diagnose motor speech disorders in children. Additional information on these tools is available in McCauley and Strand (2008) and Sayahi and Jalaie (2016). Chapter 10 provides a more detailed description of childhood dysarthria and childhood apraxia of speech.

Praxis in speech production is critically important in the diagnosis of childhood apraxia of speech, which is generally considered a disorder of praxis. One tool for the clinical assessment of praxis related to speech is the **Kaufman Speech Praxis Test for Children (KSPT**; Kaufman, 1995). This test is a norm-referenced and standardized measure designed to assess clinical characteristics of abnormal speech praxis. It was normed for the typically developing population of children as well as a population of children with speech and language disorders. The results are an overall raw score, standard score (mean, 100; SD, 15), and a percentile ranking for each of 4 subtests: (1) oral movement, (2) simple phonemic and syllabic level, (3) complex phonemic and syllabic level, and (4) spontaneous length and complexity. The subtests are numbered in terms of increased task difficulty.

An approach often used in the assessment and treatment of complex speech disorders such as those in childhood dysarthria, childhood apraxia of speech, Down syndrome, or fetal alcohol syndrome is to consider dimensions or functional subsystems of speech production. Here we consider four tests that assess component features of speech production. These tests are summarized and compared in Table 5–3, and each test is briefly reviewed in the following.

The **Motor Speech Hierarchy (MSH)** (MSH; Hayden et al., 2010; Hayden & Square, 1994) was developed as a guide for assessment and intervention within the **Prompts for Restructuring Oral Muscular Phonetic Targets (PROMPT**; Hayden et al., 2010) approach. Namasivayam et al. (2021) developed and validated a probe word list and scoring system to assess speech motor skills in preschool and school-age children with motor speech disorders. The assessment is based on the MSH and includes probe words that correspond to the seven major stages of speech motor control in the MSH: Stage I—tone, Stage II—phonatory control, Stage III—mandibular control, Stage IV—labial-facial control, Stage V—lingual control, Stage VI—sequenced movements, and Stage VII—prosody. The MSH underlies the recently published Verbal Motor Production Assessment for Children, Revised (VMPAC-R; https://vmpac-r.com/), which is designed to be used for children aged 3 to 12 years.

The **Bogenhausen Dysarthria Scales for Childhood Dysarthria (BoDyS-KiD)** (Haas, Ziegler, & Schölderle, 2021;

Table 5–3. Comparison of Four Tests for Assessing Motor Speech Disorders in Children

<table>
<tr><th>Item/Test</th><th>MSH</th><th>BoDyS-KiD</th><th>DEMSS</th><th>ProCAD</th></tr>
<tr><td>Muscle tone</td><td>Stage I—tone</td><td>—</td><td>—</td><td>—</td></tr>
<tr><td>Respiration</td><td>Stage II—phonatory control</td><td>Respiration</td><td>—</td><td rowspan="2">Low volume or loudness decay, excessive loudness, excess loudness variation, effort/audible inspiration, short breath groups, atypical voice quality</td></tr>
<tr><td>Larynx</td><td>Stage II—phonatory control</td><td>Pitch and loudness, voice quality, voice stability</td><td>—</td></tr>
<tr><td>Jaw</td><td>Stage III—mandibular control</td><td>Articulation</td><td rowspan="3">Overall articulatory accuracy, vowel accuracy</td><td rowspan="3">Imprecise articulatory contacts, consonant distortions, vowel errors, voicing errors, intrusive schwa, groping (articulatory searching), increased difficulty with multisyllabic words, difficulty with initial articulatory configurations and/or transitionary movement gestures</td></tr>
<tr><td>Lips</td><td>Stage IV—labio-facial control</td><td></td></tr>
<tr><td>Tongue</td><td>Stage V—lingual control</td><td></td></tr>
<tr><td>Velopharynx</td><td>—</td><td>Resonance</td><td></td><td>Fluctuating resonance/intermittent hypernasality or hyponasality, consistent hypernasality (with or without nasal emissions)</td></tr>
<tr><td>Movement sequences</td><td>Stage VI—sequenced movements</td><td>Articulatory rate</td><td></td><td>Increased difficulty with multisyllabic words, difficulty with initial articulatory configurations and/or transitionary movement gestures</td></tr>
<tr><td>Prosody</td><td>Stage VII—prosody</td><td>Modulation</td><td>Prosody</td><td>Slow rate, atypical stress/reduced stress, lexical stress errors, syllable segregation</td></tr>
<tr><td>Consistency</td><td>—</td><td>—</td><td>Consistency</td><td></td></tr>
<tr><td>Fluency</td><td></td><td>Fluency</td><td></td><td>Groping (articulatory searching)</td></tr>
</table>

Sources: MSH = Motor Speech Hierarchy (Hayden et al., 2010; Hayden & Square, 1994; Namasivayam et al., 2021); BoDyS-KiD = Bogenhausen Dysarthria Scales for Childhood Dysarthria (Haas, Ziegler, & Schölderle, 2021; Schölderle, Haas, & Ziegler, 2020, 2021); DEMSS = Dynamic Evaluation of Motor Speech Skill (Strand et al., 2013); ProCAD = Profile of Childhood Apraxia of Speech and Dysarthria (Iuzzini-Seigel, Allison, & Stoeckel, 2022).

Schölderle, Haas, & Ziegler, 2020, 2021) is an auditory-perceptual analysis of dysarthria in children developed for the German language. It consists of nine speech dimensions (listed in Table 5–3) and 29 individual symptoms. This tool was developed with studies of typically developing children and children with dysarthria.

The **Dynamic Evaluation of Motor Speech Skill (DEMSS**; Strand et al., 2013) was designed to assess praxis. DEMISS is dynamic in the sense that it assesses multiple attempts by a child to produce targets as the clinician incorporates cues and other strategies (e.g., slowed rate or simultaneous production) to facilitate performance. The test uses 9 different speaking tasks: CV syllables, VC syllables, reduplicated CV bisyllable, symmetric CVC, asymmetric CVC, bisyllable with repeated consonant, bisyllable with alternating consonant, multisyllabic word, and utterances of increasing length. The scoring categories vary with the utterance type but include overall articulatory accuracy, vowel accuracy, prosodic accuracy, and consistency. Overall articulatory accuracy is scored on a 5-point multidimensional scale (0 = correct on first attempt, 1 = consistent developmental substitution error without slowness or distortion of movement gestures, 2 = correct after first cued attempt, 3 = correct after two or three additional cued attempts, 4 = not correct after all cued attempts). Vowel accuracy is scored on a 3-point scale (0 = correct, 1 = mild distortion, 2 = frank distortion). Prosodic accuracy is scored as a binary judgment of correct or incorrect, and consistency is scored on a binary judgment of consistent on all trials or inconsistent on any two or more trials.

Profile of Childhood Apraxia of Speech and Dysarthria (ProCAD; Iuzzini-Seigel, Allison, & Stoeckel, 2022) was developed to facilitate the assessment of both CAS and dysarthria symptoms in children and to provide a systematic procedure for differentiating CAS and pediatric dysarthria. The assessment consists of a combined set of auditory–perceptual speech features for rating both dysarthria and CAS characteristics in published reports and current accepted features. Table 5–3 lists the components used in the assessment.

Verbal dyspraxia profile (Jelm, 2001) consists in part of tests of automatic and imitative oral-motor movements for jaw, lips/cheeks, and tongue.

Assessments of speech motor function that are out of print or otherwise no longer available include the **Apraxia Profile: A Descriptive Assessment Tool for Children** (Hickman, 1997); **Screening Test for Developmental Apraxia of Speech—Second Edition (STDAS-2**; Blakely, 2000), **Verbal Motor Assessment of Children (VMPAC**; Hayden & Square, 1999). VMPAC is now available in a revised version that is a self-scoring, on-line web application with automatic profiling and progress tracking features (VMPAC-R), as noted earlier in this section.

The assessments just reviewed focus largely, if not exclusively on speech motor function and say little about nonspeech motor performance, which is an important consideration in diagnosing the presence and severity of dysarthria. As noted earlier in this chapter, Duffy (2019) defined dysarthria as a group of neurogenic disorders characterized by abnormalities in the strength, speed, range, steadiness, tone, or accuracy of movements involved in the respiratory, phonatory, resonatory, articulatory, or prosodic components of speech production. This definition is a tall order for clinical assessment, especially because there is little agreement on how the abnormalities should be assessed. Methods of assessment for the abnormalities listed by Duffy are discussed in the following.

Strength

Muscle strength is a **muscle power function** according to the International Classification of Functioning, Disability, and Health (2001). Bohannon (2019) defined strength as "the maximum voluntary resultant output that muscles can bring to bear on the environment under a specific set of test conditions." By this definition, strength is a maximal force or power. In routine clinical examination, orofacial strength is assessed by visual observation, palpation, and force application by an examiner. In the absence of movement, the clinician can use palpation and observation to determine if the muscles of interest are active. In the presence of movement, observation can be used to estimate the proportion of an action's test range (e.g., amount of jaw opening or lateral tongue motion) that is completed. Muscle strength also can be assessed by asking a child to perform push or pull actions using the jaw, lips, or tongue. For example, the child may be asked to push his/her tongue against a tongue depressor, squeeze an object between the lips, or bite down on an object.

An instrument that permits direct and objective assessment is the Iowa Oral Performance Instrument (IOPI; Blaise Medical, Henderson, TN), which measures the pressure produced by the articulators against a pliable air-filled bulb. IOPI can be used to obtain measures of strength for lingual elevation, protrusion, and lateralization; cheek compression; and lip compression. Normative data regarding performance with the IOPI in children are available primarily for anterior lingual elevation during nonspeech tasks (Adams et al., 2013; McKay et al., 2020; Potter et al., 2009; Potter & Short, 2009; Vanderwegen et al., 2019).

Objective quantitative assessment can be valuable when conditions such as weakness or hypotonia are suspected. In healthy speakers, the muscle forces needed for speech amount to only about 20% of the maximum force capability (Netsell, 1982). However, it should be noted that young children may have only one-third of the muscle force capability of adults. Potter and Short (2009) concluded that tongue strength increases rapidly across the period of 3 to 8 years, then increases at a slower rate until reaching its maximum in late adolescence. They also noted that the IOPI standard tongue bulb could be used satisfactorily with children as young as 3 years of age.

Speed

In speech production, speed takes two different forms: (a) the number of segments produced in a unit of time (e.g., syllables/s), or (b) the time rate at which an articulator moves along a path (e.g., mm/s). Increased speed expressed in segments per time unit does not necessarily imply increased speed expressed in time rate of movement. Sometimes the relationship is inverse, because an increase in segments per unit of time often is accompanied by a reduction in the magnitude of articulatory movement and therefore a reduced time of movement (Kent & Moll, 1972; Westbury & Dembowski, 1993). In the general clinical assessment of speech, the number of segments produced in a unit of time is often determined in a task such as diadochokinesis. The measurement of speech as time rate of movement (the physical quantity of speed) requires instrumental methods that are not uniformly available in clinical settings.

Range

Range of motion (ROM) is the capability to move a structure through its complete spectrum of movements. In physical therapy and neurology, range of motion generally is assessed for joints, such as those in the limbs. Range of motion of a joint can be assessed either passively (the examiner moves the joint) or actively (the person being examined moves the joint with muscular action). Aside from the jaw, orofacial muscles do not have joints, so that range usually is assessed as the distance over which a structure is moved. In common clinical practice in speech-language pathology, range is assessed by visual observation as a child performs oral movements such as elevating and depressing the jaw, moving the tongue from side to side, and pursing the lips. Mogren et al. (2022) used a 3D motion analysis to compare ROM in children with SSD and children with typical speech development. Their results indicated that children with SSD persisting after the age of six years have more asymmetrical and more variable movement patterns in the lips and jaw during vowel production in a syllable repetition task than children with typical speech development. The differences were more pronounced in the lateral direction in both lips and jaw.

Steadiness

Steadiness is the ability to maintain a position or action over time. Steadiness can be comprised in neurological conditions such as cerebral palsy in which involuntary movements can interfere with task performance. In the clinical assessment of speech, steadiness is evaluated primarily for sustained efforts such as prolongation of a vowel or fricative. Steadiness can be assessed by auditory judgments or by instrumental methods (e.g., displays of intensity during tasks such as sound prolongation, formant patterns during sustained vowels).

Tone

Muscle tone is conventionally defined as the level of muscle contraction in a muscle at rest. A common method used in the neurological examination of muscle tone is passive movement of a limb (i.e., the clinician moves a patient's arm while in its resting state), called **passive or resting tone**. Tone also can be assessed in an active muscle, which is called **active tone.** Reduced tone is called **hypotonia** and increased tone takes the two major forms of **spasticity** and **rigidity**. Hypotonia is frequently mentioned in the literature and clinical reports on pediatric movement disorders, and it also is mentioned quite often with respect to speech disorders in the pediatric population (Chapter 11). The examination of tone is difficult with the oral and pharyngeal muscles, most of which are not easily manipulated or observed. For all its clinical importance, muscle tone is not straightforward in its assessment. Goo et al. (2018) reviewed 21 assessments that measure muscle tone for children aged birth to 12 years and concluded that the psychometric evidence was insufficient to endorse any one assessment. A few assessments had published evidence of at least validity or reliability, including three for newborns and one for infants between 2 months and 2 years. Only one assessment was recommended (with qualification) for children up to 6 years, and no assessments met criteria for children aged 7 to 12 years. It does not get better with the assessment of tone in the orofacial muscles, as discussed by Clark & Solomon (2012). Simply put, tone is not easily assessed. Objective measures can be made with two instruments, the Myotonometer™ (Neurogenic Technologies, Missoula, MT) and Myoton-3 (V6.7, 2005; Myoton AS, Estonia, EU). Reports indicate that the Myoton has better test-retest reliability than the Myotonometer™ (Clark & Solomon, 2010; Solomon & Clark, 2010) and may be more versatile in its application to different muscle groups (Clark & Solomon, 2012).

Accuracy

Accuracy is the precision of reaching a movement target, such as a vowel or consonant articulation. Common errors noted in neurology are **overshooting** (moving beyond the target position) or **undershooting** (falling short of the target position). But in speech production, accuracy takes other forms, as discussed later in the section on electropalatography. The term accuracy is used in another sense, in respect to phonemic or phonetic judgments of speech sound production (Chapter 8).

Diagnosis of Dysarthria

If dysarthria is suspected in a child, confirmatory evidence should point to specific motor disturbances that accord with Duffy's (2019) definition. These disturbances pertain to movements that are common to speech and nonspeech movements, so that both kinds of movements are relevant in an examination. Given the standard definition and criteria for diagnosis of dysarthria, it would be unusual to observe abnormalities in speech movements without similar effects on nonspeech movements. The following procedures are relevant in the assessment of dysarthria:

1. Oral mechanism examination (see Table 5–1) and Appendix B.
2. Cranial nerve examination (cranial nerves are listed in Appendix C.
3. Maximum phonation time (discussed in this chapter).
4. Diadochokinesis, both alternating motion rate and sequential motion rate (discussed in this chapter).
5. Orofacial tone (discussed earlier in this chapter).
6. Orofacial strength (discussed earlier in this chapter).

An example of an assessment that combines speech and nonspeech tasks is the pediatric Radboud Dysarthria Assessment, p-RDA (Ruessink et al., 2021). This assessment, developed for the Dutch language, consists of two observational tasks (word and sentence repetition or a reading task, and a conversation about a familiar topic), four maximum performance tasks, and two severity scales. The authors note that the p-RDA has clinical value in its assessment of functional speech in combination with maximum performance tasks, explaining that this combination is essential in addressing the five aspects of speech production (respiration, phonation, articulation, resonance, and prosody. As noted earlier in this chapter, Thoonen et al. (1996) developed a procedure for the differential diagnosis of dysarthria and dyspraxia that is based largely on maximum performance data.

Also mentioned earlier is the concept that maximum performance tests are useful in isolating subsystems of speech production and reducing the effects of cognitive and linguistic variables in speech motor performance.

Phonological Patterns

Phonological processes in typically developing speech are described in Chapter 4. The same general methods have been used in assessing delayed or disordered speech. Chapter 7 covers the general topic of phonological assessment, emphasizing phonological processes and phonological awareness.

Intelligibility and Comprehensibility

Intelligibility and comprehensibility are covered in Chapter 8. Because these topics are complex, they are given their own chapter, which discusses in some detail the various approaches that have been used for assessment and the implications of these assessments for clinical interventions.

Independent Versus Relational Assessments

As noted earlier in this chapter with respect to the phonetic inventory of babbling, it has been suggested that the two general categories of assessment are relational and independent. Relational assessments compare a child's speech with an adult or other defined standard, whereas independent assessments describe the child's speech without reference to such a standard. Relational assessments include percentage of consonants correct (PCC), phonological process analysis, phonological mean length of utterance (PMLU) (Ingram, 2002), and proportion whole-word proximity (PWP). Independent assessments include mean babbling level (MBL), syllable structure level (SSL), and word complexity measure (WCM).

Instrumental Methods

To this point, most of the assessment methods are perceptual in nature, requiring only auditory or visual examinations by the clinician. Instrumental methods, such as acoustic and physiologic measures, can confirm or extend conclusions reached through perceptual means. Furthermore, instrumental methods are increasingly used in therapy for speech disorders. Here we briefly discuss selected acoustic or physiologic methods.

Acoustic Analysis

Acoustic analysis has multiple applications in describing speech disorders. A partial list, based on Ludlow et al. (2019) is as follows.

Vowels

Potential clinical measures and features include the following: range of formant frequencies (e.g., reduced vowel space area), unusual formant shifts that might signify diphthongization or other change in vowel articulation, alterations in expected duration (e.g., lengthening of unstressed vowels, reduced contrast between lax and tense vowels) related to atypical prosody.

Stops

Potential clinical features include the following: atypical voice onset times for voiced and/or voiceless stops in syllable-initial position, multiple bursts occurring on stop release, spirantization (frication) during stop gap, absent or weak release burst for stops in syllable-initial position.

Fricatives

Potential clinical features include the following: Unusual spectral features, such as weak noise energy or atypically shaped noise spectrum, variability in spectrum over frication interval.

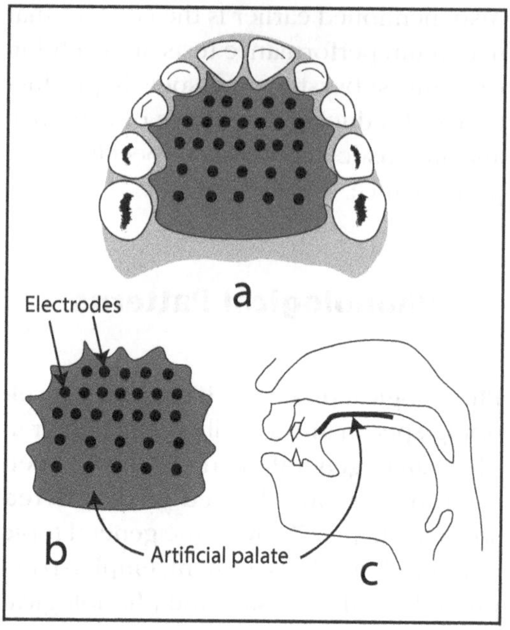

Figure 5–5. Illustration of electropalatography, showing (a) the artificial palate in the roof of the mouth, (b) the isolated artificial palate, and (c) a sagittal view of the artificial palate in position.

Electropalatography (EPG)

Electropalatography (EPG) records patterns of contact between the tongue and the palate in continuous speech, using a custom-made thin acrylic palate in whose undersurface are embedded small contact electrodes (Figure 5–5). Activations of these electrodes are mapped onto a computer display that shows changing contact patterns during speech. Limitations to this technique are (1) that the artificial palate can induce compensatory adjustments in articulation (McAuliffe et al., 2008; McLeod & Searl, 2006), and (2) that it does not reveal which region(s) of the tongue contact the palate. Spatial resolution is limited by electrode spacing, which typically is 2 to 3 mm apart. McLeod and Searl (2006) reported that wearing the appliance for about 2 hours is sufficient for acclimation. Devices currently are available from two primary sources, Articulate Instruments and SmartPalate. Their products differ mostly in the design of the pseudopalate. The SmartPalate uses 126 gold-plated palate and lip closure sensors.

EPG studies have revealed articulatory patterns that are not detected easily, if at all, by auditory-perceptual judgments. Gibbon and Wood (2002) identified atypical articulatory patterns in children with speech sound disorders. One pattern, called **drift**, is an atypical change in place of articulation during the closure for a stop consonant. The other pattern, called **undifferentiated gestures**, has increased tongue-palate contact (i.e., less precise articulation). It was observed that drift was greater for children who produced undifferentiated gestures. The authors noted that drift may reflect impaired speech motor control. Gibbon and Lee (2017a) presented EPG evidence of covert contrasts (phonetic or phonological contrasts that are not readily detected in transcription-based studies (see Chapter 4).

Ultrasound (US)

Ultrasound, also called **sonography**, creates images of internal body organs by using sound waves with frequencies higher than the upper limits of human audition. A US scanner, consisting of a console with computer and electronics, a video display screen, and a transducer (probe) that performs the scanning. The transducer emits high-frequency sound waves into the object of interest. The frequency is above the range of human hearing (hence ultra + sound). When the waves hit a boundary between water and air (or between any structures with different acoustic impedances), they are partly reflected as echoes, partly transmitted to deeper structures, partly scattered, and partly transformed to heat. The reflected waves are used to create an image on the video display. When used properly, US is safe and can be used repeatedly even with children. To scan the tongue, the probe is placed under the jaw (submental position) so that the ultrasound pulses are directed toward the superior surface of the tongue, as shown in Figure 5–6.

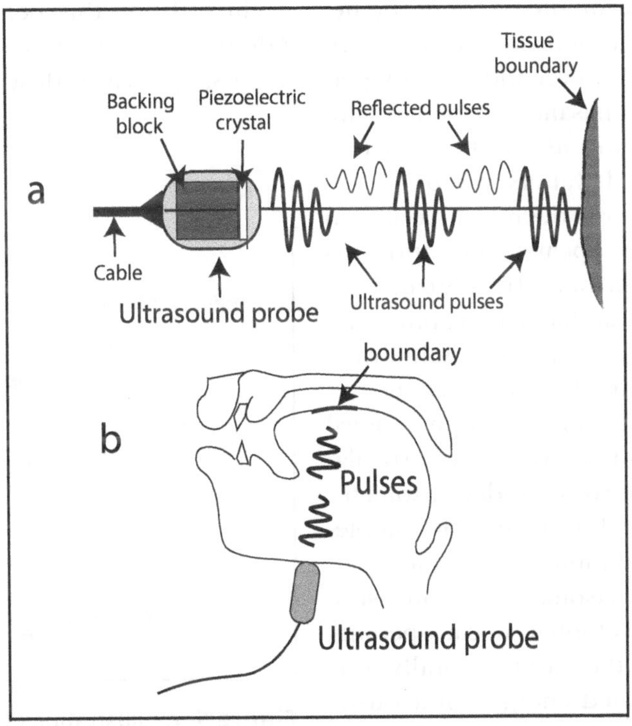

Figure 5–6. Illustration of ultrasound (US) used to study the position and movement of the tongue: (a) the ultrasound probe and the US pulses, (b) the US probe in a submental placement.

Nasometry

Nasalance is a physical measure related to the perceptual attribute of **nasality**, which pertains to the balance of oral and nasal resonance in speech production. Nasality, or nasalization, is required for the nasal phonemes that are produced with an opening of the velopharynx so that sound radiates through the nasal passages. Vowels that flank nasal consonants often are nasalized because the velopharynx is open during all or part of the vowel production. This is a common pattern of coarticulation in American English, for which vowels can be nasalized without loss of phonemic identity (this does not hold for languages such as French). Disordered or atypical resonance takes four major forms: **hypernasality**, **hyponasality**, **cul-de-sac resonance**, and **phoneme-specific nasal air emission** (as discussed in Chapter 11). However, the auditory-perceptual rating of nasality is clouded with concerns regarding its validity and reliability. Galek and Watterson (2017) concluded that, "the true degree of nasality in a speech sample appears to be capricious and difficult to quantify" (p. 429) and recommended that auditory-perceptual ratings should be accompanied by information derived from other methods, such as nasometry, aerodynamics, velopharyngeal visualization, and description of articulation errors. Here we consider nasometry as an instrumental measure that complements perceptual ratings of nasality.

The goal of nasometry is to measure the size of the velopharyngeal opening, as reflected in the ratio of orally versus nasally radiated energy (an acoustic measure), or the amount of air flowing through the nose (an aerodynamic measure). In the acoustic application, a measure call nasalance compares the magnitudes of the orally and nasally radiated sound energy (Figure 5–7). Nasalance is thought to be an acoustic correlate of perceived nasality, as has been shown in studies of the relationship between nasalance and perceptual ratings of nasality (Liu et al., 2022). The commonly used measure of nasalance is the ratio of acoustic energy at the nares (En) and the acoustic energy at the mouth (Em), as shown in Figure 5–7. This ratio, En/(En + Em), typically is expressed as a percentage, with higher values indicating larger velopharyngeal opening.

Bettens et al. (2018) offered this advice on the assessment of velopharyngeal function: "Certainly, a clinical assessment should include a nasality rating, but clinical management should not be driven exclusively by this perceptual measure. Additional information such as nasalance scores, pressure-flow measurements,

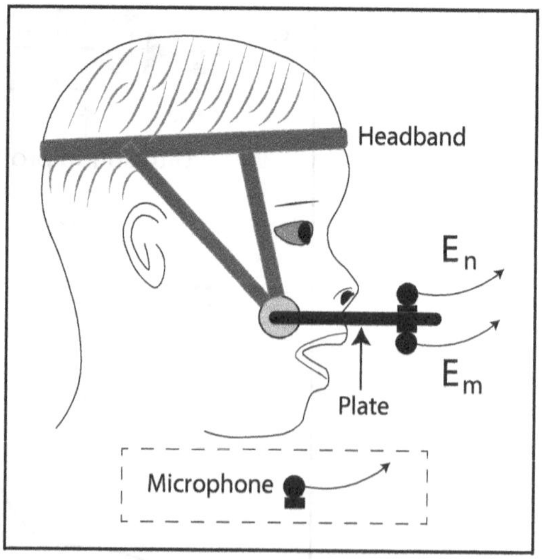

Figure 5–7. Illustration of nasometry device used to derive measures of nasalance. The device records the acoustic energy emitted from the nose (En) and mouth (Em).

velopharyngeal visualization, and the presence, absence, and type of articulation errors should always be factored into treatment decisions" (p. 429).

Aerodynamics

The aerodynamic properties in speech production include air volume, pressure, and flow. The instrumentation needed for aerodynamic assessment is not widely available but is used in specialty clinics such as centers for voice or craniofacial disorders. But a basic knowledge of aerodynamics is important to understanding speech and its disorders. Here we consider air pressure and flow. The three fundamental air pressures are shown in Figure 5–8. Atmospheric air pressure is the reference pressure in the environment. Subglottal air pressure is the pressure measured just below the vocal folds in the larynx and is essentially the same as the pressure in the lungs (called alveolar air pressure). This pressure is the driving force of speech production and typically ranges from about 6 to 10 cmH_2O (i.e., the pressure needed to balance a column of water that is 6 to 10 cm in height). Young children often have higher subglottal air pressures than adults. Intraoral air pressure is the pressure contained within the vocal tract. For voiced sounds, subglottal air pressure is higher than intraoral air pressure because a pressure difference across the vocal folds is needed to sustain vocal fold vibration. For vowels, the intraoral air pressure is equivalent to the atmospheric pressure. For voiced obstruents, intraoral air pressure is less than that for voiceless obstruents because of the pressure drop across the vocal folds. But when the vocal folds are abducted, as in the case of voiceless stops, intraoral air pressure is roughly equal to the subglottal air pressure. In recognition of their increased intraoral air pressure, the voiceless obstruents are called **pressure consonants**. Figure 5–9 illustrates how nasal and airflows can be recorded with an internally divided face mask. The respective flows are directed to a **pneumotachograph**, a device that measures continuous airflow (for details, see Ludlow et al., 2019).

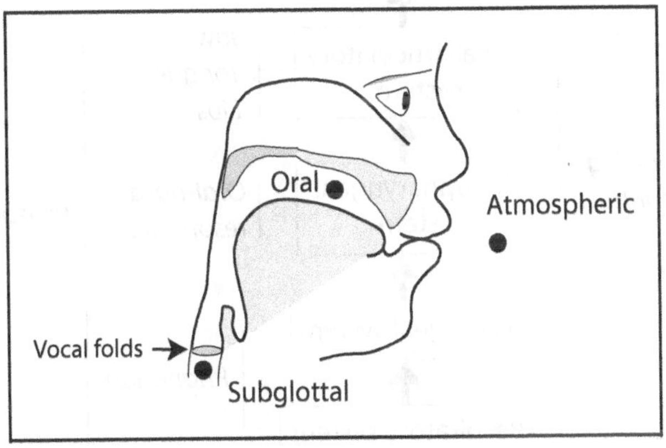

Figure 5–8. Three primary air pressures relevant to speech production: subglottal, oral, and atmospheric.

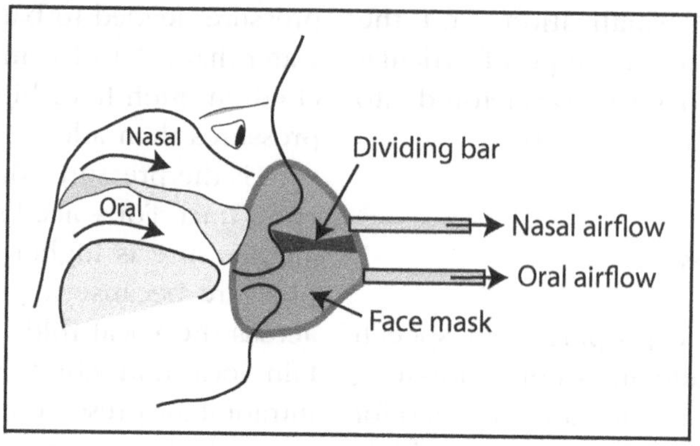

Figure 5–9. Apparatus for measurement of nasal and oral airflow. The face mask has a dividing bar that separates the two airflows.

Systems of Speech Production and Assessment Methods

This section considers various methods of assessment in a systems framework. The basic framework is illustrated in Figure 5–10 and consists of four anatomic-functional systems (respiratory, laryngeal, velopharyngeal, and oral articulatory) along with a global property of prosody that encompasses the other systems. The basic assumption is that each system can be defined in terms of its contribution to speech production using methods suitable to its examination. Figure 5–11 shows how various nonspeech or simplified speech

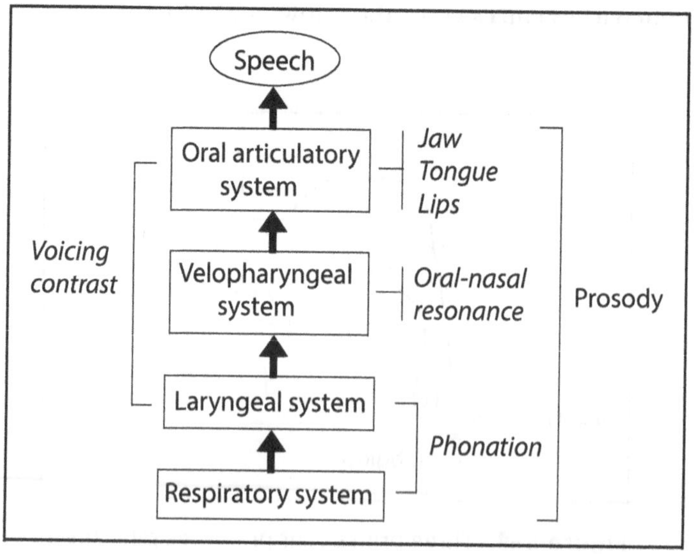

Figure 5–10. Diagram of the speech systems framework, showing the systems (regular font) and selected associated functions (italic font).

tasks relate to the systems framework. The tasks pertain to individual systems or the coordination of two systems. These tasks emphasize basic motor or physiologic functions and are relatively free of linguistic demands. Figure 5–12 illustrates how various instrumental assessments fit into the framework. For example,

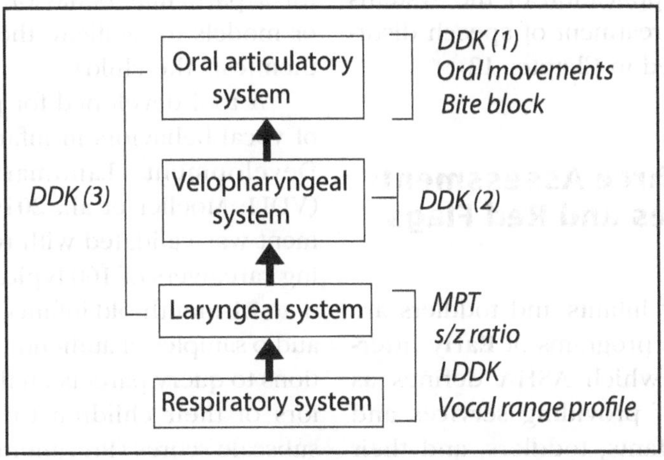

Figure 5–11. Diagram of speech system framework and associated nonspeech or simplified speech measures. DDK(1) = oral diadochokinesis for bilabial, alveolar, and velar consonants, DDK(2) = diadochokinesis for a phonetic sequence that requires velopharyngeal opening and closing (e.g., repetition of the syllable tun), and DDK(3) = diadochokinesis for syllables that vary in initial voicing contrast.

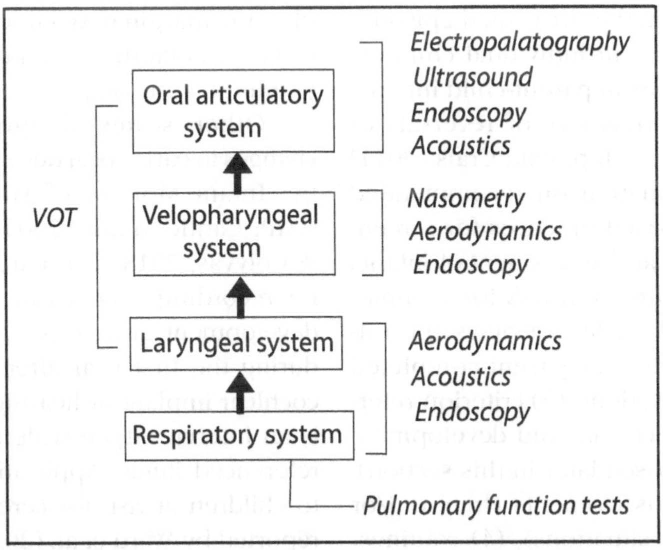

Figure 5–12. Diagram showing speech systems framework (regular font) and associated instrumental assessments (italic font).

velopharyngeal function can be assessed with the methods of nasometry, aerodynamics, and endoscopy. Information from these procedures can complement perceptual ratings of oral/nasal resonance balance. The application of the systems framework to treatment of speech disorders is discussed in Chapter 12.

Birth to Three Assessment: Milestones and Red Flags

Assessments of infants and toddlers are often related to programs of **Early intervention (EI)**, which ASHA defines as "the process of providing services and supports to infants, toddlers, and their families when a child has, or is at risk for, a developmental delay, disability, or health condition that may affect typical development and learning." It is challenging to identify children at risk for speech and language disorders because of the frequent need to use relatively unstructured tasks, the wide variability in typical development, the occasional episodes of rapid progress in individual children, cultural variations in parent-child interaction, and the possibility of reversals or slowdowns in development. Crais (2011) provided information on recommended and evidence-based practices for screening, evaluation, and assessment of infants and toddlers with, or at risk for, communication disorders. She reviews the following methods: (1) parent-completed tools and observations, (2) criterion-referenced (e.g., checklists) and developmental scales (discussed later in this section), (3) play-based assessments (free and/or structured play situations), (4) routines-based assessments (based on a child's participation in family-identified routines and activities), (5) authentic assessments (which gauge a child's functional behaviors using information from persons who interact with the child), and (6) dynamic assessments (in which a clinician tests for a particular behavior, provides cues or models to facilitate the behavior, and then tests the child).

A tool developed for parental report of vocal behaviors in infants is the Vocal Development Landmarks Interview (VDLI; Moeller et al., 2019). This instrument was validated with research involving caregivers of 160 typically developing 6- to 21-month-old infants. The VDLI uses audio samples of authentic infant vocalizations to query parents on the vocal behaviors of their children to produce three subscale scores (Precanonical, Canonical, and Word) and a total score. Scores are derived from 18 items for which the caregiver estimates the frequency of the target behavior on a 4-point Likert scale (never, rarely, sometimes, and frequently). For example, an item from the Canonical subscale is Single canonical syllables, defined as clear well-formed syllable (e.g., /ba, gi, uk/; vs. marginal syllable). The authors estimated that the VDLI takes about 20 to 30 minutes to complete.

Other scales designed to record changes in early vocal development include the Infant Monitor of Vocal Production (IMP; Cantle Moore, 2004; Cantle Moore & Colyvas, 2018) is a parent-report scale for recording changes in the early vocal development of infants with hearing loss during the first year after they receive a cochlear implant or hearing aids. The IMP is an interview-type scale of 16 criterion-referenced items. Application of the IMP to children at risk for cerebral palsy was reported by Ward et al. (2022), who found that infants identified as at-risk of cerebral palsy did not differ from age-matched peers at 6 months, but did differ at 9 and 12 months when pre-canonical and canonical babble typically appear.

Developmental milestones in communicative behavior are an important standard in clinical assessment, and these milestones have been used to identify red flags that identify children at risk for communication disorders. However, sources differ on specific milestones and the typical ages associated with them. Some examples of milestones related to speech development are compiled in Table 4–1. Among the milestones commonly recognized are the onset of babbling (at 6 to 9 months), first words (about 1 year), use of 2-word phrases (15 to18 months), and a vocabulary of 50 words (about 2 years). Red flags usually are defined as delays in reaching developmental milestones. However, red flags vary across sources. Some examples are given in Table 5–4. The recently revised CDC milestones (https://www.cdc.gov/ncbddd/actearly/milestones/index.html) do not concur in all respects with other sources and have come under criticism because they may be too lax to identify some children who are at risk.

Red flags also have been described for specific disorders, such as CAS and autism spectrum disorder. Overby et al. (2019) concluded that infants and toddlers later diagnosed with CAS were less voluble, used fewer resonant consonants (defined as phones that could be transcribed with the IPA), had a less diverse phonetic repertoire, and had delayed acquisition of resonant consonants compared to other groups in their study. Overby et al. (2020) found that infants later identified with CAS have a reduced production of canonical babbles, a later onset of canonical babbling, and reduced production of syllables per minute (reduced volubility). The authors suggested that infants with CAS may have deficiencies in vocal exploration and the production of canonical babbles, possibly due to reduced opportunities to map articulatory movements with auditory speech patterns. These features may be early indicators of problems in later speech development in CAS, such as the factors of atypical prosody, coarticulation, and consistency (Chenausky et al., 2020). With respect to autism spectrum disorder, reports indicate that children later diagnosed with this condition manifest atypical vocal behaviors in the first year of life (McDaniel et al., 2019; Roche et al., 2018; Yankowitz et al., 2019).

Table 5–4. Red Flags or Milestone References for Communication Development as Listed in Different Sources

Age in months	CDC (2022) Milestones for Red Flags	Feldman (2019) Red Flags	ASHA (2022) Red Flags
6	Takes turns making sounds with you. Blows "raspberries" (sticks tongue out and blows). Makes squealing noises.	Lack of ability to laugh, vocalize, respond to sound, participate in reciprocal vocal interactions.	Not babbling between 4 to 7 months.
9	Makes a lot of different sounds like "mamamama" and "babababababa." Lifts arms up to be picked up.	Failure to respond differentially to name or produce babble (such as baba, dada).	Making only a few sounds. Not using gestures, like waving or pointing (7 to 12 months).
12	Waves "bye-bye." Calls a parent "mama" or "dada" or another special name. Understands "no" (pauses briefly or stops when you say it).	Inability to point to objects or actions. Lack of use of gestures, such as shaking head "no." Inability to participate in verbal routines, such ability to wave to "wave bye-bye." No use of mama or dada specifically for a parent.	Saying only a few words (12 to 18 months).
15	Tries to say one or two words besides "mama" or "dada," like "ba" for ball or "da" for dog. Looks at a familiar object when you name it. Follows directions given with both a gesture and words. For example, he gives you a toy when you hold out your hand and say, "Give me the toy." Points to ask for something or to get help.		
18	Tries to say three or more words besides "mama" or "dada" Follows one-step directions without any gestures, like giving you the toy when you say, "Give it to me."	Less than 5 words beyond mama and dada. Failure to follow simple commands with gestures.	Not putting 2 words together (18 to 24 months).

Table 5–4. *continued*

Age in months	CDC (2022) Milestones for Red Flags	Feldman (2019) Red Flags	ASHA (2022) Red Flags
24	Points to things in a book when you ask, like "Where is the bear?" Says at least two words together, like "More milk." Points to at least two body parts when you ask him to show you. Uses more gestures than just waving and pointing, like blowing a kiss or nodding yes.	Vocabulary less than 50 words. No two-word combinations. <50% of utterances intelligible to unfamiliar adults.	Saying fewer than 50 words.
30	Says about 50 words. Says two or more words together, with one action word, like "Doggie run." Names things in a book when you point and ask, "What is this?" Says words like "I," "me," or "we."		
36	Talks with you in conversation using at least two back-and-forth exchanges. Asks "who," "what," "where," or "why" questions, like "Where is mommy/daddy?" Says what action is happening in a picture or book when asked, like "running," "eating," or "playing." Says first name, when asked. Talks well enough for others to understand, most of the time.	Inability to follow simple directions without gestures. No three-or-more word combinations. <75% of utterances intelligible to unfamiliar adults.	

Conclusions

1. This chapter covers an array of assessment methods, some of which are used almost routinely, others for specific purposes. For the most part, these methods require only the eyes and ears of the clinician, so that instruments are not needed. Furthermore, these methods can be used for a wide variety of clients, including those with comorbid conditions and those at different levels of development, including birth-to-three, toddlers, preschoolers, and school-aged.
2. Clinical decision making considers the purposes of the assessment and the relative value of available methods to ensure efficiency, economy, and effectiveness. Screening tests are typically brief and intended to discover if a problem exists. If a problem is identified, other tests are selected to reveal its nature and severity. A general caveat is that many of the commonly used assessments are not standardized in method and do not have adequate normative data to support confident clinical interpretation.
3. Available tests differ in several properties, including standardization, availability of normative data, and ease of administration.
4. Information obtained by a clinician's eyes and ears can be extended and enhanced by instrumental methods, which are increasingly adapted for use with children, and which create new opportunities for the examination of oral and other functions.
5. Developmental milestones for speech development give guidelines for assessing speech disorders in children.

6

ASSESSMENT OF VOICE AND PROSODY

Voice and prosody are intimately linked and are, therefore, discussed together in this chapter. Although aspects of prosody can be produced in whispered (unvoiced) speech, most descriptions of prosody rely on tasks and measures related to voiced speech (i.e., speech produced with voicing energy from the larynx that may be interrupted for voiceless segments). For example, **intonation** (the melody of voice) generally is described in terms of changes in voice pitch or its acoustic correlate, vocal fundamental frequency (f_0). Voice quality is a component of some systems of prosodic description, which compels consideration of voice in the expression of prosody. A voice quality disorder may contribute to a prosodic disorder, which may make it necessary to assess voice as part of the examination and description of a prosodic disorder. In addition, prosody can be used to design therapies for voice disorders (McCabe & Altman, 2017). Chapter 2 summarizes the typical development of laryngeal anatomy and physiology, concluding that the phonatory system has a long developmental trajectory that extends to late adolescence, especially in males. The development of prosody in children should be understood in part with reference to the anatomic and functional properties of the developing larynx.

For the purposes of this chapter, **voice** (or phonation) is defined as the production of sound by vibration of the vocal folds in the larynx. Such vibration results from an air pressure differential across the folds. In typical egressive (outflowing) airflow, the air pressure below the folds is greater than that above the folds, which induces transglottal airflow. Phonation is one of the earliest voluntary behaviors in human development, appearing in the birth cry and continuing into patterns of infant vocalization and eventually articulate speech. In connected speech, such as ordinary conversation, voicing is interrupted for voiceless sounds or for pauses, but an overall contour of pitch variation gives prosodic coherence to phrases and sentences. This coherence is described as an **intonation contour**, **pitch contour**, or **pitch pattern**. **Prosody** is a general term for the rhythm and melody of speech, usually conveyed by variations in the four dimensions of f_0, duration, intensity, and voice quality. In voiced speech, these factors relate largely, but not exclusively, to properties of phonation (i.e., laryngeal function). In classic **source-filter theory**, voice is the sound source, and the resonances of the vocal tract are the filter (Figure 6–1). The general, simplified version of this theory assumes that source and filter are independent, but it is well established that they interact in some respects (Childers & Wong, 1994). The larynx, in cooperation with the respiratory system, determines f_0, vocal intensity, and voice quality (except for oral-nasal resonance balance). These same dimensions are relevant to the classification and description of voice disorders.

Voice

This section discusses aspects of voice from a developmental perspective, with the goal of identifying changes related to gender and age in individuals under the age of 18 years. The information presented is fundamental to the understanding of system interactions in typical speech development, the assessment and treatment of dysphonia (voice disorders) in children, and the development and use of prosody. We begin with a general summary of information on pitch and f_0 followed by comments on voice quality and conclude with a review of data obtained with instrumental methods. Chapter 2 reviewed aspects of laryngeal development that are fundamental to understanding how voice changes with maturation and how it differs between boys and girls.

Vocal Pitch and f_0

Figure 6–2 shows that mean f_0 decreases with age in both boys and girls but espe-

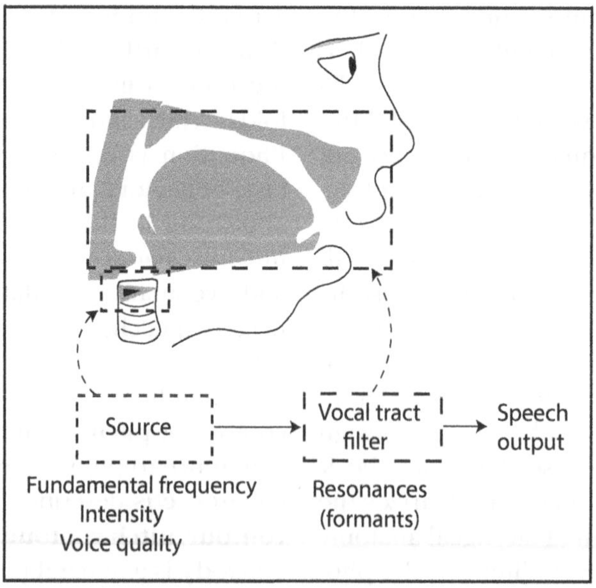

Figure 6–1. Source-filter model of speech production for vowels. The vocal folds in the larynx are the energy source and the resonances (formants) of the vocal tract are the filter function.

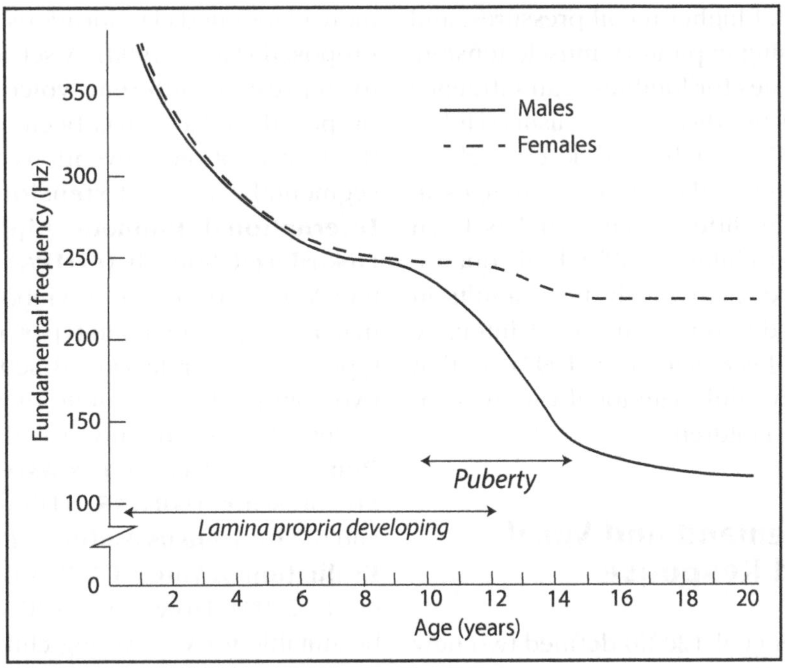

Figure 6–2. The mean fundamental frequency (f_0) of the voice from infancy to young adulthood. The values for males and females are similar until about 10 years of age, after which males have a sharp decrease.

cially for the former, beginning at the age of puberty. Before puberty, sex differences in f_0 are small and inconsistent across studies. After puberty, sex differences become large, perhaps the largest sexual dimorphism in human biology (Paus et al., 2017; Rendall et al., 1995). A speaker's vocal pitch is a primary cue that listeners use to reach decisions about the sex and age of the person who is speaking. Other developmental changes in phonation affect loudness and voice quality, as considered next.

Loudness and Vocal Effort

Loudness is an aspect of voice and prosody. It is a perceptual judgment of the magnitude of an auditory stimulus that can be expressed on a continuum from weak to strong, or soft to loud. The primary acoustic correlate of loudness is the intensity of a sound. Loudness is related to **vocal effort**, which is a multidimensional concept that enfolds different perspectives including external perception of effort with a physiological component, the experience of vocal effort, psychological effort, effort as a speech production level, and effort in terms of the communication environment conditions. E. J. Hunter et al. (2020) review the literature on vocal effort. In common use, vocal effort is defined in terms of vocal loudness and strain in voicing, so that increased effort is realized as greater loudness and/or greater strain. Speaking louder requires increased subglottal pressure, which usually is achieved in either of two major ways: (1) beginning speech at a higher lung volume, which takes advantage of higher recoil pressures, and (2) increasing expiratory muscle tension. Different cues for loudness can influence how adults use these mechanisms (Huber et al., 2005), but little is known about how children make loudness changes in response to different cues. It has been shown that children differ both quantitatively and qualitatively from adults in achieving differences in vocal intensity (Stathopoulos & Sapienza, 1993), so that results from adults cannot always be generalized to children.

Vocal Demand and Vocal Demand Response

E. J. Hunter et al. (2020) defined two new terms pertaining to use of the voice. **Vocal demand** is the vocal requirement for a given communication scenario, which is independent of the person's physiology, production technique, or perception of the scenario. **Vocal demand response** is the vocal behavior that an individual uses to respond to a perceived "vocal demand" within a communication scenario. Individuals vary in their response to specific vocal demands, and the difference in response may relate to vocal effort and vocal fatigue.

Voice Quality

Voice quality has been defined variously, but there is general agreement that it is a multidimensional perceptual attribute of voice independent of vocal pitch or loudness (Barsties & De Bodt, 2015; N. Campbell & Mokhtari, 2003; Keller, 1994; Kreiman et al., 1993). Some voice qualities that are frequently mentioned are modal, breathy, and creaky; however more elaborated classifications have been proposed (Laver, 1980). A set of symbols to represent different voice qualities proposed by Laver has been adapted to the transcription conventions for suprasegmentals in the **Extensions to the International Phonetic Alphabet for Disordered Speech (extIPA)**. This system, VoQS, arranges the symbols in three major groups: airstream types, phonation types, and supralaryngeal settings. The two commonly used auditory-perceptual scales of voice quality are the **Grade, Roughness, Breathiness, Asthenia, and Strain scale (GRBAS)** (Hirano, 1981) and the **Consensus Auditory-Perceptual Evaluation of Voice (CAPE-V)** (Kempster et al., 2009). However, CAPE-V may not be suitable for very young children, who may have difficulty producing some of the sentence material (R. B. Fujiki & Thibeault, 2021).

Voice Disorders in Children

McAllister and Sjölander (2013) reviewed data on voice quality and voice disorders in children. Some of their conclusions are as follows. Perceptual assessments of voice quality in children indicate sex differences, with boys tending to have more hyperfunctional features such as **muscle tension dysphonia** (excessive activity of the muscles and joints of the vocal mechanism) than girls and with girls having more **breathiness** (excessive air loss during phonation). Risk factors for childhood dysphonia are having older siblings, male gender, and lengthy participation in large groups. After puberty, voice disorders are more prevalent in females than males. The reasons are not entirely clear, but one possibility is that the higher fundamental frequencies of the female voice result in more trauma-inducing collisions of the vocal fold tissues. **Phonotrauma** is the term for voice use patterns that result in traumatic tissue changes of the vocal folds, such as nodules, polyps, contact ulcers, or thickening of the vocal folds. The injury can arise from excessive force in adducting the vocal folds, as may occur with frequent use of a loud voice. Phonotrauma is now preferred over terms such as vocal abuse or vocal misuse, which can carry a stigma, such as implying intentional self-harm.

The prevalence of voice disorders in children is unclear because studies are not in close agreement, with rates ranging from a low of 1.4% (Bhattacharyya, 2015) to a high of 6% (Carding et al., 2006). Voice disorders may co-occur with other communication disorders, so that voice may need to be considered in both clinical assessment and treatment of speech disorders in children and adults (St. Louis et al., 1992). Wertzner et al. (2022) reported that children with SSD had lower relative f_0 values and greater open quotient values than children without SSD. These results were interpreted to reflect inadequate f_0 adjustments to maintain voicing and less efficient voicing. Another challenge is to distinguish voice disorders from typical variations in vocal function. Murray and Chao (2021) comment that mild to moderate dysphonia may be present in children who do not have a diagnosed voice disorder, indicating that dysphonia in children is not necessarily a sign of a voice disorder per se, but rather an indication that typical laryngeal development involves transient periods of mild to moderate dysphonia.

In addition to auditory-perceptual ratings, the commonly used clinical assessments are voice handicap or voice quality-of-life rating scales and endoscopy (Campano et al., 2021; Kelchner et al., 2012), which are reviewed later in this chapter.

> Risk factors for childhood voice disorder before puberty are having older siblings, male gender, and lengthy participation in large groups. But voice disorder becomes more frequent in females than males after puberty.

Acoustic Studies

These studies reveal effects related to both age and sex. Several acoustic parameters, in addition to mean f_0, have been introduced for the study of voice for both research and clinical purposes. Most of the published data are for adults, but information on children's voices is accumulating. Different software systems and algorithms are used in voice analysis, but among the most frequently used are the Multidimensional Voice Program (MDVP™) and the Analysis of Dysphonia in Speech and Voice (ADSV™), both from Pentax Medical. Kent, Eichhorn, and Vorperian (2021) compiled MDVP and ADSV data from 12 published sources on healthy voice in children and reported additional data for 158 children with healthy voices. Acoustic parameters that decreased with age in both boys and girls were as follows: mean f_0, f_0 variability, jitter, pitch perturbation quotient, standard deviation of the low/high spectral ratio, sex-appropriate CSID, and degree of sub-harmonic breaks. Parameters with values that increased with age in both sexes were the standard deviation of CPP and the low/high ratio. A general implication of these results is that vocal behavior becomes more consistent and efficient with maturation. An important caveat is that some parameters, such as sex-appropriate CSID are based on criteria developed for adults and are not necessarily suited to children's voices. In a review of studies of children's voice, de Almeida Ramos, Souza, and Gama (2017) concluded that the acoustic measures of pitch perturbation quotient (PPQ), amplitude perturbation quotient (APQ) and the noise measures, such as NHN, change little with age in typically developing children. More consistent age-related changes are observed in mean f_0, f_0 variability, and degree of subharmonic breaks (Kent, Eichhorn, et al., 2021).

R. B. Fujiki and Thibeault (2021) studied the relationship between auditory-perceptual rating scales and objective voice measures in children aged 2.5 to 17.8 years with voice disorders. They concluded that the CAPE-V and GRBAS scales have concurrent validity but that CAPE-V ratings were more strongly correlated with acoustic and aerodynamic voice measures. They reported that the strongest correlations were between auditory-perceptual ratings of overall severity, breathiness, and strain, as well as acoustic measures of perturbation, fundamental frequency, and maximum phonation time. These results may help to design efficient and informative clinical assessments using a combination of auditory-perceptual ratings and instrumental measures.

Aerodynamic Studies

These studies have shown significant age-sex differences in several variables, including expiratory volume, expiratory airflow duration, phonation time, pitch range, and aerodynamic resistance (Weinrich et al., 2013). A measure that shows relatively consistent variations with age and sex is **laryngeal resistance (R_L)**, which is defined as the as subglottal air pressure divided by translaryngeal airflow (measurement units of $cmH_2O/L/s$) during vowel phonation. Values of R_L are shown in Table 6–1 for females and males in different age groups. The data reported for adult females by Netsell et al. (1994) differ somewhat from those reported in other studies. For example, Hoit and Hixon (1992) reported a mean value of 52 $cmH_2O/L/s$ for women aged 25 to 85 years. The values for children are considerably larger than those for adults, presumably because of differences in size and tissue properties. The significance of aerodynamic resistance in voice disorders is not clear. R. B. Fujiki and Thibeault

Table 6–1. Laryngeal Resistance in $cmH_2O/L/s$ for Females and Males in Several Age Groups

	Sex	3 to 5 yrs.	6 to 9 yrs.	9 to 12 yrs.	10 to 13 yrs.	14 to 17 yrs.	Adult
Netsell et al. (1994)	F	111 to 120	89 to 101	59 to 68	—	—	40
	M	117 to 120	91 to 99	65 to 77	—	—	34
Weinrich et al. (2013)	F	—	92.8	—	63	46.7	—
	M	—	75	—	52	40	—

(2021) found that of the various voice measures examined in their study, aerodynamic resistance was the only measure that was not correlated with any auditory-perceptual rating in either the GRBAS or CAPE-V rating scales.

Endoscopy

Endoscopy literally means "looking inside" and is performed with an instrument called an **endoscope** that permits visualization of internal cavities or structures such as the vocal tract, larynx, or velopharynx. The typical endoscope consists of a long, thin tube (either flexible or rigid) that is equipped with a light source and a video camera. Flexible endoscopes usually are preferable to rigid endoscopes for assessments of speech, voice, and swallowing, as they are easier to use and provide better comfort to the person being examined. The instrument is often inserted through the nasal passages and is, therefore, termed a **nasoendoscope**. As the tip of the tube approaches the area of interest, the image is transmitted to the camera to be viewed by the examiner. Instruments of the most recent design have a camera in the tip of the scope and have the capability of providing images of high quality of the larynx that are equivalent to, or better than, a rigid scope. Endoscopy has been used successfully with children as young as 1.7 years of age (R. R. Patel, 2018), but its use can be compromised by short phonation times or gag reflex (Wolf et al., 2005).

Voice Handicap and Voice Quality-of-Life

Commonly used clinical assessments are **voice handicap** or **voice quality-of-life** rating scales (Campano et al., 2021; Kelchner et al., 2012). The Voice Handicap Index (VHI; Jacobson et al., 1997) is a self-assessment instrument consisting of 30 statements that are scored on a Likert scale ranging from 0 to 4. It is designed to determine the severity of a voice disorder in the emotional, physical, and functional domains. A shorter version composed of only 10 statements is the Voice Handicap Index-10 (VHI-10; Rosen et al., 2004). Rating scales also have been developed for use with the pediatric population. The Pediatric Voice Outcome Survey (PVOS, Hartnick, 2002) is a four-item parental proxy questionnaire that aims to assess voice-related quality of life. The parent rates the child's speaking voice, strain, limitation in social environment, and limitations in a noisy environment. The Pediatric Voice-Related Quality-of-Life Survey (PVRQOL; Boseley et al., 2006) is a 10-item instrument adapted from the adult VRQOL instrument (Hogikyan & Sethuraman, 1999). Items in the pediatric version were structured to reflect parent proxy administration rather than self-administration. The Pediatric Voice Handicap Index (pVHI), which was derived from items in the adult Voice Handicap Index (VHI), consists of 23 items rated by the parent or other caregiver (Zur et al., 2007).

Prosody

Because prosody is for the most part expressed over sequences of words and syllables, the relevant motor control processes are aligned with phonetic, syntactic, and pragmatic variables. Wagner and Watson (2010) stated that the two aspects of prosodic phrasing (a grouping of words defined by boundaries) and prosodic prominence (the perceptual salience of a word in its context) "are influenced by linguistic factors such as syntactic constituent structure, semantic relations, phonological rhythm, pragmatic considerations, and also by processing factors such as the length, complexity, or predictability of linguistic material" (p. 905). Similarly, Speer and Ito (2009) commented that prosody "conveys a wide range of information from speaker to hearer, including the speaker's affect, illocutionary force, linguistic pragmatic intent (such as emphatic or corrective contrast), and grammatical structure, such as the location of syntactic phrasal boundaries and word boundaries" (p. 90). They went on to note that prosody provides a rhythmic scaffolding that marks important temporal locations in the speech signal. This scaffolding guides the interpretation of spoken messages and is a source of information not contained in the linguistic message itself.

Prosody entails a diverse set of issues that are being addressed in interdisciplinary research involving fields such as linguistics, psychology, neuroscience, and computer science. As Xu (2011) pointed out, a major difficulty in the study of prosody is "the lack of reference problem." That is, other than punctuation marks, orthographic representations of speech usually convey very little about prosody. Such representations are devoid of properties such as emotion, stress pattern, and speaking rate. Cole (2015) comments that prosodic annotations are usually done by experts who are trained in the use of a specific transcription method, and that transcription is difficult and tedious. This chapter highlights aspects of prosody that are most relevant to understanding speech development and its disorders.

Another name for prosody is **suprasegmental**, meaning that the variables of interest transcend individual phonetic segments. However, this does not mean that prosody and segments are completely independent. As discussed later in this chapter, prosody has effects on the segmental structure of speech. American English is considered a **stress (or stress-timed) language** in that its rhythm is determined by the opposition between strong (S) and weak (W) syllables, so that the intervals of S and W syllables are roughly constant. The S-W pattern is evident in words such as *American*, *notify*, *elaborate*, and *adjudicate*. Many words in American English can be described in terms of S-W stress patterns across words. In contrast, a **syllable-timed language** has a speech rhythm with relatively constant syllable durations. One feature of syllable-timed languages is the lack of reduced vowels. Languages commonly considered to be syllable-timed include Brazilian Portuguese, Cantonese, French, Italian, Mandarin Chinese, and Spanish. But it cannot be assumed that patterns of stress and syllable durations are straightforward and uncontroversial. As Temperley (2009) summarized the matter, "Stress has been widely studied from both experimental and theoretical perspectives, and has proven to be a subtle and complex linguistic phenomenon" (p. 75).

Languages can be divided into **tonal** and **non-tonal**, depending on whether tone is used to distinguish phonemes or words. Chinese is a tonal language, and English is a non-tonal language. In Mandarin Chinese the same sounds, as transcribed with the IPA, can be pronounced with different tones that change the meaning. For example, a sound sequence can be produced with a rising tone, a falling tone, or a flat tone, which describe different f_0 contours. English is non-tonal language because meaning is not conveyed by differences in tone. However, tone may be used for other purposes, such as expressing a speaker's emotional state. English is in the category of languages that are stress-timed and non-tonal.

Prosody usually is described in association with units that are larger than phonetic segments, units such as intonational phrases, tone units, and syllables. An **intonational phrase** is a phonological unit that (a) is the largest phonological unit into which an utterance can be divided, (b) has an intonational structure including a single most prominent point (the nucleus), and (c) it aligns with syntactic and discourse structure. A **tone unit** is the minimal unit that can carry intonation and can be as short as a single syllable but usually extends over a few syllables. The most prominent syllable in a tone unit is called the tonic syllable.

A **syllable** is an intuitive concept of a unit in speech that explains perceived linkages within a sequence of phonetic segments. Defining a syllable in perceptual, acoustic, or physiologic terms is exceedingly difficult and often runs into contradictions. Nonetheless, the concept of syllable is sufficiently useful that it is nearly ubiquitous in writings on language, and, as mentioned in various places in this book, the syllable is prominent in accounts of the perception and production of speech. The structure of a syllable is illustrated in Figure 6–3. From a structural perspective, a syllable can be defined as "a unit of speech consisting of one vowel or vowel-like element (e.g., a syllabic consonant) that may be accompanied by surrounding consonants and is used to construct words" (Shriberg et al., 2019, p. 11). Syllables are useful for many purposes, including descriptions of coarticulation, speech development, patterns of speech sound errors, and speech perception.

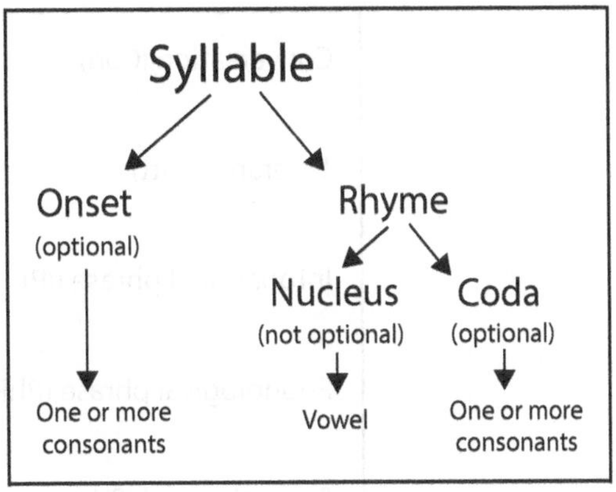

Figure 6–3. The structure of the syllable.

A hierarchy of prosody is shown in Figure 6–4, beginning with conversation at the highest level and progressively descending to the lowest level of strong and weak syllables that compose words. This hierarchy is based on the work of linguists such as Nespor and Vogel (1986) and Selkirk (1980, 1995). The basic terminology is defined as follows. Conversation, or oral communication between two people (a conversational dyad), is shaped by phenomena such as turn-taking and entrainment. **Turn-taking** in conversation and discourse is where the participants speak one at a time in alternating turns, often signaling the end of a turn with prosodic phenomena such as a pause or falling or flat intonation. **Prosodic entrainment** occurs when individuals participating in a conversation adjust their prosodic features to match one another. This adjustment is one way in which speakers establish an interactive and supportive communication, often called rapport. Such prosodic signaling can be subtle but is nonetheless influential. Conversational interactions are the context for emotional, cognitive, and social aspects of development (Hughes & de Rosnay 2006). An **utterance** is a group

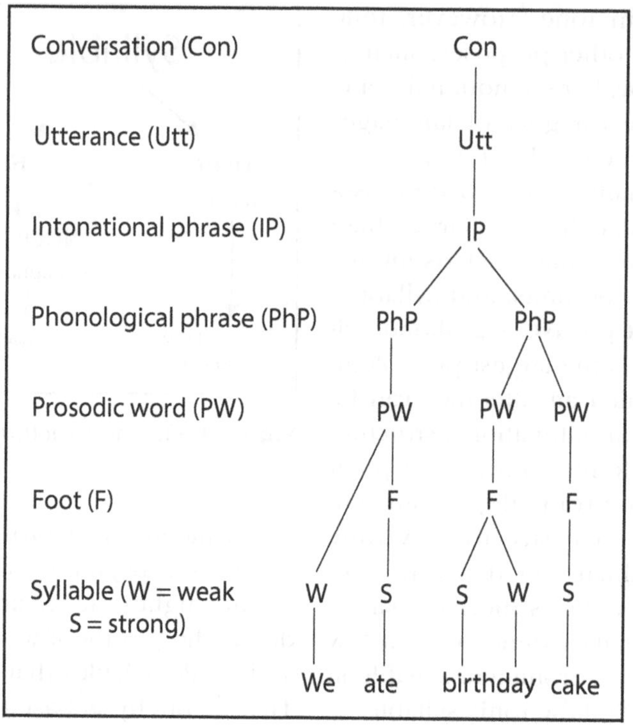

Figure 6–4. The prosody hierarchy that is often used in linguistics.

of words produced on a single exhalation and exhibiting a prosodic coherence in intonation and rhythm. It frequently corresponds to a sentence in linguistic terminology. The **intonational phrase**, as defined earlier, is the largest phonological unit into which an utterance can be divided, has an intonational structure, including a single most prominent point, and aligns with syntactic and discourse structure. The **phonological phrase** corresponds to sub-clausal noun-, verb-, and adjective-phrases in syntax and combines words and clitic groups into a single prosodic unit. The **prosodic word** carries morphological information relating to syllabification and stress placement. Prosodic words can be preceded or followed by pauses in conversation. Words are composed of a rhythmic unit called a **foot**, which represents the rhythmic structure of the word and is the unit used to describe stress patterns. A foot consists of one or more syllables and has one syllable that is more prominent than the other syllable(s) and is called the **strong (S) syllable**. It is also called the **head of the syllable**. Other syllables in the foot are **weak (W) syllables**. As noted earlier in this chapter, many words in English have alternating patterns of strong and weak syllables.

The hierarchical structure displayed in Figure 6–4 creates a rather daunting challenge for a child acquiring spoken language (and for those of us trying to understand speech development). It is not clear how a child learns the complicated framework of prosody. Tilsen (2016) proposed a means of discovery based on articulatory processes. He notes that research on speech motor control distinguishes between a mechanism that selects the movements to produce and a mechanism that controls the precise timing of movement execution. In his model, these mechanisms are called selection and coordination, respectively. Selection involves competitive control that chooses a motor plan or a set of plans from a set of alternatives, with feedback used to govern selection and deselection. Tilsen cites Lashley (1951), who theorized that representations of actions in a sequence to be performed are active in parallel before and during the production of the sequence, so that a control mechanism selects the actions in the appropriate order. Coordination complements the selection mechanism by specifying how multiple movements needed for the sequence can be performed in a precisely timed, overlapping manner. A child learning to talk deploys both mechanisms to achieve the essential operations of selecting a motor plan and executing it with the requisite accuracy.

As shown in Figure 6–5, if the phonetic segments are removed from a speech message, the remaining properties of f_0,

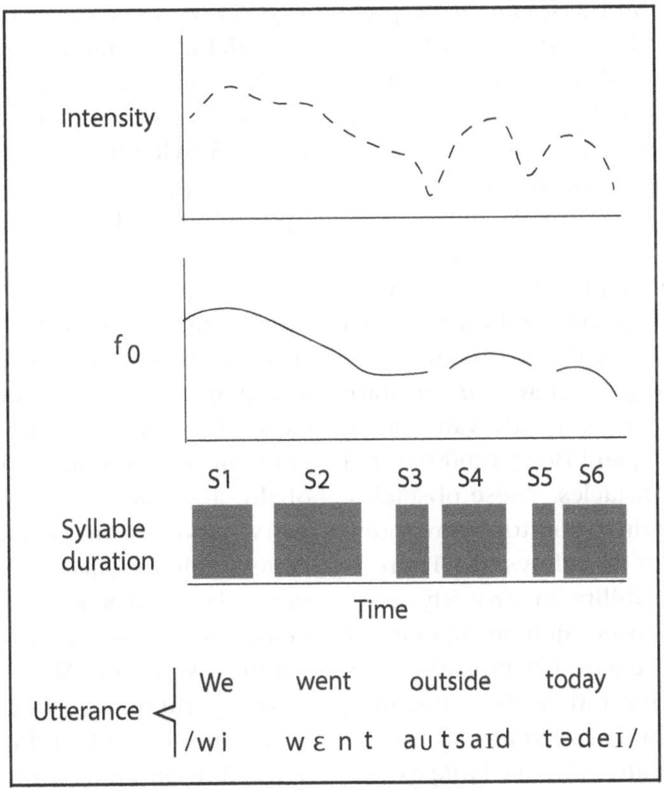

Figure 6–5. A schematic representation of the major acoustic dimensions of prosody: intensity, fundamental frequency, and duration.

intensity, and syllable duration remain in what might be considered as the prosodic skeleton of the utterance, neglecting for the moment the influence of voice quality as a fourth dimension (Campbell & Mokhtari, 2003). Prosody has been conceptualized and analyzed in different ways, and the discussion here is selective rather than exhaustive of the different approaches. In addition, various theories have been proposed to account for prosodic development in children (Kehoe & Stoel-Gammon, 1997). But the common basis of these theories is that prosody is expressed in four major ways: f_0 contour, duration, intensity, and voice quality, all of which can be studied with perceptual and acoustic methods. Peppé (2009) noted that the study and assessment of prosody is difficult because of problems in (a) isolating prosody from other domains of communication, (b) defining the relationship between prosodic phonology and atypical prosody, and (c) methods for transcription and assessment. Peppé's article is a landmark in that it illuminates several aspects of prosody in both typical and atypical speech, and it provides a framework for clinical assessment.

In discussing the potential for automated assessment of prosody, van Santen, Prud'hommeaux, and Black (2009) noted three general obstacles. These obstacles, which also pertain to auditory-perceptual assessments, are as follows. (1) There is substantial variability in prosody associated with factors such as dialect or individual differences. (2) Prosodic cues often are relative rather than absolute. For example, the cue of duration for the lexical stress status of a syllable is not associated with absolute duration but, rather, the duration in relation to speaking rate, the phonetic composition of the syllable, and the location of the syllable in the word and phrase. (3) Prosodic contrasts typically involve multiple acoustic features, such as a combination of duration, pitch, energy, and spectral balance, and the combination may differ across speakers. These factors complicate efforts to arrive at algorithmic methods for prosody assessment and they also explain the difficulty in designing a general-purpose clinical assessment.

Speech Rhythm

Speech rhythm is the temporal pattern of perceived or produced events in the speech signal. At the most basic level, the rhythm of speech is defined by the rate of syllable production, which usually is in the range of 3 to 8 syllables/s across languages, with a peak or modal rate of about 5 syllables/s (Oganian & Chang, 2019; Poeppel & Assaneo, 2020). This rate appears to be determined by the natural movement frequencies of the articulators and laryngeal structures (Peelle & Davis, 2012) and accords with the typical rate of diadochokinesis (Kent et al., 2022) as well as the optimal rate of speech comprehension (Ahissar et al., 2001). Speech rhythm is manifest in the amplitude modulation of the acoustic signal, in which the primary modulation corresponds to syllables. This modulation in adult conversational speech is not necessarily periodic in the sense of a metronome or other simple oscillator. Most approaches to studying rhythm go beyond periodicity of the simple kind, and rhythm has been defined in different ways. Turk and Shattuck-Hufnagel (2013, p. 95) commented that the definitions differ as to "whether rhythm (1) includes some aspect of periodicity in timing, (2) refers to abstract structurings of time, based on serial ordering, that reflect grouping and prominence structure, and/or (3) refers to systematic surface timing patterns determined by grouping and prominence structure as well as other factors."

Various metrics have been proposed for the study of speech rhythm, including the following (Arvaniti, 2012; Liss et al., 2009; Ramus et al., 1999):

- ΔC—the standard deviation of consonantal intervals in an utterance.
- %V—the percentage of the utterance duration taken up by vocalic intervals.
- Pairwise Variability Index (PVI)—the sum of the absolute differences between pairs of consecutive intervals (either vocalic or consonantal) divided by the number of pairs in the speech sample.
- VarcoV—standard deviation of vocalic intervals divided by the mean vocalic duration (× 100).
- VarcoC—standard deviation of consonantal intervals divided by the mean consonantal duration (× 100).
- VarcoCV—standard deviation of vocalic + consonantal intervals divided by the mean vocalic + consonantal duration (× 100).

Evidence that atypical rhythm relates to disorders of spoken language comes from studies of both children and adults. With respect to children, Ladányi et al. (2020) regarded atypical rhythm as an underlying risk factor that shares biological bases with, and may lead to, co-morbid impairments in speech and language. This formulation, called the **Atypical Rhythm Risk Hypothesis**, is grounded in the definition of atypical rhythm as a general construct covering phenomena such as impaired sensitivity to rhythm/beat/meter sensitivity, weak skills related to rhythm ability, poor dynamic attending, beat deafness, and time-based amusia. As for adults, Liss et al. (2009) concluded that rhythm metrics, mentioned earlier, can distinguish dysarthric speech from healthy speech and can discriminate among dysarthria subtypes. They also pointed out that calculation of the rhythm metrics is relatively easy and requires only a small corpus of speech material (about five sentences). However, some limitations of rhythm metrics should be noted. Arvaniti (2012) cautioned that metric scores can range substantially within a language and are influenced by methodological decisions.

Phonetic Effects of Prosody

Although prosody usually is considered in terms of variables that have effects across segments (hence suprasegmental), it also has effects on individual segments. These phonetic effects are manifest in durations, articulatory forces, spectral features, and other aspects. P. Keating (1992) wrote, "when a speaker plans for the phonetic aspects of speech production, prosodic structure organizes the treatment of possibly every feature in every segment, and the interactions of segments" (p. 122). She proposed that the interaction can be understood in large part in terms of the strength of a prosodic position and the phonetic strength of a segment in that position. Such strengthening occurs at the level of articulation, which becomes stronger or more extreme.

Many studies attest to the phonetic effects of the prosodic variables of prominence, phrasing, and surprisal (predictability). **Prominence** is the level of stress, emphasis, or focus on a syllable or word. Prominent syllables show alterations in the properties of both vowels and consonants. For example, vowels that are perceived as prominent have higher F1 frequencies and front vowels tend to be hyperarticulated (Mo et al., 2009). De Jong (1995) concluded from an x-ray microbeam study that prominence is associated with localized hyperarticulation to create increased contrastivity. These findings support the model of the **supralaryngeal implementation of prominence**, which holds that prominence affects the positions and movements of the supralaryngeal structures. **Phrasing** is the chunking or organization of a grouping of syllables or words. Phrasing is often, but not necessarily aligned with syntactic or word boundaries in an utterance. One of the most studied phenomena is **phrase-final lengthening**, in which elements at the end of constituent phrases have greater durations than those in the middle of phrases (Shattuck-Hufnagel & Turk, 1996).

Surprisal is an information-theoretic measure of contextual predictability (sometimes called **givenness**) of a linguistic unit. Units that carry a high value of surprisal are highlighted prosodically. High surprisal (lower predictability) is associated with segment lengthening, fortition, less coarticulation, and increased vowel dispersion (Malisz et al., 2018). A commonly cited example is the difference between given and new information. **Given information** is that which is assumed or supplied by the speaker. **New information** is that which is presented for the first time. For example, in the following excerpt, the word **puppy** is new information in the first sentence (and is in bold font) but given information in the following sentence (and in italic font).

> *Example:* We went to the pet store to buy a **puppy**. At first, I wanted a white *puppy,* but I fell in love with a black *puppy* and took it home.

Speech Acts

A **speech act** is an utterance defined by a speaker's intention and its effect on a listener (i.e., the action that the speaker seeks to elicit in the listener). Speech acts take many different forms and have been described in different ways (Green, 2021). Examples of speech acts are requests, warnings, commands, promises, apologies, and greetings. Speech acts also can express irony or sarcasm. For example, two different native speakers of Spanish who are learning English as a second language might say these words with entirely different meanings: "English is easy to learn." One speaker, who is adept at learning new languages, can be sincere and is pleased with his or her progress. But the other speaker, who is frustrated with the experience, uses the same words to a very different effect (irony), expressing the opposite feeling ("English is hard to learn"). Speech act theory is a relatively recent development in the study of language, but it has far-ranging applications in fields such as philosophy, linguistics, psychology, legal theory, artificial intelligence, and literary theory (Green, 2021).

"Speech act theory served to establish pragmatics as a separate area of clinical focus. It was seen as residing outside structural linguistics yet being part of communication. Once the door was open there was a rush to include other areas of communication that did not fit squarely into traditional sentence-based linguistic analyses. The other areas of pragmatics included conversation, discourse genres, social interaction, and event participation. In combination, these areas changed clinical practice so dramatically that their combined additions into assessment and intervention began to be called a 'pragmatics revolution' . . . " (Duchan, A history of speech-language pathology; https://www.acsu.buffalo.edu/~duchan/1975-2000.html)

Voice Quality

Speakers can use voice quality to mark or enhance prosody and to achieve various communication goals. A voice quality that has attracted considerable research and clinical interest is the occurrence of vocal fry at the end of utterances, which has been described as a vocal pattern in certain groups, such as young women. Wolk et al. (2012) recorded sentences read by 34 female speakers and asked two speech-language pathologists trained in voice disorders to mark the presence or absence of vocal fry. More than two-thirds of the participants used vocal fry during their readings, usually at the ends of sentences. The reasons why vocal fry is used so often are not clear, but one hypothesis is that it helps to create sociocultural bonds, as evidenced by the phenomenon of entrainment (Borrie & Delfino, 2017). Because vocal fry typically occurs at the ends of sentences, it also potentially carries information about grammatical structure and may be a cue for turn taking. However, as noted earlier in this chapter, a systematic review of the literature on vocal fry, Dallaston and Docherty (2020) concluded that the evidence on its occurrence is weak and that more rigorous investigations are needed.

Development of Prosody: General Patterns

Prosodic development has an early start, given that prosodic features are heard by the fetus (Gervain, 2018) and that features of prosody are evident in the vocalizations of infants (de Boysson-Bardies et al., 1984; Hallé et al., 1991; Prieto & Esteve-Gibert, 2018). Prosody is a major factor that shapes caregiver vocalizations directed to infants, commonly known as **infant-directed speech (IDS)** or **child-directed speech (CDS)**, which is defined as "the particular voice register observed in the majority of parents in interaction with their infants and differs from natural speech used in conversations with adults by showing exaggerated prosodic features" (Spinelli et al., 2017, p. 1). IDS is characterized by a slow rate of speech, high vocal pitch, short utterances, large vowel spaces, and enhanced prosody (Cristia, 2013; Spinelli et al., 2017). Cristia (2013) notes that "this register has the power to command infant attention; it increases arousal, enhances cognitive performance, and facilitates long-term retention of words" (p. 166). These features may facilitate the process of language acquisition (Harris, 2013), and it appears that mothers may use similar prosodic features even when addressing the fetus (Parlato-Oliveira et al., 2021).

Vihman (2018) proposed that children's initial representations of prosodic structure are based on the interaction of three types of learning during the early years of life: experience with salient elements of the ambient language, constraints associated with the developmental status of neurophysiological systems of vocal production, and memory processes that relate heard patterns to existing knowledge derived from production experience. She concluded from her data that the most crucial factor in prosodic development may be a child's experience with vocal practice as it affects memory for word forms. This conclusion is consistent with an overall theme in this book—that sensory and motor experience is fundamental to the acquisition of spoken language. How this experience is encoded and represented in neural structures is far from clear, but gathering evidence points to motor maps that are linked with sensory maps and cognitive structures. Early utterances may take the form of prosodic frames or tone units (Crystal, 1979) that are relatively stable and can gradually incorporate a diversity of phonetic segments and words. Prosodic modulation also helps children to separate units in the stream of speech, which may facilitate the learning of linguistic functions associated with each unit in a process called **prosodic bootstrapping** (L. Gleitman et al., 1988). Interventions emphasizing prosody in parental speech appear to have positive effects on infants' language development (Morningstar, 2019).

Prosodic patterns in babbling are influenced by the ambient language (DePaolis et al., 2008; Engstrand et al., 2003; Whalen et al., 1991), which indicates that infants at the prelexical stage can produce prosodic variations that are language sensitive. Identification of other aspects of prosody in early speech production becomes feasible with utterances of at least two words in length. With one-word utterances, little more than the intonational contour or intensity envelope can be assessed, but rhythm can be discerned from studies of bisyllabic or multisyllabic patterns. Language-specific rhythm begins to emerge at 12 months of age (Post & Payne, 2018). Allen and Hawkins (1979, 1980) proposed that early speech has a trochaic bias in the sense that **trochees** (strong-weak stress patterns) predominate in first words. However, Vihman et al. (1998) reported that both trochees and **iambs** (weak-strong stress patterns) were observed in their data on early word productions. Snow (1994) studied the development of two prosodic phenomena, the presence of a falling pitch contour on declarative utterances and lengthening of the final stressed syllable. Both patterns that are indicative of prosodic integration were present by the age of 2 years and became more consistent as the number of words in children's utterances increased. Rhythmic patterning in stress-timed languages such as English is still being refined at 5 years of age (Post & Payne, 2018). Further development of prosody depends on the capability to produce longer utterances, as discussed in a later section of this chapter.

Peppé and McCann (2003) identified four communication areas for which prosody has a crucial role: **interaction, affect, boundary (chunking)** and **focus**. Interaction is a pragmatic turn-taking skill that uses different boundary intonations at conversational turn-ends to indicate the response required or expected. Affect pertains to mood, emotion, or attitude. Chunking is the formation of boundary or delimitation (grouping words in prosodic units that often reflect linguistic divisions, such as the pauses between major syntactic elements of a sentence and the lengthening of clause-final words that signal a major clause boundary. Focus is a prosodic signaling of importance or emphasis in a string of words. It is also known as sentence-accent, sentence-stress, and main stress. It is assumed that all utterances have accent/stress features even in cases where focus is on the entire import of the utterance (called **broad focus,** for which accent occurs on the accent-bearing syllable of the last lexical item). **Narrow focus** (contrastive stress) shifts the accent/stress to the accent-bearing syllable of the most important word, or the contrasted syllable.

Studies of children ages 3 years and older reveal developmental patterns in the perception and production of prosody that do not reach the full range of adultlike abilities until puberty. Wells et al. (2004) concluded from a study of children aged 5 to 13 years that, "The ability to produce intonation functionally is largely established in five-year-olds, though some specific functional contrasts are not mastered until C.A. 8;7" (p. 749). In a study of children with speech and language impairments, Wells and Peppé (2003) noted that although intonation is relatively discrete from other levels of speech and language, specific areas of possible vulnerability include auditory memory for longer prosodic strings and use of prosody for pragmatic/interactional purposes.

Development of Prosody: Specific Features

As indicated in the preceding section, prosody is multidimensional, and it is important to consider how the different aspects of prosody develop in children. The following comments are directed toward this goal.

Speaking Rate and Articulation Rate

Speaking rate (or rate of speech) is regarded as a prosodic variable because it has effects that transcend syllable and word boundaries, and it is measured over a series of such units. Rate of speech is measured in two major ways. **Speaking rate** is the number of units (typically phonemes, syllables, or words) produced in a speech sample divided by the duration of the sample. Because words can be composed of varying numbers of syllables, there is not necessarily a direct correspondence between words/min and syllables/min. **Articulation rate** is the number of syllables produced in a timed speech sample after silent intervals have been removed from that sample. Because the silent intervals have been excised, articulation rate is considered a more accurate reflection of actual articulatory movements (motor function) and is not affected by variable silent intervals of different kinds. However, articulation rate is more difficult to calculate and therefore is not commonly used in clinical assessments.

Published data on children's speaking rates and articulation rates are summarized by Logan et al. (2011), who concluded that studies are consistent in reporting average rates of 2.6 syllables/s or less for 3- to 7-year-olds, and average rates between 2.7 and 3.3 syllables/s for 8- to 12-year-olds. The effect of age on speaking rate is not easy to determine, because speaking rate is strongly affected by other factors such as speaking task and emotional state. Speaking rate did not increase during the preschool years of ages 4, 5, and 6 years in the study by Walker and Archibald (2006), but it did increase in the period of 6 to 11 years of age in the studies of Kowal et al., (1975) and Sturm and Seery (2007). Articulation rates are higher than speaking rates, with average rates between 2.9 and 4.5 for 3- to-7-year-olds and 5.3 or higher for 9- to-12-year-olds. More recently, Mahr et al. (2021) reported articulation rates for a large sample ($N = 570$) of typically developing children. They concluded that articulation rate grew by 1 syllable/s over the course of 7 years, from 2.6 at 30 months of age to 3.5 at 114 months. They also noted that the growth was nonlinear, growing quickly at first and then more slowly. Comparative data for diadochokinetic rates are summarized in Chapter 4. The rates of spontaneous speech and diadochokinesis are only weakly related (Haselager et al., 1991).

Reading rates, whether silent or oral, typically are expressed in words/min. Oral reading rate in adult speakers averages about 183 words/min, compared to ranges of 175 to 300 words/min for silent reading of non-fiction texts and 200 to 320 words/min for fiction texts (with the difference being that non-fiction texts use longer words than fiction texts) (Brysbaert, 2019). Both silent and oral reading rates increase with grade level. It appears that reading rate is limited largely by visual and oculomotor factors (Seidenberg, 2017).

Speaking rate in infant-directed speech may influence language development. A slower maternal rate at 7 months of age is significantly correlated with vocabulary knowledge at two years, indicating that a slow speaking rate may benefit language learning (Ranieri et al., 2020). Adjustments in speaking rate also influence word learning in 3- to 4-year-old children (Vigliocco et al., 2020). Several studies show that speaking rate affects children's comprehension of spoken language (Berry & Erickson, 1973; Haake et al., 2014; Montgomery, 2004; N. W. Nelson, 1976). The effect is increased for children with language disorders (Guiraud et al., 2018; Montgomery, 2004). Madell (2013) summarized the matter as follows for children with typical development: 3- to 5-year-olds can process heard speech at 120 to 124 words/min., 5- to 7-year-olds at 128 to 130 words/min, and 10 to 11-year-olds at 135 words/min. But the average speaking rate in adults is 160 to 180 words/min, which creates a mismatch between children's optimal rate of comprehension and the typical speaking rate of adults. Fred Rogers, host of the popular children's television show, trained himself to speak at a rate of 124 words/min. Adults who speak to children in classrooms or clinical setting should be aware of the burdens that typical adult speaking rates place on young children. Redford (2014) reported that the perceived clarity of children's speech varies with their default articulation rates, so that that both developmental and individual differences in the temporal aspects of consonant and vowel production reflect maturation in articulatory timing control. This result supports the hypothesis that individual differences in default articulation rates are related to the maturation of speech motor skills in the sequential production of speech sounds.

Affect

Speech carries information about the speaker's emotional state ("tone of voice"), and listeners attend to this information while also interpreting the accompanying linguistic message (as discussed in

Chapter 2). But for all its importance in everyday communication, the emotional component of speech has been difficult to study, largely because of uncertainties and disagreements about how emotions are identified and classified (Adolphs, 2016; Tracy, 2014). (See Chapter 2 for deeper discussion of emotion.) Keltner et al. (2019) reviewed evidence that the voice can transmit 17 different emotions. However, it can be difficult to separate vocalizer arousal as opposed to specific emotional states, such as happiness, fear, anger, or sadness. Not surprisingly, emotional expressions are more accurately recognized from non-speech sounds (e.g., laughter, crying, moaning) than from well-formed linguistic messages (Lausen & Hammerschmidt, 2020).

Expression and recognition of emotions in the vocal signal has an early start (Y. Wu et al., 2017). The emotionally colored paralanguage of infant-directed speech is effective in gaining an infant's attention (Cooper & Aslin, 1990; Werker & McLeod, 1989). Infants respond to emotional vocal cues, and they respond in affectively appropriate ways. At the age of 4 and 5 months, infants react more positively to vocal signals with positive emotional valence than to those with negative emotional valence (Fernald, 1993; Papoušek et al., 1990). Infants of 7 months of age have differential attentional responses to verbal stimuli, depending on their emotional valence (T. Grossmann et al., 2005). Hoemann et al. (2019) emphasize the fundamental relationship between motor learning and emotional development, suggesting that infants construct an internal model that links motor activity to sensory experience during emotional events. Saarni et al. (2006) proposed a working definition of emotion that emphasizes (1) action, (2) preparation for action, and (3) appraisal of the significance or relevance in person-environment transactions. They viewed communication as a central component of action. Hoemann et al. (2019) and Saarni et al. (2006) have in common a focus on action in relation to events and environments. Cultural factors cannot be ignored, as it appears that the expression of emotion varies across cultures and situations (Mesquita, 2022).

As noted in Chapter 2, it has been reported that for speech prosody, higher performance in emotion recognition is related to better general socio-emotional adjustment in 6- to 8-year-old children (Neves et al., 2021). Grosbras et al. (2018) tested children and adolescents (ages 5 to 17) and 30 adults in a forced-choice labeling task for vocal bursts expressing four basic emotions (anger, fear, happiness, and sadness). Performance improved with age, mainly driven by increasing ability to identify anger and fear. Adult-level of performance was not reached until 14 to 15 years of age, and females had better scores than males across ages. The effect of speech and language disorders on recognition of vocal emotions is not well understood, but M. Fujiki et al. (2008) reported that children with language impairment had poorer recognition of emotions in a narrative passage than children without such impairment. It is unclear if this is a result of reduced capacity to recognize emotions or a difficulty in co-registering linguistic and paralinguistic information in a spoken message.

Content and Function Words

Every word is classified as either a **content word** or a **function word**. Content words carry information and meaning (semantic content). They are typically nouns, verbs, adjectives, and adverbs. Content words are also called "open-ended" or "open-class" words because they are frequently added to a speaker's lexicon. Function words have little semantic content but pertain to grammatical relationships among words. Included in the category of function words are auxiliary verbs, prepositions, quantifiers articles, conjunctions, and pronouns. These words are also called "closed-class" words because they are relatively fixed in number. In adult speech, content words usually carry relatively high levels of stress whereas function words are often reduced. Goffman (2004) compared articulatory movements in content and function words produced by adults and by children with typical development or with language disorder, finding that adults produced distinct rhythmic categories across the two types of words, but children did not. She also observed that children with specific language impairment differed from typically developing children in their ability to produce well-organized and stable rhythmic movements, but not in the differentiation of prosodic categories.

Declarative Versus Interrogative Contrast

A declarative sentence is a statement of fact or opinion. An interrogative sentence expresses a question. Grigos and Patel (2007), in a study of lip and jaw movements associated with the declarative-interrogative contrast, concluded that 4-year-olds modify lip and jaw movement to mark the contrast, but that these movements continue to be refined throughout childhood. This research shows the sensitivity of articulatory movements to the linguistic nature of utterances and the continuing refinement of motor skill in children's speech production.

S-W Words

Ballard et al. (2012) studied the development of lexical contrastivity for S-W (strong vs. weak) words in Australian 3- to 7-year-old children. Results indicated that typically developing 3-year-old children can manipulate vowel duration and intensity in an adult-like manner to produce S-W words. However, the children did not make effective use of f_0. The authors noted that protracted development of W-S stress production reflects physiological constraints on the production of short articulatory durations and rising intensity contours. They also recommended that it is preferable to rely on normative acoustic data rather than on perceptual judgments of accuracy. R. Patel and Brayton (2009) studied lexical stress in children aged 4, 7, and 11 years, finding that adult listeners were less accurate and more variable in identifying productions by 4-year-olds compared with the older children. The 7- and 11-year-old children differed only in identifying stress on nonfinal words. The results also indicated that duration and intensity are more reliable stress markers in a word-level picture-naming task than f_0. The authors suggested that because 3-year-old children can manipulate vowel duration and intensity in an adult-like manner to produce SW words, the inability to so may indicate impairment (as in childhood apraxia of speech or autism).

Boundary Effects

Phrase-final lengthening, as mentioned earlier in this chapter, is one of the strongest boundary or edge effects in speech production. This phenomenon appears in early speech development. Nathani et al. (2003) studied 8 normally hearing infants, aged 0;3 to 1;0, and eight deaf infants, aged 0;8 to 4;0, at three levels of prelinguistic vocal development: precanonical, canonical, and postcanonical. Phrase-final lengthening was observed at all three levels, which was taken to indicate a biological basis. The amount of lengthening decreased across the three levels. Snow (1994) showed that children of 2 years of age acquire intonational cues of boundaries before the cue of final syllable timing, indicating that final lengthening is a learned prosodic feature. He also reported that a consistent pattern of final lengthening emerged during the transition to combinatorial speech, which was interpreted as a developmental relationship between speech timing and syntax. These studies indicate that although phrase-final lengthening may have its roots in physiology, it is adapted to language learning.

Prosody and Phonological Processes

Gerken and McGregor (1988) comment that syllables that are unstressed or weak are omitted from the utterances of young children much more frequently than syllables that are stressed or strong. As noted in Chapter 3, weak syllable deletion is a commonly observed phonological processes in speech development. Gerken and McGregor describe two explanations for both this phenomenon and the related phenomenon that phrase-final syllables tend to be preserved in children's early speech development. One explanation is the stress and final syllable account, which holds that stressed syllables and phrase-final syllables have perceptual salience because of factors such as relatively long duration. The other explanation is the prosodic hierarchy account, which proposes that children omit syllables that do not readily fit into the prosodic hierarchy (as depicted in Figure 6–4). An additional possibility is that alternations of strong and weak syllables is demanding of motor control processes and that stressed syllables have an important role in specifying the motor plan of utterances.

Register or Speaking Style

Register was introduced earlier in this chapter in reference to infant-directed speech (IDS) or child-directed speech (CDS), which is a distinctive style of speech that adults often use when speaking to infants or toddlers. IDS and CDS may be regarded as special cases of a larger category called **clear speech**, in which a speaker makes a concerted effort to produce a highly intelligible message. Clear speech is contrasted with conversational speech, which is not produced with the same precision or care. When do children learn to use the clear speech register? Redford and Gildersleeve-Neumann (2009) found that adult listeners did not detect style differences in the speech of 3-year-olds but did detect these differences in the speech of 4-year-olds and 5-year-olds. Acoustic data confirmed these results. For example, clear speech in the older children was associated with shorter vowel durations and a lower fundamental frequency, but no differences in vowel formant frequencies. Syrett and Kawahara (2014) also found that preschoolers produced clear speech in a word learning task. Clear speech was characterized by vowels that were longer, more intense, more dispersed in the vowel space, and had a more expanded fundamental frequency range. These acoustic results differ from those reported by Redford and Gildersleeve-Neumann, perhaps because of differences in speaking tasks. But the central point is that preschoolers, at least those who are 4 or 5 years old, can use clear speech, a result that holds implications for intervention.

Reading Prosody

Prosody pertains to reading as well as to conversational speech. Although **reading fluency** has traditionally been defined as the ability to read rapidly and accurately, it is now recognized that prosody is also a key component. This wider view considers the communicative purpose of reading aloud and the role of the listener, as realized through prosody. Dowhower (1991, p. 166) wrote, "prosodic reading is the ability to read in expressive rhythmic and melodic patterns." She proposed six acoustic features of mature reading prosody: appropriate pausal intrusion, phrase segmentation and length, phrase-final lengthening, terminal intonation contours, and stress. Godde et al. (2020) reviewed studies of reading prosody to determine the progressive stages of reading prosody skills. Beginning in the 1st grade and continuing to adulthood, (1) reading rate increases, (2) decreases are observed in pausal intrusions and the number and duration of intra-sentencial and inter-sentencial pauses, and (3) increases are seen in the correlation with the f_0 contour in adults. Beginning in the 3rd grade, intonation develops to produce interrogative final rise and to mark focus. Beginning in the 5th grade, intensity variations appear. Reading prosody skills continue to develop into later school years, matching the protracted schedule noted in this book for other aspects of speech. It is becoming evident that prosody contributes to reading ability. Whalley and Hansen (2006) found that children's prosodic skills predicted unique variation in word-reading accuracy and in reading comprehension, even after controlling for phonological awareness and general rhythmic sensitivity.

A reading passage developed specifically for the assessment of motor speech disorders in adults is *The Caterpillar Passage* (R. Patel et al., 2013). The passage incorporates prosodic modulations in the form of contrastive sentence types (e.g., statements vs. questions) and words with emphatic stress. Powel (2006) reported that the passage has a Flesch–Kincaid grade level of 5.0, and Ludlow et al. (2019) determined a SMOG Index of 8.4 using an online source (https://readable.io/text/). There is a need to develop standardized reading passages for the assessment of prosody in children of different ages and language abilities.

Development of Prosody: Summary

Prosody develops over several years, beginning with language-sensitive patterns in babbling and extending to the acquisition of specific intonational contrasts at about puberty. Some of the major milestones in prosodic development are summarized in Figure 6–6. These milestones occur in a general context of increased speaking rate, speech motor maturation, improved auditory function, and language development. Prosody, like many other aspects of speech, has a long developmental span.

Neural Mechanisms of Prosody

Based largely on data from individuals with cerebral lesions, early theories of

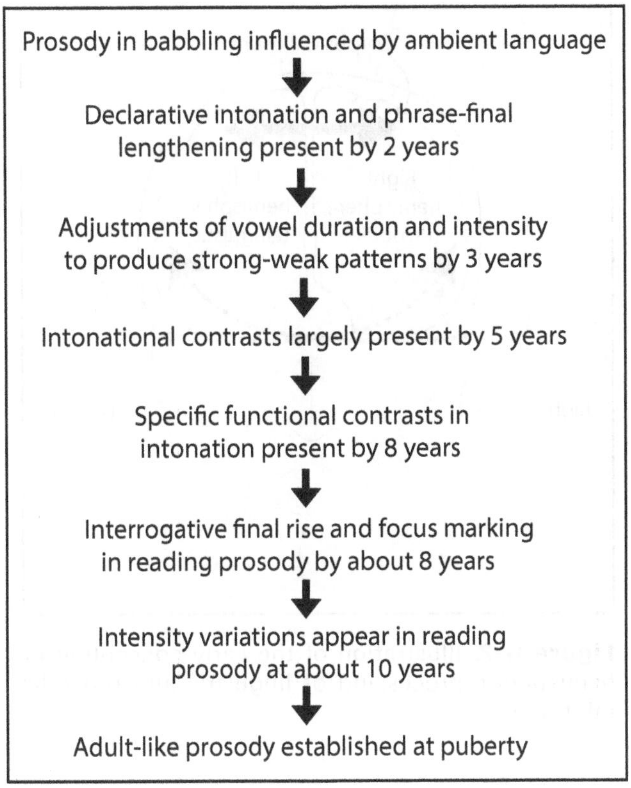

Figure 6–6. Summary of typical development of prosody production.

the neural processing of prosody focused on hemispheric specialization in which the right hemisphere was regarded as having dominance for prosody and the left hemisphere for linguistic analysis. As shown in Figure 6–7, most of the auditory nerve fibers from each ear cross over (decussate) to the opposite hemisphere. This anatomic feature is associated with the so-called **ear advantage**. In most right-handed people, phonetic analyses such as place of consonant articulation are more accurately made by the right ear (and hence left hemisphere), which is called a **right ear advantage**. However, judgments of intonation and rhythm are more accurately made by the left ear (and hence right hemisphere), which is called a **left ear advantage**. In the simple version of hemispheric specialization, it was assumed that the left hemisphere is specialized for linguistic analysis and the right hemisphere for prosodic analysis. It was commonly supposed that commissural connections, especially the corpus callosum, were responsible for integrating the information from the right and left hemispheres to yield a full linguistic-prosodic representation of the message.

The prevailing view now is that speech prosody is processed in a spatially distributed network composed of multiple areas in both cerebral hemispheres and in some subcortical structures as well (Gandour et al., 2004; Hesling et al., 2005; Liebenthal et al., 2016; Plante et al.,

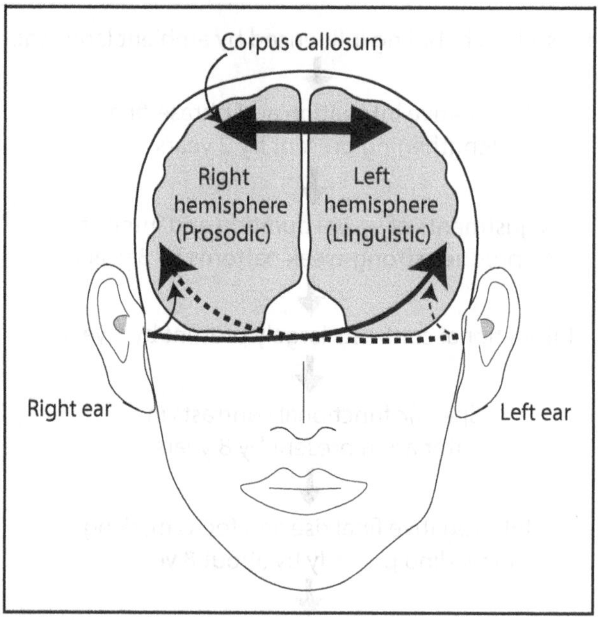

Figure 6–7. Illustration of the early conception of hemispheric processing of linguistic and prosodic information.

2006). Hesling et al. (2005) found that higher degrees of prosodic information were associated with a wider activation of the neuronal network. This result carries implications for the role of prosodic variations in speech development and for manipulation of prosody in clinical applications. For example, if increasing prosodic information activates a wider network, then more neural resources may be available for behavioral treatments. Myers et al. (2019) suggested that prosodic cues may be a foundation for neural synchronization to the speech envelope, which could scaffold linguistic processing, such as parsing a speech signal into words and phrases. Emotional prosody also seems to activate a complex neural network. Grandjean (2021) identified systems of cortical and subcortical neural networks that included perception and sound organization, related action tendencies, and associated values that integrate complex social contexts and ambiguous situations. Taken together, the results just reviewed indicate that prosody activates a widespread network of cortical and subcortical structures that have arousal and emotive capabilities.

Even if there is only a degree of imbalance between the hemispheres in processing different timescales of information, this feature can be exploited clinically, as in the case of **melodic intonation therapy (MIT)** that uses the music-like aspects of speech (melody and rhythm) to improve expressive language. Presumably, this method is effective because it stimulates a preserved function (singing) to engage language-capable regions in the undamaged right hemisphere. A music-based therapy for nonfluent aphasia was developed by Albert et al. (1993), and this method has been used with other clinical populations including childhood apraxia of speech (Helfrich-Miller, 1994; Lagasse, 2012; also see Chapter 12).

Process Analysis of Prosody

The hierarchical diagrams in Figures 6–3 and 6–4 show that prosody has a complex nature that has been described at several different levels. The diagram in Figure 6–8 takes a process-oriented view of how the components of prosody reviewed so far in this chapter come together to give final prosodic shape to an utterance. This diagram represents the basic flow of information that underlies prosody and provides an overall view of the decisions that a speaker can make to take advantage of the prosodic domain in oral communication. The highest level pertains to the language characteristics of rhythm and tone, with English being stress-timed and non-tonal. Rhythms in languages are classified as **stress-timed** (e.g., English and Dutch), **syllable-timed** (e.g., French, Italian, and Spanish), and **mora-timed** (e.g., Japanese) (Ramus et al., 1999). Most existing languages (about 60% to 70%) are tonal (Yip, 2002). These language-type features are parameters that affect the overall prosodic pattern in a native speaker. The succeeding levels in the process diagram are grammatical influences,

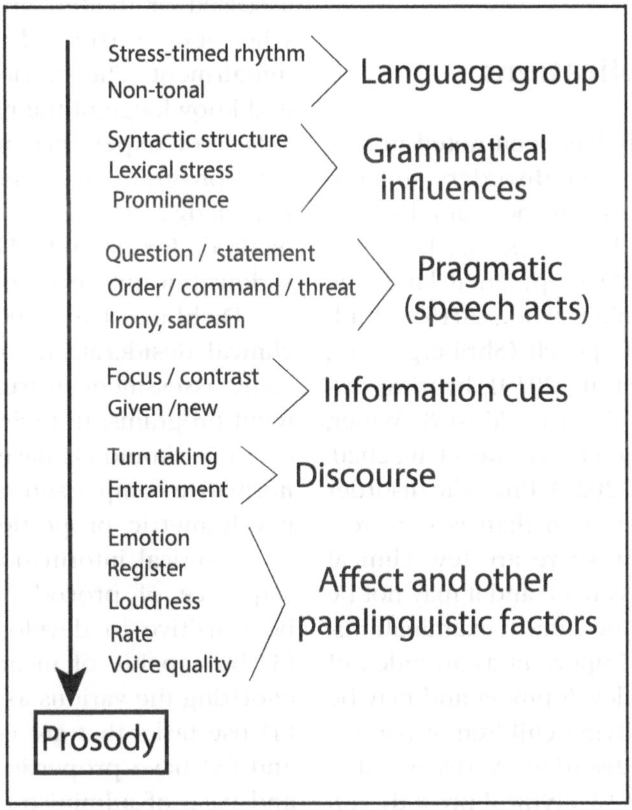

Figure 6–8. The basic flow of information that determines the prosody of an utterance in English.

pragmatic speech acts, information cues, discourse, and a variety of paralinguistic factors including affect. Some components require considerable sophistication in language use. For example, expression of irony depends not only on linguistic knowledge but also on pragmatic considerations. A competent user of language knows how to implement these different levels in speech production and to discern their effects in speech produced by others. Little wonder that prosody in its detailed nature is not rapidly acquired in childhood, or that the neural substrates of prosody are widely distributed in the CNS. Clinical assessment of the full domain of prosody is a formidable task, but tools have been developed to address some of the major aspects, as discussed next.

Clinical Applications

Atypical prosody has been noted in several communication disorders in children, including autism spectrum disorder (Asghari et al., 2021), specific language impairment or developmental language disorder (Cumming et al., 2015), childhood apraxia of speech (Shriberg et al., 2003; Terband et al., 2019), hearing disorders (Chin et al., 2012; Most & Aviner, 2009), and cerebral palsy (Mei et al., 2020; Schölderle et al., 2022). Prosodic disorder may occur more often than is now recognized, because there are few clinical tools for its assessment, and it may not be included in routine clinical examinations. Prosody can be important as an index of communicative development and may be helpful in identifying children at risk for communication disorders. As discussed in Chapters 11 and 12, atypical prosody can be a target for intervention in conditions such as autism spectrum disorder.

Peppé (2009) remarked, "Although it is impossible to speak without using prosody, it is generally allotted comparatively little time or consideration in clinical training" (p. 258). In a review of clinical assessments of prosody, Kalathottukaren et al. (2015) concluded that, "The relatively small number of tools available to evaluate prosody compared to other aspects of language indicates that, although prosody is a topic that is clinically relevant, it is often overlooked in terms of formal assessment" (p. 150). Hawthorne and Fischer (2020) surveyed 245 SLPs to assess their clinical practices for prosody and to identify potential barriers to clinical applications. Most respondents agreed that prosody was within their scope of practice, but they rarely assessed or treated prosody for clients who were considered to have prosodic impairment. The barriers included limited knowledge of the nature of prosody, a lack of experience with clients who have prosodic impairments, and limited knowledge of assessment and treatment methods for prosody. These barriers are serious but not insurmountable.

Diehl and Paul (2009) discussed the clinical desiderata of methods for prosodic assessment instruments and treatment programs. In their view, such clinical tools should (1) have a representative normative comparison sample and strong psychometric properties, (2) be based on empirical information on the typical sequence of prosodic acquisition and be sensitive to developmental change, (3) be capable of meaningfully subcategorizing the various aspects of prosody, (4) use tasks that are ecologically valid, and (5) have properties such as length and ease of administration that accommodate their inclusion in standard language assessment batteries. Adding to the challenge is that prosody is linked with a complex array of neural networks, including cortical, subcortical, cerebellar, and brainstem systems, and damage to any of these can result in dysprosody (Sidtis & Yang, 2020).

The prosody cube in Figure 6–9 is a summary of the main features that determine the prosodic pattern of an utterance. Face A of the cube pertains to pragmatic features, face B to grammatical factors, and face C to other factors such as emotion, voice quality, and speaking rate. The cube diagram illustrates the multidimensional character of prosody and helps to explain the challenges in the study of typical and atypical development of prosody. Clinical tests of prosody are considered in the next section.

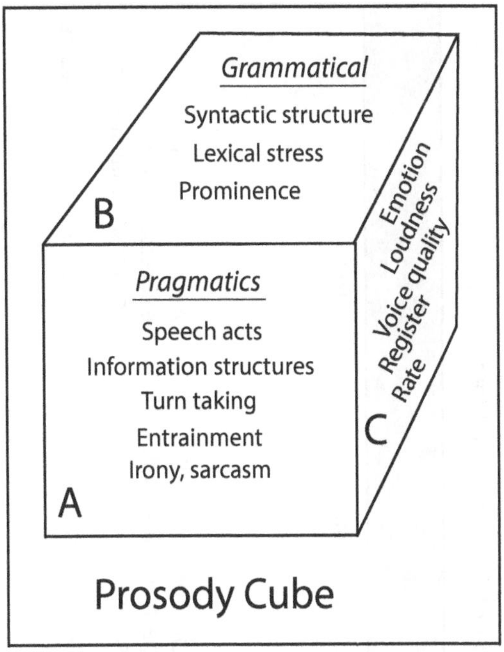

Figure 6–9. Cube diagram of the factors involved in prosody. Face A pertains to pragmatics, face B to grammatical factors, and face C to other factors.

Clinical Tests of Prosody

Clinicians seeking to assess prosody in English-speaking children might consider the instruments listed in Table 6–2 and reviewed in this section. The instruments differ in several respects, including purpose of assessment (research, clinical, or both), skills assessed (receptive, expressive, or both), target population (typical, atypical, or both), target age range, and availability of normative data.

The **Multi-Dimensional Battery of Prosody Perception (MBOPP)** (Jasmin et al., 2020) is a test of prosody perception consisting of two subtests: Linguistic Focus (a measure of the ability to hear emphasis or sentential stress) and Phrase Boundaries (a measure of the ability to hear where in a compound sentence one phrase ends, and another begins). It also permits examination of individual acoustic dimensions (Pitch and Duration), and test difficulty can be adjusted.

Profiling Elements of Prosody in Speech-Communication (PEPS-C; Peppé & McCann, 2003) is intended for use by language teachers, clinicians, and researchers to assess receptive and expressive prosody in any conditions in both children and adults. The most recent version, PEPS-C 2015 (Peppé, 2015), which supersedes previous versions, is available only for U.K. General (southern British) accent, Irish and North American (U.S. General and Canadian) accents. The test, which is not standardized, examines prosody at two different levels (functional and formal) for research and clinical purposes, using a semi-automated test battery consisting of 14 different tasks. The functional levels assessed are six primary linguistic functions conveyed by prosody: turn end, affect, lexical stress, phrase stress,

Table 6–2. Summary of Features in Several Instruments for the Assessment of Prosody in Children

Feature/ Test	MBOPP	PEPS-C	PROP	PSVP
Age	Intended for all ages, backgrounds, and ability levels, but tested on 59 adults aged 29.0±6.1 years	5 to14 years	Children and adults	3 to 81 years
Purpose	Assess receptive skills	Assess receptive and expressive skills	Describe prosodic patterns in a clinical sample	Assess voice and expressive prosody in conversational speech
Subtests	Two: One for linguistic focus and one for phrase boundaries	Six receptive, six expressive	Four prosodic patterns	Three prosody, Four voice
Aspects of prosody	Linguistic focus, phrase boundaries	Pitch direction, grammatical, affective pragmatic	Pitch, tempo, stress	Phrasing, rate, pitch, stress, loudness, laryngeal quality, resonance
Time needed	About 55 min	About 60 min	Varies with expertise in transcription	15 to 30 min to complete the PVSP from an audio recording
Comments	Stimuli are available only for UK dialect	Available only for UK General (southern British) accent, Irish and North American (US General and Canadian) accents.	Guidelines and examples of disordered prosody are provided.	Intended for clinical research, training is recommended.

Sources: MBOPP: Multi-Dimensional Battery of Prosody Perception (Jasmin, Dick, & Tierney, 2020); PEPS-C: Profiling Elements of Prosody in Speech-Communication (Peppé & McCann, 2003); PROP: Prosody Profile (Crystal, 1982); and PSVP: Prosody-Voice Screening Profile (Shriberg, Kwiatkowski, & Rasmussen, 1990).

boundary, and contrastive stress or focus. The four form tasks are two auditory discrimination tasks and two imitation tasks.

The **Prosody Profile (PROP)** (Crystal, 1982) examines expressive prosody with four subtests: intonation (nuclear pitch direction), tempo (phrasing), stress (phrasal), and strategies for producing stress. Information is included on age ranges, guidelines, and examples of impaired prosody, but normative, reliability, and validity data are not provided.

The **Prosody-Voice Screening Profile (PVSP)** (Shriberg, Kwiatkowski, & Rasmussen, 1990) is an assessment of language, speech, and prosody-voice performed on a recorded sample of conversational speech. PVSP is included in freeware titled programs to examine phonetic and phonologic evaluation records (PEPPER). The examiner codes each utterance in the sample as appropriate or inappropriate on each of 31 prosody-voice codes. The prosody component includes codes for utterances that meet criteria for inappropriate phrasing, rate, or stress. The voice component includes codes for utterances that meet criteria for inappropriate loudness, pitch, or laryngeal or resonance quality. PSVP differs from the other tests in that it assesses both voice and prosody in conversational samples. Because voice underlies many features of prosody, consideration of voice production is highly relevant to assessment of prosody. Conversation has a prima facie validity for speech examination in that it is assumed to reflect the ordinary pattern of speech communication. However, conversation can present challenges to analysis because it conflates the processes of language formulation, dyadic interaction, and speech production. Conversational samples can vary in their syntactic complexity, utterance lengths, and other features.

Prosody Assessment as a Component in Other Tests

Other assessment tools include prosody as one component but may not provide a detailed analysis of prosodic disturbances. For example, the Dynamic Evaluation of Motor Speech Skill (DEMISS; Strand et al., 2013) assesses prosody with a binary scoring (0 for correct prosody and 1 for incorrect prosody) for lexical stress errors such as segmentation, equal stress, or wrong stress. The clinician models the utterances with the appropriate lexical stress and can use cues or other facilitators as desired. Schölderle, Haas, and Ziegler (2022) included prosodic modulation as a component of the Bogenhausen Dysarthria Scales for Childhood Dysarthria, a German tool for the auditory-perceptual analysis of dysarthria in children. The three features of this component were reduced prosodic modulation, excessive prosodic modulation, and conspicuous rhythm/stress patterns.

Namasivayam, Huynh, Bali, et al. (2021) took a different perspective on prosody in their report on probe words for testing the Motor Speech Hierarchy (MSH) (introduced in Chapter 4). In their approach, prosody is both the final stage of speech refinement and the most complex system in communication. In their view, prosody is the culmination of all other speech motor stages to effect complex communications encompassing cognitive–linguistic and social–emotional contexts. According to this perspective, prosody is not simply a separate overlay on the segmental structure of speech but rather an intertwining of multiple processes in speech production (see Chapter 5 for further discussion).

Conversational Prosody

Prosody in conversation is of clinical interest because of its importance in social, cognitive, and emotional development. Individuals with communication disorders can face challenges in developing and maintaining effective conversational patterns (Borrie et al., 2015; Drosopoulou et al., 2022; Pennington & McConachie, 1999, 2001). An example noted earlier in this chapter is that when two individuals participate in conversation, they often adjust their prosodic features to match one another in a phenomenon called prosodic entrainment. Few clinical tests are designed to gauge a speaker's performance in this aspect of prosody, which is relevant to conditions such as autism spectrum disorder. Individuals with this disorder often perform well in tests of speech prosody but nonetheless are judged to have unusual expressive prosody (as discussed further in Chapter 11). A study of prosodic entrainment showed that youth with autism spectrum disorder had less conversational entrainment compared to their neurotypical peers, and sometimes even disentrained (departed from a mutual prosodic pattern) (Lehnert-LeHouillier et al., 2020). To meet the challenge of an efficient and standardized clinical assessment, Kruyt and Beňuš (2021) recommended the development of automatic methods for speech analysis and adherence to open-science principles.

Prospects for the Detailed Study of Prosody

In addition to the assessment methods reviewed to this point, other methods have potential for research and clinical applications. These are reviewed in the following.

Transcription

A group of linguists and engineers collaborated to develop a system of representation for the prosody of American English (Silverman et al., 1992). This annotation system, called **ToBI (Tones and Break Indices)** introduced an alphabet of discrete symbols to represent the different pitch accents of American English, based on sequences of symbols H (high tone) and L (low tone) and a scalar representation of the degree of separation between consecutive words (from 0 for absence of a break to 4 for a major intonation unit break. Within each pitch accent, the tone directly associated with the accented syllable of the word is marked by the diacritic [*]. In addition to break indices, boundaries are further marked by the presence of a boundary tone that can be either H (high) or L (low). In typical usage, four parallel tiers are represented: word, tone, break-index, and miscellaneous. Although ToBI was developed specifically for American English, it has become perhaps the most widely used system of prosodic representation in the world. However, its clinical application is limited because manual annotation of prosody requires both time and skill. Therefore, ToBI is used primarily in research, but it holds implications for the construction of clinically applicable tools.

Automatic Acoustic Analysis of Prosody

The interest in acoustic methods of prosodic analysis is fueled in part by dissatisfactions with perceptual analysis relating especially to the difficulty of annotation, poor reliability of some judgments, and limitations of interpretation. As already noted in this chapter, the basic acoustic dimensions of prosody are duration, vocal fundamental frequency, and intensity. Acoustic analysis is complicated in that these dimensions can be used in different combinations across speakers, and it is not always clear how acoustic measures relate to perceptual judgments of features such as intonation, volume, speaking rate, stress, and rhythm. These problems notwithstanding, methods for the automatic acoustic analysis of prosody have been developed for several different purposes including clinical applications (Patel et al., 2020) and automatic speech recognition (Ananthakrishnan & Narayanan, 2009). Acoustic analysis is readily implemented in most settings because of the ready availability of software such as Praat. Displays of acoustic measures can complement perceptual judgments and can provide visual cues for purposes such as treatment (as discussed in Chapter 12). These displays show information on the durations of words and pauses, fundamental frequency contours, and intensity envelopes.

There is, at present, no consensus on the acoustic measures that could be the core elements for analyzing prosody, but clinical research in neurodevelopmental disorders has focused primarily on speaking rate, mean f_0, variability of f_0 (e.g., standard deviation or coefficient of variation), and f_0 contour or slope. Acoustic analysis also has the potential to detect rhythmic patterns. Leong and Goswami (2015) noted that linguistic rhythms can be identified in the low-frequency statistics in the amplitude envelope of the acoustic signal, including the following frequency bands: *delta* centered at 1 to 3 Hz to detect periodicity of prosodic units, *theta* centered at 4 to 7 Hz to detect syllables, and faster modulations around 35 Hz to extract phonemic information, such as the consonant-vowel transitions in syllables). As discussed in Chapter 8, sensitivity to amplitude modulations in early life may predict important language functions such as phonological awareness.

Conclusions

1. Voice is the primary energy source of speech production, and it carries information on a speaker's age and gender, as well as being the substrate for intonational aspects of prosody. Properties of voice change during life, but some of the most dramatic changes occur during childhood and adolescence. Voice quality is a multidimensional construct that is important in assessing voice disorders and in understanding the complexities of prosody. Although some aspects of prosody can be conveyed in whispered speech, the full dimensionality of prosody is realized in voiced speech.
2. Prosody is a communication skill with complementary perceptual and expressive aspects. Competent interlocutors recognize prosodic cues in the speech of others and can produce these cues in their own speech, although the use of the cues may vary across individuals and situations. Prosody is usually considered suprasegmental in the sense that it encompasses segmental strings such as phonemes, but it has influences at all levels of speech, including articulatory movements for phonetic segments. Effects of prosody are pervasive and not

a simple overlay on the process of speech production. Aspects of prosody continue to mature until at least adolescence—a maturational trajectory like that in other trajectories in the development of speech perception and production.

3. Clinical methods for the assessment and treatment of prosodic disorders or differences have taken different approaches with respect to speech samples and measures. Normative data are generally lacking in the available tests (if normative data is defined as data obtained from a large, randomly selected representative sample from the wider population and that can be used to transform individual scores or measurements directly into standardized z-scores, T scores, or quantiles). The instruments are standardized only in the sense that the same procedures are used across individuals, but a common problem is that the procedures are not adjusted for the developmental status of the child being examined. Because the assessment of prosody can be time-consuming and not easily performed with all children (especially very young children or those with cognitive or motor limitations), there is a need for a clinical test that can be conducted efficiently with children with a range of capabilities.
4. Features of prosody vary across different speaking tasks (e.g., repetition, conversation, reading). Assessment of prosody should consider, at the minimum, the number of words or syllables in an utterance, instructions to the child, and potentially complicating factors (e.g., disfluencies, voice disorder, severe articulatory disorder).

7

ASSESSMENT OF PHONOLOGY

Phonology and phonetics are closely related. **Phonetics** deals with the description of speech sounds, including their physiologic, acoustic, and perceptual properties. Accordingly, the broad field of phonetics encompasses the subfields of physiological phonetics, acoustic phonetics, and perceptual phonetics, each of which has a sizeable literature based on laboratory methods and sets of data. Important concepts in phonetics are segments (phonemes or phonetic segments) and features (attributes such as place, manner, or voicing that can be bundled to form units such as phonemes and distinguish the sounds in a language). **Phonology** is the study of sound interrelations and functions in a certain language, that is, how speech sounds are formed into words and other language structures. Therefore, phonology is concerned with different levels of sound patterns, such as features, phonemes, syllables, and words. It is common for models of spoken language to distinguish phonetic processing from phonological processing and to propose that some kind of interface must be recognized. However, it also has been proposed that the boundary between these two processes is fluid or even nonexistent, as discussed later in this chapter. There is also disagreement regarding the status of units, such as syllables and phonemes. The perspective taken here is that these units have a descriptive and explanatory value that warrants their inclusion in a general consideration of phonetics and phonology. The ground on which we now venture is not without risk of fault or collapse, but the effort is worthwhile. Figure 7–1 builds on Figure 3–4 to show the different hierarchical levels of phonological structure, including the levels of word, syllable, stress, segment, and feature. Although not every phonological theory recognizes each of these levels, they are useful points of reference in discussing different theories and applications of phonology to speech development and disorders.

A primary concern in phonology is to identify lawful relationships in the way sounds are distributed and deployed in a particular language. It is assumed that in learning to speak, a child discovers these relationships and uses them in generalizing sound patterns for word formation, including new words to be learned. For example, if children of the age of 4 years are asked to say the plural form of a novel word like *wug*, they typically will produce the plural by adding a /z/ to the

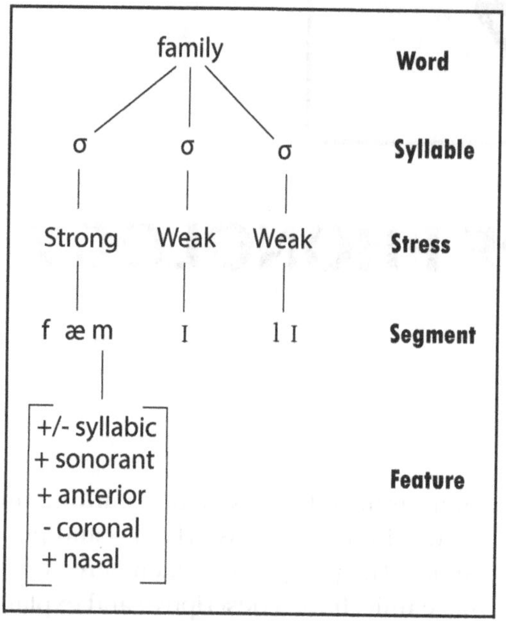

Figure 7–1. Diagram of the hierarchical levels of phonological structure, including the levels of word, syllable, stress, segment, and feature, as they apply to the word *family*.

singular form to produce /wʌgz/ (Gleason, 2019). In doing so, they demonstrate knowledge of rules or laws governing the phonological patterns of a language. This knowledge is implicit in the sense that children cannot explain the processes underlying their decision. That is, they are not likely to say something like, "The word-final consonant is a voiced stop, so the appropriate plural morpheme is the voiced alveolar fricative."

The study of speech and language disorders has carved out another branch of phonology, **clinical phonology**, which has been the subject of both journal articles (Elbert et al., 1984; Locke, 1983) and books (Ball, 2015; Elbert & Gieret, 1986; Grunwell, 1987, Klein, 1996). Clinical phonology can be defined as the application of phonological theories and methods of analysis to the understanding of speech and language disorders. As discussed in the next section, phonological theories are abundant and differ in some fundamental respects. Methods of analysis also differ across studies, but some have had a more consistent clinical application, and these are emphasized in this chapter. It is well to heed the admonition of Fey (1992) that, "adopting a phonological approach to dealing with speech sound disorders does not necessitate a rejection of the well-established principles underlying traditional approaches to articulation disorders" (p. 225). Cleaving phonology and articulation may not be straightforward in either development or disorder.

Phonological Theories

A first step in considering phonological development is to discuss the phonology of adult speakers of a language. Multiple theories of phonology have been proposed, including generative phonology, natural phonology, optimality theory, autosegmental theory, and articulatory phonology, to mention but a few (Bérce & Honeybone, 2020; Hannahs & Bosch, 2018). The abundance of theories may tell us that the problem is difficult and that different perspectives can be taken. Bérce and Honeybone (2020) regard the diversity of theories as a healthy sign, but a less sanguine view is that the application of these theories to topics, such as speech disorders, is uncertain. Speaking to this point. Balas (2007, p. 43) writes, "The usefulness of a given theoretical approach to language research is agreement on what the goals of research are. Such an agreement seems not to have been reached in phonology between formalists and functionalists who argue about the essence and role of description, explanation, and practical applications." The modern history of phonology begins with two phonological theories: generative phonology and natural phonology. Several other theories have been introduced, but the discussion here is limited to only three of these—autosegmental phonology (which introduces the concept of tiers in phonetic and phonological representation), optimality theory (which has prominence as a constraint-based theory in contemporary phonology), and articulatory phonology (which is distinct from most other theories in erasing the phonology-phonetics interface). This non-exhaustive review of phonological theories is intended only to show that very different approaches have been taken to account for the phonetic and phonological representations that underlie speech production.

Generative Phonology

In 1968, Chomsky and Halle published *Sound Patterns of English* (often abbreviated SPE), which continues to stand as one of the most influential books on phonology ever published. The first sentence of the preface modestly explains, "This study of English sound structure is an interim report on work in progress rather than an attempt to present a definitive and exhaustive study of phonological processes in English" (p. vii). SPE was innovative in several respects, but especially in its account of the surface forms of English derived from a set of distinctive features and well-defined algorithms or ordered rules that underlie **generative phonology**. SPE makes no use of syllables and represents segments (phones or phonemes) as bundles of features. Rules that operate on features are the essential innovation of this theory. The phonology is generative in the sense that it translates underlying phonological representations into surface phonetic representations by means of the ordered rules that produce only those phonetic representations that occur in English. Clinical application of generative concepts followed shortly after the publication of SPE and led to formal descriptions of phonological errors in children's speech (Compton, 1970). In her history of speech-language pathology, Duchan (n.d.) labeled the period of 1965 to 1975 as the linguistic era because of the deep influence of linguistics and psychology on the understanding of speech and language disorders.

The general form of a phonological rule is:

Structural description > structural change / _(in a specific environment)

For example, in American English, voiceless stops in the initial position of stressed words are aspirated. This regularity can be expressed as shown in Figure 7–2. The example shows the relevance of features, the process of realization or translation, and the environmental specification of rule operation. Rules of this kind are a formal statement of how an underlying representation is transformed to a surface representation that accords with the phonological patterns of the language at hand. The features in SPE are **distinctive features**, which are the basic building blocks of phonological description. These features are bundled together to form individual phonemes. For the most part, distinctive features are defined in phonetic terms and often are named after phonetic properties (e.g., [voice], [nasal], [coronal]). Typically, binary values of features are used in phonological rules. For

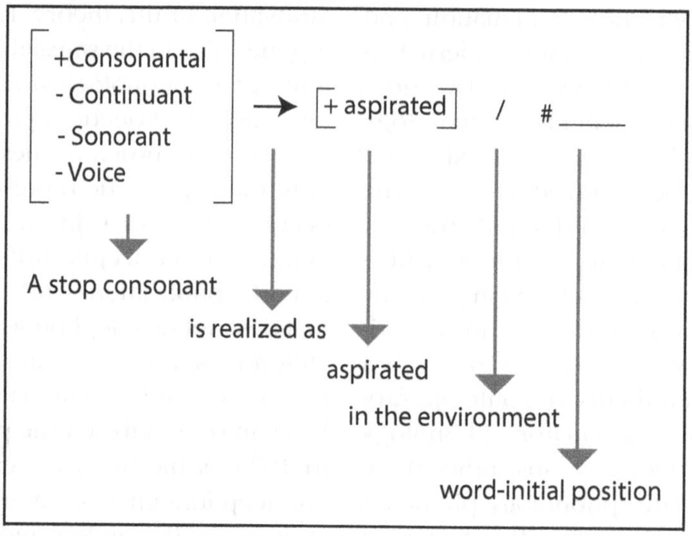

Figure 7–2. The general form of a rewrite rule in generative phonology, showing the relevance of features, the process of realization or translation, and the environmental specification of rule operation.

example [+voice] designates the presence of voicing, and [–voice] designates the absence of voicing. The universal appeal of distinctive features is that they form natural classes of sounds that are found across languages. However, there is no universal set of distinctive features agreed upon by all experts.

Distinctive features may be likened to the periodic table of elements in chemistry, which organizes all discovered chemical elements in rows (called periods) and columns (called groups) according to increasing atomic number. In similar fashion, distinctive features organize all known phonemes in the world's languages into a compact system of binary-valued items. According to Jakobson, Fant, and Halle (1963) "In the hierarchy of the sound features the distinctive features are of paramount importance" (p. 8), and "The inherent distinctive features which we detect in the languages of the world and which underlie their entire lexical and morphological stock amount to twelve binary oppositions" (p. 40). These oppositions are as follows: vocalic/nonvocalic, consonantal/nonconsonantal, interrupted/continuant, checked/unchecked, strident/mellow, voiced/unvoiced, compact/diffuse, grave/acute, flat/plain, sharp/plain, tense/lax, and nasal/oral. In short, distinctive features hold the promise of universality and economy of phonetic description.

Natural Phonology

Natural Phonology (Donegan & Stampe, 1979; Stampe, 1969) proposes that phonology is based on a set of interacting universal phonological processes that are either active or suppressed in an individual language. These processes operate on distinctive features within prosodic groups ranging in size from a syllable to an entire utterance. An important consequence of this theory is that children's speech development can be understood as simplifications derived from natural processes. Processes differ from phonological rules in three major ways: (1) processes are motivated by phonetic principles, whereas rules are not explicit in their phonetic bases, (2) processes apply involuntarily and subconsciously, whereas rules are the consequence of attending to language inputs, and (3) processes may be optional (or suppressed), whereas rules are obligatory. As the concept of phonological processes influenced the study of speech sound disorders, the zeal to distinguish phonological disorders from articulation disorders had the unfortunate consequence of dislodging them wholly or partly from their phonetic footing, leaving them as free-floating entities in an abstract phonological space. It certainly is important theoretically and clinically to recognize patterns of speech sound errors, but the existence of patterns does not imply that phonetic factors are irrelevant.

The basic model of speech production based on natural phonology is shown in Figure 7–3. The highest level pertains to the lexicon and rules, the second to prosody, and the third to processes. The processes operate on distinctive features within prosodic groups varying in size from a syllable to a complete utterance. Active or noninhibited processes operate as either fortitions or lenitions. **Fortitions** emphasize divisions within the prosodic score and enhance the clarity of intended sounds. **Lenitions** operate in a complementary fashion to promote fluency of the sequence of sounds. That is, fortitions make sounds more distinctive, and lenitions make sounds less distinctive. Phonological processes are unordered and apply simultaneously, but the output of

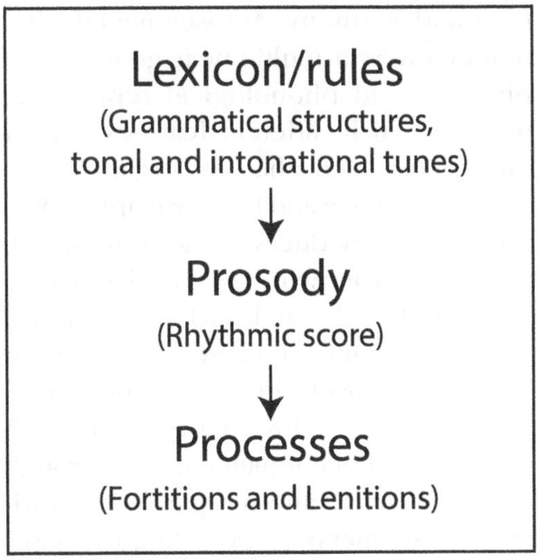

Figure 7–3. The basic model of natural phonology. The highest level pertains to the lexicon and rules, the second to prosody, and the third to processes.

one process can be input to another. An important consequence of this theory is that children's speech development can be understood as simplifications derived from natural processes.

Another version of natural phonology is based on processes of self-organization, which operate in a constructivist fashion to unify the influences of physiology, psychology, and neurology, as they underpin phonological acquisition. This theory emphasizes the interaction of genetic factors, cognitive processes, and environmental input to mold neural specialization and development of language modules (Dziubalska-Kołaczyk, 1998).

Autosegmental Phonology

The concept of autosegments was introduced by Goldsmith (1976; also see Goldsmith, 2001) with the goal of representing suprasegmental phenomena such as tone and harmony. Autosegmental phonology offers a multi-linear geometry of phonetic and phonological representations in which different features appear on separate tiers that are organized by association lines and by a principle called the Well-Formedness Condition, which entails the following: a vowel must be associated with (at least) one toneme, each toneme must be associated with (at least) one vowel, and association lines may not cross. This theory deals with phonological phenomena mainly through rules that delete and reorganize the various autosegments by adjusting the association lines that connect different tiers. As mentioned in Chapter 6, prosody is of interest in several speech disorders, but it is difficult to assess prosody across different ages of children and different levels of language ability. Autosegmental phonology and other prosody-based theories may provide helpful insights that integrate the segmental and suprasegmental aspects of speech.

Optimality Theory (OT)

Optimality theory (OT; Prince & Smolensky, 2008) abandons the rewritten rules of generative phonology and focuses instead on **constraints**, which are held to be universal but can be ranked differently across languages. Constraints determine the phonological forms of words, but they can be violated under certain conditions. A diagram of OT is shown in Figure 7–4. The basic idea is that a function called **GEN** maps a lexical form into all possible output candidates. The winning candidate or set of candidates is selected by a function called **EVAL** that examines the number of constraint violations and their

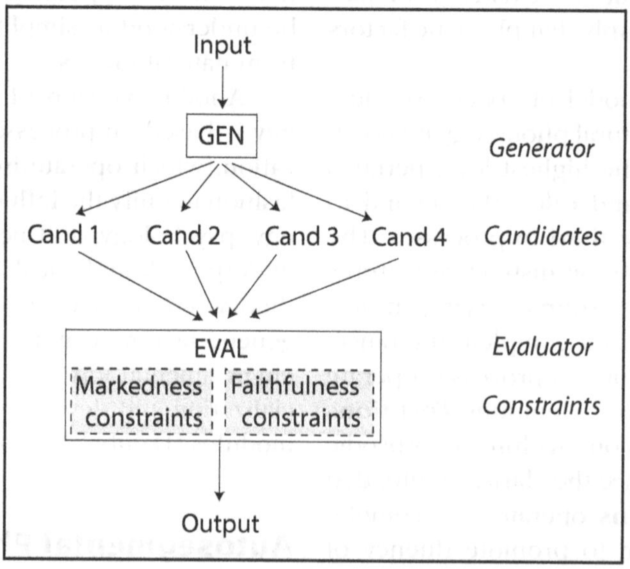

Figure 7–4. A diagram of optimality theory, showing how candidates (cand1, cand2, etc.) are generated (GEN) and evaluated (EVAL) using faithfulness and markedness constraints.

severity, as determined by the ranking in the language. The winning solution(s) might violate one or more constraints but is superior to any alternatives. Constraints are of two basic types. **Faithfulness constraints** ensure that output representations resemble input representations, that is, whatever is present in the input should also be in the output. **Markedness constraints** (also called **well-formedness** or **structural constraints**) select output forms that are unmarked in structure. Markedness is the complexity of a given structure relative to another structure, as reflected in language typologies, frequency of occurrence, and order of acquisition. Unmarked properties are the most basic, or natural, because they are present in all grammars and, therefore, have the appeal of universality.

Markedness has a complex history and is not free of controversy. Mehrdad and Ahghar (2015) summarized the matter as follows,

> The term markedness has been defined variously, but underlying all the definitions is the notion that some linguistic features are 'special' in relation to others which are more basic . . . This means that they are, in some definable way, simpler, more basic and more natural than the other members which are in turn defined as the marked member. (p. 105)

A phonetic example of markedness is that for any pair of sounds, one member is more basic, occurs with higher frequency, or is acquired earlier in development. This member is unmarked. Voiced stops are marked, and voiceless stops are unmarked. This distinction has been used in therapy for speech sound disorders by assuming that the marked member implies the unmarked member; therefore, targeting voiced stops is likely to improve production of voiceless stops even if they are not specifically included in treatment. This kind of **implicational relationship** can be extended to other speech sounds; for example, fricatives imply stops, stops in word-final position imply stops in word-initial position, and velars imply coronals. This concept is elaborated in Chapter 12 where it is applied to a complexity-based treatment for speech sound disorders. Many implicational relationships reported for children are consistent with either phonological theory or aspects of developmental phonetics. Watts and Rose (2020) caution that:

> Markedness and the implicational relationships it entails for phonological development can only be established between units which can be directly compared in terms of structural complexity . . . or, for individual phones, phonological features, or the acoustic or articulatory dimensions of speech which are involved in their production. (p. 670)

Barlow and Gierut (1999) remarked that OT "meets the three basic criteria for a viable theory of phonological acquisition: It captures common error patterns, allows for individual variation, and preserves continuity in the grammar" (p. 1494). They also comment on its clinical applicability, such as the observation of correlated error patterns. Hegde (2021, p. 317) takes a more negative view, asserting that, "there is no independent evidence for the existence of universal and innate constraints, specific language-based rankings, and the operation of GEN or EVAL."

Gestural Phonology

Gestural phonology (also called **articulatory phonology**) (Browman & Goldstein, 1992) recognizes the articulatory gesture as both a unit of phonological contrast and a characterization of the articulatory movements needed to accomplish that contrast. The basic features of this approach are shown in Figure 7–5. An intended utterance is specified as a gestural score by a linguistic gestural model. No phonemes or other segments are necessary to make this specification. As mentioned in Chapter 3, an articulatory gesture is an abstract dynamic description of a movement of one or more articulators. These gestures are the basic elements of phonology and are combined in a gestural score that specifies the temporal pattern of constricting vocal tract actions (e.g., actions of the jaw, tongue, and velopharynx). The gestural score indicates when a constriction is made, as well as the amount of constriction, so that it is essentially a blueprint of the required articulatory events. The relatively abstract information in the gestural score is transformed into actual articulatory trajectories by means of a task dynamics model (see description of system dynamics in Chapter 1), which considers the goal to be achieved in respect to the biomechanical properties of the speech production system. A striking aspect of this proposal is that it relies almost completely on dynamic descriptions, as opposed to the static concepts such as phonemes and features in traditional phonological theories. Browman and Goldstein (1992) assert that this theory can account for phenomena such as allophonic variation, coarticulation, speech sequencing errors, and aspects of phonological development. Concerning the last of these, they suggest that prelinguistic units of action in infants are formed into gestures through processes of differentiation and coordination.

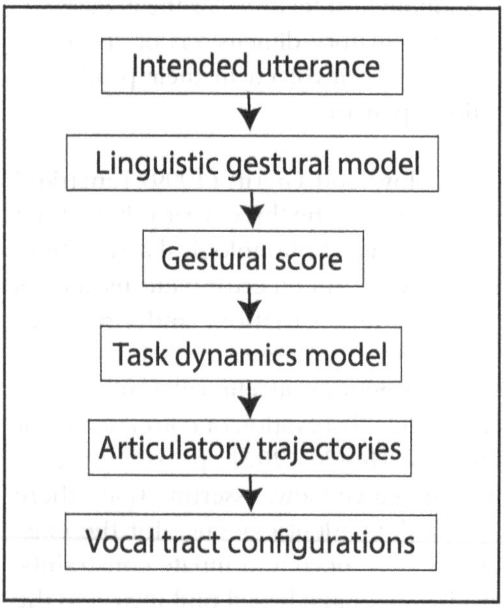

Figure 7–5. Basic components of gestural phonology.

Discussions of how gestural phonology applies to speech development and speech disorders are provided by Van Lieshout and Goldstein (2008) and by Namasivayam et al. (2020). New directions in gestural phonology are outlined by Iskarous and Pouplier (2022), who suggest that the integration of the dynamic principles of this theory into a model of utterance planning allows for prosodic specification of the timeflow of an utterance.

Phonology and Acoustics

As mentioned earlier, phonology is broadly defined as the study of the speech sounds in a language or in selected languages, and a speech sound is an acoustic and auditory event. In physics, sound is defined as a vibration that propagates as an acoustic wave, through a transmission medium of some kind, such as air or water. In perception, sound is defined as the sensation of hearing (or auditory impression). The word *phonology* is derived from a Greek word for voice or sound, and another for word or speech. The phonological theories just reviewed say little or nothing about acoustics or auditory perception, and this detachment is curious. The basic elements of a phonological theory (whether phonemes, features, gestures, or whatever) ultimately should be related to auditory experience. Distinctive features, as originally proposed (Jakobson et al., 1961), identified acoustic correlates of at least some features, but more recent phonological theories appear to stop at or before the articulatory-acoustic interface, so that acoustic phenomena and their auditory correlates are barely mentioned. There are reasons to include acoustic and auditory considerations in accounts of phonological and phonetic patterns. Neurocomputational models such as Guenther's DIVA model (Chapter 1) invoke an auditory target as the basis for learning speech sounds (Guenther, 2006; Kearney & Guenther, 2019), and it has been proposed that the "fundamental control variables for phonemic movements are multi-dimensional regions in auditory and somatosensory spaces" (Perkell, 2012, p. 382). It is possible to learn speech without auditory cues. For example, **Tadoma** is a type of tactile speech communication used by deaf and blind individuals, who place a hand over a speaker's face to monitor vibration, airflow, and articulatory movement. But the most general way of learning speech involves auditory experience, so that audition is a central factor in phonological development.

A child's phonological system at any given age is determined in part by maturation of the auditory system and the formation of neural networks that link auditory, somatosensory, motor, and linguistic representations. Perhaps a future phonological theory will be more securely planted in acoustic or auditory ground. For the purposes of this chapter, acoustic and auditory phenomena are key attributes in a child's discovery of phonological relationships. Theories of phonology developed by linguists may ignore audition but theories of phonological development in children cannot do so. Because a phonological system is learned by hearing the sound patterns of a language, auditory factors are foundational to phonological development. As reviewed in Chapter 2 and elsewhere in this book, development of the auditory system extends to at least puberty. Auditory factors are fundamental in understanding concepts such as phonological memory and phonological awareness, as discussed next.

> "Most adolescents and adults not only can use language effectively for communication and other purposes, but in addition can treat language as something that can be intentionally thought about, judged, played with, and manipulated in various ways. This ability to reflect consciously on the nature of language is called linguistic awareness or metalinguistics." (Scarborough & Brady [2002]. Toward a common terminology for talking about speech and reading: A glossary of the "phon" words and some related terms. *Journal of Literacy Research*, *34*[3], p. 312)

Phonological Processing

Chapter 3 considers the role of phonological processing in spoken language and introduces the concepts of phonological representation and phonological encoding. The present chapter continues the discussion, with the aim of describing clinical applications. Anthony and Francis (2005) identify three phonological processing abilities, as follows. (1) **Phonological memory** is the coding of information in a sound-based representation system for temporary storage (i.e., phonological representations). When we first hear a sound pattern, it is stored in this memory to be available for further processing. (2) **Phonological access to lexical storage** is retrieval of phonological codes from memory (necessary for phonological encoding of lexemes, as discussed in Chapter 3). The goal is to match the incoming sound pattern to these phonological codes. (3) **Phonological awareness (PA)** is sensitivity to the sound structure of oral language (i.e., the components needed for the assembly of phonological structures). PA is assumed to be critical for interpretation of the incoming signal and probably for the development of other skills such as reading. Anthony and Francis point out that these abilities are highly interrelated, are influential in reading acquisition, and show stable individual differences beginning in late preschool. Clinical implications are that these abilities (a) mature over a considerable period of childhood, (b) are vulnerable to developmental disruptions or irregularities, and (c) may predict problems in oral language and/or reading. As examples of disruption, children may fail to store a phonological representation in early word learning, or they may experience difficulties in retrieving a phonological representation that was correctly stored. It can be challenging to distinguish the different aspects of phonological processing. For the purposes of speech-language pathology, a fourth component should be added to those already listed, **phonological production**, which may rely to some degree on the other components but also incorporates the various processes that are needed for speech production. Phonological production basically corresponds to a phonetic transcription that reveals the sequence of sounds along with language-specific sound features.

The point of view taken here is that phonological development is an active process that builds on the capabilities and resources that are available at a particular age of development. The concept of scaffolding is applicable. A scaffold is a temporary platform from which more permanent structures are formed. Parts of a scaffold may be carried over into succeeding versions of a structure, while some parts may be discarded. This perspective is compatible with the concept of self-organization, which holds that the functional configuration in time and space of a given system emerges from the collective interactions of its individual components. As applied to phonological acquisition, this view means that phonology is not fully determined by genetic factors but by the multiple processes that operate in human development.

The next sections of this chapter consider primary clinical issues pertaining to phonology: phonological processes in children's speech, phonological memory (including the quality of phonological representation), phonological access, phonological awareness, and phonological production.

Phonological Memory

One of the most influential models of working memory was introduced by Baddeley (1986) and subsequently modified to include additional components. The main components are a phonological loop, a visuo-spatial sketchpad, an episodic buffer, and a central executive. The phonological loop consisting of a short-term store and a subvocal rehearsal process is the basis for verbal short-term memory. The visuo-spatial sketchpad processes visual and spatial information received directly through perception or indirectly through a visual image to enable storage of images of objects and their locations. The episodic buffer was added to the original model to integrate information from the phonological loop, visuo-spatial sketchpad, and long-term memory. The central executive manages information received from the phonological loop, visuo-spatial sketchpad, episodic buffer, and long-term memory. As its name suggests, this component has high-level responsibilities for functions, such as selective attention, suppressing irrelevant information, and adjustment of retrieval plans.

Figure 7–6 shows a modified and elaborated version of the model. For present purposes, the components of main interest are those pertaining to phonological memory. Phonological memory has two forms: **phonological short-term (pSTM)** and **phonological long-term memory (pLTM)**. The first of these is a type of working memory that some believe is critical in language learning as an essential step to the formation of traces in pLTM (Gathercole & Baddeley, 1993; Service, 2013). In Baddeley's (1986) model, speech accesses a phonological short-

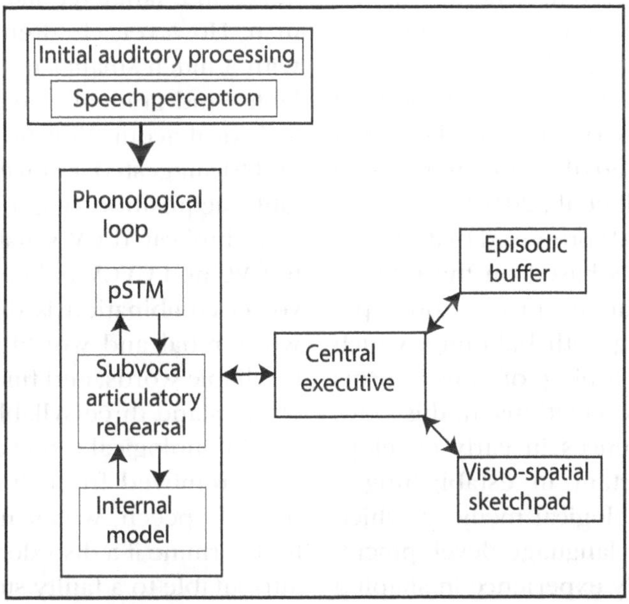

Figure 7–6. Model of working memory with the main components of a phonological loop, a visuo-spatial sketchpad, an episodic buffer, and a central executive. (Modified from Baddeley, 1986).

term store whose contents are refreshed by a rehearsal component that prevents decay of the stored items. Without such rehearsal, contents of the pSTM fade within about 2 s. The crux of this model is a **phonological loop** that consists of (1) a phonological store (pSTM) that is a temporary repository of verbal information (acting like an "inner ear"), and (2) an articulatory loop in which inner speech can reactivate the representations in the pSTM (acting like "inner speech"). Learning of words in a first or later language depends on the phonological loop to hold unfamiliar sound patterns in memory, whereas more permanent memory representations are formed in pLTM. Figure 7–6 adds two elements to the model: (1) an auditory input consisting of initial auditory processing and speech perception, and (2) an internal model to serve as the basis of subvocal rehearsal and to coordinate sensory and motor aspects of speech production, whether covert or overt (see Chapter 3 for discussion). Studies indicate that the left supramarginal gyrus is a critical node of the STM network and preserves temporal order of verbal and nonverbal elements (Guidali et al., 2019; Savill et al., 2019).

Vihman (2022) proposed that phonological memory is based on the interaction of perceptual and production experience, beginning with babbling, which mediates the mapping of novel forms onto lexical representations. In this view, language experiences in early development are important in establishing a competent phonological memory, which is critical to later language development. The value of early experience in shaping phonological memory has been demonstrated in studies of different language learning populations, such as children with cochlear implants, children with developmental language disorder, and internationally-adopted children (Delcenserie et al., 2021).This perspective is also supported by studies showing that phonological working memory is related to the activity of cortical structures that canonically underlie speech perception and production (Perrachione et al., 2017). These cortical areas, which show increasing activation with increases in the load of phonological memory, are the bilateral superior temporal gyrus, inferior frontal gyrus, and supplementary motor area. The concept of a syllabary is closely linked with phonological memory, if it is assumed that syllables are stored as units. The core syllables in a syllabary consist of early-acquired, high-frequency syllables that are contained in a network of syllabic neighbors (Cholin, 2008). Schiller et al. (1996) estimate the number of core syllables to be about 500, compared to the total number of 11,000 to 12,000 syllables in a language like English or German. However, children probably begin with a much smaller number of core syllables and gradually add to that number as lexical acquisition proceeds. Jacobson (1968) suggested a universal order of syllable acquisition beginning with single or reduplicated CV syllables, proceeding to CVC and CVCV (where the consonant-vowel combination is different), then to word-initial and word-final clusters and bisyllabic words, and finally to additional clusters and three-syllable words.

Phonological representation is somewhat removed from the actual production of speech, which makes it difficult to determine if a disordered production is attributable to a faulty storage of the representation or to some other disturbance, such as impaired retrieval of the PR or a problem in motor planning that converts the PR to motor commands. The **quality**

of representation (QPR) task (Sutherland & Gillon, 2005) presents children with pictures of different multisyllabic words and asks them to judge whether the words are produced correctly or incorrectly by selecting a mark on a computer screen. Because no verbal response is required, the task focuses on receptive ability and reduces the influence of productive abilities.

Phonological memory is a factor (among many) in **fast mapping**, or the ability to map words to referents in the world, often with even a brief exposure to the word (Carey & Bartlett, 1978; Dollaghan, 1985; Vlach & Sandhofer, 2012). Phonological memory is also involved to some degree in **extended mapping** (Carey, 2010), or the eventual alignment of the new word in the child's lexicon. Much of the research on this topic has focused on retention of linguistic and nonlinguistic information, but Vlach and Sandhofer (2012) presented data showing that word learners forget word mappings at a rapid rate that parallels functions of domain-general memory processes. They contend that memory processes are critical to word learning and that forgetting supports extended mapping by promoting the memory and generalization of words and categories.

Phonological Access to Lexical Storage

Lexical access is accomplished when sensory information (e.g., auditory or visual information) is matched to a lexical representation. Taft (1986) concluded that the access code for activating lexical information differs between spoken word recognition and printed word recognition. In the former, the code is the first few phonemes regardless of syllable structure, whereas in the latter, the code is the first (orthographically defined) syllable. For spoken word recognition, listeners try to determine the initial sound sequence as a first step in deciding which word was produced. Various theories have been advanced to explain this process in detail, but the basic point is that we do not need to hear the entire acoustic pattern of a word to activate access to the lexicon. **Cohort theory** (Marslen-Wilson, 1984), for example, proposes that when we hear the first 200 ms of a word, we activate a cohort of possible word candidates. As we hear progressively more of the word, we deactivate candidates that no longer match the acoustic pattern until only one candidate remains. Word recognition uses both segmental and suprasegmental (prosodic) information, as reviewed by McQueen (2007).

Phonological Awareness (PA)

Phonological awareness (PA) can be defined as sensitivity to the sound structure of a language. There is growing agreement that phonological awareness is a single, unified ability that is manifest in different skills throughout a child's development. PA often is described as an umbrella term that embraces the different skills, or as a continuum showing the developmental sequence of the skills. A diagram of PA in Figure 7–7 shows its different components, including a pyramid of six different developmental levels of phonemic awareness. The crux of PA is the recognition that oral language can be divided into smaller components that are subject to various manipulations. These smaller components include (1) syllables, (2) onsets and rhymes of syllables, and

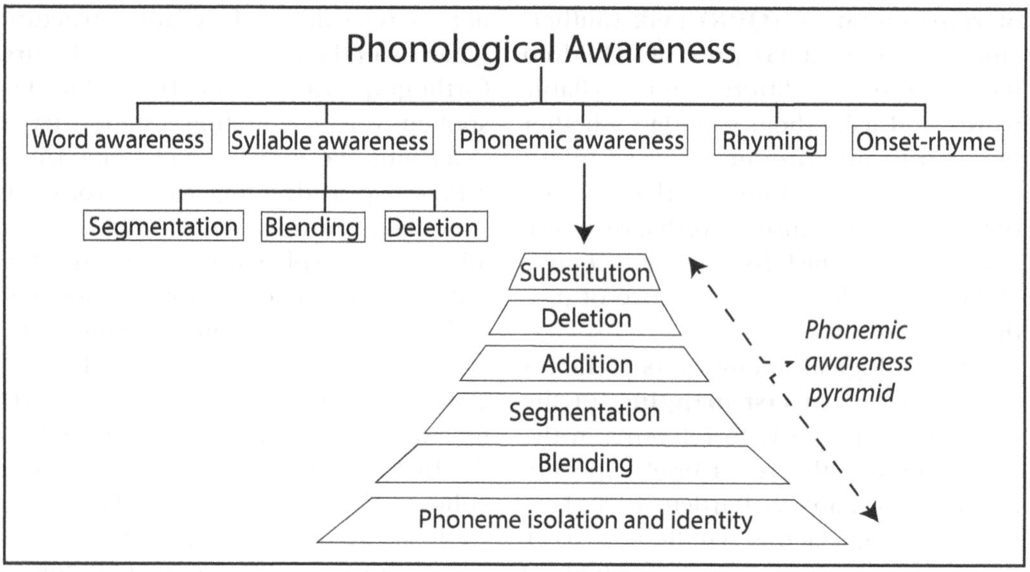

Figure 7–7. Components of phonological awareness (PA).

(3) phonemes. Whatever the status of these elements in phonological theories, they have operational value in assessing and treating PA. The concept of the syllable is introduced in Chapter 3, and syllable structure is illustrated in Figure 3–6. The words **rhyme** and **rime** are similar, but they have different meanings. *Rime*, derived from the Germanic *rim*, identifies a part of a word that has a particular spelling, beginning with a vowel and ending before the next vowel in the word. For example, the words *big*, *dig*, and *fig* share the rime "ig." The initial sounds /b/, /d/, and /f/ are onsets. A *rhyme* is a correspondence of sounds between words. If two words contain similar sounds usually at the end of the words, they are said to rhyme. For example, the words *tore*, *door*, *four*, and *nor* all rhyme but do not contain the same rime. As children develop PA, they show the ability to recognize words that rhyme or possess alliteration (repetition of the same initial sound), to parse a sentence into words, to identify the syllables in a word, and to blend and segment onsets and rhymes. PA is the most demanding and last to develop capability. This capability includes being able to blend sounds into words, break words into their component sounds, and delete, exchange, or otherwise manipulate the sounds in spoken words.

PA is usually assessed by asking a child to detect a sound or to manipulate sound patterns in larger units, such as syllables or words. PA develops in a fairly ordered pattern that has two major characteristics (Anthony & Francis, 2005). The first is an increasing gradation in phonological sensitivity: children detect or manipulate syllables before onsets and rimes, and they can detect or manipulate onsets and rimes before individual phonemes within intrasyllabic word units. That is, development proceeds from larger units to smaller units. The second is that children can detect words that are similar or dissimilar in sound pattern before they can manipulate sounds within words, and they can blend phonological information before they can segment phonological information of the same linguistic complexity (Anthony et al., 2003). The three main methods of assessing PA are norm-referenced, criterion-referenced, and curriculum-based (Taylor, 2000). Assessments in these methods are reviewed by Sodoro et al. (2002). Examples of specific phonological tasks are as follows:

Word awareness: How many words are in this sentence? "I will sit down." (Correct response: 4).

Rhyme: Do these words rhyme? "big, dig." (Correct response: Yes)

Syllable blending: I am going to say a word in parts. Listen: win . . . dow What word did I say? (Correct response: window)

Syllable segmentation: Can you tell me the two parts of the word "window?" (Correct response: win . . . dow)

Syllable deletion: Say "window" without the "dow" (Correct response: win)

Onset-rime: What word do these sounds make? /b/ – /ee/ (Correct response: bee). How about /s/ – /up/? (Correct response: soup)

Poor skills of PA have been associated with a variety of disorders, including the following: omissions and atypical speech errors in children with speech sound disorders (Brosseau-Lapré & Roepke, 2019; Holm et al., 2008), CAS (McNeill et al., 2009), developmental language disorders (Thatcher, 2010; Vukovic et al., 2022), dyslexia (Dodd & Gillon, 2001), and ASD (O'Brien et al., 2022). PA potentially draws on several different cognitive, sensory, and motor resources that may be variably affected in these disorders. Predictors of PA in children include auditory processing ability (Eccles et al., 2021; Jain et al., 2020), receptive vocabulary and nonword repetition (Erskine et al., 2020). In turn, PA has been shown to predict development of language skills in areas such as word recognition and spelling (Hulme & Snowling, 2009).

Phonological Production

Phonological production is the output of the phonological system. It integrates aspects of phonological memory, access, and awareness, together with the processes involved in formulating a phonological sequence that is converted to speech movements. The output can be regarded as resembling a phonemic or phonetic transcription, but with prosodic details that are often neglected in such transcriptions.

Phonological Processes in Children's Speech Production

Chapter 4 discusses how phonological processes are used to describe typical speech production in children. The usual explanation given for these processes is that they are simplifications that children employ as they attempt to produce adult-like speech. This assumption is fundamental to natural phonology, reviewed earlier in this chapter. Persistence of a process beyond the typical age of suppression (disappearance) is often taken as evidence of a delay in speech development.

Some children with speech sound disorders produce speech with atypical phonological processes, that is, processes that are not observed at any stage of typical speech development. These atypical processes potentially indicate disorder rather than delay because they deviate from the typical developmental pattern. Dodd (2011) identified several atypical processes including: backing of bilabial and palatal stops, deletion of initial consonants in words or syllables, substitution of stops by fricatives, clusters marked by bilabial fricatives, vowel errors, pervasive sound preferences, intrusive vowels, and extensive assimilation. The departure of these processes from the typical pattern would seem to require an explanation other than the usual assumption of simplification that is invoked to explain typical processes. Some atypical processes violate the assumption of simplification (e.g., backing of bilabial stops, deletion of initial consonants, and substitution of stops by fricatives). Atypical speech errors have been associated with poor skills of phonological awareness (Brosseau-Lapré & Roepke, 2019; Preston & Edwards, 2010; Preston et al., 2013), which may indicate that these errors arise in a faulty phonological representation, a possibility considered in more detail later in this chapter. At the minimum, phonological process analysis is a summary of patterns of speech sound errors. Whether it succeeds as an explanatory vehicle is open for debate.

A clinical index based on phonological processes is the **Phonological Density Index (PDI)**, which is calculated by counting the number of process applications in each word of a speech sample, adding the values obtained, and dividing the resulting sum by the total number of words in the sample (Edwards, 1992). PDI has been used as a measure of severity of a speech disorder (van Borsel & D'haeseleer, 2019; Wertzner et al., 2007). Because the PDI is based on an overall count of processes, it does not assign different weights to these processes.

Rapid Autonomized Naming (RAN)

Rapid automatized naming (**RAN**, also called **rapid automatic naming** or **rapid serial naming**) is the ability to quickly name aloud objects, pictures, colors, or symbols (e.g., letters or digits). Therefore, it is a task that combines retrieval and productive abilities associated with a visually presented stimulus (Norton & Wolf, 2012; Scarborough & Brady, 2002). Some authorities view rapid automatized naming as focusing on phonological retrieval, but others regard it as encompassing a set of skills that are needed for reading. Variations in rapid automatized naming time in children provide a strong predictor of their later ability to read and are independent from other predictors, such as phonological awareness, verbal IQ, and existing reading skills. Närhi et al. (2005) concluded that rapid autonomized naming is influenced by phonological skills, processing speed, motor dexterity, and verbal fluency. They also noted that tasks used to assess rapid autonomized naming vary in their properties according to both the stimuli and the arrangement of the tasks. Several commercial RAN tests are available, and they generally show four types of items: objects, colors, letters, and numbers. The typical procedure is to show small sets of items in the same category on a single page (e.g., five small squares of several different colors). It is important to select stimuli that are familiar to the child and within the child's lexicon.

Nonword Repetition (NWR)

A task often used in phonological assessment is the nonword repetition test (NWRT), a speaking task in which children are asked to repeat phonetic sequences, often but not necessarily multisyllabic, that are not recognizable words in the language (e.g., the nonword or nonsense word /taʊf/ for speakers of English). Nonword repetition tests include the Children's Test of Nonword Repetition (CNRep; Gathercole & Baddeley, 1996; Gathercole et al., 1994), Nonword Repetition Test (NRT; Dollaghan & Campbell, 1998), Syllable Repetition Test (SRT; Shriberg et al., 2009), Late-8 Non-word Repetition Task (L8NRT; Moore et al., 2010), a prosodically controlled word and nonword repetition task for 2- to 4- year-olds (Roy & Chiat, 2004), and the Crosslinguistic Nonword Repetition framework, which includes three tests that vary the phonological characteristics of nonwords (Chiat & Polišenská, 2016). Children with several types of communication disorders may have deficits in nonword repetition that are related to factors, such as auditory temporal processing, phonological short-term memory, lexical knowledge, and output processes (Archibald & Gathercole, 2006).

Erskine et al. (2020) found that PA was predicted by a measure of speech production and a measure of phonological processing derived from NWR. The implication is that NWR accuracy is an implicit measure of phonological skills foundational to later PA at an age when explicit PA tasks are not suitable. Furthermore, as Coady and Evans (2008) remark, "because the task taps so many underlying skills, it is a powerful tool that can be used to identify children with language impairments" (p. 1). The clinical utility of NWR extends to other clinical populations as well, as discussed in the following.

CAS. Rvachew and Matthews (2017) found that the SRT combined with other measures revealed three patterns in children with CAS: (1) deficits in phonological planning, (i.e., low memory scores on the SRT and high word inconsistency), (2) deficits in motor planning, (i.e., low transcoding scores on the SRT and prosodic errors), and (3) other profiles (i.e., primary deficits in the domain of phonology or language rather than speech production). Peter et al. (2018) reported that adults with either dyslexia or probable CAS had persisting deficits in NWRT, with disproportionately more sequencing than substitution errors.

Developmental Fluency Disorder. Gerwin et al. (2022) concluded that children with developmental fluency disorder with or without concomitant communication disorders had more errors on syllable onsets, more errors on the first and fourth syllable of the four-syllable nonwords, and more substitution errors than children without a fluency disorder. Children with a fluency disorder who had concomitant speech sound and/or language disorders had more omission and migration errors than children without a fluency disorder or children with a fluency disorder without concomitant speech sound and/or language disorders. Smith et al. (2012) found that children who stutter and have concomitant speech or language disorders had more errors in nonword repetition than typically developing children, but children who stutter and do not have other speech or language disorders were as accurate as typically developing children in this task. However, these children had atypical articulatory movements, indicating the presence of speech motor control difficulties.

Developmental Language Disorder (DLD). Reduced performance on NWR tasks has been reported for children with DLD (Archibald, 2008; Graf Estes et al., 2007; Jackson et al. 2019; Pigdon, Willmott, Reilly, Conti-Ramsden, & Morgan, 2020). A meta-analysis by Graf Estes et al. (2007) revealed that, for monolingual children, nonwords that are best suited to discriminate between typically developing children and children with DLD are word-like, longer, and articulatorily complex. An appealing aspect of NWRTs is that they potentially can be used with children who have different language backgrounds. Studies support this possibility, but some cautions should be observed. A systematic review and meta-analysis indicated that NWRT has value in identifying DLD in monolingual and bilingual children, but the test materials should be selected in keeping with the children's language background and combined with other assessments (Schwob et al., 2021). A meta-analysis indicated that diagnostic accuracy of the NWRT in bilingual children accuracy ranged from poor to good, and that quasi-universal tasks (i.e., those with phonotactic constraints across multiple languages) had better diagnostic accuracy and resulted in less misidentification of children with typical language than language-specific tasks (Ortiz, 2021).

Speech Sound Disorder (SSD). Children with SSD are less accurate than typically developing children in nonword repetition tasks (Martikainen et al., 2021; Munson et al., 2005; Pigdon, Willmott, Reilly, Conti-Ramsden, Liegeois, Connelly, & Morgan, 2020). Munson et al. compared the performance of children with SSD and TD children on the production of low- and high-frequency diphone sequences. Both groups were less accurate in producing low-frequency sequences than high-frequency sequences. Although the children with SSD were less accurate overall, they did not show a marked disadvantage for the low-frequency sequences compared to the TD children. The magnitude of the frequency effect correlated with vocabulary size but not measures of speech perception and articulatory ability, which was interpreted to mean that the production difficulty associated with low/frequency sequences is related more to vocabulary growth rather than to articulatory or perceptual abilities. The authors explained the results of their study as follows:

> Phonological acquisition involves not only the development of well-practiced articulatory and acoustic–auditory representations but also the emergence of a symbolic representation that links both of these primary phonological representations to each other as well as to representations of other types of linguistic knowledge in the lexicon. (p. 77)

It is becoming clear that multiple factors contribute to NWR performance in both TD children and children with SSD. Farquharson et al. (2021) commented that children with SSD are a complex and heterogeneous group, and that many different factors account for their reduced ability to perform phonological tasks such as NWR. Pigdon, Willmott, Reilly, Conti-Ramsden, and Morgan (2020) also pointed to the multidimensional nature of the nonword repetition task and presented evidence of the contributions from phonological memory, word reading, speech sequencing, and oromotor control.

Model of Phonological Processing in Children

This section is an overview of children's phonological processing as it relates to speech and language disorders. It presents a version of what could be called "performance phonology," that is, a phonology that is oriented to the operations that are involved in the perception and production of phonological patterns from a developmental perspective. The discussion is keyed to Figures 7–8 and 7–9. Figure 7–8 is a diagram of the various processes involved in producing a word or nonword utterance. These processes are contained in the three shaded blocks in the illustration: Perception, Representation, and Phonetic-Motor. Perception has the components of initial auditory processing and speech perception. Representation has the components of phonological representation (for both words and nonwords) and semantic representation (for words but not nonwords). Phonetic-Motor has the components of phonetic encoding (with access to a syllabary) and motor planning/programming (with access to an internal model of speech production). The boundaries of the blocks should not be considered as impermeable, as some components, such as the syllabary, can relate to more than one block.

Each component of the diagram in Figure 7–8 is vulnerable to disruptions

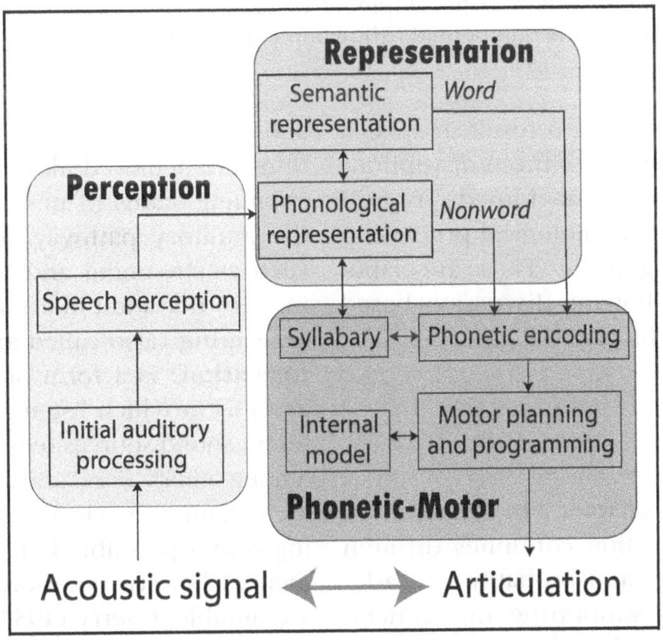

Figure 7–8. Diagram of the various processes involved in producing a word or nonword utterance. The processes are contained in the three shaded blocks: Perception, Representation, and Phonetic-Motor.

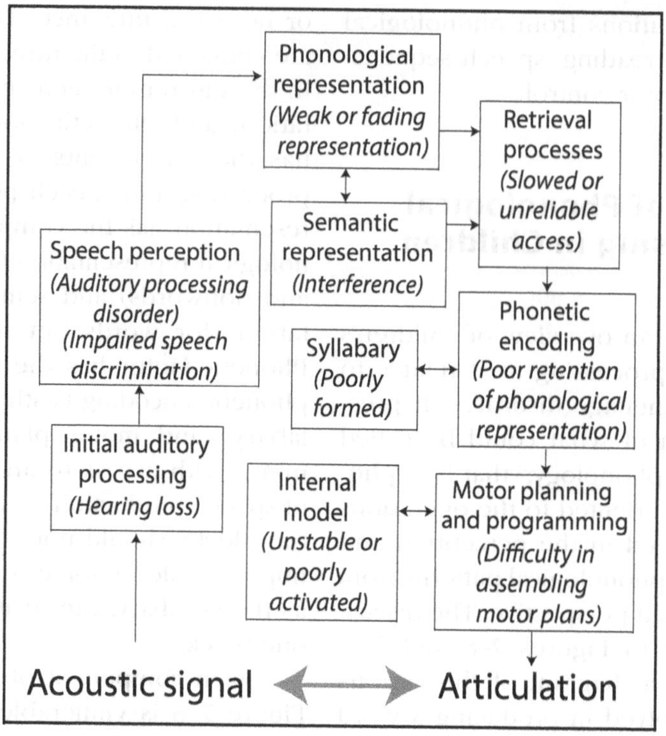

Figure 7–9. Examples of disruptions and weaknesses that impede typical development of phonological processing using the components shown in Figure 7–8.

or weaknesses that can result in speech disorders. Examples of these disruptions and weaknesses that impede typical development of phonological processing are shown in Figure 7–9. These are elaborated in the following discussion based on the shaded blocks in Figure 7–8.

Perception

It was noted in Chapter 2 that maturation of auditory function continues through at least puberty and probably into adolescence. Data supporting this conclusion are from studies of psychoacoustics, speech perception, and phonological processing. Maturational aspects of audition are summarized in Table 7–1, which shows the ages at which adult-like functions are achieved along with the corresponding status of neural maturation of the auditory pathway. Some functions, such as streaming and backward masking, are not adult-like until adolescence. **Streaming** (also called **auditory stream formation**) is a form of auditory scene analysis in which listeners parse out different sound sources (e.g., one voice from among other voices) and assigns appropriate meaning to selected sources. Streaming is indispensable in listening environments where two or more sound sources are audible. Cherry (1953) described the **cocktail party problem** as the ability to listen selectively to one among several competing voices. As applied to children, we might call this phenomenon the **play-**

Table 7–1. Maturation of the Auditory Pathway Based on Age at Which Adult-Like Functions Are Achieved and Maturation of Neural Processes

Age Group	Adult-Like Auditory Function Achieved	Status of Neural Maturation
Infancy	High-frequency detection Frequency discrimination	Axons appear in the white matter of the temporal lobe, radiating into the deeper cortical layers 4, 5, and 6.
Preschool age	Loudness perception	Progressive maturation of the thalamocortical projections, and of the longer-latency Pa and P1 evoked potentials Mature axons appear in cortical layers 2 and 3.
Early school age	Low-frequency detection Intensity discrimination Maximal sensitivity for stimuli of 2 and 4 kHz	
Middle school age	Maximal sensitivity for stimuli of 0.4 and 1 kHz	Density of axons in cortical layers 2 and 3 is similar to that of young adults.
Teen age	Auditory scene analysis (streaming) Backward masking	The adult waveform complex of the cortical auditory evoked potential (CAEP) is achieved between 14 and 16 years of age but variability continues to decrease during adolescence.

Sources: Fiori (1972), Fitzroy et al. (2015), Litovsky (2015), and Pasman et al. (1999).

ground problem, in which a child distinguishes another child's voice from among many. In the case of a speech signal, coherence is maintained through various cues, such as linguistic structure, speaker-specific formant patterns, and intonational continuities in the utterance. The processes involved in streaming are illustrated in Figure 7–10. These processes can operate in either bottom-up or top-down directions and are critical to the ability to identify sound sources and maintain coherence of a signal attributed to an individual source. **Backward masking** is the masking of an auditory stimulus by another stimulus that occurs immediately after it. Backward masking requires temporal processing of information relating to signal/masker delays and is a useful index of the maturation of temporal processing ability. In general, the auditory functions that are last to mature are those pertaining to temporal information processing (and which are central to complex signals such as speech). Research has shown that this kind of processing can be impaired in children who have a variety of speech and language disorders.

Table 7–1 gives a general indication of auditory-perceptual development, but it should be noted that (a) there are wide variations in developmental patterns across individual children (Moore et al., 2011) and (b) attentional processes

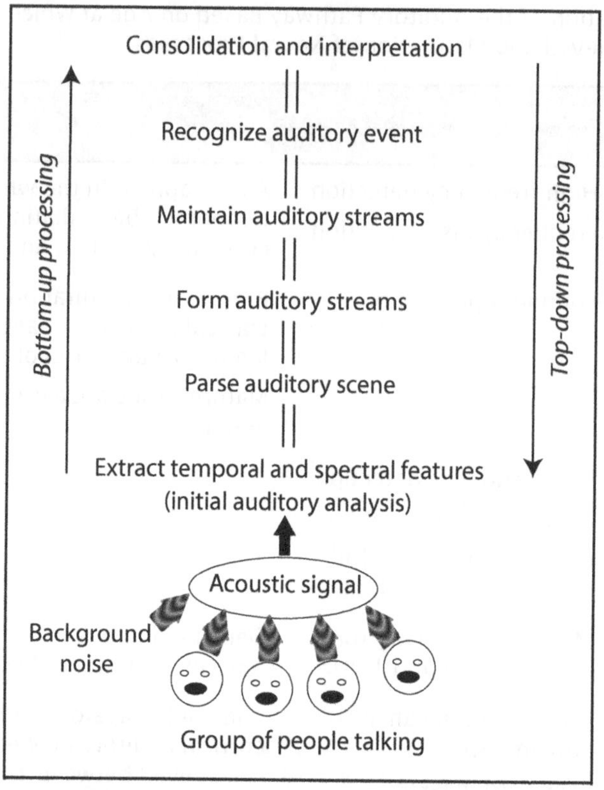

Figure 7–10. Processes involved in auditory streaming. These can operate in either bottom-up or top-down direction.

rather than sensory limitations per se may account for some aspects of typical development (Price & Moncrieff, 2021). Richardson et al. (2004) reported that individual differences in auditory tasks based on differences in the rise time of the amplitude envelope explained significant variance in phonological processing, leading to the inference that amplitude envelope cues are critical to forming well-specified phonological representations that include rhythmic and syllable-level information. Accumulating evidence points to the importance of temporal auditory processing to support speech and language development. Neural processing occurs at several levels of the auditory pathway, including subcortical structures. For example, Banai et al., (2009) show that reading and phonological processing are related to subcortical auditory encoding of timing and harmonics.

Representation

The core elements of this component are phonological and semantic representations, which interact, especially when they are linked to a common lexical element. The phonological representation can work independently to produce nonwords or novel words. The syllabary, which usually is assumed to be located between the levels of phonological and phonetic encoding, is a store of the syllables that occur with high frequency in a language. The syllabary is advantageous in speech production because it contains precompiled motor programs that permit rapid articulation with minimal demands on computation (Cholin, 2008). As a child's lexicon grows, it becomes advantageous to retrieve syllable-sized elements to form words. But the syllabary also is useful for words that are new and do not have a secure phonological or semantic representation.

Phonetic-Motor

This component pertains to the production of speech patterns, but it is the product of the components of perception and representation. The production of speech is inevitably influenced by how speech is perceived and represented. The Phonetic-Motor component consists of operations of phonetic encoding and motor planning/programming, which translate a phonological representation into patterns of speech movements (not only articulation in the usual sense of supra-laryngeal adjustments but also adjustments at the respiratory and laryngeal levels for aspects of prosody). As discussed in Chapters 2 and 4, the anatomic and physiologic maturation of the systems of speech production extends up to at least adolescence, and refinement of speech motor control is similarly protracted. General assessment methods, as covered in Chapter 5, can be used to detect the presence and severity of impairments in the phonetic-motor component.

Clinical Assessment Guidelines

The preceding discussion identifies the basic issues to be addressed in clinical assessment: phonological memory, phonological access, phonological awareness, and phonological production. These are interactive processes, and it is not easy to isolate any one of them. Nor is likely that any single test will provide satisfactory information for all of them. In clinical assessment, these usually are components in a broad spectrum, as summarized in the following description of articulatory/phonological assessments.

Fabiano-Smith (2019) listed ten components of an evidence-based protocol for assessment. Each of these, along with some additions, is briefly discussed in the following. The discussion is keyed to information presented in other chapters.

Detailed case history. This typically includes a child's health history along with information on the child's family and life circumstances. It can be important to obtain information on risk factors and associated health problems (discussed in Chapter 11).

Speech sample. Stoel-Gammon and Stone (1991) recommended that the child's language level be considered in collecting and analyzing a sample and in interpreting the results. If the child has age-level language abilities, then it is appropriate to use a sample consisting of both a single-word test and a running speech sample (also called a connected speech sample). Both independent and relational analyses can be used. If the child has delayed expressive language and a small productive vocabulary, then it is advisable to use a sample of spontaneous productions that should be analyzed with respect to sound classes and syllable and word shapes (a phonological process analysis is inappropriate). The results should be interpreted with consideration of the child's language level. In general, the size and sophistication of the phonological system varies with the size of the child's vocabulary and the number of word combinations the child uses. If a child has delayed language and is within the first 50-word stage of expressive vocabulary, a limited phonological system is likely. As noted in Chapter 5, a connected speech sample of at least 75 to 100 words is needed for the analyses that are most common in clinical assessment.

Routine assessments. These are discussed in Chapter 5 and include speech mechanism (oral peripheral) examination, selected motor assessments, and articulation tests, as appropriate for an individual child and assessment goals.

Phonetic inventory. Discussed in Chapter 5.

Consonant accuracy. Discussed in Chapter 5.

Error patterns (e.g., SODA). Discussed in Chapter 5.

Phonological pattern analysis. Discussed in Chapter 5 and the present chapter. Stoel-Gammon and Stone (1991) recommended that a child's phonological system be considered in its entirety, with attention to the presence or absence of sound classes and syllable shapes rather than on individual sounds. This point could be extended to consider co-occurring auditory and motor skills, which can interact with phonology.

Measures of whole-word proximity. Discussed in Chapter 5.

Phonological memory, access, and awareness. Discussed in this chapter.

Nonword Repetition. Discussed in the present chapter. Several tests are available and can be selected with consideration of child characteristics such as age, language ability, and language background.

Stimulability. Discussed in Chapters 5 and 9.

Voice and prosody. Discussed in Chapter 6. These aspects are not always noted in assessment protocols, but they can be important in describing the full character of a speech disorder, especially in conditions such as ASD and Down syndrome.

Intelligibility and/or comprehensibility. These, along with other global properties such as naturalness and accentedness are discussed in Chapter 8.

Conclusions

1. Several phonological theories have been introduced within the field of linguistics. These theories differ in several important respects, but one feature in common is that they say very little about acoustic, auditory, or motor factors that are critical

to phonological development in children. Clinical assessment would benefit from a more performance-oriented phonological framework.

2. The main aspects of phonology considered in this chapter are phonological memory, access to phonological patterns in memory, phonological awareness, and phonological production (output to the speech production system). Each of these plays a role in phonological development and each is susceptible to weakness or error in children with speech disorders. Because they interact with one another, it can be difficult to isolate their effects on speech disorders.
3. Phonological development and phonological disorders can be understood in terms of models of spoken language (discussed in Chapter 3) and neural networks serving speech perception and production.
4. Several different methods can be used to assess aspects of phonological processing in children. Some are suitable for children as young as 2 to 3 years of age, whereas others can be used with older children who have more mature language abilities.

8

ASSESSMENT OF INTELLIGIBILITY, COMPREHENSIBILITY, AND OTHER GLOBAL FEATURES

The production of fluent, intelligible speech is a supreme motor behavior that is unique to humans. Vocal behavior is shared by many species, but human speech is in a class by itself. Certainly, speech is more than a motor behavior, but motor activity is the means to the accomplishment of speech that is intelligible and comprehensible, two major global aspects of speech communication. Additional global properties of speech are accuracy, listener effort, communicative efficiency, fluency, naturalness, and accentedness, each of which has been the subject of research in typical and atypical speech. These variables determine functional communication, that is, communication that serves functions related to daily living and other pursuits (Figure 8–1). They give perspective to the study of speech in various populations, including individuals with typical speech, those with speech disorders, and those learning a second language. Because these terms generally lack a standardized definition and because they can overlap with one another in some respects, this chapter begins with a set of definitions and then proceeds to methods of assessment for each global property.

Definitions of Speech Intelligibility and Comprehensibility

These terms do not have a standard definition across specialties such as speech-language pathology, second-language learning, psycholinguistics, or speech technologies such as automatic speech recognition. The definitions used in this book pertain mainly to speech disorders and reflect the literature in that field.

Pommée et al. (2022) provide definitions of intelligibility and comprehensibility that are useful for clinical purposes. Pommée et al. defined **intelligibility** as the "reconstruction of an utterance at the

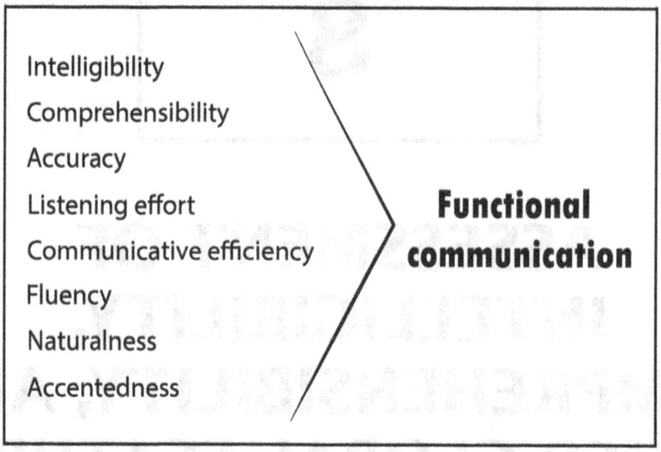

Figure 8–1. Diagram showing elements that contribute to functional communication.

acoustic–phonetic level, intelligibility-related information is thus carried by the acoustic signal (i.e., intelligibility focuses on signal-dependent information)" (p. 31). This definition may not cover all circumstances, for example, when a clinician uses visual information that accompanies a client's spoken message. It is well established that speech perception can be accomplished with auditory-visual integration, as in the McGurk effect (McGurk & MacDonald, 1976), which shows that speech perception is not exclusively auditory but can include processing of cross-modality components even when the auditory information is intact (Alsius et al., 2018). A more general definition of intelligibility is, therefore, the reconstruction of an utterance at the phonetic level, relying on signal-dependent information from available sensory channels. A narrow definition pertains only to acoustic information, and a somewhat broader definition adds the possibility of visual cues, such as facial expressions and gestures. The basic elements of speech intelligibility are represented by the dark shaded area in Figure 8–2. Intelligibility cues can be acoustic and/or visual. Much of the research on intelligibility in speech disorders relies on recordings of the acoustic signal, but a smaller number of studies have used video recordings in which acoustic and visual cues are available.

Pommée et al. define **comprehensibility** as the "reconstruction of a message at the semantic–discursive level, subsequent to the acoustic–phonetic reconstruction" (p. 31). With these definitions, intelligibility is regarded as a component of comprehensibility, with the latter requiring acoustic–phonetic decoding but also signal-independent, contextual elements such as the linguistic or non-verbal context. Comprehensibility is represented in Figure 8–2 as the light shaded area that contains within it the darker shaded area of intelligibility. Intelligibility is necessary to some degree but not sufficient to ensure comprehensibility. In one of the first reports on this concept as it relates to a communication disorder, comprehensibility was operationally defined as "the extent to which a listener understands utterances produced by a speaker in a communication context" (Barefoot

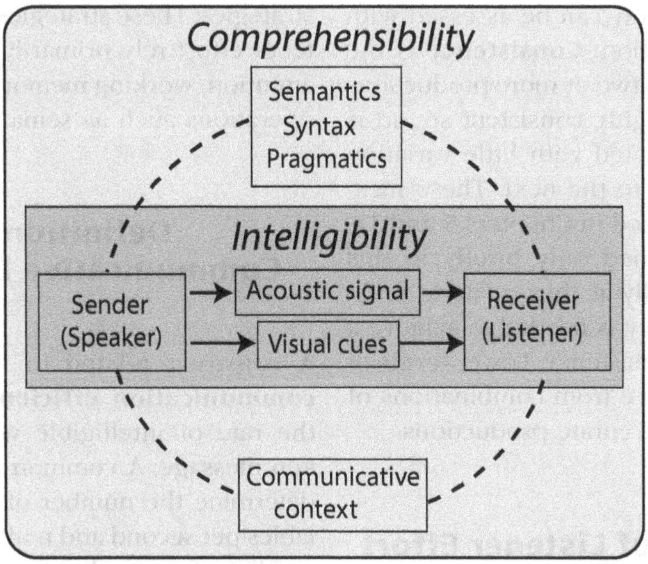

Figure 8–2. Diagram of factors contributing to speech comprehensibility, which includes speech intelligibility (dark shaded area) and the elements shown in lighter shading.

et al., 1993). In a study of 41 deaf young adults, these authors concluded that comprehensibility can be evaluated reliably and that it is associated with both speech intelligibility and language proficiency. Yorkston et al. (1996) considered the concept of comprehensibility as it applies to dysarthria, noting that the main distinction between intelligibility and comprehensibility is that the former relates to signal-dependent information (the acoustic signal of speech) whereas the latter incorporates signal-independent information (syntax, semantics, and physical context). Comprehensibility also has been defined in terms of listeners' judgment as to how challenging it is to comprehend an utterance (Derwing & Munro, 2005). These definitions converge on the basic concept that comprehensibility is based to some degree on speech intelligibility in the narrow sense of signal-specific acoustic information; on information from other senses (especially visual information regarding gestures and facial expressions); by higher-level linguistic knowledge relating to semantics, syntax, and pragmatics; and to situational factors that define the communicative context.

Definition of Speech Accuracy

Speech accuracy is the correspondence between a speech target (usually a phoneme or a word) and the production of that target by a client, as discussed in Chapter 5. The term *accuracy* also has been used in relation to variability or consistency of production, as in the case of repeated productions of a target. This book distinguishes between accuracy and consistency. A highly accurate production is one that closely matches a defined target, such as a sound segment. Accuracy defined in this way can be assessed with a single production. **Consistency** is the variability across two or more productions of a target. A highly consistent sound is one that is repeated with little variation from one token to the next. These measures are discussed in Chapters 5 and 11, and are mentioned only briefly in this chapter, especially as they relate to intelligibility. Accuracy is needed to achieve a high level of consistency. Lower levels of consistency derive from combinations of accurate and inaccurate productions.

Definition of Listener Effort

Listening (or listener) effort is generally defined as the attention and cognitive resources (e.g., working memory and semantic integration) needed to understand a speech signal. Much of the research on this topic pertains to degraded listening environments, especially the presence of noise or other disruptions. Peelle (2018) wrote that, "functional brain imaging reveals that the neural resources required to understand degraded speech extend beyond traditional perisylvian language networks, most commonly including regions of prefrontal cortex, premotor cortex, and the cingulo-opercular network" (p. 204). Listener effort is an important consideration when speech production is affected by bilingualism or dialect (Van Engen & Peelle, 2014) or speech disorder (Fletcher et al., 2022; Landa et al., 2014; Whitehill & Wong, 2006). Listener effort is distinct from intelligibility and comprehensibility because a speech message may have various degrees of intelligibility or comprehensibility depending on the success of a listener's cognitive strategies. These strategies involved in listener effort rely primarily on motivation, attention, working memory, and cognitive operations such as semantic integration.

Definition of Communicative Efficiency

A construct related to intelligibility is **communication efficiency**, defined as the rate of intelligible words in a spoken message. A common procedure is to determine the number of intelligible syllables per second and multiplying the proportion of correctly transcribed syllables with speech rate in syllables per second. Speech rate is more easily measured than articulation rate and allows for the effects of reduced communication rate through both slowed articulation and dysfluent speech (Haas et al., 2022). Efficiency is proportional to the number of intelligible words in a specified interval of time.

Definition of Fluency

The American Speech-Language-Hearing Association defines **fluency** as the continuity, smoothness, rate, and effort in speech production (https://www.asha.org/practice-portal/clinical-topics/fluency-disorders/). Fluent speech is free of interruptions, has smooth transitions across segments and syllables, has a normal or typical rate, and is produced without exceptional effort. Each of these terms must have their own definition to give a full understanding of speech fluency. Interruptions are breaks in the continuity of a speech pattern and can take several forms, including, silent or vocalized pauses; repetitions of sounds, syllables, or words; or prolongations of sounds. Smooth transitions are movements of normal duration between sound elements. Normal rate is a rate that is typical of a conversation or reading task for a given age of speaker. Effort is the energy expenditure in a motor task. Assessment of fluency is discussed in Chapter 5 and fluency disorders in Chapter 11.

Definition of Naturalness

Perhaps no concept in the study of speech communication has been as difficult to define as **naturalness**. Several definitions have been proffered and they vary considerably in their characteristics (Klopfenstein et al., 2019). Despite the definitional uncertainty, the concept of naturalness is pervasive in the study of both human and machine speech. With respect to neurogenic communication disorders, Yorkston et al. (1999) wrote that, "Speech is natural if it conforms to the listener's standard of rate, rhythm, intonation, and stress patterning, and if it conforms to the syntactic structure of the utterance being produced" (p. 464). This is rather a tall order, given that it encompasses just about every aspect of speech. Stepp and Vojtech (2019) wrote that, "Speech naturalness is a global descriptor that integrates the effects of numerous perceptual cues of speech into one overarching measure. As a global measure, it captures a wide range of individual features across a broad range of communication disorders" (p. 1777). In the area of speech synthesis, naturalness often is defined in terms of being "humanlike," which, along with intelligibility, is the holy grail of machine-generated speech. An additional source of confusion is that several other terms have been used almost interchangeably with naturalness, including bizarreness, acceptability, and normalcy (Klopfenstein et al., 2019). It might be asked if naturalness is an independent dimension, distinct from other dimensions such as intelligibility. The answer appears to be in the affirmative, given indications of dissociation between naturalness and intelligibility in the study of both human and machine speech. It appears that the hallmark of speech naturalness is typicality, the quality of being typical or representative of most speakers in a particular population. In evaluating text-to-speech systems, a typical procedure is to determine mean opinion scores (MOS) for judgments of naturalness on a scale between 1 (worst) and 5 (best), often with no definition of naturalness so as not to bias the listener.

Definition of Accentedness

Accentedness is the degree to which a listener judges L2 speech to differ from that of a typical native speaker (Munro & Derwing, 1995). It has been shown that even heavily accented speech can be highly comprehensible and intelligible (Luchini, 2017; Nagle & Huensch, 2020). Therefore, accentedness is distinct from intelligibility and comprehensibility, although interactions are possible. As discussed in Chapter 10, accentedness can be a major concern with individuals who are learning English as a second language and may be a focus of intervention even if speech is intelligible and comprehensible.

Assessing Intelligibility

Both speaker and listener characteristics must be considered in assessments of intelligibility and comprehensibility. For optimal communication, speakers and listeners should share language in its various facets, including phonetic, semantic, and syntactic. As discussed later in this chapter, many different approaches have been taken to assess intelligibility. Some authors recognize two major approaches: objective and subjective (Hustad & Borrie, 2021). In this view, objective approaches typically quantify intelligibility in terms of units of some kind (phonemes, syllables, words, or sentences) correctly transmitted. Judgments take the form of a transcription (e.g., orthography, broad phonetic transcription, narrow phonetic transcription, or forced-choice recognition of target items). Subjective approaches generally use listener ratings of the degree of perceived intelligibility in tasks such as direct magnitude estimation, equal appearing interval scales, percentage of speech that is understood, or visual analog scales.

A caveat to these definitions should be noted. All judgments of speech by a listener are influenced by individual characteristics such as familiarity with a speaker, the dialect used by a speaker, experience with different groups of speakers, attention, and other factors. Fletcher and Galt (1950) proposed a proficiency factor *P* to account for differences in intelligibility related to factors such as differences in the communication skills of talkers/listeners, dialectal differences between talkers and listeners, and practice effects. The value of *P* is a product of the proficiency of the talker and the proficiency of the listener. *P* has a maximum value of 1 in the ideal communicative setting, in which talker and listener are familiar and well-practiced and there are minimal obstacles to communication.

Studies of the intelligibility of adults with dysarthria have revealed substantial differences among listeners, with familiarity often being highly influential (DePaul & Kent, 2000; Hirsch et al., 2022; Tjaden & Liss, 1995a, 1995b). The same result holds for children's speech intelligibility. A study of audience response system-based evaluation of children's speech revealed that judgments obtained from individual listeners lacked adequate reliability but data from a listener panel achieved a satisfactory result (Strömbergsson et al., 2020). There is at present no truly objective measure of intelligibility for clinical use if objective is defined as a measure that is not influenced by human experience or personal standards. Intelligibility is a cognitive construct and is not objective in the sense of laboratory techniques such as blood tests, spirometry, or measures of weight and height. Furthermore, intelligibility scores can differ significantly across different measurement approaches (Johannisson et al., 2014). Speech comprehensibility also relies on cognitive capabilities related to individual judgment and experience. For present purposes, objective assessment is a term reserved for technological methods, as described next.

Objective approaches, sometimes referred to as **objective intelligibility measures (OIMs**; Tang et al., 2018), are algorithmic estimates of speech intelligibility and are the subject of modern developments in speech technology. OIMs have the potential advantages of speed, economy, automation, reliability, and repeated application (Feng & Chen, 2022). The two main categories of OIMs are intrusive and nonintrusive, which differ on the need for a reference signal. Intrusive approaches are reference-based methods that are based on a clean speech or noise sample for reference. Nonintrusive approaches do not require such a reference and would be highly useful for speech disorders. Feng and Chen (2022) identified three main types of nonintrusive approaches: traditional or heuristic (feature-based) approaches, statistical or data-driven methods that typically use machine learning and deep learning models, and neurophysiological measures that integrate neuroimaging or oculometric techniques. This is an active field of research and development, and it may lead to truly objective measures of speech intelligibility.

Various approaches have been used to assess the intelligibility of children's speech (Allison, 2020; Hustad & Borrie, 2021; Kent et al., 1994), which gives clinicians considerable latitude in selecting a specific method for their clients. Intelligibility is a major consideration in both assessment and treatment of speech disorders, as it may be the most critical aspect of successful communication. Direct assessment of intelligibility is one of the most frequently used clinical assessments for children with speech disorders (Skahan et al., 2007). Lousada et al. (2014) concluded that intelligibility is a more stringent measure of change compared with other commonly used measures of severity. The following decisions are needed to perform an assessment of intelligibility. These decisions are summarized in the following.

1. What are the materials to be used? Some possibilities are syllables, words, sentences, and conversation, which can be used in various combinations.
2. Who will make the assessment and under what conditions? Some possibilities are (a) the clinician performs the assessment with recorded speech samples, (b) the clinician judges the intelligibility in a face-to-face setting, and (c) a person unfamiliar with the child performs the assessment either face-to-face or from recorded speech samples, and (d) a listener panel performs the assessment from recorded speech samples. The first two of these are commonly used clinically, whereas the last two are more common in research.
3. What type of assessment will be used? Possibilities are shown in Figure 8–3. These are considered next.

Parental Report

The Intelligibility in Context Scale (ICS; McLeod et al., 2012) appears to be the most used scale for parental reports on children's intelligibility. The ICS consists of seven items for which parents consider their child's speech intelligibility over the past month and estimate the degree to which the parents themselves and the six other types of communication partners understand the child using a 5-point interval scale (1 = never, 2 = rarely, 3 = sometimes, 4 = usually, 5 = always). Data have been reported on cross-language use, validity, and reliability (McLeod, 2020; McLeod et al., 2015) as well as applications to speech disorders associated with cerebral palsy (Soriano et al., 2021), cleft lip or palate (Seifert et al., 2021), and velopharyngeal insufficiency (Hosseinabad et al., 2022). Lagerberg, Anrep-Nordin, et al. (2021, p. 884) stated,

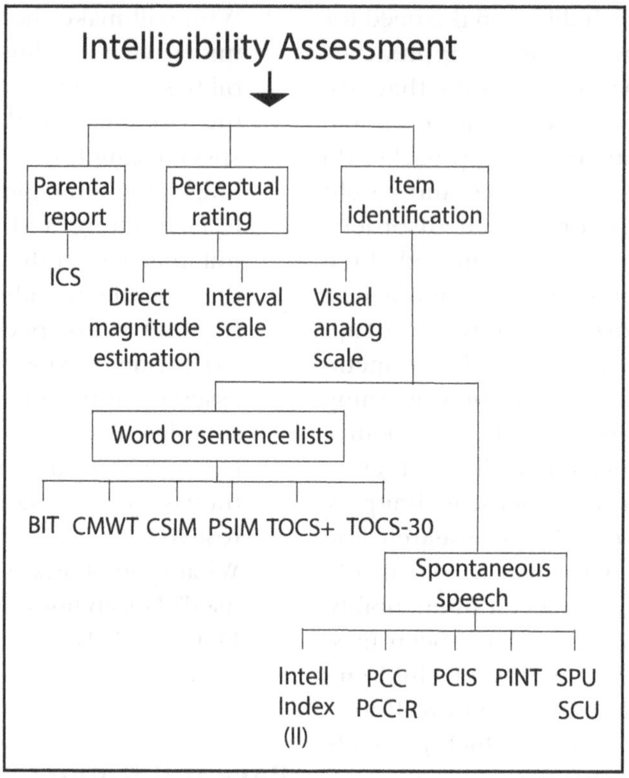

Figure 8–3. Major choices in intelligibility assessment of children's speech.

"ICS provides a measure that cannot be equated with intelligibility in a narrow sense. This confirms McLeod's (2012) suggestion that the ICS should primarily be used as a screening material to identify children in need of further investigation; it does not in itself provide a valid measure of intelligibility. For this purpose, the ICS should be used in combination with methods assessing other aspects of intelligibility."

Judgment by Clinician or Other Adult

The two main ways of measuring intelligibility are rating scales and item identification. These are discussed in relation to Figure 8–3, which serves as a decision-making chart.

Rating Scales

As mentioned in Chapter 5, speech intelligibility appears to be a prothetic rather than metathetic attribute, so that the method of direct magnitude estimation (DME) is more appropriate than equal-appearing interval scales, such as the Likert scale. However, interval scales are widely used in numerous clinical specialties, which is testimony to their ease of application. A basic decision in using interval scales is selecting the number of scale values. As discussed in Chapter 5, even if 7 points of gradation represents a limiting value in human decision-making, it is necessary to use a scale of more than 7 points to achieve that level of performance. Research has shown that increasing the number of scale points results in a closer approach to the underlying distribution, and hence normality of interval scales. Wu and Leung (2017) recommended that practitioners in social work should use 11-point Likert scales from 0 to 10, which they considered to be a natural and easily comprehensible range.

A general practice is to attach verbal descriptors to the numerical values on an interval scale, which assists raters in making their judgments. An example follows.

1. Speech is impossible to understand.
2. Speech is mostly impossible to understand.
3. Speech can be understood about half the time.
4. Speech can be understood most of the time.
5. Speech can be understood all the time.

The gradations of such a 5-point scale may not be fine enough to detect small differences in intelligibility that reflect increasing severity of a disorder or improvements related to maturation and/or treatment. However, the scale may be adequate for purposes such as screening to determine if reduced intelligibility reaches the level of clinical concern.

With the visual analog scale, ratings are made by placing a mark on a vertical or horizontal line. There is limited research on the relative merits of interval scales and VAS for ratings of speech intelligibility, but Xue et al. (2021) concluded that VAS is as reliable and valid as the measure of words accurately produced. However, they also comment that the rating task may not provide sufficient information for in-depth diagnosis and detailed analysis in research and clinical practice.

Item Identification

The typical procedures for item identification are based on transcriptions of spoken messages. The transcriptions can be orthographic or phonetic, depending on the skills and experience of the listener, and on the objectives of analysis. An advantage of orthographic transcription is that it can be performed by individuals who have not received training in phonetics. Orthographic transcription is the "gold standard" for measuring intelligibility (Duffy, 2013; Miller, 2013; Stipancic et al., 2016). However, Abur et al. (2019) commented that this method is not always optimal in clinical practice because of a clinician's previous exposure to a client's speech, the time constraints in the clinical setting, limited access to needed resources, and the cost of implementation. Transcription certainly can be demanding of time and effort, so the critical question is whether the information gained justifies the efforts to obtain it. Another important question is how to handle items that are unintelligible. One solution is to analyze only the intelligible items, but this discards part of the data. Alternative methods are discussed next for samples of spontaneous speech in which listeners have open responses in the form of transcription of some kind.

Spontaneous Speech

Item identification for conversation or spontaneous speech relies on transcription, either orthographic or phonetic, with the goal of determining the proportion of words that can be correctly identified by a listener. The speech sample can be obtained through conversation with the child, description of pictures or objects, story retelling, or any other method that elicits multiword utterances. Because intelligibility increases with the number of presentations of the sample (Lagerberg et al., 2015), this number should be reported in clinical assessments.

Several different indices have been introduced, as summarized in the following.

1. Percentage of Consonants Correct (PCC) or percentage of consonants correct–revised (PCC-R) (Shriberg et al., 1997a) (discussed in Chapter 5)
2. Intelligibility Index–Original (II-O; Shriberg et al., 1997b) groups unintelligible syllables into words.
3. Intelligibility Index–1.25 (II-1.25; Flipsen, 2006) calculates the number of unintelligible words and assumes that, on average, words in children's speech include 1.25 syllables.
4. Intelligibility Index–PS (II-PS; Flipsen, 2006) allows speakers to serve as their own control in that the average number of syllables per word in the intelligible portion of the sample is taken as an estimate of the number of words in the unintelligible portion.
5. Intelligibility Index–Age Normalized (IIAN; Flipsen, 2006) calculates age-normalized values for syllables per word to estimate the number of unintelligible words.
6. Intelligibility Index–All Syllables (II-AS; Lagerberg et al., 2014) counts the number of syllables for both the intelligible and unintelligible sequences and uses the calculation:
   II-AS = [Total number of syllables in transcribed words]/[total number of syllables in the sample] × 100
7. The Percentage of Intelligible Correct Syllables (PICS) is calculated by dividing the number of accurately produced syllables by the total number of syllables produced (accurate, inaccurate, and unintelligible). A similar measure, PINTS, is the proportion of intelligible syllables.
8. Syllables correctly understood (SCU; Lagerberg, Holm, et al., 2021) is determined by counting the number of syllables transcribed by the listener (i.e., perceived as understood) and dividing by the total number of syllables in the transcript (i.e., both the transcribed syllables and the unintelligible syllables). The fraction is multiplied by 100 to obtain percentage of syllables perceived as understood (SPU intelligibility score). The SCU-based intelligibility score is calculated by checking the listener transcripts against the master transcript, which has the number of correct syllables (assuming that the master transcript consists of the target words). The number of correct syllables for each speech sample and listener is divided by the total number of syllables (i.e., including both transcribed syllables and the 0 s) in each listener transcript and multiplied by 100. The result is an intelligibility score expressed as the percentage of syllables correctly understood (SCU).

Word or Sentence Lists

In this approach, listeners select the word or sentence that is presented. The speech material is known and structured, thereby avoiding the problem of unknown items that may occur with spontaneous speech. It is assumed that a child is attempting to produce the target word or group of words modeled by the examiner or other person, associated with a picture or object, or both. Examples of these assessments are shown in Figure 8–3 and Table 8–1. Single word tests offer the advantage of general application, including very young children or children with severe communication difficulties. As Allison (2020) points out, word identification approaches give a measure of intelligibility that is sensitive to change over time, which makes them suitable to track functional progress in therapy. However, unlike sentence tests they are not suitable to assess prosody or multisyllable sequencing abilities (Klopfenstein, 2009). Care should be taken with sentence tests to be sure that the materials do not exceed a child's verbal memory capability.

Developmental Reference Data

Table 8–2 lists reference data from several sources on speech intelligibility for typically developing children. Recent data indicate that children do not achieve 100% intelligibility until the age of about 6 years, compared with the often-cited age of 4 years from Coplan and Gleason (1988), and a similar result from Chin et al. (2003). The variability in the data reflects differences in methods and criteria across studies. Hustad et al. (2021) suggested the following guidelines in assessing the intelligibility of multiword utterances for unfamiliar listeners, based on data for the lowest performing participants in their study: by 4 years, children should be at least 50% intelligible, (b) by the 5 years, children should be at least 75% intelligible, and (c) by just over 7 years, children should be 90% intelligible. Gordon-Brannan and Hodson (2000) proposed that any child older than 4 years with an intelligibility percentage below 66% should be considered as a potential candidate for intervention. Developmental variations in intelligibility are relevant to AAC applications using children's speech. Drager and Finke (2012) reported considerable variation in the intelligibility of digitized children's speech and recommended that clinicians and parents who select child speakers for AAC devices with digitized speech should carefully consider the speakers used for recording digitized speech output and the speech characteristics of the individual speaker.

Factors Involved in Speech Intelligibility

Whatever method is used to estimate speech intelligibility, the final score or rating can be associated with several underlying features or processes, and which are the subject of this section. The basic question is: How can differences in speech intelligibility be explained? Conceivably, two different children could receive the same estimate of intelligibility (for example, 75%) but not have the same factors that account for reduced intelligibility.

Phonological and Linguistic Factors

Hodson and Paden (1981) compared the phonological processes exhibited by children who differed in intelligibility. The speech of most of the unintelligible children was characterized by one or more of

Table 8–1. Basic Features of Speech Intelligibility Tests for Children

Test/Feature	Speech Material	Target Population	Elicitation Method	Listener Task
BIT (Ertmer, 2010, 2011; Osberger, 1994)	Four lists of 10-sentences each, with simple syntax and words of one or two syllable familiar to children	Children with cochlear implants	Auditory model accompanied by objects or pictures	Transcription
Computer-mediated single-word test (Zajac et al., 2012)	50 monosyllabic words	Children with cleft lip and/or palate	Repetition after examiner	Transcription
CSIM (Morris & Wilcox, 1999)	Single words	School-aged children	Repetition after examiner	Multiple choice
PSIM (Morris et al., 1995)	Single-word, multiple-choice.	Preschool children	Repetition after examiner and picture naming	Multiple choice
TOCS+ (Hodge & Gotzke, 2014)	Sentence test composed of vocabulary and morphosyntax appropriate for children with developmental language ages between 3 to 7 years and with a mean length of utterance ranging from utterance (MLU) ranging from 2 to 7 words	Children aged 3 to 7 years	Direct imitation of prerecorded auditory models, which are presented with representative photographs and text	Orthographic transcription
TOCS-30 (Hodge, 2003)	TOCS-30 consists of 30 items (31 English words as one item has two words) that sample 53 consonant targets, 33 vowel targets, and 33 syllable targets.	Preschool children with severe speech and expressive language delay	Picture naming and repetition of auditory model	Transcription
Weiss Intelligibility Test (Weiss, 1982)	Single words and spontaneous speech (about 200 words)	Children and adolescents	Picture naming	Transcription

Table 8–2. Intelligibility Scores for Typically Developing Children as Reported by Five Sources

Age in Years	Coplan & Gleason (1988)	Chin et al. (2003)	Hustad et al. (2021)	Weiss (1982)	Wild et al. (2018)
1	25%	—	—	—	—
2	50%	54%	—	26% to 50%	—
3	75%	72&	50%	71% to 80%	—
4	100%	95%	75%	—	—
5	—	96%	—	—	76% to 81%
6	—	99%	—	—	—
7	—	—	100%	—	>90%

the following processes: final consonant deletion, syllable reduction, fronting of velars, backing, glottal replacement, and prevocalic voicing. The first two of these relate to syllable shapes, the next three relate primarily to place of articulation, and the last to voicing. Weston and Shriberg (1992) found that children's intelligibility was associated with utterance length and fluency, word position, intelligibility of adjacent words, phonological complexity, syllable structure, and grammatical form. Another way of measuring the severity of phonological disorders is the phonological density index (PDI). For this, the total number of phonological processes (defined as any systematic simplification of a sound class calculated and divided by the number of words analyzed in the sample).

Acoustic Factors

Intelligible speech is an aggregate of acoustic and other cues. In everyday conversations, the cues are embedded in the acoustic signal, in facial expressions and gestures, and in the communication setting (e.g., objects in the visual surround). The identification of correlates has been hindered by the fact that intelligibility has multiple cues that can have redundant or complementary effects and may be differently weighted by different listeners. Therefore, it can be misleading to assert specific acoustic correlates of intelligibility for any group of speakers. Hazan and Markham (2004, p. 3117) commented that, "There is also evidence that high intelligibility can be achieved by different talkers through a combination of different acoustic-phonetic characteristics, and that there are no acoustic-phonetic characteristics that consistently lead to high intelligibility." However, certain acoustic features have been reported frequently enough that they are strong candidates for future research and clinical application. A good basic reference is Pommée et al. (2021), who reviewed the acoustic correlates of speech intelligibility in healthy individuals. The authors concluded that no single acoustic feature predicted speech intelligibility to an appreciable degree but the following features emerged as being linked to sub-lexical speech intelligibility ratings: (a) for vowels, steady-state F1 and F2 measures, F1 range, /i/-/u/ F2 difference, F0-F1 and F1-F2 differences in selected vowel pairs, the vowel space area, the mean amount of formant movement, vector length and spectral change measure; (b) for consonants, the centroid energy and the spectral peak in the [s]-sound, as well as the steady-state F1 offset frequency in vowels preceding [t] and [d]. Some of the same features have been identified as correlates of intelligibility in children with speech disorders, as considered next.

Vowel Space Area (VSA), as defined in Chapter 3, is a measure of the area enclosed by the three or four corner vowels. This measure is relatively easy to make and is applicable to a wide range of speaker ages, given that vowels are among the earliest speech sounds to be acquired. The clinical value of VSA in the study of children's speech has been reported in several studies reviewed by Vorperian and Kent (2007), which generally show that reduced VSA is correlated with reduced speech intelligibility. Reduced VSA is interpreted to reflect a reduced range of articulatory positions for vowels, or what has been termed the articulatory working space. This relationship is depicted in Figure 8–4, which shows a formant graph and a corresponding articulatory graph. Reduced VSA can result from a contraction affecting all four corner vowels or a reduction in either the F1 or F2 dimension. Reduction of the F2 difference between front and back vowels has been reported in Down syndrome and cerebral palsy.

When speakers are asked to speak clearly to enhance their intelligibility, expansion of the VSA is commonly observed. Similar expansion has been reported for infant- or child-directed speech. Syrett and Kawahara (2014) reported that children's production of clear speech, compared to conversational speech, had vowels that were lengthened, more intense, more dispersed in the vowel space, and

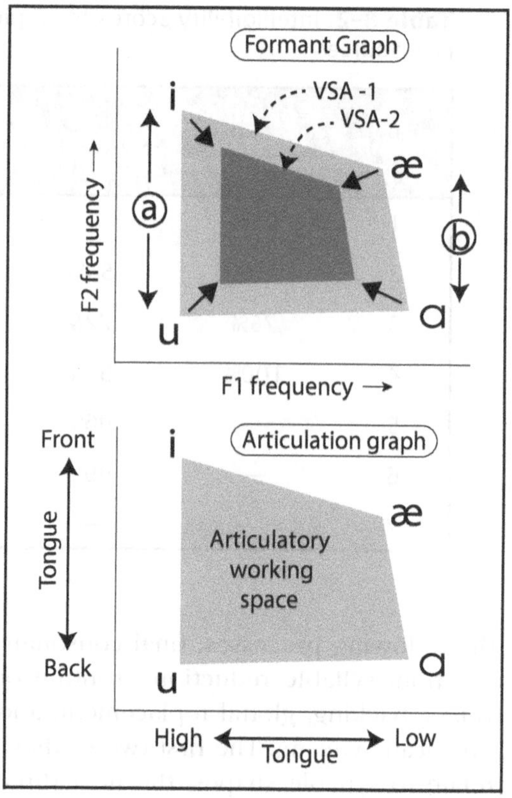

Figure 8–4. Vowel formant frequency patterns related to speech intelligibility. Top portion (Formant Graph) shows vowel space area (VSA) as the area contained within the vowel quadrilateral. As the corner vowels are centralized (shown by the arrows), VSA is reduced. VSA-1 is the original area, and VSA-2 is the reduced area. Also shown are (a) F2 differences between /i/ and /u/ and (b) F2 differences between /ae/ and /a/. Bottom portion (Articulation Graph) shows the articulatory dimensions (tongue height and advancement) related to the formant graph.

had a greater range of vocal fundamental frequency.

Visual Factors

Viewing a speaker can enhance a receiver's ability to understand the spoken message. The McGurk effect (McGurk & MacDonald, 1976) demonstrates that visual cues can sometimes override acoustic cues in making phonetic decisions, and visual cues can be particularly helpful in difficult listening conditions, such as a noisy background. Training to make optimal use of visual cues for speech perception is the basis of **speech reading** (also called **lip reading**), a method of oral communication that relies on communication strategies to compensate for auditory information that is reduced or lost because of hearing loss or noise in the environment. Speech reading uses visual cues from a speaker's face, gestures, posture, and body language.

The wearing of face masks during the Covid pandemic demonstrated the importance of visual cues in speech communication. Face masks were associated with reduced speech intelligibility in various settings, including classrooms (Bottalico et al., 2020) and laboratories (Cohn et al., 2021; Kim & Thompson, 2022). Face masks reduce both auditory and auditory-visual recognition of consonants (Lalonde et al., 2022) and perception of intonational and emotional prosody (Sinagra & Wiener, 2022). The use of clear speech or transparent masks is beneficial (Lalonde et al., 2022; Yi et al., 2021).

Assessing Comprehensibility

Comprehensibility has been measured in three main ways: global ratings, orthography-based measures, and questions regarding message content (Dagenais et al., 2011; Yoder et al., 2016). These are discussed in the following.

Global Ratings

In making global ratings, listeners use a rating scale to judge the overall comprehensibility of a spoken message (Yoder et al., 2016). Interval scales appear be commonly used, but ratings could also be obtained with visual analog scales. It is important that instructions to the raters are clearly specified. A general instruction such as "How well do you understand the message" may not be sufficient to distinguish intelligibility from comprehensibility.

Orthography-Based Measures

As the name suggests, orthography-based measures are derived from orthographic transcriptions of speech samples. Kwiatkowski and Shriberg (1992) used a measure based on the proportion of word attempts fully glossed by a listener. A limitation of this method is that it can be extremely difficult to identify how many words are attempted in highly incomprehensible speech. Another orthography-based measure of speech comprehensibility that has been used in research is the proportion of utterance attempts that orthographers fully gloss from a conversational language sample (Yoder et al., 2016). This approach recognizes that semantic, grammatical, and terminal prosody information can be used to segment utterances, Yoder et al. (2016, p. 461) wrote, "Reasonable guesses at particular words that are inaccurately produced are supported by access to visual and auditory contextual information. Thus, the proportion of utterance attempts fully glossed might be a useful measure of comprehensibility."

Questions Regarding Message Content

This method was used by Dagenais et al. (2011) in a study of dysarthric speech produced by four young men with traumatic brain injury. Although this approach has advantages in potentially separating speech intelligibility from comprehensibility, its use in clinical settings requires the participation of listeners who are naïve to the speech materials used in testing.

Assessing Accuracy

Commonly used accuracy measures are percent consonants correct (PCC and PCC-R) and percent vowels correct (PVC), or a rating on a scale (Jing & Grigos, 2022). PCC and PCC-R are discussed in Chapter 5. These measures are sometimes considered as proxies of speech intelligibility, but speakers can have notable inaccuracies without sacrificing intelligibility. In clinical usage, accuracy often pertains to whether a production is considered correct according to the standards of a given language, dialect, or speech community. An alternative to PCC or PCC-R is the Weighted Speech Sound Accuracy (WSSA; Preston et al., 2011). WSSA compares an adult target form with the word form produced by a child. It differs from PCC or PCC-R in that it gives a differential weighting to error types. For example, heavy weighting is given to phoneme omissions and unusual changes in manner, place, and voicing, whereas a lighter weighting is given to common substitutions.

As noted earlier in this chapter, the term accuracy also has been used in relation to variability of production, in which case the appropriate measures can be data on rate of correct production, variation in acoustic variables, or some other index of stability.

Assessing Listening Effort

"To start with a question, how do you connect the following group of measurements: EEG spikes, Cortisol levels, Chromogranin A, Reaction times, Infra-red spectroscopy, Driving simulators, Questionnaires, Pupil diameter, Response times, Fatigue scales, Functional MRIs and Skin conductance?" (Shields et al., 2022, p. 114). The answer given by Shields et al. is that all of these have been used as proxy measures of listening effort. Alhanbali et al. (2019) argued that traditional measures of listening effort reflect multiple underlying dimensions. They concluded that there is no "gold standard" measure of listening effort and that different measures should not be used interchangeably. In speech-language pathology, listening effort has been assessed with interval scales (Nagle & Eadie, 2018), direct magnitude estimation (Cote-Reschny & Hodge, 2010), visual analog scales (Nagle & Eadie, 2018; Whitehill & Wong, 2006; Wilson et al., 2020), or response time (Cote-Reschny & Hodge, 2010).

Assessing Communicative Efficiency

Communicative efficiency is typically measured as the number of intelligible syllables or words produced in 1 s. There are few reports on the developmental pattern of communicative efficiency. In a study of typically developing German children, Schölderle et al. (2021) reported median values in syllables/s as follows: 3 years—2.36, 4 years—2.95, 5 years—3.43, 6 years—3.82. 7 years—4.14, 8 years—4.39, and 9 years—4.6. If these results apply to other languages, then the developmental pattern is one of monotonically increasing values from 3 to 9 years, over which the median rate nearly doubles.

Assessing Fluency

It is not the purpose of this chapter to discuss fluency disorders in detail, but rather to note that observation of disfluencies can be part of a speech assessment and may identify children at risk for a fluency disorder. The fluency disorders of stuttering and cluttering are discussed in more detail in Chapter 10. Schölderle et al. (2021) suggested that several communication-related parameters (e.g., intelligibility, articulation rate, fluency, and communicative efficiency) should be combined for an assessment of a child's ability to communicate through speech. This perspective is adopted here. Disfluencies in either children or adults do not necessarily lead to a diagnosis of stuttering. Disfluencies are commonly noted in the speech of individuals considered to have typical speech production (Bortfeld et al., 2001; Fox Tree, 1995) and are common in children as young as 2 years of age (Yairi, 1981) and in preschoolers aged 44 to 64 months (Yaruss et al., 1999). Yairi (1981) studied the spontaneous utterances of 33 2-year-old children and concluded that there was large individual variability, with many children being only infrequently disfluent. The most common type of disfluency was repetition of short segments, one syllable or less. Although Yairi did not observe a sex difference in disfluencies, Tumanova et al. (2014) found that boys produced more non-stuttered disfluencies than girls. These authors also noted that parental concern for stuttering is strongly associated with the frequency of stuttered disfluencies.

Yaruss and Pelczarski (2007) and Clark et al. (2017) discuss the primary methods that speech-language clinicians can use to document children's speech fluency and communication skills. These methods are listed below, along with examples of relevant clinical tests and other materials.

1. Caregiver interview (see Clark et al., 2017, for details).
2. Assessments of impairment of stuttering (speech surface behaviors) through tests such as the Stuttering Severity Instrument-3 (Riley, 1994), Test of Childhood Stuttering (TOCS; Gilliam et al., 2009), and informal frequency counts (Yaruss, 1998).
3. Assessments of activity limitation, participation restriction, and both personal and environmental factors with tests such as the Behavioral Assessment Battery (BAB; Brutten & Vanryckeghem, 2006) and the Overall Assessment of the Speaker's Experience of Stuttering–School-Age (OASES-S; Yaruss & Quesal, 2006).
4. Related aspects of speech and language.
5. Portfolio assessments.

Assessing Naturalness

The predominant method of assessing naturalness in both human and machine speech is a rating scale, typically an interval scale. In studies of machine speech, such as text-to-speech synthesis, naturalness is generally determined from a mean opinion score (MOS) based on ratings using a 5-point scale between 1 (worst) and 5 (best), with "no definition of what "natural" means, nor a provision of context within which the sample occurs, out of concern that it may prime the listeners" (Shirali-Shahreza & Penn, 2018, p. 347). Ratings of naturalness have been applied to several clinical populations, including motor speech disorders (Yorkston et al., 1999), developmental stuttering (Martin et al., 1984), and augmentative and alternative communication (Ratcliff et al., 2002). Studies indicate that speaker characteristics such as age and gender may affect ratings of speech naturalness (Coughlin-Woods et al., 2005; Merritt & Bent, 2020). Stepp and Vojtech (2019) concluded that there is substantial, although not complete, agreement that speech naturalness is a metathetic dimension (i.e., being substitutive and qualitative, rather than additive and quantitative). This conclusion is consistent with the perspective that naturalness is a global property encompassing many component variables that vary in their psychometric features. An implication is that research on objective correlates, such as acoustic measures, is complicated by the potentially large number of variables to be addressed.

Assessing Accentedness

Accentedness has been assessed most often with interval scales and less often with direct magnitude estimation and sliding scales (Jesney, 2004; Poljak, 2019). The usual procedure is to ask native speakers to judge speech samples using a Likert-type scale, the ends of which are labeled with something like "no foreign accent" and "very heavy foreign accent." The number of scale values ranges from three to ten, with a recent trend toward use of a nine-point scale (Jesney, 2004).

ICF-CY Considerations

As noted in Chapter 1, the International Classification of Functioning, Disability and Health: Children and Youth Version (ICF-CY) is a conceptual framework for measuring health and disability factors at the individual and population levels. The global properties reviewed in this chapter are potentially relevant to considerations of the domains of body functions and structures, activity, and participation. However, measurements of communication do not always fit well with the ICF-CY framework (Barnes & Bloc, 2019), there are conceptual differences in the use of this framework as it relates to speech-language pathology (Kwok, Rosenbaum, & Cunningham, 2022), and commonly used clinical measures are not adequate to address the main domains of the ICF-CY (Kearney et al., 2015). Alignment of speech-language pathology with the ICF-CY is a work in progress. McCormack et al. (2009) is a landmark in providing a systematic review of the association between childhood speech impairment and participation across the lifespan.

Conclusions

1. The global properties of speech include intelligibility, comprehensibility, accuracy, listening effort, communicative efficiency, fluency, naturalness, and accentedness. These can be used individually or in various combinations to describe

speech development or the effects of a speech disorder, dialect, or other aspects of speech production. These properties can overlap to some degree, but they are complementary in creating a profile of speech communication. In general, these global properties index the success or ease of a communicative exchange, which makes them of high interest.

2. These properties are potentially dissociable in an individual speaker. For example, a speaker may be judged to be highly intelligible but also judged to have a heavy accent, which increases the level of listening effort.
3. The lack of standardized definitions and methods of assessment hinders clinical applications and cross-disciplinary usage for both human and machine speech.
4. Clinicians and others can choose among different assessment approaches, but interval scaling appears to be the most popular method and the most easily implemented in clinical settings. However, visual analog scales are increasingly used. Both interval scaling and visual analog scales rely on listener judgements, which are susceptible to several factors that can affect validity and reliability.

9

PRINCIPLES OF MOTOR DEVELOPMENT AND MOTOR LEARNING OF SPEECH

A major theme of this book is that speech production is a motor activity and therefore should be understood in part through motor concepts and principles. All behavior is motor behavior, and every act of speech is a motor act. Even inner or covert speech (discussed in Chapters 3 and 4) may rely on motor representations and experience. This chapter develops the theme more fully and examines the increasingly important domain of motor learning. Motor behavior is a physiological process in which motor, sensory, and cognitive factors contribute to the acquisition of motor skills. This process is supported by the maturation of both neural control and the peripheral effectors (sensorimotor systems).

Motor control is defined as the processes in the central nervous system (CNS) that produce purposeful, coordinated movements. Although motor control includes both voluntary movements and reflexes, the emphasis in this chapter is on the former (oral reflexes are discussed in Chapter 2). Voluntary motor control involves the following major steps.

1. Identify the task to be performed. Sensory information on the current state of the motor system (e.g., the positions of the articulators) is used to select or formulate a movement plan that is suited to the task goal.
2. The plan is coordinated within the CNS to send instructions to the motor neurons in the brain stem and spinal cord to activate synergies that offer efficiency and economy of movements.
3. Sensory feedback from the movement is supplied to the CNS, which can (a) modify the plan during its execution, (b) confirm that the goal was achieved, and (c) store the information to prepare for future performance of the same task-goal combination.

As Mulder (2007) points out, motor control is not accomplished with a rigid hierarchically organized system, but rather with a heterarchical process involving the continuous interaction of motor processes with cognitive and perceptual processes. This perspective, as applied to the assessment of speech production, means that motor function is interwoven with perception and cognition. That is, motor control is not an isolated component but one that is highly interactive with other aspects of human experience.

Motor learning is defined as a process that results in relatively permanent changes in motor behavior due to experience. The changes usually are rooted in functional and/or structural changes in the CNS, such as the formation of neural networks specific to a motor task. Motor learning in children is achieved on the maturational substrate of motor development, aspects of which are discussed in Chapter 2. A classic conception of the stages of motor learning was formulated by Fitts and Posner (1967). Basic features of this stage model are depicted in Figure 9–1. The three stages (cognitive, associative, and autonomous) differ in their demands on cognitive effort and attention, the speed and efficiency of movements, and the variability of movement performance. The cognitive stage typically requires instructions (e.g., verbal description and modeling) on how to perform the movements, the associative stage relies on training sessions that provide practice opportunities, and the autonomous stage benefits from cues that optimize performance. This final stage achieves rapid, efficient, and accurate performance in a nearly automatic fashion (i.e., requiring little cognitive effort). The Fitts and Posner stage model applies

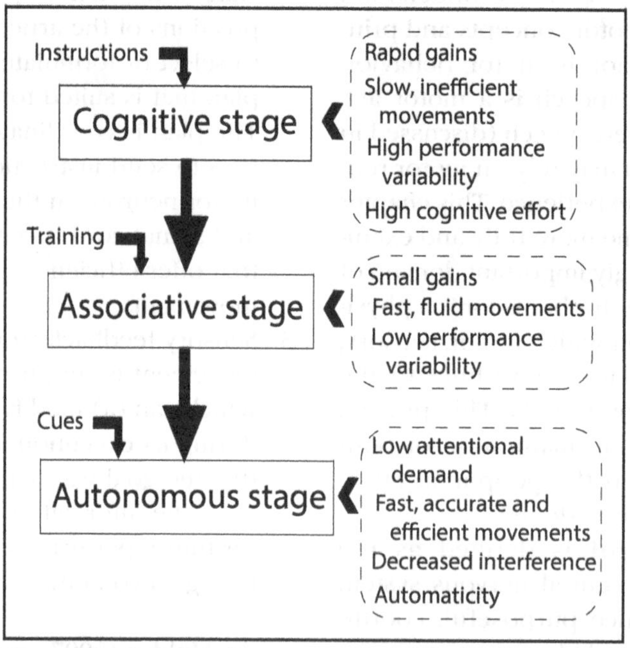

Figure 9–1. Basic features of the Fitts and Posner (1967) stage model of motor learning. The three stages (cognitive, associative, and autonomous) differ in their demands on cognitive effort and attention, the speed and efficiency of movements, and the variability of movement performance.

to a large range of movement skills and has been highly influential in the literature on motor control.

Contemporary Motor Development Research

Motor development is an active area of research as reflected in a steep increase in the annual number of motor-learning publications for preschoolers and school-age children (Xu et al., 2022). Research on general motor development has strongly influenced the study of speech motor development, and parallels are examined in this chapter. Whitall et al. (2020) described contemporary research on motor development with respect to three general areas.

(1) A **developing systems approach** considers development in terms of interacting systems (e.g., cognitive, perceptual, linguistic, motor, etc.) that combine to produce behavioral patterns that change over time. This approach owes much of its inspiration to the work of Thelen (2000). Supporting evidence comes from a systematic review of motor learning in children, which concluded that "The main results indicated that learning occurs based on experiences (cognitive, perceptual, motor, linguistic, neuronal, organic and cultural) and requires processes of adaptation, stabilization, and maturation of brain synchronization of vestibular, perceptual and visual processes" (p. 312). The impact of this approach on the understanding of speech development is noted frequently in this book with examples of sensory, cognitive, linguistic, motor, and emotional interactions.

(2) A **developmental motor neuroscience** approach unites the study of motor development with the methods and theories of modern neuroscience and seeks to understand how the brain controls movement across developmental time. A sub-branch that might be called "developmental speech motor neuroscience" is reflected in recent research that describes neural circuits associated with speech development, beginning with preverbal vocalizations such as babbling. This perspective is a recurring theme in this book, which reports on progress toward the developmental neuroscience of speech.

(3) A **developmental health approach** emphasizes the use and promotion of motor skills to support and enhance health across the lifespan. This concept also has been used to signify a developmental perspective on health and well-being. Speech and language development are core features of well-being in children and therefore deserve consideration in education and health policies at the national and local levels.

Neural Systems for Motor Control

The neural organization of motor control is coming under new understanding through advances in brain imaging, neurocomputational modeling, and behavioral studies. Some central issues are summarized in the following.

Motor Control Has a Cognitive Investment

There is a close link between mental representations and the execution of motor actions, such that mental representations guide both the biomechanical parameters of a movement and the overall structure of the action (Land et al., 2013). Diagrams of the production of spoken language, such as those in Chapter 3, may convey the false impression that motor control is far removed from cognition and that only higher-level linguistic operations are tied to cognition. To the contrary, motor control is aligned with cognitive operations throughout human development. Cortical area M1, classically associated with voluntary motor control, is activated by cognitive functions such as motor imagery and working memory, emotion/empathy, and language (Tomasino & Gremese, 2016).

Cerebro-Cerebellar Circuits

The cerebrum and the cerebellum are close partners in motor control and motor learning. There is evidence to show that the cerebellum can copy the dynamics of the cerebral cortex to predict the state of the cerebral cortex and therefore enable rapid and stable operations in motor control and cognitive processing (Tanaka et al., 2020). Cerebro-cerebellar loops are fundamental to motor learning and motor control by establishing internal models of motor actions.

Variability of Movements

Movements are inherently variable, and this variability reflects the neural system's active exploration to optimize motor plans (Krakauer et al., 2019). Even neurologically healthy adults performing a well-learned motor task can exhibit variability in movements. This variability is now regarded not as noise but rather as purposive efforts to ensure that movements are effective and adaptive.

A challenge to both research and clinical applications is to distinguish healthy variability from atypical variability that reflects disorders in motor and/or cognitive processing. Studies on speech motor development are converging on several important conclusions. First, variability in speech motor performance decreases with age, but an initial phase of this reduction is reached at about 9 to 11 years of age (Sadagopan & Smith, 2008; Whiteside et al., 2003). Sadagopan and Smith (2008) suggested that by the age of about 9 years, children begin to plan the timing of sentence internal phrases with adult-like pre-speech processes that continue to mature through late adolescence. Sosa (2015) noted that phonemic variability was prevalent in typically developing 2- and 3-year-olds and even in the oldest children in the sample, concluding that, "Clinicians should use caution in interpreting the presence of intraword variability as indicative of specific subtypes of speech disorder" (p. 24).

Architecture of Motor Control: Hierarchy and Modules

Merel et al. (2019) identified six key principles of hierarchical motor control, as follows: (1) Information factorization means that different types of information are sent to different subsystems of motor control, which allows for factored learning that economizes the role of experience and affords reusability across contexts. This principle has important implications for speech because of its plurimodal feedback possibilities that can be differentially used during learning and interference. (2) Partial autonomy of subsystems means that lower-level subsystems can function somewhat independently, with modulation from higher-level subsystems. This principle allows for robustness and reduced demands on higher centers in managing motor control. (3) Amortized control means that movements that have been performed successfully many times are compressed into a form that permits rapid and certain reproduction. An example in speech is the preparation of motor commands for syllables that are repeatedly used in speech production. (4) Modular objectives means that specific subsystems can be recruited to achieve specific objectives that are distinct from, but related to, the global task objective. Modules, as defined in Chapters 1 and 4, distribute responsibilities of motor control to different components of a hierarchically organized system. (5) Multi-joint coordination means the selection of frequently used combinations of muscle groups. Speech is a multi-articulate motor behavior that can be effectively performed by the selection of synergies (also called coordinative structures) that are based on movement experiences. (6) Temporal abstraction means that timing patterns can be defined in a relatively coarse timescale. Such a timescale would be useful in speech to align features in the segmental and suprasegmental domains.

Motor Perspectives on Speech Development and Speech Sound Acquisition

According to Adolph and Hoch (2019), the acquisition of motor skills requires and reflects the basic psychological functions of **embodiment, embedding, enculturation**, and **enabling**. Each of these functions can be related to **speech motor skill development (SMSD)**, as discussed in the following.

SMSD is **embodied,** insofar as possibilities for action are based on the status of the speech production system at a given point in development. According to the theory of embodiment, behavior is shaped by the physical properties of the body (the characteristics of the sensorimotor system), the structure of the task, and relevant physical properties of the environment (Steels & De Boer, 2008). Dynamic systems theory (Chapter 1) takes the same view. Chapter 2 reviews relevant developmental phenomena in the maturation of the physical apparatus of speech which factor into embodiment. Developmental functional modules in infant vocalizations (Kent, 2021, 2022; discussed in Chapter 4) are predicated on the principle that vocal development can and should be understood with respect to the biological status of the infant. The function of embodiment is also relevant to understanding speech disorders. For example, a child with cerebral palsy has motoric limitations that are represented in the neural representation of movements, including sensory consequences of atypical movements (Neilson & O'Dwyer, 1984), and a child with cleft palate has structural limitations that affect oral/nasal resonance balance and its effects on articulatory proficiency (Oren et al., 2020; Zajac, 2015). Embodiment is a property of the individual speaker and is based on current developmental status. The relevance of the concept of embodiment to neurogenic communication disorders is discussed by Ahlsén (2008) and is a ripe concept for future exploration.

SMSD is **embedded** in that variations in the environment create and constrain possibilities of vocal activity. An important environmental condition in speech development is the ambient language, which has effects beginning in the fetal stage and continuing through development, as discussed in Chapter 4. Also important is the nature of the interaction between caregiver and child, such as the frequency of vocal examples and exchanges. The effects are evident in both the sensory domain (particularly the auditory representation of speech) and the motor domain (such as the establishment of a language-specific articulatory setting, as discussed in Chapter 1).

SMSD is **enculturated** in that social and cultural factors have a molding influence on the perception and production of speech as well as progress in overall language development. Fluent native speech is adapted to the speech community of the individual, taking on aspects of acoustic-phonetic features, prosody, and voice quality. Ramírez-Esparza et al. (2014, p. 880) concluded that, "the social context and the style of speech in language addressed to children are strongly linked to a child's future language development." Enculturation is highly evident in studies of bilingualism and dialect (Chapter 10).

SMSD is **enabling** because the maturation of speech motor ability opens the way to language development, social interaction, and educational experiences in a variety of settings. The enablement is best understood as a cascade of developmental advances. These advances are put at risk in children who have difficulties producing intelligible speech. Speech is a gateway to many social, educational, and recreational opportunities available to children.

Motor Control of Skilled Movements: Basic Problems and Principles

SMSD requires the coordination of motor activity in the respiratory, laryngeal, and supralaryngeal systems, each of which has its own complex arrangement of components. Because the movements are largely invisible to the unaided eye, the detailed study of speech movements is challenging to say the least. But technological advances have greatly enhanced the ability to determine developmental changes in speech motor control and the implications of these changes for speech motor learning.

For the sake of discussion, let's assume that about 100 muscles are used in producing speech. Let us further suppose that each muscle can be in the binary state of either contracted or relaxed (of course, muscle activation is much more complex than that because of possible gradations of contraction). Even with the severe simplification of two possible activation states for each muscle, the number of possible patterns of motor activation is 2^{100}, or more than one nonillion. That is more activation patterns than we have neurons. This calculation poses problems for a theory of motor control that proposes that speech is controlled by detailed motor programs that are assembled in the central nervous system. Those of us who study speech—and the child who is learning to talk—must find ways of simplifying the challenge of motor control. This does not mean that motor programs should be abandoned but rather that motor programs should be conceptualized in ways that make the control problem tractable.

A further problem is that that a given movement goal can be achieved in different ways. For example, the relatively simple goal of closing the lips for a sound like /p/ can be accomplished with differing combinations of lip and jaw movement. The different patterns of movement that achieve the same goal have motor (or functional) equivalence. Bernstein (1967) called this challenge the degrees of freedom problem and it applies to just about all skilled movements, but especially to multi-articulate systems such as speech. In Bernstein's view, an effective motor control strategy reduces the degrees of freedom to simplify the specification of movement patterns.

Principles of Motor Learning (PLM)

Motor learning, or **Principles of Motor Learning (PLM)**, refers to a relatively permanent change in the ability to perform a motor skill achieved through practice or experience. Motor learning is different from simple **motor performance**, which is the act of executing a motor skill that results in a temporary change rather than a lasting one. Contemporary theories of motor learning usually incorporate a systems' view of distributed control in the nervous system so that skilled movement results from the interaction of multiple systems working in concert to solve a motor problem. Motor learning is not simply learning to activate a muscle or even a group of muscles. A particular emphasis in the systems' perspective is that it can account for flexible and adaptive motor behavior. Flexibility and adaptability are features that are critical to both motor development and clinical intervention. Principles of motor learning have had a broad impact, being used in diverse specialties such as occupational therapy (Zwicker & Harris, 2009, neurorehabilitation (Kitago & Krakauer, 2013), physical therapy (Kafri & Atun-Einy, 2019), and speech-language pathology (Maas et al., 2008).

Motor learning is closely related to concepts in **neuroplasticity**, which is defined as "the ability of the central nervous system (CNS) to change and adapt in response to environmental cues, experience, behavior, injury or disease" (Ludlow et al., 2008, p. S241). Cramer et al. (2008) commented that, "Neuroplasticity occurs with many variations, in many forms, and in many contexts. However, common themes in plasticity that emerge across diverse central nervous system conditions include experience dependence, time sensitivity and the importance of motivation and attention" (p. 1591). Berlucchi and Buchtel (2009) review the historic roots of the concept of plasticity and suggest that the term *plasticity* is "appropriate only when the system achieves a novel function by transforming its internal connectivity network or by changing the elements of which it is made" (p. 318). Studies of animals and humans have demonstrated that neural changes and adaptations are facilitated by incorporating several principles in training or rehabilitation. These principles include: (1) usage enhances function (not just "use it or lose it" but "use it and improve it"), (2) plasticity is experience specific (i.e., it builds on discrete behaviors), (3) repetition in the form of extensive and prolonged practice is important, (4) intensity (continuous training over long periods) is needed to achieve optimum results, (5) training should be salient and relevant to the goals to be achieved (task specificity), (6) transference can occur in the sense that plasticity following training in one function may enhance related behaviors, (7) interference can occur in the sense that plasticity can alter neural function in ways that interfere with certain behaviors or skills. Many of these principles apply to the following discussion of motor learning, which, after all, seeks to make long-term changes in the neural systems of movements.

A maxim in neuroscience is that "neurons that fire together, wire together" meaning that when different neurons are activated in concert to complete a task, their connections are strengthened. As a result, networks or linkages are established that are ready for the next performance of the task.

Task Specificity, Generalization, and Task Potency

A basic tenet of research on neuroplasticity and PLM is that training should be specific to the task skills to be acquired. In other words, "motor skills are specific and only superficially resemble other similar skills or variations of the same skill" (Shea & Kohl, 1990, p. 169). This principle of **task specificity** has been emphasized in studies of speech motor control (Bunton, 2008; Rochet-Capellan et al., 2012; Tremblay et al., 2008; Wilson et al., 2008) and has been used to question, if not refute, the use of nonspeech oral movements in speech therapy (Forrest, 2002; Lof & Watson, 2010). However, taken to its extreme, task specificity implies that there is no benefit to motor learning from any task other than the individual task to be learned. This position runs counter to two important concepts in motor learning. One concept is the **variability of practice hypothesis** that proposes that experiences with task variations are critical to developing the memories (schemata) used in response production and learning (Schmidt, 1975; Shea & Kohl, 1990). The other concept is **motor generalization**, the ability to apply what has been learned in one context to other contexts. Generalization can be beneficial (enabling transfer of skill or knowledge) or detrimental (creating interference with learning of a novel task).

Speech-language therapy is replete with clinical protocols based on the concept of generalization. For example, a common strategy to treat /s/ misarticulation is to begin with production of the stop /t/. The two sounds /s/ and /t/ are not identical in their production, but there appears to be benefit in a treatment protocol that uses production of /t/ as a foundation for the correct production of /s/. Accounts also attest to the value of similar, but not identical, tasks in treating rhotic misarticulations. (Preston, Benway, et al., 2020). The principle of task specificity should not neglect either the demands of the task to be learned nor the capabilities of the learner.

It may be more useful to consider **task potency** rather than task specificity. The term *task potency* was introduced in a study of neural networks associated with different cognitive tasks (Chauvin et al., 2019). For present purposes, task potency is defined as the relative advantage or relationship between two motor tasks. With this definition, task potency represents a continuum of similarities or differences, as opposed to the seemingly bipolar nature of task specificity (either a task is specific, or it is not). Task potency is compatible with the concepts of variability of practice and generalization (both transfer and interference) and can be used to design interventions for speech disorders.

Implicit Versus Explicit Learning

Kleynen et al. (2014) distinguish these two types of learning. **Explicit motor**

learning is learning that relies on verbal knowledge of movement performance. It incorporates cognitive operations within the learning process and requires involvement of working memory. In contrast, **implicit motor learning** is accomplished with no or minimal increase in the verbal knowledge of movement performance (e.g., facts and rules) and without awareness. Intervention strategies designed to provide high conscious awareness of how motor behavior is accomplished are in the domain of explicit motor learning. Intervention strategies that lead to low conscious awareness of how motor behavior is accomplished are in the domain of implicit motor learning. A review of motor learning in children with developmental disorders indicated that implicit paradigms are at least as effective as explicit paradigms of motor learning (van Abswoude et al., 2021). However, the authors note the need for additional research with better methodological quality. The relative advantage of one form of learning over another may depend on child characteristics. For example, Torres-Moreno (2022) concluded from a systematic review of motor learning in children that explicit instructions, which require a theoretical verbalization of motor action, present a greater benefit for children with high motor skills, whereas implicit instructions present a greater benefit for children with low motor skills.

Phases of Motor Learning

Motor learning can be assessed in three major phases: **acquisition, retention**, and **transfer** of skills. Acquisition is the initial practice or performance of a skill to be acquired (or modified control of a previously learned motor skill). For example, the initial practice may focus on a particular syllable or syllable sequence that we want a child to learn. Decisions about the nature of this practice are reviewed later in this chapter. Retention is the ability to demonstrate attainment of the skill after an interval in which the task is not practiced. An example is production of the target syllable or syllable sequence after playing a game or some intervening activity. What we seek to know is if the motor skill has the desired degree of permanence. Transfer is performance of a task that resembles the original task practiced in the acquisition phase but differs from it in some well-defined aspect(s). For example, we could assess a child's ability to produce a syllable that has the same syllable structure as the target syllable but differs in its phonetic constituents or in its position in a prosodic pattern. Transfer can greatly enhance the benefit of motor learning because the skill generalizes to related tasks or targets. It is important to note that the ability to perform a motor skill within a single session or even a series of sessions does not suffice to show that the skill has been learned.

A skill is learned when retention and/or transfer of that skill can be demonstrated. Sometimes, a skill can be quickly acquired but not retained or transferred. A faster rate of skill acquisition does not necessarily mean better retention. As illustrated in Figure 9–2, the learning pattern shown by the dashed line has a rapid acquisition but poor retention and transfer, whereas the learning pattern shown by the solid line has a slower rate of acquisition but better retention and transfer. All three phases of motor learning should be considered in a treatment program. Although rapid acquisition of a motor skill can be rewarding, the ultimate goals of retention and transfer may not be satisfied.

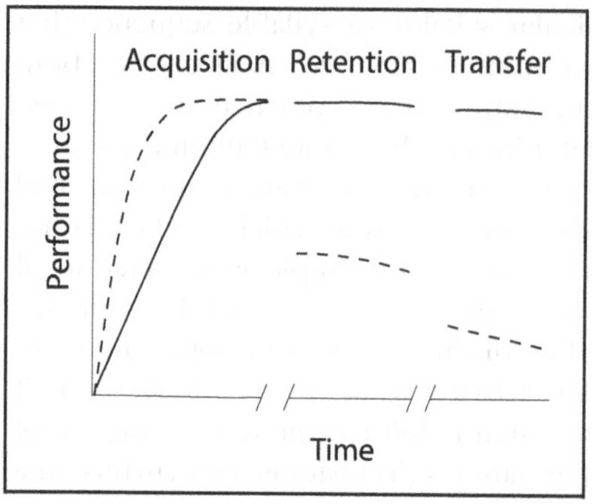

Figure 9–2. Hypothetical example of motor learning in which performance varies over the stages of acquisition, retention, and transfer. Rapid acquisition of a motor skill does not guarantee retention or transfer of the skill.

PLM Framework: Components and Clinical Applications

Researchers and clinicians from many different specialties recommend using a systems model of motor control that incorporates neurophysiology, biomechanics, and motor learning principles based on interactions among the client, the task, and the environment. We now turn to specific components of PLM and the relevance of these components to clinical interventions for speech disorders in children.

Motor Imagery (Mental Practice)

As mentioned in Chapter 1, evidence shows that simply imagining a movement, or observing another person perform that movement, can influence motor performance and learning. **Mental practice**, also known as **mental rehearsal** (Ruscello & Shelton, 1979), involves mentally focusing on the skill and imagining the performance of that skill. Ruscello and Vallino (2014) noted that mental practice is thought to assist in the development of the cognitive component of motor learning. The term **motor imagery**, as frequently used in cognitive science and neuroscience, can be defined as a dynamic state in which representations of a motor act are rehearsed in working memory in the absence of overt motor behavior (Decety, 1996). Motor imagery involves motor preparation, which is accomplished by processing or transferring a motor act from long-term to working memory (Farah, 1984). The motor image has interesting properties, including an attentional component and the opportunity to inspect the image to compare its details with other percepts or to give a verbal report on the imagined sensations (Munzert et al., 2009). A potential obstacle to the general use of imagery with young children is that they may not understand what it means to imagine a movement and may not have the ability to examine or report on their mental representations. Toys, puppets, and computer animations may be helpful in prompting a child to imagine the act of speaking. Apps can be used for the same purpose. Motor imagery has been used in neurorehabilitation for conditions such as stroke, where it is the basis for action observation therapy and embodiment (Maier et al., 2019). Therapeutic application to children' speech disorders has not been extensively reported.

Modeling of Motor Behavior

Motor imagery, as discussed above, depends on a model of the behavior to be performed. **Modeling**, or **demonstration**, is commonly used in teaching motor skills. Bandura's (1986) **Social Cognitive Theory**, among the most influential papers on modeling, proposes that acquisition of a modeled behavior depends on cognitive processes including attention, coding, and rehearsing the essential features of the action to be performed. A cognitive representation of the motor pattern both guides performance of the action and serves as a reference goal to which performance is compared. The bulk of the research on modeling pertains to motor skills that can be observed as body movements.

The literature on speech sound acquisition and disorders focuses mainly on phonemes or phonetic segments, the particles of speech. In contrast, the literature on motor learning pertains mostly to visually guided limb movements or whole-body movements. Speech consists of movements that, for the most part, are auditorily guided. That is, speech typically is learned in reference to the auditory events associated with movements of the speech production systems. Speech movements are largely hidden from view, so that modeling is largely auditory but may use selected visual cues (e.g., lip or jaw movements) and tactile cues (as in some therapy approaches discussed in Chapter 12). Modeling of speech can be enhanced by using methods such as clear speech or amplification. **Clear speech** (discussed in Chapters 7 and 11) is a deliberate effort to increase speech intelligibility by altering prosodic and articulatory patterns. Clear speech, as compared with conversational speech, has the following acoustic properties: increased mean and range of vocal fundamental frequency, longer phoneme durations, increased amplitude modulation, larger vowel spaces, increased energy in higher-frequency regions, and more phoneme insertions (e.g., schwa). The benefits of clear speech on intelligibility are evident in the auditory, visual, and audiovisual modalities (Gagné et al., 2002).

Auditory discrimination is commonly used as a component in therapy for speech disorders (Chapter 12) and is justified by research showing the importance of auditory-motor associations in typical and disordered speech production (Shiller & Rochon, 2014; Terband et al, 2014). **Amplification** can be used to increase the audibility of speech sounds and is used as part of auditory bombardment in therapies such as the cycles approach (Hodson & Paden, 1991). (A later section offers related information on aspects of modeling of speech.) In speech therapy, modeling is an essential component of imitation, as discussed next.

Imitation

Imitation (reproduction of a modeled behavior) is commonly used as part of the treatment for speech disorders and for disorders such as aphasia, autism spectrum disorder, and specific language impairment. The essential components of imitation are joint attention, a model to be imitated, representation of the model in short- and possibly long-term memory, translation of the stored representation into a motor plan for reproduction of the stimulus, and execution of the motor plan. Imitation is an integrated sensorimotor activity based on a dyad of model and imitator. The model can be strictly auditory, strictly visual, or auditory-visual. The modeled behavior can be verbal or nonverbal, and within each, different levels of challenge can be incorporated.

For example, verbal imitation can apply to individual syllables, nonwords, single words, or combinations of syllables or words. Some children do not readily participate in imitation tasks, in which case alternative methods are used, such as providing access to AAC, minimizing pressure to speak, imitating the child, augmenting auditory, visual, tactile, and proprioceptive feedback, and avoiding emphasis on nonspeech-like articulator movements (focus on function) (DeThorne et al., 2009). The role of imitation in treating speech disorders in children has been discussed by Bradford-Heit and Dodd (1998), Eikeseth and Nesset (2003), and Gill et al. (2011).

Imitation has been related to the concept of **mirror neurons**. A mirror neuron fires during both observed and self-produced actions, a phenomenon that may underlie an action-perception linkage. The name is derived from an analogy to a mirror that reflects the behavior that is observed. This tantalizing discovery has prompted hypotheses (and even well-developed theories) that mirror neurons serve vital functions in the development of spoken language and in the perception of speech. The relevance of mirror neurons to speech and language disorders has been noted in both scientific and lay literature. For example, mirror neurons have been linked to imitation in infants (Simpson et al., 2014), imitative disturbances in ASD (Williams et al., 2001), therapies for stroke (Small et al., 2012), and the ontogeny and phylogeny of brain and language (Stamenov & Gallese, 2002). However, the attraction of the concept has faded somewhat in the face of criticisms of methodology and interpretation (Heyes & Catmur, 2022; Hickok, 2014; Holt & Lotto, 2014). The mirror is not cracked but is somewhat cloudy.

> "Since their discovery much has been written about these neurons, both in the scientific literature and in the popular press. They have been proposed to be the neuronal substrate underlying a vast array of different functions. Indeed, so much has been written about mirror neurons that last year they were referred to, rightly or wrongly, as 'The most hyped concept in neuroscience.'" (Kilner, J. M., & Lemon, R. N. [2013]. What we know currently about mirror neurons. *Current Biology, 2*[23], R1057–R1062. https://doi.org/10.1016/j.cub.2013.10.051)

Focus of Attention

According to Wulf et al. (2010), research on the role of the performer's focus of attention repeatedly show that instructions inducing an **external focus** (directed at the movement effect) are superior to those promoting an **internal focus** (directed at the performer's body movements). They assert that an external focus facilitates automaticity in motor control and promotes movement efficiency. However, both types of focus may have roles in motor learning. For example, in treating speech sound disorders, it may be helpful to focus on articulatory movements before focusing on an external focus, such as the auditory target. It is also possible to alternate the foci, which may have the benefit of aligning the external and internal aspects of a movement.

Context of Movement

The **context of a behavior** affects motor performance and motor learning, either by facilitation or interference. With respect to speech sounds, facilitation can be defined as "a relative improvement in judged adequacy of sound production, determined by phonetic factors such as word position, stress, and neighboring sounds" (Kent, 1982, pp. 66–67). Examples of context effects on speech sound production are discussed in Curtis and Hardy (1959), Hoffman et al. (1977) and Kent (1982). In a review of studies, Stilp (2020) identified a common theme in which acoustic differences between contexts and targets are perceptually magnified, so that contrast effects facilitate perception of target sounds and words. Prosody can exert similar effects. For example, stressed words have different movement profiles than unstressed words, and this difference can be exploited in speech treatments (see Chapters 7 and 11 for discussion). Context, then, has both perceptual and motor aspects that can influence the production of speech sounds.

Task Decomposition

In some situations, it may be desired to decompose a complex task into smaller or simpler parts. **Decomposition** involves breaking down a movement into its parts, training a part separately, and then reintroducing that part into the whole movement with the goal of improving the primary task. Wightman and Lintern (2017) identified three ways in which a task can be decomposed during training: segmentation, fractionation, and simplification. Fractionation decomposes components of a task that are simultaneously produced into independent subcomponents. In speech treatment, fractionation decomposes articulatory adjustments that are simultaneous in the original speech task. An example is isolated practice with elevation of the tongue tip for a child who has difficulty with lingua-alveolar sounds like /s/. Experience in making the isolated movement may provide the motoric foundation for production of the phoneme target. Segmentation divides the task into a series of spatial or temporal components that have identifiable boundaries. For example, in speech treatment, an isolated phone can be practiced in isolation before it is placed in syllabic or word context. Simplification makes the motor task easier by adjusting characteristics of the task. An example from speech treatment for the /s/ sound is to begin with production of the stop /t/, which is similar in place of articulation to /s/.

Amount of Practice (Intensity)

Studies of motor skill acquisition have demonstrated the importance of **intensity of practice**. As noted in Chapter 3, children learn skills such as walking and talking through ample practice, with successes and failures. Acquisition of a motor skill takes effort, and sustained practice is the means of establishing accurate, reliable, and flexible motor control. In a study of intervention for children with cleft palate, children receiving high-intensity intervention made gains in 2 weeks of therapy that were equal or superior to the gains made by children who received 10 weeks of low-intensity therapy (Alighieri et al., 2021). Allen (2013) reported that a multiple oppositions approach for treating speech sound disorders in preschool children was more effective with a more intensive dose frequency. In a review of published studies, Kaipa and Peterson (2016) concluded that higher treatment intensity was better than lower treatment intensity for treating childhood apraxia of speech and speech sound (phonological) disorders.

Type of Practice

There are two major types of practice. **Mass practice** has short time intervals between trials or sessions. For example, if the skill to be learned is correct production of the fricative /s/, mass practice might involve consecutive trials, one following another in short order. In **distributed practice**, trials or sessions are separated by longer time intervals than in mass practice. This type of practice also may include intervening activities, such as focusing on another goal of therapy. Sessions of mass and distributed practice can be alternated as needed.

Another aspect of practice is giving the learner a measure of self-control, or autonomy. **Self-controlled practice** that includes feedback and model demonstrations controlled by the learner is more effective than externally controlled practice conditions (Wulf et al., 2010). An interesting result of this research is that self-control learners prefer and choose feedback mostly after successful trials. In a review of studies on self-control, Sanli et al. (2013) concluded that self-controlled practice promotes feelings of autonomy and competence, which support the psychological needs of the learner and result in long-term changes in behavior. Wulf (2007) suggested that self-control enhances the learner's motivation and leads to deeper information processing and improved retention and transfer. Most of the research has been done with adults, but the benefits of self-controlled practice may apply as well to children and may offer advantages in motivation and reward.

Practice Variability (Constant Versus Variable)

Constant practice is repeated practice of the same target in the same context, for example, production of the liquid /ɹ/ in the word *road*. **Variable practice** is practice in which the target and/or context are changed between trials. For example, practice on the /ɹ/ may alternate with practice on another sound, such as /l/, or the phonetic context may change from a back vowel like /o/ in *road* to a front vowel like /i/ in *read*. Both types of practice are relevant in treating speech disorders. For example, constant practice may be beneficial in early stages of treatment to ensure that a child has established the basic spatiotemporal properties of a movement. Variable practice could then be introduced to provide opportunities for learning adaptive, context-sensitive motor control.

Practice Schedule

The two main schedules are blocked and random. In **blocked practice**, the same target or targets are practiced in the same order. An example of /ɹ/ treatment is repeated production of the word *red*. In **random practice**, the target (or its context) changes between trials. An example is a trial structure such as the following word sequence: *red, read, road, red*. Both types of practice may be used in designing a treatment program, for example, by using blocked practice in early stages to ensure stability of the basic motor act and by using random practice in later stages to encourage adaptive and flexible motor control.

Feedback Type

Feedback is information on motor performance that helps the learner to make any needed adjustments. Wulf et al. (2010) pointed out that in addition to its informational function, feedback has motivational properties that can influence learning. They note that feedback after successful trials and social-comparative (normative) feedback indicating a better-than-average performance have a positive effect on learning. As noted earlier in this chapter, learners involved in self-control practice prefer positive feedback. This is not to suggest that negative feedback should never be used, but rather that the advantages of positive feedback should be recognized.

Feedback falls into major classes, intrinsic and extrinsic feedback. **Intrinsic feedback** is provided by the sensory systems (visual, auditory, proprioceptive, vestibular, and cutaneous). Speech generates multimodal feedback, and the combination of different types of feedback varies with the sound being produced (Figure 9–3). **Extrinsic feedback** (also known as augmented feedback) is supplemental information given to the client about the task performance. The two major types of extrinsic feedback are **Knowledge of Results (KR)** and **Knowledge of Performance (KP)**. KR relates to the outcome or goal, such as whether a speech sound is produced correctly. KP relates to the movement pattern that is used in reaching the goal. It has two types: **internal focus of attention** and **external focus of attention**. **Attentional focus** is the target or location of an individual's attention in relation to the performance environment or task. An internal focus in speech production is directed toward components of articulatory movements, to encourage conscious awareness of how an individual is performing. An external focus is directed toward the end goal, such as perception of a speech sound. KP provides more detailed information than KR, such as advising a child to maintain the tongue contact for /s/ for a longer time and to try to get the feel of this tongue position. Instrumental methods can be used

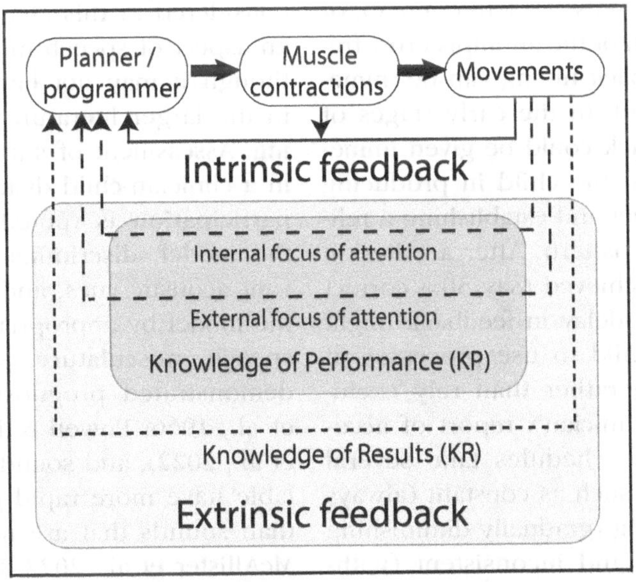

Figure 9–3. Diagram of the feedback channels in motor learning and performance, showing intrinsic feedback and extrinsic feedback (knowledge of performance and knowledge of results).

to provide KP that is not readily available from perceptual information. Extrinsic feedback can be linked with intrinsic feedback to integrate their influences.

Wulf and Lewthwaite (2016) proposed a motor learning theory called Optimizing Performance through Intrinsic Motivation and Attention for Learning (OPTIMAL), which integrates evidence from various lines of research showing the importance of motivation and attentional focus in motor performance and learning. According to this theory, motor performance and learning are facilitated in practice conditions that (a) enhance expectancies, (b) support autonomy, and (c) provide external focus of attention.

Frequency and Timing of Feedback

Frequency is simply the amount of feedback in relation to task performance. For example, feedback can be provided for every attempt (100% frequency), about half of the attempts (50% frequency), or about one-tenth of the attempts (10% frequency). Feedback timing can be immediate or delayed. In the early stages of therapy, feedback could be given immediately to assist the child in producing the correct target and establishing a reliable reference pattern. After a criterion of success is achieved (say 50% correct productions), a delay in feedback might encourage a child to use processes of self-monitoring rather than rely exclusively on the clinician's report of accuracy. Feedback schedules take several different forms such as constant (always provided), fading (gradually diminishing with practice), and inconsistent (without fixed schedule). The optimal schedule may depend on the characteristics of the client, the learning goal, and the task requirements. Rather than adopt a fixed schedule for a treatment, it may be advantageous to begin with a high frequency of feedback and then gradually decrease the frequency as the child gains proficiency with the task.

> Speech generates several different kinds of sensory feedback, including auditory, kinesthetic, tactile, and barometric. The roles of these different kinds of feedback are adapted to phases of motor learning and the relative availability of feedback in each modality. Errors identified through sensory feedback are used to refine internal models of motor control.

Stimulability

Stimulability, the ability to produce a speech sound correctly when a model is provided (Powell & Miccio, 1996), is considered in this chapter because it is an aspect of speech motor control, even though it may not have direct parallel in the larger literature on motor learning. Assessment of stimulability is done in a clinician-child dyad, and the child's participation is rooted in attention to the model, discrimination of the relevant acoustic cues, and reproduction of the model by appropriate control of the speech musculature. Stimulability has demonstrated prognostic value (Irwin et al., 1966; Powell & Miccio, 1996; To et al., 2022), and sounds that are stimulable have more rapid gains in therapy than sounds that are nonstimulable (T. McAllister et al., 2022; Powell & Miccio, 1996; Rvachew, 2005). It is one of the most frequently used components in the clinical assessment of speech sound disorders (Farquharson & Tambyraja, 2019). Modeling (discussed earlier in this chapter) is an important aspect in assessing stimulability. Lof (1996) reported that factors associated with stimulability were articulation visibility, child's age, family's socioeconomic status, and child's overall imitative abilities.

Compensatory and Adaptive Movements

In physical therapy, compensatory or adaptive movements are used in the rehabilitation of patients who have experienced conditions such as amputations, paralysis, or trauma. A **compensatory movement** is an alternative motor pattern that is suited to a client's individual capabilities and limitations. Compensatory articulations in speech-language pathology are encountered most often in children who have velopharyngeal dysfunction such as cleft palate (a condition discussed in Chapter 11). Henningsson et al. (2008) described three types of compensatory articulations in individuals with cleft palate: (1) abnormal backing of oral articulatory targets to a post-uvular place (i.e., place of production posterior to the anomaly in the vocal tract), resulting in sounds such as the glottal stop /ʔ/, pharyngeal fricative /ʕ/, and laryngeal fricative /h/); (2) articulations produced at the velopharyngeal port taking the form of phoneme specific nasal emissions, also called posterior nasal fricatives; and (3) backed place of production within the oral cavity, resulting in the voiceless mid-dorsum palatal stop /c/, voiced mid-dorsum palatal stop /ɟ/, and voiced velar nasal fricative /ŋ/. These compensatory articulations can be ingrained in speech motor behavior and therefore can be difficult to treat even after velopharyngeal function has been improved by surgery or prosthetics.

Compensatory articulations also have been observed in children with severe speech-sound disorders who have a normal velopharyngeal function. These articulations replace oral fricatives, typically sibilants, (Howard, 2004; Kjellmer et al., 2021; Oren et al., 2020; Trost, 1981; Zajac, 2015). Glottal stop substitutions also have been described as non-developmental phonological processes in children with hearing loss (Eriks-Brophy et al., 2013). It has been shown that at least some compensatory articulations can be modified though motor learning. Kjellmer et al. (2021) reported that a motor-based, hierarchically structured intervention is effective in remediating active nasal fricatives substituting /s/ in children who have normal palatal functioning.

Memory Consolidation

Memory consists of at least three distinct processes known as encoding (getting information into a form suitable for memory), consolidation (storing and integrating memories), and retrieval (recalling stored representations). **Memory consolidation** is the process that transforms new and somewhat labile memories into stable representations that are integrated into the system of pre-existing long-term memories. This process depends on elapsed time and can be influenced by sleep, which appears to assist consolidation. Sleep dependency is observed when post-learning sleep leads to improved performance or qualitative changes in memory compared with a wake interval of equal length. The learning of motor skills, including speech, depends in part on acquiring stable memory traces for motor gestures (van Zelst & Earle, 2021).

Memory consolidation involves at least two distinct processes. First, synaptic consolidation is achieved by localized changes to synaptic strength, including both changes to membrane potentials and new dendritic growth. Second, systems consolidation is the reorganization of information from short-term to long-term store, a process that reflects how new, episodic information is gradually integrated with preexisting declarative knowledge, so that the new information does not simply overwrite the old. Sleep may facilitate consolidation by allowing for an integration that is not always easily accomplished during a conscious state. The role of sleep as it relates to memory and learning in speech-language pathology is discussed by Morrow and Duff (2020).

Speech Motor Control Compared to Other Human Motor Skills

There is much to be learned from the general study of motor control that is relevant to understanding the motor control of speech. Principles of motor learning can apply across types of motor skills, including those in speech. But certain differences between speech and nonspeech motor behaviors should be kept in mind. First, speech is tied to language, which endows it with cognitive elements that are unlike those in most other motor behaviors, with some exceptions such as manual communication used in American Sign Language. Second, speech is learned and maintained by reference to its auditory patterns. Aside from music, few other motor behaviors are so keenly registered to audition. Third, as pointed out by Grimme et al. (2011), speech is unusual in its rapid, task-dependent compensatory reactions to perturbations. Fourth, speech involves very fast rates of movement that underlie the ability to produce 150 words/min in ordinary conversation (super-fast talkers can manage 600 words/min; Ludlow et al., 2019). In comparison, the fastest typists can produce about 90 words per minute and American Sign Language is produced at rates of about 150 signs per minute (Bellugi et al., 1988). Speech and signing are among the fastest discrete motor performances in human behavior, and both serve the important function of communication.

Care should be taken in generalizing results from studies of skeletal muscles to the craniofacial muscles, especially when the latter are purposed to speech movements. The muscles of speech are unique in their genetic, developmental, functional, and phenotypical properties (Kent, 2004). The complex musculature of speech consists of several different structural-functional groups, including (a) joint-related muscles of the jaw, (b) sphincteric muscles of the lips, pharynx, and velopharynx), (c) the muscular hydrostat of the tongue, (d) muscles specialized for vibration and airway valving in the larynx, and (e) the muscles that inflate and deflate the lungs. In addition, these muscles have a highly heterogeneous muscle fiber composition that may be suited to the demands of speech motor skills.

Clinical Considerations for Speech Disorders in Children

Studies on motor learning for speech have been conducted primarily, but not exclusively, with healthy adults and with adults who have neurological impairments. A much smaller literature is devoted to children who are either typically developing or have communication disorders, and it should not be assumed that motor learning in children is the same as in adults. As reviewed in Chapter 2, children differ from adults in several ways that affect the processes of speech production. It may prove beneficial to work toward a speech motor learning theory for children that intertwines developmental processes in the neural, musculoskeletal, sensory, hormonal, and psychological domains. Children learn the motor control of speech with a biological system that is undergoing changes in size, configuration, and tissue properties. At the same time, they are expected to make advances in language, emotional processing, and social interactions.

Examples of studies that applied PLM to children's speech are CAS (Maas et al., 2014; Strand, 1995; Strand et al., 2006), cerebral palsy (Korkalainen et al. 2023), cleft palate (Hanley et al., 2023), and speech sound errors (Ruscello & Vallino, 2014; Skelton & Richard, 2016). However, PLM is not always consistently followed, which complicates interpretation of the data. Moreover, it can be argued that PLM is a set of principles and not a set of specific strategies that are rigidly applied across clients and therapeutic goals. It is especially important to recognize that much more is known about the application of PLM to adults rather than children. As shown in Figure 9–4, motor learning

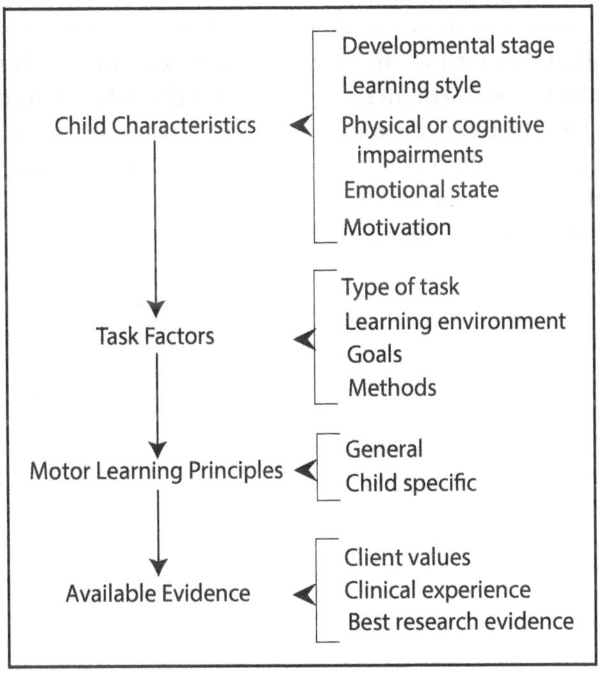

Figure 9–4. Diagram of the overall decision-making process, beginning with factors relating to an individual child, proceeding to task factors, and culminating with motor learning principles and available evidence.

is one component of an overall decision-making process, beginning with factors relating to an individual child, proceeding to task factors, and culminating with motor learning principles and available evidence. Motor learning can be used with a variety of different treatment strategies specific to speech disorders (as considered in Chapter 12). The transdisciplinary application of PLM reflects its generality.

Conclusions

1. Concepts and theories of motor learning are broadly applied across clinical specialties and their effectiveness has been demonstrated in numerous studies, mostly with adults. Most of the research on motor learning involves motor skills that are essentially an end in themselves (e.g., athletic performance, manual dexterity). But speech movements are purposed to linguistic and emotional expressions, so that speech motor control is intimately linked with high-level cognitive processes. Because speech motor control is based on sensory, cognitive, linguistic, and other factors, it cannot be easily isolated from these influences, which are critical to the learning and refinement of motor skills.
2. The musculature of speech production differs in important ways from the skeletal musculature, which implies that speech motor control should be understood with due consideration of its specialized nature.
3. A treatment based on motor learning principles should consider several factors relating to modeling, observation, imaging, imitation, focus of attention, practice, and feedback.
4. Motor learning has broad clinical application and is not restricted to the disorders commonly placed in the category of motor speech disorders. Furthermore, motor learning can be used in combination with various therapies (Chapter 12).

10

BILINGUALISM AND DIALECTS

Chapter 1 touched on the different types of developmental speech disorders and variations, and this chapter and the following chapter continue and deepen the discussion. The objective is to identify the major types of disorders and other conditions or variations and to describe the speech characteristics in different populations. As noted in Chapter 1, classifications are a work in progress, so what is presented here reflects contemporary knowledge that may well be modified in the future. Terminology is adapted to changes in sociocultural factors and preferences. Speech and language can be sensitive issues regarding membership in linguistic and cultural communities, which entails a nuanced recognition of how terminology fits groups of people.

Delay Versus Disorder Versus Difference

Deviations in speech from the norms of the dialect and speech community are usually categorized as one of three major groups: **delay**, **disorder**, or **difference** (or combinations of these three).

Delay is defined as development that is slower than is typical for a comparison group, such as same-aged peers. Frequently, delay is recognized when developmental milestones are not reached at the expected age. An important and defining feature of delay is that it follows the normal or typical pattern but at a slower rate. The patterns of typical development summarized in Chapter 5 are the basis for identifying delay and can be the framework for intervention that follows the typical course of development (e.g., treating error sounds in the approximate order of their mastery in typically developing children). An important caveat is that typical development is not fixed to a calendar that applies to all children. Many developmental processes, especially those in speech and language, are highly variable across children with respect to their onsets and rates. Some children utter their first words before one year of age, others at closer to two years, but both groups can end up with highly intelligible speech. The issue is not simply a matter of relative timing of landmark events but, in some rare cases, whether a landmark event occurs at all. For example, crawling is a typical landmark in the development of locomotion, but some children do not crawl and nevertheless go on to age-typical walking (Størvold et al., 2013). Studies of early speech production in typically developing children have shown substantial variability (McGillion et al., 2016; Vihman, 1993), and this variability must be considered in using developmental landmarks as guidelines in clinical assessment.

A **disorder** is defined as a pattern that deviates from the normal or typical pattern and is not only a delay in reaching milestones. Identification of a disorder presumes knowledge of typical development and often points to errors that are exceptional or idiosyncratic. A disorder in the strict sense of the word is a pattern that is characteristic of a different developmental trajectory, possibly including speech sound features that are not observed in typical development. A possible semantic confusion is that the general category of children's speech disorder, as typically used, includes both delay and disorder. The same is true of the term phonological disorder, which is often used as a general category that includes both phonological delay and phonological disorder, which comprise the two largest subgroups of children with speech sound disorders (Waring et al., 2022).

A **difference** is a departure from the normal or typical pattern that usually is associated with sociolinguistic factors, such as bilingualism. However, as mentioned earlier, a difference can occur in combination with a delay or disorder, for example, a child who is learning English as a second language may also have a speech disorder. The word *difference* is frequently used but is not without criticism because some authors believe that it implies inferiority or other negative status (Yu et al., 2022). If a person is described as "different" the connotation under certain circumstances can be offensive or exclusive. But because the word *difference* is well established in the literature (Kester, 2014; Stockman, 2010) and there does not appear to be a widely recognized alternative, it is used here, with the caveat that it may not be as neutral as intended and probably should be replaced. (For a perspective on this issue, see Grover et al., 2022.) Children learning English as an L2 may exhibit speech characteristics derived from their first language, and it can be difficult to distinguish a possible disorder or delay from the effects of the L1. That is, some features of the L1 may affect L2 learning in a way that may resemble either a delay or disorder. This clinical challenge is often framed as a matter of separating difference from disorder, but Oetting et al. (2016) suggested that disorder within difference is a better formulation. That is, a child learning an L2 contends with differences between the L2 and the L1, so that any effects of a delay or disorder exist within the context of the L1–L2 differences. This issue has been addressed in technical reports of the American Speech-Language Association (1983, 1985, 1998), and these reports offer general guidelines for clinical services and professional preparation. Figure 10–1 represents the potential overlap or interaction among difference, disorder, and delay. An individual child might be classified as having a difference, a disorder, a delay, or any combination of these three. Characterizing difference is a first step in meeting the challenge of determining if delay or disorder is present. The following sections address this problem by considering several aspects of L1 and L2 acquisition.

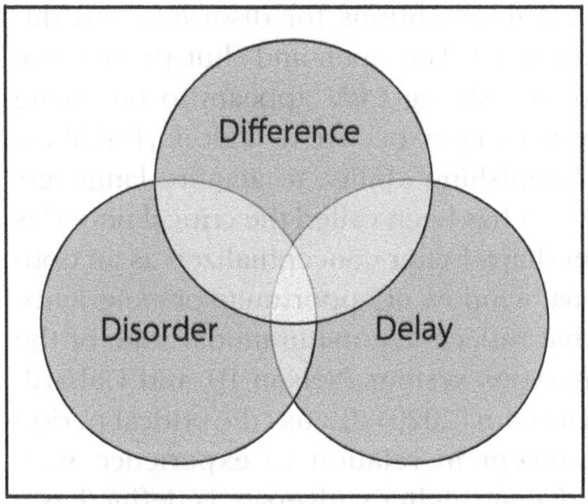

Figure 10–1. Venn diagram of clinical populations presenting with SSD. The intersecting circles show the possible combinations of disorder, delay, and difference.

Critical Period for Language Acquisition

In studies of development, a **critical period** is generally defined as a maturational interval during which crucial experiences exert their maximal effect on development or learning. A **critical period in language acquisition**, as proposed by Penfield and Roberts (1959) and Lenneberg (1967), has been highly influential in understanding age-related limitations on language learning. Although critical periods have been proposed for other sensory and motor processes (Hensch, 2004), language is one of the few complex cognitive systems for which a critical period has been a centerpiece of scientific literature (Werker & Hensch, 2015). The **critical period hypothesis (CPH)** has been applied to both the first or native language (L1) and to subsequently learned languages (L2). This is not to claim that L1 and L2 acquisition are based on the same processes. L1 typically is learned by exposure—children receive considerable language input during their early development. In contrast, L2 usually is learned by attention, effort, and direct instruction, as in taking a course on a foreign language. Research on CPH is clouded by methodological problems that hinder confident conclusions. The generally accepted understanding is that acquisition of L1 is best accomplished by the age of puberty, so that the critical period of language acquisition begins at about the first year of life (given the perceptual attunement discussed in Chapter 2) and extends to the age of about 12 years. This hypothesis was compatible with the theory of universal grammar (Chomsky, 1986), which states that there is an innate and defined set of mechanisms (**language acquisition device**) that enables children to learn, develop, and understand language. The acquisition of L1 is based on these mechanisms. Another language may be acquired later in life, but fluency (in the sense of native-like language) is likely to be compromised (e.g., it will be spoken with an accent that reflects features of the L1).

The CPH is the subject of considerable research and debate, and only a few highlights of the controversy are noted here. On the assumption that a critical period exists (and there is by no means agreement on this point; Azieb, 2021; Bialystok & Kroll, 2018; Flege, 2019; Redmond, 1992; Vanhove, 2013), there are differences of opinion on its age of application. As noted earlier, it is often stated that the critical period of language acquisition closes at puberty (about 12 years of age), but in a large study of nearly 700,000 native and non-native English speakers, it was concluded that the ability to learn grammar is preserved until the age of 17.4 years and then declines (Hartshorne et al., 2018). Alternatives to the strict form of the CPH have also been proposed, including the possibilities of a sensitive or optimal period (meaning that certain maturational stages afford *relative* advantages in language learning) or multiple critical periods with their own time scales (meaning that language acquisition is related to different skills or processes that have their own developmental schedules). Multiple critical periods could be successive, with one following another, or they could be overlapping, in which one critical period is largely contained within another (Reh et al., 2020). Friedmann and Rusou (2015) concluded from a review that included studies of **feral children** (children who have lived in isolation from human contact from an early age) that the critical period for syntax closes at about the first year of life (the age at which infants lock on to the phonetic properties of their ambient language). Generally, these different approaches share the assumption that there are maturational limits on the ability to learn a language, but they differ in some respects, such as whether the period of language acquisition is sharply defined or is one of gradually diminishing capability, and whether the critical period can be reopened by interventions. As mentioned in Chapter 1, evidence is mounting that language is malleable to some degree throughout life. Thiessen et al. (2016) proposed that processes of language acquisition, especially the role of statistical learning, are continuous, rather than discontinuous, across the lifespan. They explain acquisition in terms of experience, age differences in input, and maturational changes in the cognitive architecture of learning. This proposal has implications for language acquisition, language instruction, and interventions for disorders and differences. The open-and-shut perspective of the strong CPH appears to be giving way to a perspective of lifelong, but likely diminishing ability, to acquire language. What has been called the critical period is perhaps better conceptualized as an optimal window of opportunity or experience that reflects the maturational state of the nervous system. Nelson III and Gabard-Durnam (2020) discuss the critical period concept in relation to experience with adversity, where adversity is defined as a violation of the expectable environment in the form of hazards (biological, psychosocial, or both) that exert negative effects on development. In their view, critical periods of brain development correspond to heightened neuroplasticity that encodes the expectable environment, that is, the environment most suited to typical development. Risk factors, such as those discussed in Chapter 11, are examples of adversity in speech and language development.

Since its earliest formulation, CPH has been linked with maturational changes in the brain, for example, the hypothesis that neural plasticity diminishes in adults. The exact mechanisms are uncertain, but possibilities include stabilization of neural networks (Kuhl et al., 2005), the balance between excitatory and inhibitory processes that determine the onset of plasticity and molecular brakes that determine its offset (Werker & Hensch, 2015), and processes involving cortical disinhibition and thalamic adenosine (Patton et al., 2019). As shown in Figure 10–2, neuroplasticity may be shaped by brakes that operate during early development (a period of immaturity in which neural networks are initially forming) and later development (a period of consolidation or stabilization of the net-

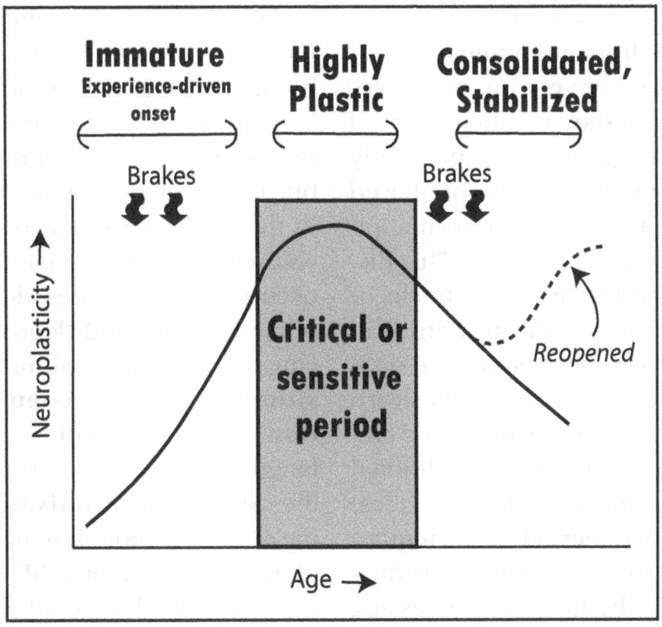

Figure 10–2. Diagram of a critical period in a developmental process. The critical period, shown as a shaded box, is the interval of maximum plasticity. Brakes operate on either side of the critical period to reduce plasticity. The dotted line indicates the potential for reopening the window of flexibility.

works). The critical period occurs during the interval of maximal plasticity. The dotted line in Figure 10–2 represents a potential reopening of the critical period (enhanced neuroplasticity). Some of the proposed biological mechanisms of neuroplasticity hold promise for enhanced language learning by pairing sounds with the activation of neuromodulatory circuits involved in attention. In a review of the literature on neuroplasticity related to second language learning, Li, Legault, and Litcofsky (2014, p. 301) concluded that, "second language experience-induced brain changes, including increased gray matter (GM) density and white matter (WM) integrity, can be found in children, young adults, and the elderly; can occur rapidly with short-term language learning or training; and are sensitive to age, age of acquisition, proficiency or performance level, language-specific characteristics, and individual differences." In their introduction to a special issue of the *Journal of Phonetics*, de Leeuw and Celata (2019) comment that, "native phonetic and phonological domains are malleable throughout the lifespan in the context of bilingualism" (p. 88). Neuroplasticity is a general phenomenon that applies to the processes of spoken language, including auditory processing (Whitelaw & Yuskow, 2006), learning L2 phonology (Heidlmayr et al., 2021), motor skill learning (Dayan & Cohen, 2011), and vocabulary in L2 learning (Isel, 2021). This topic is developed further in a later section on bilingualism. Neuroplasticity has profound implications for treating speech and language disorders in both children and adults.

Critical periods are not unique to biological systems, as they can be observed in artificial learning systems, apparently owing to fundamental constraints based on learning dynamics and information processing (Achille et al., 2017). This discovery shows that the first few epochs of training a neural network are critical in creating strong connections that are optimal in representing the input data distribution. After these connections are created, they change little during additional training. The full understanding of critical periods (or sensitive periods) may require an appreciation of principles of information processing whether this processing is accomplished by biological or artificial systems. Knowledge of these principles could lead to effective interventions based on information structures. It is important to note that individual differences are prominent in studies of L1 acquisition, and these differences should be considered in drawing inferences regarding critical periods or any other developmental theory. Kidd et al. (2020) stated that any theory of language acquisition should consider intrinsic differences in neurocognitive learning mechanisms, the communicative environment, and developmental cascades in which emerging linguistic skills depend critically on previously acquired foundational abilities. As discussed later in this chapter, individual differences are similarly prominent in the acquisition of another language.

Bilingualism

Bilingualism is an increasingly important feature of the U.S. population. It is estimated that in 2019 about 45% of people born in the U.S. are bilingual (Zeigler & Camarota, 2019). In the narrow sense, bilingualism is the ability to speak two languages. The ability to speak more than two languages is called **multilingualism**, but the term *bilingualism* is often used in the same sense and is not necessarily restricted to two languages. Bilingualism occurs in several types, depending on the relative timing and degree of use of the languages involved. **Simultaneous acquisition** (also called **compound acquisition**) is the acquisition of two or more languages at the same time in a person's life. **Successive acquisition** is the learning of two or more languages at different phases in a person's life (e.g., one language may be learned during early childhood and another in adulthood). **Coordinate bilingualism** is the equal use of two or more languages, and **subordinate bilingualism** is the predominant use of one language over another. **Natural acquisition** is learning a language without formal instruction, which is the way that most people learn their L1. **Guided acquisition** is learning a language with formal instruction, as in the case of taking a foreign language course. **Symmetric acquisition** is learning several languages with the same, or almost the same, proficiency. **Asymmetric acquisition** is the dominance of one language over another (or others) in the learning process. **Additive bilingualism** is learning a second language that does not interfere with the learning of a first language, so that the languages are learned about equally. **Subtractive bilingualism** is learning a second language that interferes with the learning of a first language, so that the second language often replaces the first language. Bilingualism, then, is a multifaceted topic that encompasses a wide range of language characteristics and experiences.

The term **heritage language** identifies languages other than the dominant language (or languages) in a specific social context. Fishman (2001) notes three kinds of heritage languages spoken in the U.S. An **immigrant heritage language** is a language spoken by immigrants arriving in the United States after it became an independent country. An **indigenous heritage language** is a language of the peoples native to the Americas, many of which are now extinct or spoken by very few (e.g., elders in a speech community). A **colonial heritage language** is a language of the various European groups that first colonized what is now the U.S. and continues to be spoken here. Examples are Dutch, German, Finnish, French, Spanish, and Swedish.

A U.S. census report (Dietrich & Hernandez, 2022) provides data on the languages spoken at home for the population aged five years and older. The ranked percentages (out of 100%) for the most frequently used languages were as follows for 2019:

Spanish (61.6%)

Chinese (including Mandarin and Cantonese) (5.2%)

Tagalog (including Filipino) (2.6%)

Vietnamese (2.3%)

Arabic (1.9%)

French (including Cajun) (1.7%)

Korean (1.6%)

Haitian (1.4%)

Russian (1.4%)

Hindi (1.3%)

German (1.3%)

Selected Models of Bilingual Language Learning

Bilingualism is the ability to use two or more languages in everyday life. This section summarizes four influential models of bilingual language learning.

The **speech learning model (SLM)** (Flege, 1995) proposes that during the first exposure to a foreign or second language (L2), listeners automatically relate the sounds in that language to their L1, a process called interlingual identification. Learning of the L2 sounds then depends primarily on the perceived relationship between each L2 sound and the closest sound in the L1, as well as the quantity and quality of the L2 input. Sounds that are similar in L1 and L2 present the greatest difficulty because the L2 sounds tend to be perceived as the nearest L1 sound (called equivalence classification). A revised version of the model, **speech learning model-revised (SLM-r)**, holds that the phonetic categories in the L1 and L2 subsystems interact dynamically and are updated to accommodate changes in the statistical properties of the input distributions defining L1, L2, and composite L1-L2 categories (Flege & Bohn, 2021).

The perceptual assimilation model (PAM; Best, 1994) states that adults perceive unfamiliar non-native phones in relation to articulatory similarities/dissimilarities to phonemes and contrasts in their native language. That is, PAM accounts for the influence of native-language attunement on speech perception in adults and infants. An implication of this model and the SLM model for the assessment of children's speech is that it is important to compare the sounds in L1 and L2 (contrastive analysis). PAM has been extended to learning of a third language (L3), with the assimilation of some

L3 sounds to both L1 and L2 categories (Wrembel et al., 2019).

The **Bilingual Processing Rich Information from Multidimensional Interactive Representations (PRIMIR)** (compare with the monolingual PRIMIR described in Chapter 2) is a model of bilingual phonological acquisition that was formulated to consider the sources of transfer and deceleration in bilingual speech (Curtin et al., 2011; Fabiano-Smith et al., 2015). This model consists of three representational spaces that are formed during phonological acquisition. The general perceptual space stores information about the acoustic features in the speech signal that a child hears. Within this space, similar sounds cluster together to form perceptual categories that lack phonemic status. The word space consists of words, that is, sequences of speech sounds, associated with a given referent (e.g., house). Finally, the phoneme space is a store of phonemes identified by mutual consideration of the general perceptual space and the word space. Transfer results from clustering of information from two languages within the representational spaces.

The **Automatic Selective Perception (ASP) model** (Strange, 2011) considers speech perception to be a purposeful, information-seeking activity in which adult listeners focus on the most reliable acoustic parameters that identify phonetic segments and sequences in their native language. This strategy, which relies on over-learned routines of selective perception, allows the rapid and robust detection of L1 phonetic contrasts even in difficult listening conditions or when attention is drawn elsewhere. However, late second language (L2) learners must devote attentional resources to extract information needed for non-native phonetic contrasts.

Individual Differences in L2 Learning

Individual differences in language learning have sparked decades of research in efforts to understand why some people are better than others in learning a second language (Dörnyei, 2014; Ehrman et al., 2003; Pawlak, 2021). Variables that have been investigated include learning styles, learning strategies, affective variables, motivation, age, gender, and cultural background. Differences in language learning also may be affected by individual differences in auditory and motor abilities. With respect to individual differences in audition, G. R. Kidd et al. (2007) identified a general auditory ability and four specific abilities (loudness and duration overall energy discrimination, sensitivity to temporal envelope variation, identification of highly familiar speech and nonspeech sounds, and discrimination of unfamiliar simple and complex spectral and temporal patterns). With respect to motor skill learning, Anderson et al. (2021) emphasized in their review of the literature that motor learning, performance, and transfer are highly specific and individualized. These authors note that aptitude-treatment interactions hold important implications in understanding the effects of cognitive and affective aptitudes, and personality characteristics. For example, learners classified as high ability tend to respond better to learning environments with low structure (e.g., affording a high degree of independence and autonomy during learning; variable and random practice). In contrast, low ability learners tend to respond better to highly structured learning environments (e.g., constant and blocked practice). These observations are relevant to designing the optimal structure of motor learning, as discussed in Chapter 9. The importance of individual differences in relation to training method has been shown in a study of the acquisition of a novel phonological contrast (Perrachione et al., 2011). An implication is that no single method is optimal for all individuals, and training should be selected in accord with the characteristics of the learner.

Factors that might affect L2 learning are shown in Figure 10–3, which elaborates on the model of Atkinson and Shiffrin (1968). The physical signal of speech is processed by the sensory system which transfers information to a sensory memory, which is a relatively faithful representation of the physical signal but is affected by limitations in sensory acuity (e.g., immaturity or pathology). Next in line is short-term memory (also known as working memory), which relies on attention to select important aspects of the information in sensory memory and subsequently on maintenance rehearsal to ensure that the memory trace is robust. Maintenance rehearsal may draw on relevant articulatory information to establish sensory-motor associations. This operation is similar to the phonological loop proposed by Baddeley (1992). Reference to articulation is potentially based on

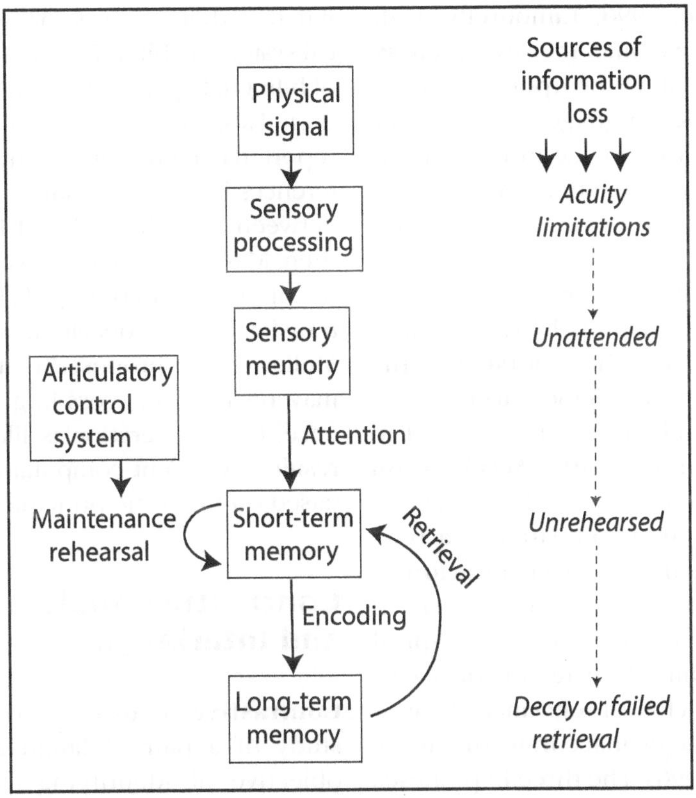

Figure 10–3. Factors that may affect L2 learning. The right side of the figure lists sources of information loss that may affect the learning process.

inner or covert speech (Marvel & Desmond, 2012) and not necessarily on overt articulatory behavior. Information in short-term memory is used to create representations in long-term memory, with retrieval mechanisms operating between short-term and long-term memories. The right side of Figure 10–3 indicates sources of information loss that may affect learning of L2.

Acceleration, Deceleration, and Transfer in Bilingual Phonological Development

Phonological development in bilingual children may reflect three primary effects (Fabiano-Smith & Goldstein, 2010; Paradis & Genesee, 1996; Tamburelli et al., 2014). **Transfer** (sometimes called **cross-linguistic transfer)** incorporates an element from one language into another, such as when a phoneme in L1 transfers to production of utterances in L2. Transfer can be positive or negative. **Positive transfer** is the application of an L1 element to L2 learning when that element is in fact appropriate to L2 (resulting in **facilitation**). **Negative transfer** is the application of an L1 element to L2 learning when that element is not present in L2 (resulting in an **error**). **Acceleration** is the earlier emergence of an element in a bilingual child compared to a typical monolingual peer. **Deceleration** is the delayed emergence of an element in a bilingual child compared to a typical monolingual child. Transfer and deceleration have high clinical relevance because they can result in inaccurate diagnosis (Dodd et al., 1996). The three hypotheses just noted were introduced by Paradis and Genesee (1996). In their article, deceleration was called delay. These hypotheses resonate in recent studies of bilingualism, and they serve as a framework for understanding language interactions (Core & Scarpelli, 2015; Fabiano-Smith & Barlow, 2010; Hambly et al., 2013). Hamby et al. (2013) conducted a systematic review of speech acquisition in bilingual infants and children (where one language was English). A generally consistent finding across the reviewed studies was evidence for transfer between the two phonological and language systems, including positive and negative transfer of features from L1 to L2, as well as from L2 to L1. Positive transfer occurred more often with increased age and length of exposure to the L2. The authors noted that the current trend in research is to investigate how phonological systems interact, rather than whether there are one or two phonological systems in bilingual children. In a study of bilingual Spanish-English speaking children, Fabiano-Smith and Goldstein (2010) reported evidence of both transfer and differences in accuracy, but not acceleration, between monolingual and bilingual children. Marecka et al. (2020) concluded that the phonology of bilingual children shows transfer but not deceleration in their L1. Müller (2017) proposed that deceleration may result from cross-linguistic interference, but acceleration is likely to be the result of efficient computation that is not based on linguistic principles.

Contrastive Analysis and Interlanguage

Contrastive analysis is the systematic study of a pair of languages with the objective of identifying structural differences and similarities between them. This method has been widely used in **second language learning (SLA)** and has applications in speech-language therapy

(McGregor et al.,1997). Contrastive analysis requires specification of the properties of the two languages, which in SLA are often called the *first language* and the *target language*. As applied to phonology, this kind of analysis typically entails determining the phonetic inventory of each language and the phonological patterns of word production. This parallel description of the languages gave rise to the **contrastive analysis hypothesis**, which holds that elements that are similar between L1 and L2 will be learned more easily than elements that are dissimilar. However, judgments of similarity or dissimilarity can be challenging, and even when elements appear to be similar in two different languages, there may be subtle differences. For example, the base-of-articulations hypothesis holds that languages may have different articulatory settings that reflect the settings of the most frequently occurring segments and segment combinations (Honikman, 1964; Bradlow, 1995). The articulatory settings may be optimal for a particular language or dialect and could be a factor in the fluent production of that language or dialect (Gick et al., 2004; Ramanarayanan et al., 2014; Wieling & Tiede, 2017; Wilson & Gick, 2014). The contrastive analysis hypothesis has been questioned because it fails to make accurate predictions of the various kinds of errors that occur in L2 learners (Perkins & Zhang, 2022).

An alternative view is that of **interlanguage**, the evolving system of rules in L2 learning that result from various processes and influences, including the influence of L1 (transfer), contrastive interference from L2 (target language), overgeneralization of newly encountered rules, and rules that are not present in either L1 or L2 (Eckman, 2014). As shown in Figure 10–4, interlanguage overlaps with L1 (native language) and L2 (target language) but may have its own unique features. Compared to the contrastive analysis hypothesis, the hypothesis of interlanguage is a more nuanced, idiosyncratic, and dynamic representation that enfolds factors such as speaker age, experiences, and cognitive constructions.

Bilingual Advantage

Although much has been written on the difficulties of L2 learning, a countervailing view is that bilingualism affords certain

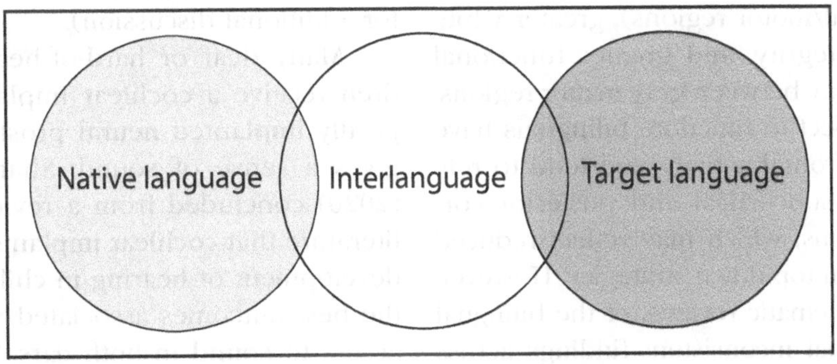

Figure 10–4. Relationships between a native and target language in L2 learning. Interlanguage contains elements that are not present in either the native or target language.

advantages in both nonlinguistic and linguistic aspects of cognition (Spinu et al., 2018). Bilingualism may have positive effects on several aspects of nonlinguistic cognition, including multitasking, selective attention, cognitive function, and delayed onset and slower rate of decline in dementia as compared to monolinguals. Bilingualism also could enhance aspects of linguistic processing, such as manipulating discrete phonemic units, novel word acquisition, and vowel space restructuring when learning novel accents. Choo, Smith, and Lee analyzed data from the U.S. National Survey of Children's Health for years 2007, 2011–2012, 2016, and 2017, and concluded that bilingual children aged 12 to 17 were less likely to be identified with a speech disorder compared to their monolingual peers. Spinu et al. (2018) hypothesized that the bilingual advantage may arise from a more efficient coupling of sensory and cognitive functions and that echoic memory may help in the remapping between existing mental representations of sounds and existing articulatory command configurations. Grundy et al. (2017) reviewed differences in neural structure and function between monolinguals and bilinguals. With respect to structural differences, bilinguals have greater gray matter volume (especially in perceptual/motor regions), greater white matter integrity, and greater functional connectivity between gray matter regions. With respect to function, bilinguals have reduced frontal activity and tend to rely more on subcortical and posterior cortical regions. which may reflect reduced reliance on top-down strategies. However, recent systematic reviews of the bilingual effect reveal inconsistent findings across studies and the likely influence of moderators such as socioeconomic status (Giovannoli et al., 2020; Gunnerud et al., 2020).

Sign Languages and Bimodal Bilingualism

A signed modality of language, such as American Sign Language (ASL), achieves communication by means of a gestural medium used principally by the deaf community and their caregivers and teachers. The signs are specific handshapes and movements that are often accompanied by facial expressions and body movements. Children learn natural sign languages on roughly the same time scale as children learning spoken languages if they have access to fluent adult signers from birth (Lillo-Martin & Henner, 2021). It has been suggested that manual signs may assist development of communication not only in deaf and hard-of-hearing children, but also typically developing children (Goodwyn et al., 2000) and children with neurodevelopmental disorders such as Down syndrome and ASD (Özçalışkan et al., 2017). However, it also has been argued that early use of sign language may interfere with the development of spoken language. Pontecorvo et al. (2023) review studies on this issue and conclude from their own studies of vocabulary development that acquisition of sign language does not harm spoken vocabulary acquisition. (See Hall, Hall, and Caselli, 2019, for additional discussion).

Many deaf or hard-of-hearing children receive a cochlear implant, a surgically implanted neural prosthesis that gives a sense of sound. Sharma et al. (2020) concluded from a review of the literature that cochlear implants promote development of hearing in children with the best outcomes associated with early access to sound in both ears. They also note that the benefits can be limited by social determinants of health that hinder needed support and by medical comorbidities that complicate care and outcome. Behavioral therapy such as auditory-verbal therapy is needed to ensure the optimal results of a cochlear implant (Binos et al., 2021; Noel et al., 2023; Thomas & Zwolan, 2019). Auditory-verbal therapy is an early intervention program that teaches hearing-impaired children to listen and speak using their residual hearing, along with the auditory stimulation provided by the regular use of hearing aids, cochlear implants, or FM devices. The Cochlear Implant Alliance Task Force (Warner-Czyz et al., 2022) stated that speech, language, and listening therapy are an essential component of (re)habilitation pre- and post-implantation.

Bimodal bilingualism is achieved by individuals who are capable of both sign language and spoken language, as in the case of deaf children who have deaf, signing parents and receive both cochlear implantation and bilingual language experience (Goodwin & Lillo-Martin, 2019). These children develop some, but not necessarily equal, proficiency in both signed and spoken language. Speech, while signing, called simultaneous communication (SimCom), differs from speech only in having a slower speech rate, lower lexical richness, and lower syntactic complexity (Rozen-Blay et al., 2022).

Accent and Dialect

Variation occurs within a given language, especially in the form of accent and dialect. **Accent** is the characteristic pattern of pronunciation of a language associated with a particular nation, geographic region, social class, or other group of speakers. Accent is the way in which words are pronounced and is satisfactorily studied by phonetic methods, such as transcription or acoustic analyses. (It should be noted that the word *accent* is also used to denote the emphasis on a syllable or word in speech, usually by increased stress or altered pitch.) Accentedness is considered in Chapter 8 as a global concept that is complementary to intelligibility and comprehensibility, noting that a person's speech can be highly intelligible but still have an accent. Furthermore, it has been shown that listeners can adapt to speech patterns that deviate substantially from the pronunciation norms in the native talker community, sometimes even within a single listening session (Bradlow & Bent, 2008). **Dialect** is a form of a language that is specific to a particular geographical region or a group of people. It includes accent as a component but goes further in having possibly distinctive patterns of grammar, vocabulary, syntax, and common expressions. Typically, speakers of different dialects of a language are mutually intelligible although there may be instances of failed communication. Estimates of the number of different regional dialects spoken in the United States vary across studies according to methodology and other factors. The number of dialects differs across sources, as shown by the following examples.

1. Three dialects: Northeast, South, and Midwest/West (Clopper & Pisoni, 2006).
2. Six dialect regions: Northeastern, Inland North, Midlands, Southern, North Central, and Western (Labov et al., 2006).
3. 24 dialects: too numerous to be listed here (Wilson 2013).
4. 30 dialects: too numerous to be listed here (Fluency Corp, 2020).

Dialects have been classified with different terms. The term **standard dialect** has been used by some writers to identify the dialect that predominates in written form, often in a wider region than that of the dialect itself. In other words, this dialect has been highly codified in grammar and usage, so that it prevails over other dialects. One problem with this definition is that some languages do not have a written form but nonetheless can have a standard dialect. A similar term is **mainstream dialect**, which identifies a dialect used in formal contexts, such as school, workplace, and public broadcasting. This dialect also may be reflected in standard orthography (i.e., written versions of the language). Both standard and mainstream are used to indicate the predominant dialect in a country or other region. It often is used in teaching reading, which reinforces its usefulness. Alternative dialects are known by names such as **nonstandard**, **nonmainstream**, or **vernacular**. The term *substandard* is avoided because of its negative connotations.

Dialect is to some degree gender dependent. Gender is not a dichotomous variable but rather a complex social construct that is subject to modification (Schilling-Estes, 2002). In a study of Southern and Midland dialects of American English, Clopper and Smiljanic (2011) observed significant effects of talker gender on the distributions of pitch accents and phrasal-boundary tone combinations. These results indicate that features of regional and gender identity are encoded partly in prosody, which motivates closer study of the prosodic aspects of dialect to complement the more frequently studied variations in vowel production. It also appears that dialect use in children can be affected by both SES and gender (Washington & Craig, 1998).

Sociolect and Idiolect

Other variations in speech patterns should be noted. A **sociolect** is a speech pattern common to a specific social class. An **idiolect** is the manner of speaking of an individual person, that is, patterns of speech that mark our individuality within a speech community. Therefore, an individual speaker has both a dialect and an idiolect—and sometimes a sociolect. Examples of sociolect are discussed in the following.

Uptalk is a prosodic feature often associated with the speech of young people, especially females. Cruttenden (1997, p. 99) defined uptalk (also known as **high rising terminal, HRT**), as the use of "high-rise on declaratives where no questioning seems to be involved." In other words, a pitch rise occurs at the end of declarative sentences where a pitch fall is usually expected. This feature is by no means unique to North America, as it has been noted for speakers in Australia, Britain, Ireland, and New Zealand, among others. It may have a social function such as group identification. Another phenomenon that usually occurs at the end of utterances is vocal fry, the lowest voice register that is usually characterized by a low fundamental frequency and relatively high perturbations (jitter and shimmer). Other names for vocal fry are pulsatile, laryngealization, pulse phonation, creak, croak, popcorning, glottal fry, glottal rattle, glottal scrape, strohbass glottal fry, and vocal roll. Much has been written about the use of vocal fry in both the scientific and popular press, often emphasizing its occurrence in young female adults (Fessenden, 2011; Pointer et al., 2022; Wolk et al., 2012). However, a review of the literature did not reveal consistent data on this vocal behavior, indicating that further research is needed (Dallaston & Docherty, 2020).

As mentioned in the discussion of bilingualism, it has been proposed that bilinguals may construct an interlanguage that combines features of both L1 and L2, along with features that may not be present in either language. Perhaps there is also an *interlect,* or a dialect representation that combines features of the mainstream dialect and the native dialect, along with features that may not appear in either of these dialects. Such a proposal is consistent with idiosyncratic differences in dialect use that result from cognitive processes in individual speakers.

Commonly Encountered Dialects

In addition to regional dialects, other dialects are specific to groups of people based usually on country of origin or genetic origin. Attention is given here to two main dialects.

African American English

The distinctive speech patterns of certain groups of African Americans have been labeled by linguists as **African American English (AAE)**, **African American Vernacular English (AAVE)**, **Black English**, or **Ebonics** (Rickford, 1996). This dialect is characterized by several types of variation, including lexical, phonological, vowel, grammatical, prosodic, and pragmatic (Charity, 2008). Assessments of articulation or phonology should be done with recognition of consonantal and vowel variations that often occur in AAE (Bailey & Thomas, 2021; Bland-Stewart, 2005; Charity, 2008; Craig et al., 2003). Some examples are as follows:

Postvocalic consonant deletion: [m aʊ θ] produced as [m aʊ]

Consonant substitution: final [θ] produced as [f] in the word *mouth*

Consonant substitution: Initial [ð] produced as [d] in the word *they*

Final consonant reduction in clusters: [h æ n d] produced as [h æ n]

Final consonant devoicing: [b æ d] produced as [b æ t]

Deletion of /l/: [h ɛ l p] produced as [h ɛ p]

Deletion of [ɹ]: [k ɑ ɹ] produced as [k ɑ]

Consonant cluster movement: [æ s k] and [æ k s]

[ɛ] – [ɪ] merger before nasal consonants: [p ɛ n] produced as [p ɪ n]

Monophthongization of dipththongs: [t aɪ m] produced as [t ɑ m]

Syllable deletion: [b ɪ k eɪ m] produced as [k eɪ m]

Besides differences in phonetic inventory, phonotactic differences affecting syllable and word structure are influential (Pearson et al., 2009). Discovery of such differences requires more than a standard test of articulation, which typically is restricted to a small number of words with limited variability in syllable structure.

Spanish-Influenced English

English dialects of native speakers of Spanish have been termed **Chicano English**, **Mexican-American English**, **Hispanic English**, **Spanish-Influenced English (SIE)**, or **Spanglish**. Whatever name is used, these dialects are widely spoken because Spanish speakers are now the largest group of immigrants to the U.S. mainland. Hispanics are also the largest minority group in the U.S., numbering over 40 million. The six major dialects of Spanish speakers in the United States are: Mexican and Southwestern United States; Central American; Caribbean, Highlandian; Chilean; and southern Paraguayan, Uruguayan, and Argentinean (Dalbor, 1980).

Spanish presents interesting challenges in learning English as a second language because it has similarities to English but also differences. Both Spanish and English have roots in the Indo-European language family, but Spanish differs from English because of unique features in its historical development and influences. Native speakers of Spanish who are learning English are likely to demonstrate both negative and positive transfer. Goldstein (2001) describes phonetic differences between SIE and mainstream English. Spanish rhythm has been traditionally classified as syllable-timed, whereas English is regarded as stress-timed (see Chapter 6). Spanish and English differ in their vowel repertoires, with Spanish having six vowels and no lax vowels, compared to 20 vowels including lax vowels in English. Spanish has a smaller number of fricatives (three) compared with six in English. Spanish consonant phonemes not found in English include / x r ɾ ɲ /. Spanish syllables are of three types. The most commonly occurring are direct or open syllables that have either a consonant preceding a vowel, as in [sa pa to] meaning *shoe*) or a syllable that contains only a vowel, as in ([a zul] meaning *blue*). Indirect or closed syllables have a vowel that precedes the consonant, as in [kam po] meaning *field*). Mistas or compound syllables contain elements of both direct and indirect syllable structures, as in [fras ko], meaning *jar)*. Gildersleeve-Neumann et al. (2008) compared speech development in three groups of children: monolingual English children, English–Spanish bilingual children predominantly exposed to English, and English–Spanish bilingual children with relatively equal exposure to the two languages. The results showed a higher English error rate in typically developing bilinguals, including the application Spanish phonological properties to English.

Core and Scarpelli (2015) noted two major obstacles in assessing dialect in bilingual children. First, there are few standardized, norm-referenced tests of speech ability for bilingual children (McLeod & Verdon, 2014). Second, for tests that have published norms (Bilingual English-Spanish Assessment [Peña et al., 2014] and the Contextual Probes of Articulation Competence–Spanish [Goldstein & Iglesias, 2006]), the norms do not consider factors such as age of acquisition, relative exposure, or proficiency level in each language. Another factor is the possibility of dialect differences within a bilingual population, such as the differences between General Spanish dialect and the Puerto Rican dialect of Spanish (Goldstein & Iglesias, 2001). Burrows and Goldstein (2010) investigated the use of whole word measures, such as phonological mean length of utterance (pMLU) and the proportion of whole-word proximity (PWP) as complements to more traditional phoneme-based assessments. In a study of African American and Hispanic children from low-income families. Finneran et al. (2020) reported cultural-linguistic influences on performance on the Peabody Picture Vocabulary Test

(PPVT-4). This result indicates the need to consider the characteristics of test instruments relative to the background of the tested individuals.

> "So, what's the difference between a language and a dialect? In popular usage, a language is written in addition to being spoken, while a dialect is just spoken. But in the scientific sense, the world is buzzing with a cacophony of qualitatively equal 'dialects,' often shading into one another like colors (and often mixing, too), all demonstrating how magnificently complicated human speech can be. If either the terms "language" or "dialect" have any objective use, the best anyone can do is to say that there is no such thing as a "language": Dialects are all there is." (McWhorter, J. [2016, January]. What's a language, anyway? *The Atlantic*. https://www.theatlantic.com/international/archive/2016/01/difference-between-language-dialect/424704/)

Accent Modification

Accent modification (also called by a host of other names, including **accent addition, accent coaching, accent reduction, accent elimination, accent expansion, foreign accent modification, pronunciation instruction)** is training designed to alter patterns of regional dialects or foreign accents so that the speaking pattern conforms more closely to those of a target community, such as a new country of residence. A related term is **dialect shifting**, defined as "the act of interchanging between two dialects depending on the social or cultural context and can increase students' awareness between their native dialect, such as AAE [African-American English], and academic dialects, such as MAE [Mainstream American English]" (Byrd & Brown, 2021, p. 140). Dialect shifting is often combined with contrastive analysis as a means of learning the relationships between the dialects at hand.

The diversity of names for dialect training or instruction reflects the controversies that surround it. Accents are not necessarily undesirable, and efforts to eliminate or modify them sometimes confront serious issues about individual liberty and social identity. As stressed in Chapter 8, accentedness does not equate to reduced intelligibility or comprehensibility. Therefore, it is not necessarily a hindrance to communicative success. However, an accent sometimes can interfere with communication, in which case training to modify may be warranted. Accents can contribute to difficulties in learning to read given that instruction in reading is often based on Mainstream American English (Brown et al., 2015) and dialect is associated with literacy (Gatlin & Wanzek, 2015). The decision on whether to modify an accent is more easily made with adults, who usually have the capacity and autonomy needed for such a decision. Accent modification for children is a very different and complicated matter. It is conceivable that a child could receive such training unintentionally if the child is enrolled in therapy for a speech or language disorder. For example, a clinician may not have the requisite knowledge of a child's native language to distinguish an accent from a disorder and may focus treatment on speech patterns that are linked to the native language. It can be advantageous if the clinician speaks the native language of the child, but this is often not the case. Dialect training focuses on perception or production, or both. Errors in L2 learners' speech production errors can result from either perceptual or production errors (e.g., non-native-like timing of gestures), and it appears that perception and production have partly independent representations (Huensch & Tremblay, 2015). Perceptual errors may be overcome by the principles of perceptual learning. (Goldstone, 1998; Samuel & Kraljic, 2009). Goldstone (1998) described four mechanisms of such learning: develop a novel detector, improve differentiation of cues, improve the unitization or integration of cues, and assign different attentional weights to the cues. In concluding their review of the literature on perceptual learning, Samuel and Kraljic (2009, p. 1217) stated, "the perceptual system is aggressively opportunistic in its adaptation to the environment in which it must operate." This opportunism is fertile ground for dialect training. Production training may be based on several different approaches, including articulation or phonological training (Tessel & Luque, 2021), and motor learning (Ojakangas, 2013). (Motor learning is discussed in Chapter 9.) Schmidt and Sullivan (2003) concluded from a national survey that the five most common treatment goals for accent modification were: rhythm/intonation, vowel contrasts, consonant contrasts, sentence stress, and phoneme articulation (in other words, nearly all aspects of speech production).

Accent poses several challenges to the practice of speech-language pathology, including the following: (1) Are there special considerations for students who have an accent and are enrolled in academic programs in communication sciences and disorders? (Levy & Crowley, 2012.) (2) Do students who aspire to be speech-language pathologists hold attitudes or beliefs regarding dialect that might hinder their effectiveness? (Easton & Verdon, 2021; Hendricks et al., 2021.) (3) What factors should be considered in designing instructional programs to ensure competence in multicultural service delivery, including dialect training? (Foote & Thomson, 2021; Rosa-Lugo et al., 2017; Schmidt & Sullivan, 2003; K. E. Smith et al., 2022.) (4) How can professional practice accommodate newly emerging dialects (e.g., the Spanish dialect emerging in the American South)? (Wolfram et al., 2004.)

Code Switching and Diglossia

These phenomena may be observed in some bilingual individuals. **Code switching** is an alternation between languages or dialects. For example, a bilingual individual may switch between languages, sometimes mixing their features, or an individual may switch between African American Dialect and Mainstream American Dialect depending on the communicative setting. Other terms are **code-meshing** and **translanguaging**, which are preferred by some authors because they are more consistent with the fluid and adaptive use of language (Lin, 2013). Gross and Kaushanskaya (2022) distinguished **cross-speaker switching** (the child's response is in the opposite language from the conversation partner) from **intrasentential code-switching** (the child integrates both languages within a single utterance). **Diglossia** is the use of two languages (or two varieties of the same language) under different, usually compartmentalized, conditions within a community of speakers. It is often reported for languages that have distinct "high" and "low" (colloquial) varieties, such as Arabic. (Note: The same word is sometimes used to mean bilingual.)

The Biology and Sociology of Ancestry, Race, and Ethnicity

Genetic ancestry is a concept in genetics that describes the architecture of genome variation between populations. This term is preferred over racial or ethnic labels (Fujimura & Rajagopalan, 2011), but the term *ancestry* itself may carry over outdated concepts of race and ethnicity (Ross & Williams, 2021). The growing consensus is that race is a social construct rather than a biological attribute. Studies of race and ethnicity are fraught with methodological problems with potentially misleading and even harmful consequences. Genetic ancestry is thought by some to be more securely based on biological principles and may provide information relevant to functional differences, including speech differences among different communities of speakers. If genetic differences exist in craniofacial and vocal tract features, these differences should be considered in research and clinical services. Imaging and cephalometric studies have revealed some differences in craniofacial anatomy among groups differing in genetic ancestry (Durtschi et al., 2009; Farkas et al., 2005, 2007). Moreover, specific variations in the anatomy of the vocal tract associated with genetic ancestry have been reported, for example, differences in vocal tract length and volume (Xue & Hao, 2006), and velopharyngeal anatomy (Kollara et al., 2016; Xue & Hao, 2006). Acoustic studies of adults of different genetic ancestries have shown differences in vowel formant frequencies (Andrianopoulos et al., 2001; Mayo & Grant, 1995; Mayo & Manning, 1994) and in features of sustained vowel phonation (Walton & Orlikoff, 1994). Certainly, more data are needed to make a definitive statement of genetic ancestry differences for both sexes, but reports published to date indicate the possibility that such differences may be needed to establish suitable normative reference values for vocal tract dimensions, acoustic measures of speech, and perhaps other descriptions of speech output. Ching et al. (2021) offer important perspectives and caveats on this topic.

Environmental factors are potentially an aspect of genetic ancestry, and it can be challenging to distinguish genetic from environmental influences. There is evidence that environmental variations, such as climate and weather, diet, and language spoken by a group of people can influence articulatory and even anatomic aspects of speech production. Buretić-Tomljanović et al. (2007) reported data showing that body height and craniofacial features may be associated with geographic, climatic, or dietary distribution, or with the variability of different climatic characteristics. Variations in craniofacial features could have an influence on vocal tract anatomy. Everett et al. (2015) found that data on vocal fold physiology predicts that climatic factors constrain the use of phonemic tone, supposedly because aridity places pressures on vocal fold function. Similarly, Everett (2017) concluded that languages in arid regions use fewer vowels than languages in more humid regions.

Cultural and Linguistic Diversity

Cultural and linguistic diversity is a rapidly changing landscape, with new information disseminated through publications, workshops, and online resources. Sensitivity to cultural and linguistic diversity is apparent in several domains, including educational programs, research funding, clinical services, and advocacy. The American Speech-Language-Hearing Association has developed advocacy and informational materials on several topics, including:

1. Issues in Ethics: Cultural and Linguistic Competence (https://www.asha.org/practice/ethics/cultural-and-linguistic-competence/)
2. Accent Modification (https://www.asha.org/practice-portal/professional-issues/accent-modification/)
3. Bilingual Service Delivery (https://www.asha.org/practice-portal/professional-issues/bilingual-service-delivery/)
4. Cultural responsiveness (https://www.asha.org/practice-portal/professional-issues/cultural-responsiveness/)

Another valuable resource is a report of the Multilingual and Multicultural Affairs Committee of the International Association of Communication Sciences and Disorders (Scharff Rethfeldt et al., 2020)

Standardized testing can have undesired consequences when used with cultural and linguistic groups for whom the tests are not suited. Standardized tests are typically normed with a majority population and may not represent other groups, even relatively large ones, by population. Nair et al. (2023) discuss how standardized testing often resides in a medical model of disability that can pathologize cultural and linguistic variations.

Conclusions

1. Spoken language is a multifaceted phenomenon shaped by age, gender, linguistic background, social networks, and other factors. The speech of an individual speaker may reflect influences of a dialect, sociolect, and idiolect. These influences add distinctiveness and group membership to speech patterns.
2. The diagnostic triad of disorder, delay, and difference is important in clinical services, but the word *difference* may carry negative connotations. Terminology is in flux and may well be revised in the future. But the basic issue is that influences of a native language may affect a second language in ways that can be confused with presence of disorder or delay.
3. The critical period of language acquisition for either L1 or L2 appears not to be simply open-and-shut, but rather variably open with maximum plasticity between the ages of about one year to puberty. Besides neural maturation, the critical period is affected by attentional processes and the information structure available to the individual. There may not be a single critical period but several different critical periods that pertain to different aspects of language.
4. Bilingualism is increasingly important in speech-language pathology. Learning a second language may

involve creation of an interlanguage that shares properties of both L1 and L2, along with other features that may not be part of either of those languages.

5. Bilingualism in itself does not appear to put children at risk for speech disorders, but bilingualism combined with other risk factors (e.g., comorbidity and male gender) may present some degree of risk.
6. Dialect, a form of a language specific to a particular geographical region or a group of people, includes accent as one component but encompasses other factors as well. Dialect modification should be undertaken with full consideration of potential consequences, including those that may be harmful to an individual's self-esteem or social setting.
7. Contrastive analysis is one step in understanding the relationships between a native and second language, but it may fail to identify some important differences.
8. The constructs of race and ethnicity are losing favor, at least in some circles, and are being replaced by the construct of genetic ancestry. But contemporary literature shows that ancestry itself is controversial.

11

CLINICAL POPULATIONS AND CONDITIONS

This chapter considers specific clinical populations and conditions in which speech disorders often occur. Because the nature of the speech disorder is rooted in part in the characteristics of the clinical condition, each condition is summarized as it relates to problems in speech production and other aspects of communication. Speech disorders are secondary to, or comorbid with, a variety of pathologies, and this chapter gives a selective discussion of disorders and conditions that are likely to be encountered by speech-language pathologists.

Etiologies: Functional, Organic, and Multifactorial

The three broad etiological classes of speech disorders are **functional**, **organic**, and **multifactorial** (or complex), as shown in Figure 11–1. According to the American Speech-Language-Hearing Association (n.d.) "Speech sound disorders can be **organic** or **functional** in nature. Organic speech sound disorders result from an underlying motor/neurological, structural, or sensory/perceptual (e.g., hearing loss) cause. Functional speech sound disorders are idiopathic—they have no known cause." In other words, a disorder is considered organic if a biological basis can be identified. If not, then it is functional (although it may be an organic disorder awaiting discovery of its pathophysiological basis). As research continues to find genetic contributions to many different disorders, it would not be surprising if a disorder that is now regarded as functional is ultimately reclassified as having at least a partially organic basis. A multifactorial or complex disorder, from the perspective of genetics, results from the contributions of multiple genomic variants and genes in combination with the influences of the physical and social environment. Communication disorders that have been considered to have a multifactorial basis include developmental language disorder (Mountford et al., 2022), stuttering (Smith & Weber, 2017), and voice disorders (Altman et al., 2005). This list is likely to grow.

The terms *functional* and *organic* have longstanding presence in medicine, but they are coming under question as

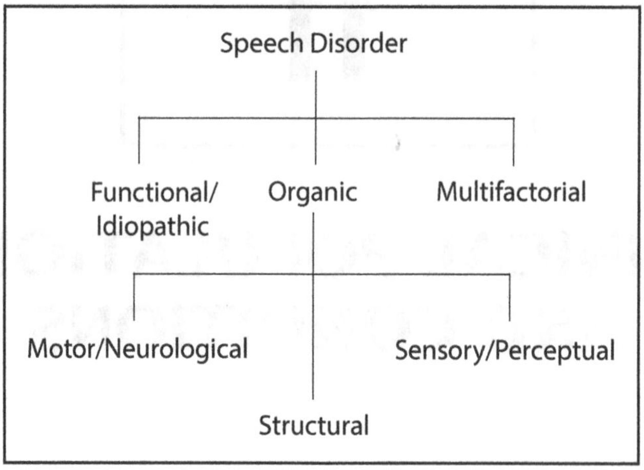

Figure 11–1. Three broad etiologic classifications of speech disorders in children.

to their validity and value in specialties such as neurology and psychiatry. Bell et al. (2020) comment that the distinction between these terms often rests on an implied model of "zero sum" causality, which invites classification of syndromes into discrete and dichotomous categories of organic versus functional. Such a view is not consistent with the contemporary understanding of neuropsychiatric disorders as resulting from a dynamic interaction between personal, social, and neuropathological factors. Bell et al. wrote, "the interaction between neurocognitive capacity, perception, affect, action, and context is perhaps one of the central assumptions of the neurocognitive sciences" (p. 6). This statement applies to many communication disorders, including some of the speech disorders covered in this book. Even when a frank organic etiology is identified (as in the case of a craniofacial anomaly such as cleft palate), the effects on communication often must be understood in a larger constellation of personal and social factors. Organic disorders may very well have a functional overlay, so that organic and functional factors interact.

How then should functional disorder be defined and used? Little is gained by defining functional as synonymous with idiopathic. If the intent of a diagnosis is to say that no cause is evident, then it simply should be called idiopathic (although this term may be meaningless to many in the lay public, so that preference may be given to a plain language version such as, "unknown cause" or "we do not know"). The word *functional* has currency in the field of neurology. A **functional neurological disorder (FND)** is a medical condition in which there is a problem with "the functioning of the nervous system and how the brain and body sends and/or receives signals, rather than a structural disease process such as multiple sclerosis or stroke" (National Organization for Rare Disorders). According to Duffy (2016) and Maurer and Duffy (2022), functional speech and voice disorders are defined as acquired psychogenic or functional disorders that are a subtype of functional neurologic disorders or functional movement disorders. The authors also note that functional disorders can be challenging to diagnose. If the term functional disorder in relation to speech disorders in children is retained, it should denote disorders related to environment or experience (e.g., limited exposure to language and limited stimulation to speak), or specific learning difficulties.

The main etiologic categories of organic disorders are motor/neurological (e.g., dysarthria and apraxia), structural (e.g., congenital anomaly or trauma), and sensory/perceptual (e.g., hearing loss). This tripartite conception does not readily accommodate evidence pointing to genetic, metabolic, or hormonal factors that can predispose to a disorder or lead directly to a disorder. Multifactorial etiology is likely to be increasingly recognized in communication disorders, but it does not always yield a simple understanding of a disorder. Multiple interacting factors can make it difficult to identify the optimal timing, goal, and method of intervention. In addition, communications disorders are often comorbid with other childhood conditions (Pinborough-Zimmerman et al., 2007).

Genetics and Genomics

Substantial progress has been made in identifying the genetic pathways that underlie speech disorders. The literature is too vast to be reviewed in this chapter, but highlights of important discoveries are noted. Important points of progress are the identification of (1) chromosomal anomalies that usually arise from alterations in the DNA containing chromosomal regions identified by karyotype analysis, and (2) multifactorial disorders that often involve multiple genes and environmental interactions. A seminal paper by Fisher et al. (1998) identified the genetic basis for the speech and language disorder in the KE family, a large three-generation pedigree in which this disorder is common. The phenotype affects nearly all aspects of speech and language. The effects on speech include severe orofacial dyspraxia and reduced intelligibility. The genome-wide search for linkage in this family conducted by Fisher et al. (1998) revealed the genetic origin on a region on chromosome 7, which is responsible for the autosomal dominant monogenic trait. Many subsequent reports have confirmed and extended this work to establish the genetic and genomic bases of speech and language disorders. A notable advance was the identification of the FOXP2 gene, a forkhead gene mutated in both the KE family and an individual known as CS (Lai et al., 2001). These discoveries stimulated excitement in the popular media, which heralded the idea of a "language gene."

The current view is that the genetic basis of language most likely involves multiple genes in a complex architecture. FOXP2 is relevant especially because it is a transcription factor, that is, a protein that binds to and controls genetic information within cells, thereby regulating expression of other genes. However, many different genes are implicated in various speech and language disorders (Hunter, 2019) and other neurodevelopmental conditions (Den Hoed & Fisher, 2020). Den Hoed and Fisher (2020, p. 103) note that "gene-driven studies show blurring of boundaries between diagnostic categories, with some risk genes shared across speech disorders, intellectual disability and autism." They pointed to the importance of regulatory genes that are co-expressed in early human brain development as playing a role in different neurodevelopmental disorders. Similarly, Guerra and Cacabelos (2019) commented that many speech and language disorders may reflect neurodevelopmental processes in which molecular mechanisms and pathways interact, so that these disorders may be comorbid with other disorders unrelated to communication. Kaspi et al. (2022), who proposed that some cases of CAS are a critical clinical indicator for single gene disorders, nonetheless wrote "our findings support the increasing overlap between genes conferring risk for a range of neurodevelopmental disorders including CAS, epilepsy, ASD and intellectual disability." (p. 16). As for CAS itself, studies indicate that regulatory genes in the embryonic brain have an important role (Eising et al., 2021), that a novel neural phenotype distinct from FOXP2 involves disruption of the dorsal language stream (Liégeois et al., 2019), that it is often a sporadic monogenic disorder that is highly genetically heterogeneous (Hildebrand et al., 2020), and that it may be explained in part by its effects on auditory-motor integration that could influence feedback and feedforward control of speech production (Zhang et al., 2018).

> "Indeed, the thinking now is that unravelling speech is essential for making progress on the greater challenge of language evolution, which is a highly complex phenotype that must involve multiple genes in combination with the development of motor vocalization skills. The evolution of vocalization and complex language must have proceeded in tandem generating interactive selective pressures for both domains." (Hunter, 2019, p. 3)

The genetic and genomic landscape is rapidly changing, and anything written here runs the risk of eventual, if not immediate, revision. It is a tall order for SLPs or many other clinical specialists to follow progress in this highly active area of research, but it is likely that genetic and genomic advances will have a profound effect on the understanding of many disorders of speech, language, and hearing. The summary discussion here is by no means exhaustive and is intended simply to point out the relevance of genetic and genomic studies to disorders commonly encountered by SLPs. Another helpful resource is the article by Patil et al. (2014) that summarizes chromosomal and multifactorial genetic disorders that have manifestations in oral structure and function.

Another strategy for phenotype identification is the use of **phecodes,** a high-throughput phenotyping tool based on ICD (International Classification of Diseases) codes that can achieve rapid determination of case/control status of thousands of clinically meaningful diseases and conditions (Bastarache, 2021). Phecodes were originally developed for phenome-wide association studies to scan for phenotypic associations with common genetic variants, but more recently they have been used to support a wide range of phenotyping methods using electronic health records (EHR) data, including the phenotype risk score. Pruett et al. (2021) found that highly enriched phecodes included codes related to childhood onset fluency disorder, adult-onset fluency disorder, hearing loss, sleep disorders, atopy, a multitude of codes for infections, neurological deficits, and body weight.

Risk Factors for Speech Disorders in Children

A **risk factor** is any condition, circumstance, or characteristic that increases the likelihood of developing or acquiring a disease or disorder. Table 11–1 summarizes studies of risk factors associated with children's speech disorders. The studies involve children from several different countries, including the U.S., Australia, China, India, Pakistan, Serbia, and Turkey. Accordingly, the identified risk factors may be universal and are not restricted to any one language or nation. In compiling the table, efforts were made to include studies that focused on speech disorders, but it was not always possible

Table 11–1. Risk Factors Identified for Speech Disorders in Several Studies

Risk Factor/Source	1	2	3	4	5	6	7	8	9	10	11	12	13	14
Caesarean section	X													
Congenital anomaly				X						X				X
Consanguinity				X										X
Hearing loss	X							X		X				
Inadequate stimulation				X		X						X		X
Low parental education		X	X	X	X	X								X
Maternal age >35 years						X								
Maternal health, medication	X													
Multilingual family environment	X			X										
Oral habits (sucking and pacifier use)							X		X	X	X		X	
Positive family history	X	X	X	X	X		X		X	X	X	X	X	
Prenatal or perinatal problems	X		X	X			X		X		X		X	X
Prenatal drug or alcohol exposure													X	
Screen exposure	X													
Seizure disorder				X										X
Sex (male)		X			X			X	X	X	X	X		
Socioeconomic status			X		X	X								
Temperament								X			X			

Sources: 1—Bogavac et al. (2019); 2—Campbell et al., (2003); 3—Çiçek et al. (2020); 4 -Delgado et al. (2005); 5—Eadie et al. (2015); 6—Fan et al. (2021); 7—Fox, Dodd, & Howard (2002); 8—Harrison & McLeod (2010); 9—Hoque et al. (2021); 10—Kumar et al. (2022); 11—Molini-Avejonas et al. (2017); 12—Mondal et al. (2016); 13—Silva et al. (2013); 14—Sunderajan & Kanhere (2019).

to exclude language disorders because of variations in participant recruitment and description. Among the most frequently reported risk factors are some that are relatively immutable (male sex, positive family history, consanguinity, and some congenital anomalies) and others that are potentially modifiable through appropriate intervention (low parental education, inadequate stimulation, hearing loss, oral habits, and pre- and peri-natal problems). Chapter 2 reviewed factors that appear to be associated with male sex as a risk factor for communication disorders. Further research is needed to show how risk factors interact. For example, it could be hypothesized that the risk of a speech disorder is amplified by the combination of male sex, positive family history, and inadequate stimulation. Some support for this hypothesis comes from studies such as that of Campbell et al. (2003), who found that a male child with positive family history and a mother with low education was 7.71 times as likely to have a speech delay as a child without any of these factors. Choo et al. (2020) concluded that bilingualism alone is not a risk factor for speech disorders, but it combined with male gender and comorbidity to constitute a risk.

Risk factors should be considered in designing prevention and treatment programs, as discussed in Chapter 12. Because some risk factors can be eliminated or moderated, attention to these factors may help in preventing a disorder or in facilitating treatment. When multiple risk factors are present, early intervention may be warranted to ensure the most favorable outcomes. It also can be helpful to identify protective factors that operate in a child's environment. A **protective factor** is a condition or attribute that reduces or buffers the effects of risk, stress, trauma, or other negative condition. Protective factors are strengths that mitigate the potential harm associated with risk. For example, Harrison and McLeod (2010) noted that protective factors included a child's temperament and maternal well-being. Discovery of protective factors could be an important asset to treatment planning.

Speech Biomarkers

According to the Biomarker Working Group (U.S. Food and Drug Administration, & National Institutes of Health, 2016), a **biomarker** is "a characteristic that is measured as an indicator of normal biological processes, pathogenic processes or responses to an exposure or intervention." A digital biomarker is defined as "a characteristic or set of characteristics, collected from digital health technologies that is measured as an indicator of normal biological processes, pathogenic processes, or responses to an exposure or intervention, including therapeutic interventions" (U.S. Food and Drug Administration, 2020). Speech has been investigated as a biomarker primarily because the speech signal may give insights into neural processes and because aspects of speech may assist in the diagnosis of types of speech disorders.

Robin et al. (2020, p. 99) commented, "Speech represents a promising novel biomarker by providing a window into brain health, as shown by its disruption in various neurological and psychiatric diseases." They note that valuation steps for speech-based digital biomarkers can be based on the recent V3 framework (Goldsack et al., 2020). The V3 framework consists of three components of evaluation for digital biomarkers: verification, analytical validation, and clinical validation. Verification pertains primarily to the suitability and integrity of speech recordings, including assessment of the quality of speech recordings and determining the effects of hardware and recording conditions. Analytical validation includes confirming the accuracy and reliability of data processing and computed measures, with consideration of test-retest reliability, demographic variability, and comparison of measures to reference standards. Clinical validity is chiefly concerned with verifying the correspondence of a measure to clinical outcomes, such as diagnosis, disease progression, or response to treatment. A Work Group on Neuroimaging Markers of Psychiatric Disorders (Botteron et al., 2012) proposed that a promising biomarker should have two or more independent well-powered studies providing evidence of sensitivity and specificity at least of 80%.

Ramanarayanan et al. (2022) review progress in the development of speech biomarkers and discuss examples of application to specific speech disorders, mainly in adults. Biomarkers for children's speech have been proposed for CAS (Chenausky et al., 2020; Peter et al., 2018; Shriberg et al., 2003; Shriberg et al., 2017). These are discussed in the section on CAS. Cortese et al. (2023) describe potential biomarkers for neurodevelopmental disorders in children, with a focus on neuroimaging data.

Speech Disorders in Children

This section provides an overview of conditions and clinical populations in which speech disorders are either defining characteristics or are frequently observed. For each condition or population, the summary includes a basic description along with a summary of the associated speech disorder. The first item is speech sound disorders, which accounts for most of the speech disorders in children. The remaining clinical populations are listed alphabetically. Some of the included clinical conditions are primary causes of speech disorders, but two or more can occur in combination to contribute to the full expression of a speech disorder. For example, a child may have both a hearing loss and a malocclusion that may be involved in a speech sound disorder.

Speech Sound Disorders (SSD)

This term subsumes the categories of articulation and phonological disorders. As noted in Chapter 1, the distinction between these two is not always clear, which is why some authors bundle them into a single category of either articulation/phonological disorders (APD), phonological/articulatory disorders (PAD), or speech sound disorders (SSD). The latter term is used here, despite some definitional problems discussed in Chapter 1. SSD constitutes about 31% of the caseloads of pediatric speech-language pathologists in the United States (American Speech-Language-Hearing Association, 2021) and 92.6% of school-based clinicians work with children's speech sound production (American Speech-Language-Hearing Association, 2015). Therefore, these disorders are of high clinical significance. Ireland et al. (2020) review evaluation and eligibility requirements for children with speech sound disorders in the United States based on federal requirements, state and local requirements and guidance, other sources of guidance such as professional associations, and research. McLeod and McCormack (2007) discuss the application of the ICF and ICF-children and youth for children with speech disorders, emphasizing the importance of recognizing not only Body Functions but also Activities and Participation, Environmental and Personal Factors to design a holistic treatment.

According to the *Diagnostic and Statistical Manual of Mental Disorders* (5th ed., *DSM–5*, American Psychiatric Association, 2013; First, 2014), there are four criteria for Speech Sound Disorder (previously known as Phonological Disorder):

1. Persistent unintelligible speech consisting of phoneme addition, omission, distortion, or substitution, which interferes with verbal communication.
2. Interference with social participation, academic performance, or occupational performance (or any combination thereof).
3. Symptom onset is during childhood.
4. Symptoms cannot be accounted for by another medical or neurological condition, including TBI (Traumatic Brain Injury).

The *DSM-5* criteria are highly oriented to speech segments such as phonemes and do not mention problems in other domains of speech production, such as voice or prosody. The web site of the Royal College of Speech and Language Therapists asserts that, "Speech sound disorders is a term used to cover difficulties that some children have with their articulation, phonological and/or prosodic development" (https://www.rcslt.org/speech-and-language-therapy/clinical-information/speech-sound-disorders/). This definition accords with the definition of speech sound given in Chapter 1: A speech sound is a unit in the acoustic signal of speech, with the duration of the unit ranging from a phonetic segment to a larger prosodic unit, depending on the purpose of the analysis.

As mentioned briefly in Chapter 1, different classification systems have been developed for speech sound disorders in children. Several of these systems are summarized in the following.

1. The psycholinguistic framework of Stackhouse and Wells (1997) was developed not so much as a classification system but rather as a means of profiling the disorder in individual children. It is based on a developmental model that considers abilities (input, representation, and output) with respect to phases of development (prelexical, whole word, systematic simplification, assembly, and metaphonological).
2. Dodd's Model for Differential Diagnosis (MDD; Dodd, 2014; Ttofari Eecen et al., 2019) is based on a descriptive-linguistic approach and consists of three major types and associated subtypes: phonetic (subtype: articulation disorder); phonemic (subtypes: phonological delay, consistent atypical phonological disorder, inconsistent atypical phonological disorder, and motor planning, programming, and execution (subtype: CAS). Geytenbeek (2019) remarked that this classification system is theory-driven and has strong construct validity.
3. Speech Disorders Classification System (SDCS; Shriberg et al., 2010) is based on the behavioral

phenotype of a child's speech and etiological background. The SDSC recognizes several subtypes of SSD classified with respect to the four levels of etiological processes (distal causes), speech processes (proximal causes), clinical typology (behavioral phenotypes), and diagnostic markers (critical signs of phenotype). It is illustrated in Figure 11–2.

4. Articulatory phonology approach (Namasivayam et al., 2020) advocates the description and analysis of SSD based on articulatory phonology (called gestural phonology in Chapter 7). Articulatory phonology discards the traditional phonology-phonetics interface and proposes that gestures are the basic elements common to both types of description. Namasivayam et al. explain speech sound errors in terms of the development, maturation, and combinatorial dynamics of articulatory gestures. They note that many speech sound errors could reflect compensatory strategies to enhance the stability of the speech motor system. Examples of these strategies are as follows: decreasing speech rate; increasing movement amplitude; bracing; intrusion gestures; cluster reductions; deleting segments, gestures, or syllables; and increasing lag between articulators. The authors also suggest that children with SSDs are at the low end of the continuum of speech motor skill and that the differences between the subtypes of SSD could result from different strategies to cope with motor skill deficiencies.
5. Process-oriented profiling (Diepeveen et al., 2022) resulted from a study of 4- to 7-year-old Dutch children with SSD using a broad test battery analysis. Cluster analysis revealed three subgroups that differed significantly on intelligibility, receptive vocabulary, and auditory discrimination but not on age, gender and SLPs diagnosis. These clusters identify three

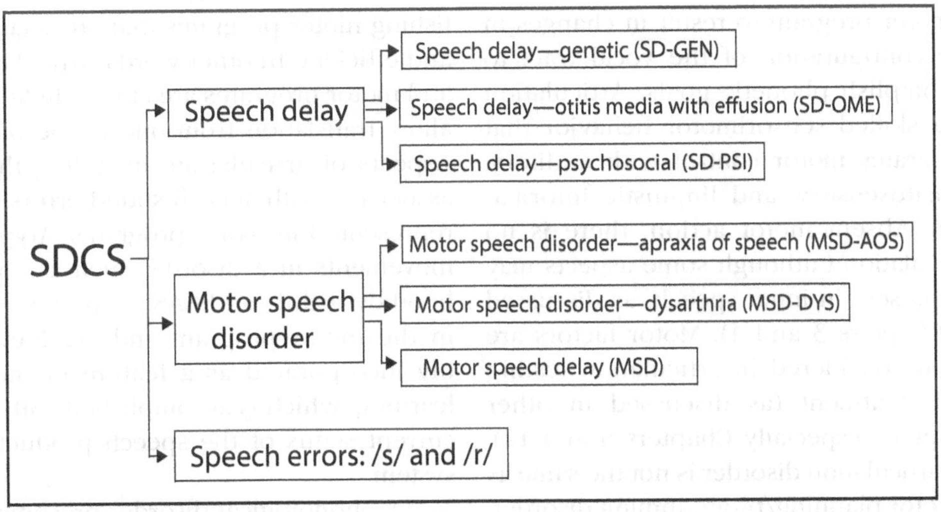

Figure 11–2. The Speech Disorders Classification System (SDCS; Shriberg et al., 2010).

specific profiles: (1) phonological deficit; (2) phonological deficit with motoric deficit; (3) severe phonological and motoric deficit. The authors concluded the different profiles of SSD reflect a spectrum of degrees of involvement of different underlying problems.

Because identification of subgroups of children with SSD can hold implications for assessment and treatment, as well as the fundamental understanding of the disorder, it is important to delineate and compare the characteristics of proposed subgroups. Waring and Knight (2013) noted that the first three classification systems listed above have in common a recognition of three subgroups of disorder: articulation-based, motor planning/programming, and phonological (characterized primarily by simplification processes). The following discussion considers possible subgroups in more detail, using the categories proposed by Waring and Knight (2013).

Articulation-based disorder implies errors at the articulatory level. Articulation can be defined as the execution of a motor program to result in changes in the configuration of the vocal tract to accomplish phonetic goals. Articulation is a skilled sensorimotor behavior that integrates motor control with auditory, somatosensory, and linguistic information. Absent motor action, there is no articulation (although some aspects may be present in inner speech, as discussed in Chapters 3 and 4). Motor factors are often considered in articulation testing and treatment (as discussed in other chapters, especially Chapters 5 and 12). An articulation disorder is not the same as a motor planning/programming disorder, but principles of motor learning (Chapter 9) may still apply, and motor factors are often considered in the assessment and treatment of speech sound disorders and in training for accent modification. For example, McAuliffe and Cornwell (2008) applied principles of motor learning in treatment of a lateralized /s/.

Motor planning/programming disorder is not easily defined but most discussions center on problems in the selection and sequencing of units of some kind (e.g., phonemes, phonetic segments, articulatory gestures). The plan or program is a relatively abstract level that can be translated to articulatory actions but does not in itself fully specify these actions. The usual assumption is that performance of a motor plan or program is accomplished by further processing of motor control operations to determine the details of articulatory movements (as discussed in Chapter 3). For convenience and simplicity, the following discussion uses the term motor program to include both planning and programming aspects. Motor programs are established through experience and practice, which means that the performance of articulatory movements is one factor in establishing motor programs that are accurate and efficient. In other words, articulation and motor programs are closely linked to allow translation from one to the other. Aspects of articulation, including those associated with speech sound errors, are represented in motor programs. Atypical movements in a disorder such as childhood dysarthria and CAS are represented in the motor program and are inevitably incorporated as a feature of motor learning, which is accomplished with the current status of the speech production system.

A phonological disorder presumably excludes explanations at the articulatory or motor programming levels. An example often given of a phonological error is simplification (discussed in Chapter 7). However, phonology has a motor component in that phonological patterns are rooted in part on motor or physiological factors that are often invoked to explain limitations in speech production. Some examples of motor factors in individual phonological patterns are as follows. Final consonant devoicing is linked to a physiological process in which the vocal folds tend to abduct, and subglottal air pressure typically declines at the end of an utterance. This effect applies to all syllable-final consonants, which invites the interpretation that it is a property of phonology in which classes of sounds are affected similarly, but the underlying principles lie in speech physiology and motor control. Weak syllable deletion reflects a limitation of speech motor control (and perhaps auditory temporal processing) that hinders production of brief elements in a motor sequence. Similarly, consonant cluster reduction could result from motoric limitations in the sequencing of articulatory movements. Stopping could result from a difficulty in producing fricative sounds that require precise articulation to generate an interval of turbulent noise. These examples show that an abstract phonological process, such as final consonant devoicing, may be explained at the level of speech production and perception. That is, final consonant devoicing happens for a reason, and the reason is found in the physiology of speech production. As mentioned in Chapter 7, physiological factors are implicit in Stampe's theory of natural phonology.

The concept of simplification as the basis for phonological processes needs to be examined to ensure that it is not simply reification (i.e., a process in which an abstract notion is considered a concrete object or event). McReynolds and Elbert (1981) commented on the need to establish reasonable quantitative and qualitative criteria for the identification of phonological processes to distinguish them from surface forms. Adherence to such criteria is rare. To make simplification more than a name, it is necessary to describe its nature. A common approach is to assume that a child's speech patterns are the result of constraints or filters that reduce the adult target to a form that is within the sensory and motor capabilities of a child. Constraints and filters as a means of suppression are usually passive in nature. An alternative view is that a child is a constructive agent who is deliberate and intentional in learning to speak, taking advantage of available resources. The general study of motor development for behaviors such as locomotion, reaching, and grasping rarely appeals to the concept of simplification to explain why motor patterns change over time. A more productive approach has been dynamic systems theory, which considers the developmental status of the child with respect to properties such as size or mass, muscle strength, and muscle synergies. According to this view, the child is a builder and not a suppressor. Namasivayam et al. (2020) discuss the possibility that apparent simplifications such as cluster reduction are the consequence of attempts to establish motor stability.

The intent of these statements is not to deny a level of phonology in speech production, but rather to say that phonology in many respects has a phonetic or motor foundation. In this vein, Ohala (1990) wrote that "phonology and phonetics are not mutually autonomous or independent whether as parts of the speech universe or as disciplines" (p. 154). The lack of autonomy applies to the learning of speech production, so that atypical motor patterns inevitably influence phonological representation, however that representation is established. A difficulty is that the term *motor disorder* in respect to speech disorders often is taken to mean dysarthria, childhood apraxia of speech, and perhaps speech motor delay. However, more subtle motor disorders may result in faulty or inefficient motor learning. Moreover, principles of motor learning may have a general application to both disorders and differences that come to the attention of a speech-language pathologist. As discussed in Chapter 9, principles of motor learning are applied to a variety of speech disorders and can be used in connection with different treatments.

To be sure, description of phonological processes may hold clinical value. Miccio and Scarpino (2008) note that describing errors as phonological processes satisfies a need to recognize multiple errors. They also noted that phonological assessments used in clinical practice have varying numbers of processes used to describe children's speech patterns. This lack of uniformity is bothersome and reinforces the need to establish qualitative and quantitative criteria for identification of processes. It should also be recognized that phonological processes are not the only means of recognizing and categorizing multiple errors, as this goal can be achieved by sensory and motor considerations, as described earlier in this section. Many phonological processes are rooted in the physiology of speech production. Process analysis may yield important insights. For example, Dodd (2011) described atypical phonological processes that could be used to identify children with disordered, as opposed to delayed, speech development. The atypical processes (those not observed at any stage in typically developing children) included: backing of bilabial and palatal stops, word or syllable initial consonant deletion, substitution of stops by fricatives, clusters marked by bilabial fricatives, vowel errors, pervasive sound preferences, intrusive vowels, and extensive assimilation. It has been suggested that atypical speech sound errors reflect problems at a linguistic representational level, and these errors may reveal how phonological information is organized or represented (Dodd et al., 1989; Preston & Edwards, 2010). Waring et al. (2022) noted that phonological development is influenced by several domain-general cognitive processes, including phonological working memory, ability to revise faulty underlying representations, rule abstraction, and cognitive shift.

Children with SSD exhibit substantial heterogeneity. For example, Tambyraja et al. (2023) concluded from a study of 157 school-aged children receiving school-based speech therapy that the children had a range of phonological processing difficulties, particularly on the measure of verbal short-term memory. Although no specific skill differentiated children with and without reading difficulties, the children classified as poor readers on the word-decoding measure had more widespread difficulties, even when language ability was controlled.

Adenotonsillar Hypertrophy

Adenotonsillar hypertrophy is enlargement of the lymphoid tissue in the pharynx, including both the palatine tonsils and the pharyngeal tonsil (adenoid), usually resulting from viral or bacterial infections, allergies, or exposure to chemicals or other agents. As discussed in Chapter 2, the velopharyngeal anatomy undergoes changes in early childhood as age-related lymphoid hypertrophy increases the likelihood of a restricted airway, especially during the age period of 3 to 5 years. Diseases and other conditions can exacerbate the condition, with adenotonsillar hypertrophy potentially affecting sleep breathing, swallowing, mastication, and speech. Serious enlargement may limit movements of the tongue and interfere with normal velopharyngeal valving needed for nasal and non-nasal sound contrasts. Gargano et al. (2022) reported that 40% of the children with adenotonsillar hypertrophy in their study had phonetic-articulatory disorders, with 75% having interdental sigmatism (frontal lisp) and all children having hyporrinophony (altered oral-nasal resonance).

Scales have been developed for visual examination of the supralaryngeal airway, with the two most common scores being the Mallampati (Mallampati, 1983) and Friedman (Friedman et al., 2002). Mallampati scoring is divided into four classes based on the visibility of the base of the uvula, faucial pillars, and soft palate: class 1, full visibility of all three structures; class 2, visibility of hard and soft palate, upper portion of tonsils and uvula; class 3, visibility of soft and hard palate and base of the uvula; and class 4, visibility of hard palate only. Friedman classification evaluates tonsillar size, with scores divided into 4 classes: grade 1+, the tonsils are hidden within the tonsillar pillars; grade 2+, the tonsils extend to the tonsillar pillars; grade 3+, the tonsils extend beyond the pillars but do not reach the midline; and grade 4+, the tonsils extend to, or beyond, the midline.

Surgical remedy is either total tonsillectomy or intracapsular tonsilltomy (partial tonsillectomy). The effectiveness of such surgery for speech problems has been reported in several studies (Abdel-Aziz et al., 2019; Lundeborg et al., 2011; Maryn et al., 2004). However, a rare complication of such surgery is altered speech, especially nasal resonance (Maryn et al., 2004; Stewart et al., 2002; Witzel et al., 1986), which may require palatoplasty and/or speech therapy.

Ankyloglossia (Tongue Tie)

The anatomic feature of ankyloglossia (*ankylo-* meaning bent, hooked, fused, fixed, or closed; *glossia* meaning tongue) mentioned and illustrated in Chapter 2, is a condition in which the tip of the tongue is tethered to the floor of the mouth. If in fact the tongue tip is anchored in such a way that it does not move freely for purposes of speech articulation or other oral behaviors such as swallowing, this condition is of concern to speech-language pathologists and other specialists. Among the possible consequences of ankyloglossia are difficulties with breastfeeding, including poor latch, maternal nipple pain, mastitis, poor weight gain and early unnecessary weaning. Accordingly, ankyloglossia has been of particular interest to physicians and lactation consultants.

The literature on ankyloglossia does not yield an entirely clear picture on prevalence, functional effects, or treatment outcomes. Prevalence data are highly variable, ranging from 0.3% (Çetinkaya et al., 2011) to 16% (Ngerncham et al., 2013). In a systematic review and meta-analysis, Hill et al. (2021) concluded that the overall prevalence of tongue-tie was 8% (95% CI 6–10%, $p < 0.01$), with a prevalence of 7% in males and 4% in females. Prevalence was greater with a standardized assessment tool compared to visual examination alone. Hill et al. (2021) noted that the assessment tools currently available do not have adequate psychometric properties. Similarly, Segal et al. (2007) concluded that there is no well-validated clinical method to diagnose ankyloglossia, and Walsh and Tunkel (2017) commented that available evidence is insufficient to formulate definitive practice guidelines. Katz et al. (2020) conducted a Delphi study to formulate a definition of ankyloglossia. The result recognizes two separate pathways for identifying a newborn with this condition. One pathway is based on a single pathognomonic anatomic feature, while the other specifies a single functional deficit that is accompanied by at least 2 of 12 other diagnostic items (functional, anatomic, or behavioral). A surgical remedy for ankyloglossia is **tongue-tie division** or **frenotomy**. Available evidence indicates that frenotomy is effective in reducing breastfeeding difficulties and nipple pain at least in the short term (Bruney et al., 2022; O'Shea et al., 2017; Webb et al., 2013). Fortunately, complications or negative outcomes appear to be rare.

The effects of ankyloglossia on speech production are unclear. A systematic review (Webb et al., 2013) reported on the efficacy of tongue-tie division for breastfeeding problems but was inconclusive regarding speech articulation. In a clinical consensus statement, Messner et al. (2020) concluded that ankyloglossia typically does not affect speech, and they commented that even speech sounds with substantial tongue elevation, /l/ and /r/, and protrusion, /ð/ and /θ/, generally can be produced in the presence of significant tongue tip restriction. Salt et al. (2020) found little evidence that tongue tie affects speech articulation in children. However, Baxter et al. (2020) reported that after tongue-tie releases paired with exercises, the majority of 37 children in their study had functional improvements in speech, feeding, and sleep. Wang et al. (2022) concluded from a systematic review that the quality of evidence was generally low and that there was no clear connection between ankyloglossia and speech disorders. Zhao et al. (2022) concluded from a randomized trial that for children aged 2 to <3 years of age, there were no statistically significant differences between surgical intervention and no surgical intervention groups for tongue appearance, tongue mobility, speech production, and intelligibility. However, for children in the groups of 3 to <4 and 4 to <5 years, the surgical intervention group showed significant improvements in speech production and intelligibility compared to the no surgical intervention group. The authors concluded that the optimal timing range for surgical intervention is 4 to 5 years.

Similar controversy applies to the superior labial frenulum (also known as the maxillary labial frenulum), which attaches the upper lip to the anterior surface of the maxillary gingiva. In a study of 100 newborns, Santa Maria et al. (2018) reported that some degree of superior labial frenula attachment was present in all babies. The authors noted that the Kotlow grading scale of attachment had poor intra- and interrater reliability. It was concluded that, "Given the lack of knowledge surrounding the function of the upper frenulum, the ubiquity of its presence, and level of attachment in most infants, the release of the superior labial frenulum based on appearance alone cannot be endorsed at this time" (p. 5).

Attention Deficit/ Hyperactivity Disorder (ADHD)

Attention-deficit/hyperactivity disorder (ADHD) is among the most common neurobehavioral problems in children between 6 and 17 years of age. It has an estimated prevalence of 11% of children and almost 5% of adults in the U.S. (CDC, 2017). ADHD is recognized as a heritable, chronic, neurobehavioral disorder characterized by hyperactivity, inattention, and impulsivity. It has three main subtypes: predominantly hyperactive impulsive, predominantly inattentive, and a combination of the first two subtypes. Etiology is not well understood, but studies indicate that the primary areas showing deficits include the prefrontal cortex, caudate, and cerebellum, which form a neural network that regulates attention, thoughts, emotions, behavior, and actions (Sharma & Couture, 2014). Both pharmacologic and nonpharmacologic treatments have been developed (Sharma & Couture, 2014; Zecker, 2004). Medications approved by the Food and Drug Administration (FDA) comprise stimulants (amphetamines and methylphenidate) and nonstimulants (atomoxetine and extended-release clonidine and guanfacine) (Cortese, 2020; Sharma & Couture, 2014). Behavioral interventions include video games (Penuelas-Calvo et al., 2020). The Food and Drug Administration (FDA) approved a game-based digital therapeutic device (EndeavorRx) to treat ADHD in the pediatric age group of 8 to 12 years of age, especially for the inattentive or combined-types of ADHD in children with an attention issue. As noted by Pandian et al. (2021), this is the first game-based therapeutic device to gain approval by the FDA for any type of condition.

Disorders of speech and/or language are not among the factors needed for a diagnosis of ADHD, but research has shown a high prevalence of communication disorders among children with ADHD (Al-Dakroury, 2018). Although language impairment has been emphasized as an associated or comorbid communication disorder (Lewis et al., 2012), there are indications that speech disorders should also be recognized. ADHD has been associated with difficulties in auditory processing of speech and nonspeech signals (Blomberg et al., 2019; Jafari et al., 2015), speech production assessed by correct syllables per second and overall speech rate (Etter et al., 2021), speech problems at age 9 years (Cervin, 2022), vocal hyperfunction (Barona-Lleo & Fernandez, 2016), and stuttering (Healey & Reid, 2003). McGrath et al., (2008) found that individuals with both speech sound disorders and language impairment had increased rates of ADHD symptomatology compared to individuals with language impairment only.

Autism Spectrum Disorder (ASD)

ASD is a group of neurological and developmental disorders with an onset in childhood and persisting throughout life. According to the *DSM-5*, people with ASD have (1) difficulty with communication and interaction with other people, (2) restricted interests and repetitive behaviors, and (3) symptoms that hurt the person's ability to function properly in school, work, and other areas of life. The Centers for Disease Control and Prevention estimated that autism affects 1 in 59 children in the United States. The Autism and Developmental Disabilities

Monitoring Network 2016 (Maenner et al., 2020) reported an ASD prevalence of 18.5 per 1,000 (one in 54) children aged 8 years, and ASD was 4.3 times as prevalent among boys as among girls. ASD includes conditions formerly known as Asperger's syndrome, childhood disintegrative disorder, and pervasive developmental disorders. The severity of the disorder varies greatly, and many reports distinguish between high- and low-functioning individuals with ASD. Etiology is heterogeneous, and studies indicate an increased offspring vulnerability to ASD through advanced maternal and paternal age, valproate intake, toxic chemical exposure, maternal diabetes, enhanced steroidogenic activity, immune activation, and possibly altered zinc–copper cycles, and treatment with selective serotonin reuptake inhibitors (Bölte et al., 2019). The relative contribution of genetic versus environmental factors is uncertain but results from a study of twins indicated that genetic factors had a consistently larger role than environmental factors (Taylor et al., 2020). This finding means that environmental factors are unlikely to explain the apparent increase in the prevalence of ASD.

According to Mody and Belliveau (2013),

> A failure to develop language is one of the earliest signs of autism. The ability to identify the neural signature of this deficit in very young children has become increasingly important, given that the presence of speech before five years of age is the strongest predictor for better outcomes in autism. (p. 157)

Gillon et al. (2017) reported survey results from SLPs indicating that the typical age at diagnosis of ASD is 3 to 4 years of age across most countries. This age of diagnosis delays early intervention, which motivates efforts to identify earlier signs and symptoms of the disorder. Progress in identifying behavior and neuroimaging biomarkers of ASD is summarized by Hiremath et al. (2021).

Speech characteristics of ASD are not always easily distinguished from co-occurring problems with language or cognition. Furthermore, it is not always easy to identify individuals with ASD from perceptual judgments of their speech samples (Dahlgren et al., 2018). The discussion in this chapter focuses on speech, voice, and prosody to the degree that they can be isolated from other features. Mounting evidence indicates that infants at risk for ASD exhibit atypical characteristics in the early stages of vocal development. Studies of infants have focused on babbling, especially volubility and characteristics of canonical babble (see Chapter 4 for definitions and reviews of typical development). Low volubility, delay in emergence of canonical babble, and/or low rates of canonical babble have been reported in infants at risk for ASD (Chenausky et al., 2017; Patten et al., 2014; Plate et al., 2022; Yankowitz et al., 2022). However, other studies failed to find clear and consistent differences in babbling between infants at risk for ASD and typically developing infants (Garrido et al., 2017). The safest conclusion is that infant vocalizations should be considered in a larger developmental context and should not be regarded as sufficient in themselves to diagnose ASD. Aside from the possible value of early vocalizations in diagnosing ASD, these behaviors are important in characterizing the natural history of the communication disorder. For example, limitations in babbling could be an early manifestation of a speech disorder.

Atypical vocalizations may be a general indication of neurodevelopmental disorders and, therefore, should be recognized in strategies of early detection and intervention.

Atypical features of speech observed in some children with ASD during the toddler and preschool years include reduced verbal output (Moffit et al., 2022), delayed phonological development and atypical phonological processes (Wolk & Brennan, 2013), speech sound disorders (reviewed in Broom et al., 2017), ratio of syllabic versus nonsyllabic vocalizations (Tenenbaum et al., 2020), vocal stereotypy (D. Wang et al., 2020), and atypical prosody (Schoen et al., 2011). Atypical prosody has long been recognized as a feature of ASD (Baltaxe & Simmons, 1985), but descriptions are inconsistent (McCann & Peppé, 2003). A likely source of the discrepancies is variability in methodology and the difficulty of using any given tool across ages and severity of the communication disorder in ASD. Auditory-perceptual methods have been predominant, but acoustic methods also have been used in a few studies. Research has established that atypical prosody appears in infants and toddlers (Schoen et al., 2011) and school-aged children (Nakai et al., 2014). Several studies reported flat or monotonous intonation, restricted use of pitch and volume, abnormal vocal quality, and atypical stress patterns (Nakai et al., 2014; Rapin & Dunn, 2003; Shriberg et al., 2001; Tager-Flusberg, 1981). These studies point to a general prosodic insufficiency. However, contrary descriptions have been reported in many other studies showing that individuals with ASD have high pitch values, large pitch ranges, and high pitch variability (Asghari et al., 2021; Diehl & Paul, 2013; Lyakso et al., 2021; Sharda et al., 2010). These results are consistent with a general description of prosodic excess. It is possible that atypical prosody in ASD can take different forms, with the most frequent pattern being one of exaggerated intonation on a foundation of high vocal pitch.

In a systematic review and meta-analysis, Asghari et al. (2021) concluded that a higher mean pitch, larger pitch range, high pitch variability and longer voice duration are the prosodic features that most reliably distinguish individuals with ASD from typically developing individuals. But a systematic review and meta-analysis concluded that no single feature serves as an acoustic marker of ASD, although relatively consistent findings have been reported on mean pitch and pitch range (Fusaroli et al., 2017). MacFarlane et al. (2022) differentiated children with and without autism using a combination of automated language measures and automated voice measures. The language measures were more effective for children with ASD who were younger, had lower language skills, and shorter activity time, whereas the voice measures were more effective for children with better language profiles. Cross-linguistic studies have potential to identify universal features of ASD. Examples of such features are rhythm (Lau et al., 2022), higher pitch and longer pauses (Fusaroli et al., 2022), and increased pitch variations (F. Chen et al., 2022). These features pertain to voice and prosody, which are prominent in descriptions of speech production in ASD.

High mean pitch and large pitch range are possibly parameter values of voice and prosody that serve as settings and boundaries for more refined measures of prosody, such as pitch contours and interactions of intensity, duration, and pitch. Why should mean pitch and pitch range be affected in ASD? At the basic physiological level, pitch is determined by the size of the laryngeal tissues, but there do not seem to be differences in laryngeal size between persons with or without ASD. Vocal pitch (or its physical correlate, fundamental frequency) is controlled mainly by two intrinsic laryngeal muscles, the cricothyroid and thyroarytenoid, both of which are innervated by laryngeal motor area in the primary motor cortex (M1). Among primates, cortical representation of vocalization is unique to humans. It has been proposed that the pitch features in ASD reflect those of infant-directed speech (also known as "motherese" or "parentese"), which typically has elevated pitch and exaggerated pitch contours (Sharda et al., 2010). According to this explanation, children with ASD incorporate aspects of infant-directed speech into their own vocalizations. However, this interpretation is contrary to reports that individuals with ASD, together with their first-degree relatives, exhibit reduced verbal entrainment and even disentrainment (Patel et al., 2022).

An alternative view of the voice-prosody profile in ASD is an over-activation of the laryngeal muscles to overcome difficulties in neural control of the speech apparatus. These difficulties may arise from disharmonies of activation in cortical and subcortical regions. Schoen et al. (2011) concluded that a misalignment of vocalizations to the duration, pitch, and phonotactic properties of the ambient language could explain the suprasegmental features in ASD. In a study of neural activation for speech production, Pang et al. (2016) reported differences between children with ASD and typically developing children in activation magnitude and peak latencies in several cortical areas including the primary motor cortex (Brodmann Area 4), motor planning areas (BA 6), temporal sequencing and sensorimotor integration areas (BA 22/13) and executive control areas (BA 9). The authors suggested that significant functional brain differences between these two groups on these simple oromotor and phonemic tasks indicate that these differences in neural activation could be foundational and may contribute to language deficits in ASD. Difficulties in audio-vocal integration may be another neural feature of ASD. Patel et al. (2019) reported that individuals with ASD as well as their parents had atypical response onset latencies during tasks of speech production, a finding that was interpreted to indicate underdeveloped feedforward systems and neural attenuation in detecting audio-vocal feedback. The studies of Pang et al., and S. P. Patel et al. are consistent with the hypothesis that individuals with ASD overdrive the laryngeal system in attempts to coordinate the receptive and expressive aspects of speech by enhancing feedforward and feedback signals. High mean pitch and wide pitch range are evidence of laryngeal hyperfunction. These features may contribute to difficulty in production of stress contrasts. Studies show that this difficulty pertains to the production and perception of emphatic stress and lexical stress (Paul et al., 2005; Shriberg et al., 2001). However, atypical prosody may not be uniform across subgroups of ASD. Peppé et al. (2011) suggested that impairment in prosodic skills may be a reliable indicator of autism spectrum subgroups. Perceptual factors also should be recognized. Y. Chen et al. (2022) concluded from a systematic review and meta-analysis that individuals with ASD show enhanced pitch perception and differ from neurotypicals in their developmental trajectories of auditory pitch perception. The neural correlates of pitch processing are not fully understood, but it has been proposed that pitch processing in the auditory cortex is hierarchical, with pitch initially extracted in the auditory cortex of both hemispheres, followed by processing of long-term variations with a possible hemispheric bias (Yuskaitis et al., 2005).

Until recently, atypical articulation was not noted as a common feature of ASD. The perspective appears to be changing. Chaware et al. (2021) concluded from a systematic review and meta-analysis that significant speech errors in ASD include errors of articulation, phonology, expressive language, and receptive language. They also concluded that most speech errors were due to impairment of local oral sensory-motor disturbance, incomplete motor planning, and poor oral neuromuscular coordination. Lau et al. (2023) reported findings that atypical articulatory timing is a feature of ASD and may relate to the prosodic and pragmatic language differences characteristic of ASD. Some of the articulatory differences are rather subtle and may have been missed in earlier accounts that emphasized prosodic characteristics, which may have been more salient than errors of articulation.

Limited progress has been made in the assessment and treatment of the speech and language disorders associated with ASD. Broome et al. (2017) concluded from a systematic review that studies do not give clear guidelines for best practice in the speech assessment of children with ASD. Holbrook and Israelsen (2020), in a review of studies on speech prosody intervention, concluded from the limited evidence that interventions that directly target prosody over a relatively long time can result in improvements.

Cerebellar Mutism (CM), Cerebellar Mutism with Dysarthria (CMD)

Cerebellar Mutism or **Cerebellar Mutism with Dysarthria** is a transient loss of speech usually caused by surgical removal of a tumor in the cerebellum or posterior fossa, most often in children. It is also called post-operative cerebellar mutism syndrome (pCMS). Other symptoms that occur in some individuals are ataxia, mood changes, impaired swallowing, and impaired vision (Noris et al., 2021). Cerebellar tumors are the most common form of brain tumors in children (Paquier et al., 2020), with cerebellar mutism occurring in between 20% and 38% of individuals undergoing such surgery (Cobourn et al., 2020). Causes other than surgery include trauma, degenerative disease, cerebellitis (inflammation of the cerebellum), hemorrhage (internal bleeding) in the brain, embolism, or a tangled congenital arteriovenous malformation. Chewing and swallowing difficulties (dysphagia) can be associated with mutism. Speech may be recovered after a week and up to several years, but the usual pattern is for some speech to appear 48 hours postsurgery and nearly complete recovery of speech within 7 to 8 weeks. Dysarthria may persist in about 80% of the affected individuals, and low muscle tone (muscular hypotonia) is typical. Speech problems include difficulties in initiating speech and articulation that is slow with imprecise coordination and hypernasality. Voice can be hoarse (harsh whispery), and suprasegmental aspects of speech are often poorly controlled, with variability in intonation and lexical stress. Common features include distorted vowels (71%), slow speech rate (71%), voice tremor (57%), and monotone (57%) (Catsman-

Berrevoets & Patay, 2018). Language deficits are possible, particularly in patients who undergo radiotherapy. Postoperative speech and communication difficulties, sometimes called cerebellar speech, may be observed even when mutism does not occur. Surgical risk factors for cerebellar mutism include brainstem invasion, fourth ventricle invasion, superior cerebellar peduncle invasion, a diagnosis of medulloblastoma, left-handedness, and a vermis incision (Pettersson et al., 2021). A possible risk factor for CMS is preoperative language impairment, which may be manifest as reduced spontaneous language, decreased MLU, and word-finding difficulties (Di Rocco et al., 2011). Pharmacological treatments that may reduce and mitigate symptoms in the acute phase of CMS include fluoxetine, bromocriptine, zolpidem, midazolam, delorazepam, and risperidone (Noris et al., 2021).

In addition to mutism, children who undergo surgery in the region of the posterior cranial fossa are at risk of several other conditions, including cranial neuropathies, corticospinal damage, cerebellar ataxia and related motor disorders, neuropsychiatric and cognitive changes (Cámara et al., 2020; Schmahmann, 2020). Generally, children who do not develop post-surgical mutism are less likely to develop these conditions (Cámara et al., 2020).

Mutism and dysarthria may give insights into the role of the cerebellum in speech production and its development in children (cerebellar development is summarized in Chapters 2 and 12). The mutism would seem to reflect a total breakdown in the motor processes of speech, but the spontaneous recovery in most individuals implies that the neural damage can be repaired to a considerable degree, sometimes with surprising rapidity. These clinical features may be the consequence of damage and restoration of the internal model in speech production. The initial damage disrupts the model, or access to it, so that speech loses its foundation of motor control. Recovery could be the consequence of reconstructing the internal model or improving access to it. The nature of an internal model is dynamic in that it is continually seeking to establish sensorimotor linkages that optimize the motor control of speech.

Cerebral Palsy

Cerebral palsy (CP) is a nonprogressive neuromuscular disorder caused by damage to the brain that occurs before, during, or shortly after birth (Rosenbaum et al., 2007; Sadowska et al., 2020). The prevalence of CP has been estimated to be between 1.5 and 2.5 per 1,000 live births. CP is the most common cause of motor disability in children and may be accompanied by disturbances of sensation, perception, cognition, behavior, and communication. Estimates of communication impairment vary widely, from 30% to 90% but recent data tend to fall in the higher range. Several different classifications of CP have been proposed, including severity level, topographical distribution, and gross motor function. About 80% of children with CP have motor involvement, typically classified as spastic, dyskinetic, or ataxic. The most common form is spastic cerebral palsy, which is characterized by increased muscle tone. But because many children exhibit both spasticity and dystonia, mixed presentations are often seen. Less common forms are nonspastic cerebral palsy characterized by decreased or fluctuating muscle tone. The traditional approach to classifying limb distribution for the hypertonic (primarily spastic) form of CP recognizes hemiplegia, diplegia, and quadriplegia/tetraplegia (and occasionally triplegia). However, questions have been raised as to the inter-rater reliability of these classifications.

Both positive and negative signs are observed in CP. The primary positive signs are hypertonicity and dyskinetic movements (motor signs of increased activity). Negative signs (features of decreased or insufficient activity) include weakness, poor selective motor control, ataxia, and apraxia/developmental dyspraxia. Several classification and rating systems have been developed, including the Gross Motor Function Classification System (GMFCS; Rosenbaum et al., 2008) for ambulatory function, the Manual Ability Classification System (MACS; Eliasson et al., 2006) for upper extremities, and the Communication Function Classification System (CFCS; Hidecker et al., 2011) for communication skills.

Indications of a speech disorder in CP may appear in the first year of life. Levin (1999) noted that 1-year-old infants with CP often had delayed onset of canonical babbling, restricted phonetic repertoires, and only monosyllabic utterances. Ward et al. (2022), using the Infant Monitor of vocal Production (IMP; Cantle Moore & Colyvas, 2018) found that vocalizations of infants identified as at-risk of CP were like those of age-matched peers at 6 months of age, but group differences emerged at 9 and 12 months, the period when precanonical and canonical babble typically emerge (as discussed in Chapter 4). Long and Hustad (2023) observed prolonged rates of marginal syllable forms that could be indicative of speech motor impairment. These studies indicate the importance of early vocalizations in identifying children with CP at risk of speech disorders.

The typical type of speech impairment in CP is dysarthria but the differential diagnosis of dysarthria in CP is problematic. Schölderle, Haas, and Ziegler (2021) point out that the consequences of the dysarthria pathology interact with developmental speech features and are not as clear-cut as the dysarthrias in adults. Lust et al. (2014) noted persistent motor planning deficits for nonspeech movements in children with CP, and it would not be surprising if this feature applies to speech as well as nonspeech movements (as discussed in Chapter 5). Schölderle et al. (2022) identified four speech features as especially relevant in differentiating between children with dysarthria and children with typical speech (in decreasing order of their relative importance): atypical rhythm/ stress pattern, hypernasality, strained–strangled voice, and reduced articulation. It is notable that these features pertain to all or most of the speech production subsystems (prosody, voice, resonance, and articulation). The pervasive effects of CP on speech production would have profound effects on internal models or any other conception of speech motor control that assumes availability of a stable reference for controlling movements.

These pervasive effects also pose challenges for the assessment of speech functions in CP given the likelihood of multiple dimensions of speech disorder. Allison et al. (2021) found that SLPs are less reliable in judgments of phonetic accuracy and hypernasality of children with dysarthria than for children with typical speech development, and that reduced speech sound accuracy in children with CP may interfere with reliability of SLPs' perceptual judgments. Long et al. (2022) reported that early speech performance is highly predictive of later speech abilities, and recommended speech therapy for children with any level of speech impairment at age 4 years. Dysarthria is common in CP, but it is not the only speech disorder. Mei et al. (2020) reported that for a community sample of 84 children with CP aged between 4;11 and 11;6 that 82% had delayed or disordered speech production. Of the 64 children with verbal capability, 78% had dysarthria, 54% had articulation delay or disorder, 43% had phonological delay or disorder (43%), and 17% had features of CAS or mixed presentations of these conditions. Speech intelligibility was most affected in the children with dysarthria and features of CAS. Soriano and Hustad (2021) concluded that children with CP often have nonverbal cognitive impairment that co-occurs with language and speech motor impairment.

Acoustic and kinematic studies of speech production in CP are relatively few, but progress is notable. Allison and Hustad (2018) found that two acoustic measures, articulation rate and the F2 range of diphthongs, distinguished between children with CP from typically developing children with a high level of accuracy. Allison et al. (2022) reported that sequence duration and number of cycles in the DDK task (discussed in Chapter 5) have potential value as sensitive measures for detecting speech motor involvement in CP. Chen et al. (2010) reported that children with CP have high values of the spatiotemporal index (STI) and high variability of utterance durations. Acoustic studies have shown reduced vowel space (Mou et al., 2019) and a constricted and creaky vocal quality due to lower spectral tilt and greater noise (Nip & Garelik, 2021). These studies confirm auditory-perceptual assessments in showing widely distributed effects of CP on the speech production system.

Medical interventions include selective dorsal rhizotomy for reducing muscle spasticity and Botulinum toxin type A (BoNT-A), which is the most widely used medical intervention in children with cerebral palsy (Multani et al., 2019). The benefits of this intervention are not entirely clear, especially for long-term use. Multani et al. noted that clinical trials generally have used a single injection cycle, which is insufficient to judge the ratio of benefit and harm. Outcomes are usually reported in terms of changes in muscle tone and few studies have reported on functional improvements. Multani et al. comment that a possible negative outcome is loss of contractile elements with replacement by fat and connective tissue. De Beukelaer et al. (2022) report a reduced cross-sectional muscle growth six months after BoNT-A injection in children with spastic CP. Additional research is needed to make an informed judgment on benefit-harm ratio in this form of pharmacologic treatment.

Limited data are available on behavioral interventions for the speech disorder in CP. Pennington et al. (2020) noted that two types of therapy for speech disorders in CP have been most often reported. These are the Lee Silverman Voice Therapy (LSVT; discussed in Chapter 12) in the U.S. and the Speech Systems Approach in the UK. The approaches have in common a focus on breath support by targeting speech loudness. The Speech Systems Approach also targets speaking rate. Another recently developed approach is the Speech Intelligibility Treatment (SIT), a dual-focus speech treatment that targets increased articulatory excursion and vocal intensity (Levy et al., 2021). Korkalainen et al. (2022) reported a systematic review of eight motor speech interventions for children with CP that had sufficient detail for an evaluation of quality, efficacy, inclusion of motor learning components, and ICF-CY levels. The quality of evidence for these interventions ranged from moderate to very low, with SIT/mSIT having a moderate level of evidence with some nonindependent replication across two RCTs. The quality of all the other interventions ranged from low and very low. LSVT LOUD had a series of small studies and one independent replication. Similar limitations are seen in the use of general motor interventions in physical therapy. Baker et al. (2022) reported only low-quality evidence that task-specific motor training and constraint induced movement therapy (CIMT) improves motor function of infants and toddlers with CP.

Childhood Apraxia of Speech (CAS)

CAS has been defined as "a neurodevelopmental disorder with heterogeneous communication and other comorbid manifestations" (Stein et al., 2020). The disorder was termed **developmental apraxia of speech** in the initial description by Yoss and Darley (1974). An influential description of CAS is an ASHA technical report (American Speech-Language-Hearing Association, 2007):

> Three segmental and suprasegmental features that are consistent with a deficit in the planning and programming of movements for speech have gained some consensus among investigators in apraxia of speech in children: (a) inconsistent errors on consonants and vowels in repeated productions of syllables or words, (b) lengthened and disrupted coarticulatory transitions between sounds and syllables, and (c) inappropriate prosody, especially in the realization of lexical or phrasal stress. Importantly, these features are not proposed to be the necessary and sufficient signs of CAS.

The last statement in the quoted material does not always receive the attention it deserves, which is unfortunate given the difficulties in diagnosis of the condition. Murray et al. (2021) remarked on the lack of evidence-based diagnostic guidelines, criteria, or markers for differentiating CAS from other speech sound disorders in children. Some authorities regard CAS as a motor speech disorder in which children experience difficulties in planning, coordinating, sequencing, and producing speech sounds even in the absence of weakness, incoordination, or tone. The most frequently mentioned features of the disorder include inconsistent sound production, vowel errors, prosodic abnormalities, groping articulation, and slow rate. Sayahi and Jalaie (2016) concluded from a systematic review that clinical markers of CAS were, in decreasing order of mention: inconsistency, vowel errors, prosodic abnormalities, difficulty in complex sequences, consonant and syllable omission, inadequate diadochokinetic profile, groping, intelligibility, limited phonetic repertoire, and reduced expressive language. This impressive listing of diverse features of the disorder illustrates its profound effects on speech and the potential overlap with other speech disorders, including dysarthria. Similarly, Malmenholt et al. (2017) reported survey results indicating that the seven top features that SLTs reported as typical for children with CAS were: inconsistent speech production (85%), sequencing difficulties (71%), oromotor deficits (63%), vowel errors (62%), voicing errors (61%), consonant cluster deletions (54%), and prosodic disturbance (53%). Chenausky et al. (2020) conducted a factor analysis of speech features in CAS and concluded that the results aligned with the three consensus criteria for CAS from the American Speech-Language-Hearing Association: inappropriate prosody, disrupted coarticulatory transitions, and inconsistent errors on repeated tokens. They also noted that a high loading of the syllable segmentation sign on the inappropriate prosody factor agrees with the use of a pause-related biomarker for CAS. Murray et al. (2023) determined the reliability of expert diagnosis of CAS, concluding that intra-rater reliability was acceptable (85% agreement) but that inter-rater reliability on the presence or absence of CAS was poor as both a categorical diagnosis and on a continuous scale of "likelihood of CAS" scale.

The labels used in describing the salient features of CAS deserve further comment, as follows.

Inappropriate Prosody

This feature is often associated with syllable segregation and atypical lexical stress. Syllable segregation is defined as an inappropriate pause between syllables within a word and is thought to reflect difficulty in transitioning between syllables (Brown et al., 2018; O'Farrell et al., 2022). Therefore, pause duration is a basis for detecting syllable segregation. Perceptual studies indicate that adult listeners detect syllable segregation with an accuracy of about 80% at pause durations of between 85 to 125 ms (Brown et al., 2018; O'Farrell et al., 2022). These results hold the implication that acoustic displays can be used to confirm the physical basis of the perceived phenomenon of syllable segregation. Atypical lexical stress was proposed as a marker for CAS by Shriberg et al. (2003), who defined a composite marker called the lexical stress ratio that combined acoustic measures of frequency, intensity, and duration. Subsequent studies showed reduced temporal control for lexical stress production in CAS, even for productions judged to be perceptually accurate (Kopera & Grigos, 2020) and prospects for an automated lexical stress classification tool (McKechnie et al., 2021).

Lengthened and Disrupted Coarticulatory Transitions

This label pertains to the transitions between sounds or syllables. Unfortunately, the descriptor "coarticulatory" implies that listeners can detect coarticulation. To the contrary, coarticulation in speech production is not easily studied with perceptual methods. Farnetani and Recasens (2010) wrote on coarticulation that "these effects are usually not audible, which is why their descriptive and theoretical study in various languages became possible only after physiological and acoustical methods of speech analysis became available and widespread during the last 40 years" (p. 316). Inspired in part by the influential work by Kozhevnikov and Chistovich (1965), coarticulation has been studied largely by instrumental rather than perceptual methods. Evidence of coarticulatory abnormalities in CAS has been derived almost entirely from a small number of acoustic and kinematic studies (Maassen et al., 2001; Nijland et al., 2002).

Many of the phenomena listed in the category of lengthened and disrupted coarticulatory transitions perhaps are more properly called difficulties in sequencing. In this respect, it is interesting that Murray et al. (2015) concluded that "polysyllabic production accuracy and an oral motor examination that includes diadochokinesis may be sufficient to reliably identify CAS and rule out structural abnormality or dysarthria" (p. 43).

Inconsistent Errors on Repeated Token

Inconsistency of errors has been distinguished from variability of speech production. McIntosh and Dodd (2005) define these terms as follows.

> Variability is defined as productions that differ, but can be attributed to factors described in normal acquisition and use of speech. Inconsistency is speech characterized by a high proportion of differing repeated productions with multiple error types that include errors at both the phonemic (e.g. fronting of velars, /h/ deletes word initially) and syllable level (e.g. syllable deletion or addition). (p. 10)

Betz and Stoel-Gammon (2005) noted the lack of standardized definitions of error inconsistency and proposed three formulas for different aspects of articulatory error consistency:

1. proportion of errors: [number of errors/number of total productions] × 100,
2. consistency of error types: 1–[number of different error types/number of erred productions] × 100), and
3. consistency of the most frequently used error type: [number of productions of the most frequently used error type −1]/[number of erred productions −1] × 100).

These different formulas address different aspects of error inconsistency, thereby revealing the complexity of the concept. Also important is the definition of error. The usual procedure is to use the SODA (substitutions, omissions, distortions, additions), but there is some difference of opinion on the category of distortions, which often require narrow phonetic transcription for their representation. Severely unintelligible speech can pose challenges to both phonemic and phonetic transcription. Iuzzini-Seigel et al. (2017) concluded that although speech inconsistency is a core feature of CAS and can help to distinguish between CAS and speech delay, the sensitivity and specificity of this factor depend on the stimuli. Preston et al. (2021) concluded that the Maximum Repetition Rate of Trisyllables (MRR-Tri) identified more children as having sound sequencing errors indicative of CAS than the Syllable Repetition Task (SRT).

Variability and inconsistency can be assessed with different methods. Terband, Namasivayam et al. (2019) advised as follows on the use and value of perceptual, acoustic, and kinematic studies of CAS:

> The three types of measurement procedures should be seen as complementary. Some characteristics are better suited to be described at the perceptual level (especially phonemic errors and prosody), others at the acoustic level (especially phonetic distortions, coarticulation, and prosody), and still others at the kinematic level (especially coarticulation, stability, and gestural

coordination). The type of data collected determines, to a large extent, the interpretation that can be given regarding the underlying deficit. (p. 2999)

Case and Grigos (2020) concluded from a review of kinematic studies that children with CAS have atypical patterns of movement and timing even within perceptually accurate speech. This conclusion means that variability in CAS is not equivalent to that observed in typically developing children and deserves consideration as a potential marker of the disorder. This variability is not perceptually detectable by even the most discriminating SLPs and brings into question the classification of inconsistent errors versus variability in CAS. A reasonable conclusion from the literature is that children with CAS demonstrate a high degree of kinematic variability that combines with, and in some cases may give rise to, phonemic errors identified perceptually. To the extent to which difficulty with motor planning/programming is the core of CAS, data and explanations at the motor level are needed for its accurate diagnosis and treatment. As Terband et al. (2019) noted for CAS, there is risk of conflating the type of data with the level of explanation. If data are confined to a relatively high level of phonology, then the disorder may be conceptualized chiefly as a phonological impairment. But if data from different levels are integrated, then CAS comes into relief in its full complexity.

An Integrated View of CAS

Chilosi et al. (2022) address major challenges to the diagnosis of CAS, three of which are considered here. First, isolated CAS accounts for only a fraction of the total number of children diagnosed with CAS. Most children with CAS have complicated profiles of comorbidity (e.g., CAS comorbid with language impairment, intellectual disability, attention deficit and hyperactivity disorder, or ASD). Second, multidimensional diagnostic and clinical management is needed for CAS. Chilosi et al. point specifically to the high frequency of language impairment, which may be a central factor in designing a personalized treatment approach. Third, speech motor deficits appear to be common across different comorbidity profiles. These deficits included syllable omissions, inaccuracy, and inconsistency, especially in multisyllabic productions. In addition to disorders of speech and language, children with CAS have also been shown to have atypical performance on nonverbal tasks, especially those that involve sequencing of motor behaviors or implicit learning (Bombonato et al., 2022; Iuzzini-Seigel, 2021).

Childhood Dysarthria

The diagnosis of dysarthria is discussed in Chapter 5, where it was noted that there is no widely accepted system for the classification of childhood dysarthrias. Iuzzini-Siegel et al. (2022, p. 926) follow Duffy (2020) in defining dysarthria as "a neuromuscular disorder of motor execution resulting from abnormalities to the strength, range of motion, tone, or precision of movements required for appropriate control of the speech subsystems (i.e., articulatory, respiratory, phonatory, resonatory, and prosodic)." As mentioned in Chapter 5, the restriction of the definition to specify execution is questionable given the possibility (if not inevitability) of motor program deficits associated with faulty motor learning of speech production in the face of abnormal sensory and motor function. Dysarthria in children, whether linked to a congenital condition or acquired during development, affects the fundamental processes of speech motor learning. A further difficulty is the challenge of assessing the supposed abnormalities of strength, range, tone, and precision, for which few standardized methods are available (see Chapter 5). In short, there is a lack of well-defined standards for the clinical assessment of dysarthria in children.

Studies on dysarthria in children are predominantly focused on cerebral palsy (discussed in this chapter). This focus is understandable given the high likelihood of speech disorders in cerebral palsy, but it neglects other sources of childhood dysarthria, such as acquired brain injury (ABI) related to conditions such as cerebrovascular accident, brain tumor, and traumatic brain injury. ABI is major cause of disability in children, and dysarthria is a common and often persistent aspect of the condition (Morgan & Vogel, 2008). Acquired dysarthria also may occur in neuromuscular disorders. Kooi-van Es et al. (2020) reported that dysphagia and dysarthria were present in almost all of 14 diagnostic groups of pediatric neuromuscular disorders in their sample, with a pooled overall prevalence of dysarthria of 31.5%. The current literature offers few guidelines for the assessment and classification of acquired dysarthria in children. There is little assurance that classifications of acquired dysarthria in adults can be used confidently with children.

Cleft Palate

Cleft palate is a congenital condition in which the lateral plates of the palate fail to fuse during embryonic development, leaving a medial fissure in the palate, and sometimes involving one or both sides of the upper lip, into the nostril(s). The fissure may be complete, with the cleft extending from the lip, through the intervening structures of the hard palate, to reach the uvula at the end of the soft palate (**complete or total cleft palate**). A less-than-complete cleft palate may result in a cleft (bifid, split) uvula or may involve any combination of the soft palate, the hard palate, or the alveolar ridge (an **incomplete, partial, or subtotal cleft palate**). The cleft may be on only one side of the mouth (a **unilateral cleft palate**) or on both sides (a **bilateral cleft palate**). Chapter 2 includes illustrations of types of cleft. Bilateral cleft palate occurs when the two lateral halves of the hard palate fail during embryonic development to unite with the nasal septum. Cleft palate is the most common craniofacial malformation in humans. The results of a systematic review by Salari et al., (2021) indicate that the global prevalence in 1,000 live births is 0.33 for cleft palate, 0.3 for cleft lip, and 0.45 for cleft lip and palate. Cleft palates without cleft lips are more frequent in girls and cleft lips with or without cleft palates are more frequent in boys. Associated problems of children with a cleft palate and/or cleft lip include early difficulties with feeding, a greater susceptibility to ear infections and hearing impairment, and dental anomalies in the eruption, number, position, and shape of teeth. A **submucous cleft palate** (also called an **occult cleft palate**) results from incomplete fusion of the muscles within the soft palate. This condition occurs in about 1 in 1,200 children and often is identified late in development, mainly through presence of a bifid or wide uvula and symptoms of velopharyngeal insufficiency (such as hypernasal speech and Eustachian tube dysfunction) (Reiter et al., 2010).

Speech problems in children with a cleft palate arise mainly from difficulties in achieving an effective seal between the oral and the nasal cavity, causing hypernasality and an inability to produce adequate intraoral air pressure for pressure consonants. The intelligibility of front oral consonants (oral labial, labiodental, dental, alveolar, postalveolar and palato-alveolar stops, fricatives, and affricates) in cleft palate speech may consequently be affected and the development of appropriate language skills delayed. Individual speech sounds may be produced with atypical articulation, including compensatory articulations described in Chapter 9. Surgery is the standard treatment for improving palatal form and function, but repair is challenging and can have significant complications, such as speech disorder and maxillary growth deficiency (Naidu et al., 2022). In a study of comparative outcomes using the objective methods of nasopharyngoscopy and nasometry (see Chapter 3), Kara et al. (2020) concluded that the 18th month is a cutoff time in palatal repair for improved speech results. By the time of repair, many children may have developed compensatory speech patterns that continue to affect post-surgery intelligibility, which prompts the need for speech-language therapy. Because SLPs may not always have substantial experience with craniofacial anomalies, such as cleft palate, Baigorri et al. (2020) developed a module training series for craniofacial assessment and treatment. This resource is recommended to those who would like to supplement their knowledge in this area of practice. Interventions for speech disorder include a linguistic-phonological approach (Alighieri et al., 2020) and motor learning approaches (Alighieri et al., 2021; Hanley et al., 2022).

Developmental Coordination Disorder (DCD)

Developmental Coordination Disorder (DCD) is a developmental disorder of motor coordination. According to the *International Statistical Classification of Diseases and Related Health Problems* (10th ed.; *ICD-10*; World Health Organization, 2016), specific developmental disorder of motor function is defined as

> A disorder in which the main feature is a serious impairment in the development of motor coordination that is not solely explicable in terms of general intellectual retardation or of any specific congenital or acquired neurological disorder. Nevertheless, in most cases a careful clinical examination shows marked neurodevelopmental immaturities such as choreiform movements of unsupported limbs or mirror movements and other associated motor features, as well as signs of impaired fine and gross motor coordination.

DSM-5 criteria for diagnosing DCD are a combination of the following at around 5 years of age: (1) motor coordination below what would be expected for chronological age and exposure to motor activities, (2) movement qualities including clumsiness, slowness or inaccuracy, which impact daily living skills, school productivity, leisure and play, (3) symptoms which began in the developmental period, and (4) symptoms that cannot be explained by other conditions such as an intellectual disability or other neurological conditions with motor impairments. Subara-Zukic et al. (2022) concluded from a systematic review and meta-analysis that the most profound deficits were in: voluntary gaze control during movement; cognitive-motor integration; practice-/context-dependent motor learning; internal modeling; more variable movement kinematics/kinetics; larger safety margins when locomoting, and atypical neural structure and function across sensorimotor and prefrontal regions. Similar symptoms are seen in dyspraxia, which creates some difficulties in definition of the disorder and steps to accurate diagnosis (Wasserman & Wasserman, 2023). Prevalence estimates of DCD range from 2% to 20% of children, with 5% to 6% being most often reported (Blank et al., 2019).

DCD can be associated with atypical performance of complex speech gestures (Ho & Wilmut, 2010) and with a diagnosis of CAS (Duchow et al., 2019; Hodge, 1998; Iuzzini-Seigel, Moorer, & Tamplain, 2022; Licari et al., 2021). These associations raise questions regarding the etiology and presentation of CAS in the presence of DCD. Missiuna et al. (2002) give guidelines for the role of SLPs in recognizing and referring children at risk for DCD.

Down Syndrome (DS)

DS (Trisomy 21) is the most common chromosomal anomaly, as well as the most common form, of intellectual disability, occurring in about 1 in 700 to 800 births (Sherman et al., 2007). It is characterized by the presence of all or a portion of a third chromosome 21. DS is one of the most complex genetic conditions that is survivable, having multiple effects on body systems and organs (Lagan et al., 2020; Roizen, 2010). It is both a neurodevelopmental and neurodegenerative condition because neural effects are present at birth (Patkee et al., 2020; Shiohama et al., 2019; Vacca et al., 2019) and additional neural changes may occur later in life in the form of early Alzheimer's disease (Snyder et al., 2020) and Down syndrome disintegrative disorder (Rosso et al. 2020). The life expectancy of people with DS has increased from less than 20 years to nearly 60 years over the last two generations, primarily due to improved health care (Bittles et al., 2007).

Communication disorders are common, and reduced speech intelligibility can be a persistent problem (H. N. Jones et al., 2019; Kent & Vorperian, 2013; Kumin, 1994; Wild et al., 2018). Kumin (2006) commented that, "Reduced speech intelligibility is a widespread problem for children with Down syndrome that has been documented in the literature in clinical case studies, surveys, and reports" (p. 10). In a survey of 228 parents of individuals with DS, speech was identified as being in the top four of 16 areas needing further research and the second area of greatest parental interest, behind only cognition (White et al., 2022). The speech disorder often involves all subsystems or aspects of speech production, including respiration, phonation, articulation, resonance, and prosody (Jones et al., 2019; Kent & Vorperian, 2013). Phonological profiles in DS reflect both delayed and atypical patterns of development (Diez-Itza et al., 2021; Stoel-Gammon, 2001). Diez-Itza et al. suggested that phonological-lexical asynchronous development in DS may be explained in part by phonological memory deficits (Laws & Gunn, 2004). It has been estimated that approximately 90% of children aged birth to 5 years receive speech therapy services (E. King et al., 2022). A high prevalence of hearing loss and abnormal middle ear status has been reported in children with DS (Nightingale et al., 2017), which points to the need for audiologic assessment and appropriate treatment of hearing loss.

Craniofacial and laryngeal anomalies in individuals with Down syndrome (DS) have been linked with difficulties in speech, swallowing, sleep apnea, and other airway functions. Commonly occurring craniofacial anomalies include relative macroglossia (a normal-size tongue confined to a small oral cavity), shortened midface skeleton with smaller facial height, maxillary hypoplasia (including a short and narrow palate), mandibular hypoplasia, and dental malocclusion (Achmad et al., 2021; Díaz-Quevedo et al., 2021; Kaczorowska et al., 2019; Sforza et al., 2012; Suri et al., 2010; Uong et al., 2001). Laryngeal dysmorphologies include laryngomalacia (collapse of supraglottic structures during inspiration, causing stridor) and tracheal stenosis (Mitchell et al., 2003). Several of these features are illustrated in Figure 11–3. A common functional abnormality is hypotonia of both the oral (Dodd & Thompson, 2001) and vocal musculature (ventricular as well as true vocal folds) (Novak, 1972; Pebbili et al. 2019). Hypotonicity may be associated with reduced force capability (Zarzo-Benlloch et al., 2017). The constellation of atypical speech features is not invariant across individuals but is often widely distributed across the laryngeal, articulatory, resonatory, and prosodic subsystems (Jones et al., 2019; Kent & Vorperian, 2013; Kent et al., 2021). The speech disorder has been described as dysarthria, childhood apraxia of speech, or a combination of these (Rupela & Manjula, 2010; Rupela et al., 2016; Vorperian et al., 2023; Wilson et al., 2019). The presence of a dysarthric

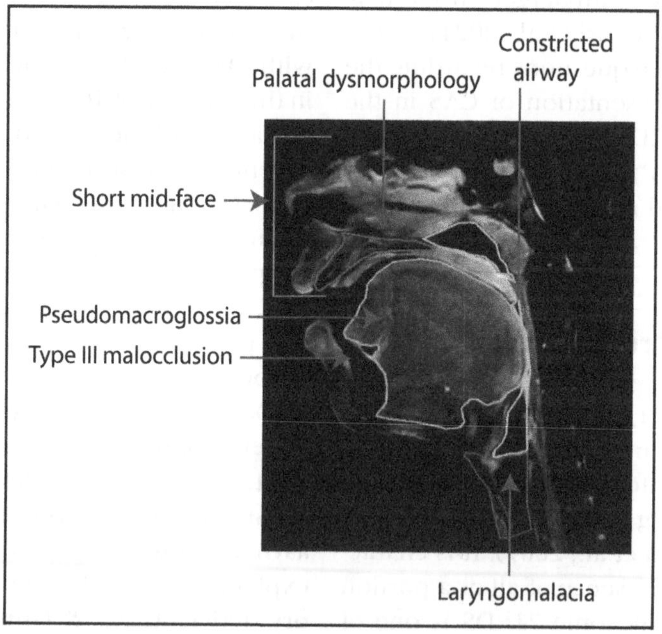

Figure 11–3. Frequently occurring anomalies of the vocal tract and related structures in children with Down syndrome.

component is indicated by evidence of reduced tongue and lip strength (Farpour et al., 2021; Zarzo-Benlloch et al., 2017). It also has been suggested that the speech disorder in DS may be a disorder-specific profile related to the combined effects of hypotonia, dysarthria, disordered motor programming, phonological disorder, and craniofacial dysmorphology (Vorperian et al., 2023). The complexity of the speech disorder may reflect maldevelopment of the cerebrum, cerebellum, and brainstem (Patkee et al., 2020; Shiohama et al., 2019; Vacca et al., 2019).

There is no standardized approach to treating speech disorders in DS. In their systematic review and meta-analysis of communication interventions in DS, Neil and Jones (2018) remarked that, "Few interventions were tailored to the needs of the Down syndrome behavior phenotype" (p. 1). However, promising behavioral treatments for the speech disorder include intensive treatment with LSVT LOUD (Boliek et al., 2022; Langlois et al., 2020; Mahler & Jones, 2012), biofeedback with ultrasound (Fawcett et al., 2008), and electropalatography (Page & Johnson, 2021; Wood et al., 2019).

Fetal Alcohol Spectrum Disorders (FASD)

Fetal alcohol spectrum disorders (FASD) are a group of conditions that result from alcohol exposure to the fetus during prenatal development. This exposure commonly occurs when alcohol in the mother's blood is transmitted to the fetus through the umbilical cord. The effects vary among affected individuals but often include altered physical development and problems with behavior and learning, such as cognitive-linguistic impairments, hearing disorders, social-behavioral issues, poor executive function, growth deficiencies, and dysmorphic facial and skeletal features. The five disorders that comprise the spectrum are fetal alcohol syndrome (FAS), partial fetal alcohol syndrome (pFAS), alcohol-related neurodevelopmental disorder (ARND), a neurobehavioral disorder associated with prenatal alcohol exposure (ND-PAE), and alcohol-related birth defects (ARBD). These five conditions have the common etiology of prenatal exposure to alcohol, which is highly teratogenic to a fetus. (*Teratogenic* is an unfortunate word that literally means monster-producing, from the Greek word for monster, *teratos*. It is now defined as relating to embryonic or fetal malformations). Prenatal exposure to alcohol has effects that are wide-ranging and irreversible. Increased exposure to prenatal alcohol exposure is associated with increased incidence and severity of FASD, but it appears that there is no amount of alcohol that can be consumed safely during any part of pregnancy. Simply put, alcohol is toxic to fetal development.

Terband et al. (2018) concluded that the speech impairment in boys with FASD results from effects on multiple subsystems, including craniofacial anatomy (heightened palate), auditory discrimination, oral motor control (especially involving the tongue), and speech motor planning/programming. However, the features varied considerably across affected individuals. Some features may have a common embryonic origin in malformations of the first and second branchial arches and may have similar developmental vulnerability to toxic insult. Specific oral motor deficits appear to contribute to communication disorders in young speakers with FAS. Bollinger and Dembowski (2019) identified a motoric component as evidenced by: (1) inconsistencies in phonological findings (i.e., variability in articulation abilities across individuals, and inconsistent phoneme production in multiple attempts by individuals), and (2) deficiencies in oral-motor control as suggested by the VMPAC Focal Oromotor Function subtest (Hayden & Square-Storer, 1999). A review of longitudinal studies indicated that prenatal exposure to alcohol was associated with delays in receptive and expressive communication up to 36 months of age and that contextual risk factors had a significant effect on language development (Hendricks et al., 2019). Blanck-Lubarsch et al. (2019) concluded that children with FAS need interventions such as speech treatment, ergotherapy, and physiotherapy to ensure optimal development.

Structural and functional characteristics of hearing are often affected in individuals with FASD. A systematic review and meta-analysis (Cheung et al., 2021) revealed that the most common structural features were microtia, railroad track ear, and misplaced ear. The most common functional ear abnormalities were chronic serous otitis media, abnormal auditory filtering, and unspecified conductive hearing loss. A review of human and animal research revealed four types of hearing disorders associated with FASD: (1) delayed auditory maturation, (2) sensorineural hearing loss, (3) intermittent conductive hearing loss due to recurrent serous otitis media, and (4) central hearing loss (Church & Kaltenbach, 1997). However, hearing loss per se is not the only auditory problem, as suprathreshold effects have been reported. McLaughlin et al. (2019) found that listening difficulties in the absence of hearing loss are prevalent across the entire fetal alcohol spectrum. They reported atypical auditory behavior among 80% of children with FASD and noted that the prevalence did not vary by FASD severity or hearing status but was positively correlated with attention-deficit/hyperactivity disorder.

Fluency Disorders

A **fluency disorder** is a disruption in the flow or rhythm of speech production, often taking the form of hesitations, repetitions, prolongations, or other interruptions. The two major clinical types of fluency disorder are stuttering and cluttering. Stuttering that appears in childhood (typically between 3 and 5 years of age) is called **developmental stuttering** or **childhood onset fluency disorder.** (Neumann et al., 2017, suggest the term **originary neurogenic non-syndromic stuttering**). The *DSM-V* defines childhood-onset fluency disorder as a disturbance in the normal fluency and time pattern of speech that is inappropriate for the individual's age and persists over time. This childhood disorder should be distinguished from acquired adult forms such as neurogenic or psychogenic stuttering. Developmental stuttering is a complex, multifactorial neurodevelopmental disorder (Chang et al., 2019) with an incidence in young children of about 8% (Yairi & Ambrose, 2013). Of these, approximately 20% develop lifelong chronic stuttering. Factors that predict recovery are diverse and not easily determined (Einarsdóttir et al., 2020). Sugathan and Maruthy (2021) identified predictive factors as being phonological abilities, articulatory rate, change in the pattern of disfluencies, and trend in stuttering severity. Singer et al. (2020) found predictive factors to be age at stuttering onset, frequencies of stuttering-like disfluencies, speech sound accuracy, expressive and receptive language skills, male gender, and family history of stuttering. Heritability estimates for fluency disorders range from 40% to over 80% (Neumann et al., 2017; Polikowsky et al., 2022). Developmental stuttering can co-occur with other communication disorders and syndromes discussed in this chapter (e.g., Down syndrome, Fragile X syndrome). Basic approaches to assessing fluency are discussed in Chapter 5.

Cluttering is the other main type of fluency disorder in children. According to the website of the International Cluttering Association (ICA; https://sites.google.com/view/icacluttering/home), cluttering is a fluency disorder characterized by a rate that is perceived to be abnormally rapid, irregular or both for the speaker (although measured syllable rates may not exceed normal limits). These rate abnormalities are further manifest in one or more of the following symptoms: (a) an excessive number of disfluencies, the majority of which are not typical of people who stutter; (b) the frequent placement of pauses and use of prosodic patterns that do not conform to syntactic and semantic constraints; and (c) inappropriate (usually excessive) degrees of coarticulation among sounds, especially in multisyllabic words. The website also cautions that the definition is a work in progress. In a concise review of the complex literature on cluttering, Duchan and Felsenfeld (2021) noted that cluttering has been categorized in different ways, including a type of articulation disorder, a type of language disorder, and a type of fluency disorder. It is now generally classified as a fluency disorder, and Duchan and Felsenfeld concluded that the defining features include the presence of excessive normal disfluencies, particularly repetitions; a fast or irregular speaking rate; excessive coarticulation; and anomalies in pause placement, syllable stress, and/or speech rhythm. They also comment that cluttering is often thought to be a heritable motor speech disorder of unknown pathophysiology.

The etiology of developmental stuttering and cluttering remains elusive, but a synthesis of neuroanatomic and neurofunctional studies by Chang et al. (2019) indicated deficits in the neural circuits involved in "planning and execution of self-initiated, intrinsically timed sound sequences" (p. 575). These circuits include (1) auditory-motor areas primarily in the left hemisphere and (2) basal ganglia-thalamocortical loop and cerebellar pathways. It has been reported that individuals who stutter are more variable in speech movements than individuals who do not stutter, even for utterances judged to be fluent (Namasivayam & Van Lieshout, 2011; Wiltshire et al., 2021), which may indicate that stuttering is associated with a pervasive motor variability that interferes with precisely timed performance. Further insights into etiology may come from comparisons to other conditions. For example, childhood fluency disorder and Tourette's syndrome have several features in common: onset in childhood, male to female ratio of 4:1, favorable response to dopamine antagonists, and exacerbation by dopamine agonists (Maguire et al., 2020). Several different treatments are available. Neumann et al. (2017) concluded from their review of studies that Lidcombe therapy and the indirect treatment approach have the strongest evidence for preschool children, but for children aged 6 to 12 years no treatment had strong evidence.

Fragile X Syndrome

Fragile X syndrome is a genetic disorder that is the most common type of inherited intellectual disability in males, as well as a major cause of intellectual disability in females. The genetic basis is usually a mutation in the FMR1 gene in which a DNA segment, called the CGG triplet repeat, is expanded. This expansion or atypical repetition inactivates the FMR1 gene, preventing the formation of a protein called Fragile X mental retardation protein. The condition, which occurs in all racial and ethnic groups, affects about 1 in 4,000 males and 1 in 8,000 females. Males are more severely affected because they possess a single X chromosome. Individuals with Fragile X often have cognitive impairment, attention deficit disorder, attention deficit hyperactivity disorder, autism spectrum disorders, social anxiety, poor eye contact, sensory disorders, and increased risk for aggression. Weaknesses are often observed across all language and literacy domains compared to typically developing peers of the same chronological age (Finestack et al., 2009). Physical features of the body are variable and may include large ears, long face, soft skin, and large testicles (macro-orchidism), and various connective tissue disorders. Affected individuals are often sociable and friendly. Common strengths include excellent imitative abilities and strong visual and long-term memory. Fragile X is strongly associated with autism spectrum disorder, with 16% to 47% of those with Fragile X satisfying diagnostic criteria for autistic disorder, with a consensus estimate of 20% to 30% (Kover & Abbeduto, 2010).

Effects on speech are evident in infancy as a delay in onset of canonical babbling and a lower canonical babbling ratio (Belardi et al., 2017) and lower volubility (Roche et al., 2018) compared to typically developing infants. Barnes et al. (2006) reported on oral structures and functions in boys with Fragile X, noting for structure that 75% of the boys scored in the atypical range for lip relationship, teeth occlusion, and palatal vault height. For tongue and velopharyngeal functions, boys with Fragile X scored lower than typically developing boys. These results point to both structural and motor function that could contribute to problems with speech articulation and other oral functions. Reduced speech intelligibility has been reported for boys with Fragile X (Barnes et al., 2009; Schmitt et al., 2020). Schmitt et al. (2020) suggested that the intelligibility deficit is related to reduced prespeech activity and increased frontal gamma power prior to speech production, which could indicate disruption of coordinated prespeech activity between frontal and temporal cortices. Also common to Fragile X are fluency disorders, especially cluttering (Bangert et al., 2022; Van Borsel et al., 2008) and repetition or perseveration (Finestack et al., 2009; Martin et al., 2012). Childhood apraxia of speech has been reported in some individuals (Spinelli et al., 1995).

Hearing Disorders

By the age of 18 years, hearing loss affects nearly 1 in every 5 children in the United States and can have serious consequences on quality of life and a child's participation in education, social activities, and other pursuits (Lieu et al., 2020). Congenital hearing loss is the most frequently occurring birth anomaly, with a prevalence of 2 to 3 cases per 1,000 newborns (Vohr et al., 2008). Genetic etiology accounts for at least 50 % of cases of permanent hearing loss in childhood (Kral & O'Donoghue, 2010). Congenital sensorineural hearing loss can be either nonsyndromic (70%) or syndromic (30%) (Tanna et al., 2021), with inheritance patterns of autosomal recessive (approximately 75% to 80%), autosomal dominant (about 20%), X-linked (less than 2%), and mitochondrial (about 1%) (Sheffield & Smith, 2019). Environmental causes of hearing loss in children include hypoxia, hyperbilirubinemia, very low birth weight, ototoxic medications, and bacterial or viral infections (with the cytomegalovirus being the most common congenital infection and a relatively common etiology of hearing loss) (Roizen, 2003).

Conventional classification of hearing impairment recognizes degrees of hearing loss:

- Slight impairment is a loss of 15 to 25 dB.
- Mild impairment is a loss of 26 to 40 dB.
- Moderate impairment is a loss of 41 to 55 dB.
- Moderate to severe impairment is a loss of 56 to 70 dB.
- Severe impairment is a loss of 71 to 90 dB.
- Profound impairment is a loss greater than 90 dB.

It was once thought that mild hearing loss and unilateral hearing loss have relatively minor effects on child development, but it is now recognized that these conditions can have important consequences and, therefore, merit serious attention. Mild hearing loss can affect speech perception in noisy environments and cognitive abilities underpinning language and reading (Moore et al., 2020). Unilateral hearing loss (UHL) is defined as having normal hearing in one ear, and hearing loss of any degree, type, or configuration in the other ear. If UHL is severe-to-profound, it is called single-sided deafness (SSD) (Vila & Lieu, 2015). UHL and SSD interfere with sound localization, speech in noise understanding, spatial awareness, ease of listening, and spoken language development (Bagatto et al., 2019; R. Bell et al., 2022; Fitzpatrick et al., 2019; Hearnshaw et al., 2019; Lieu, 2004; Rohlfs et al., 2017). Accordingly, hearing specialists give priority to identifying such losses and advising on interventions (Bagatto, 2020). As noted in Chapter 2, there may be a critical or sensitive period (and perhaps several such periods) of auditory development, which underscores the need for intervention.

Otitis media (OM) (introduced in Chapter 2) has long been suspected of interfering with speech and language development, but studies do not give a clear picture of the degree of risk associated with this form of auditory pathology. OM presents clinically in different ways, including a transient occurrence as acute otitis media (AOM) and OM with effusion, or a persistent occurrence as recurrent AOM (rAOM) and chronic suppurative otitis media (CSOM). It is estimated that 80% of young children, primarily between the ages of 6 and 24 months, experience at least one OM episode and many have multiple recurrences each year (Mason et al., 2022). Studies of the associations between OM and the development of speech and language have given mixed results. Conclusions from meta-analyses and reviews rate the association as follows: none to very small negative (Roberts et al., 2004), generally negative (Sagr & Sagr, 2021), and negative (Homøe et al., 2020). However, definite conclusions cannot be drawn because the relevant studies often had mixed results, and the effects of other variables, such as socioeconomic status and other health conditions were not always controlled. The evidence is sufficiently strong to warrant close observation of children with OM, especially when it has recurrent or chronic occurrence. It has been reported that OM can affect auditory temporal processing (Khavarghazalani et al., 2022) and features of infant vocalizations, including the onset of canonical babbling (Lohmander et al., 2021).

Auditory processing is critical to speech development, as considered in Chapters 7 and 12. Auditory discrimination is one of the most commonly used approaches in the treatment of speech disorders. Auditory processing skills mature over an extended period of life and do not reach adult-like levels until adolescence (Chapters 2 and 12).

Hypotonia

Hypotonia is generally defined as reduced resistance to passive range of motion (phasic tone), or a loss of postural control. It may or may not be accompanied by weakness. In evaluating infants with suspected floppy infant syndrome, Peredo and Hannibal (2009) suggest that a "more useful definition of hypotonia is an impairment of the ability to sustain postural control and movement against gravity" (p. e66). Hypotonia is not a diagnosis per se but rather a neurological sign that is present in a variety of medical and neurodevelopmental disorders and is usually assessed in trunk and limb muscles, and the skeletal craniofacial muscles. Hypotonia in infants and young children is associated with four broad categories of pathology: the CNS, the peripheral nerves (motor and sensory), the neuromuscular junction, and the muscle. Hypotonia of central (CNS) origin accounts for the great majority of cases (Harris, 2008). Central hypotonia is often observed as a feature of neurodevelopmental disorders, including congenital blindness, autism spectrum disorder, intellectual disability, Down syndrome, Fragile X syndrome, Prader-Willi syndrome, cerebellar mutism and dysarthria, some types of cerebral palsy, neurofibromatosis type 1, and as many as 500 different genetic conditions (Lisi & Cohn, 2011). Therefore, hypotonia is frequently encountered in conditions that are associated with problems in speech development, and it is possible that hypotonia is at least a partial explanation for speech disorders in these populations. However, the role that hypotonia plays is not clear.

Latash et al. (2008) remarked that hypotonia does not have a clear definition, a transparent interpretation of underlying mechanisms, nor a universally accepted method of measurement. As noted in Chapter 5, assessing tone in the speech musculature poses special challenges. It is difficult to perform tests of passive range of motion for the articulators except for the mandible. Specialized instruments for measurement of tone are not generally available to speech-language clinicians, and the effects of hypotonia on speech production are not well established. Assessment of hypotonia in the speech musculature apparently is performed mostly with impressionistic methods rather than quantitative tools. It has been recommended to use rapid genome or exome sequencing as a first-line testing option for NICU patients with unexplained hypotonia (Morton et al., 2022). Despite the difficulties in assessment, hypotonia cannot be dismissed as a contributing factor to motor problems with speech or other motor systems. It can be an early sign of neurodevelopmental disorders including cerebral palsy (Krustev et al., 2000) and autism spectrum disorder (Gabis et al., 2021). It is also frequently reported in Down syndrome, fetal alcohol spectrum, and other congenital conditions.

Inherited Metabolic Disorders (IMD)

These disorders (also known as **hereditary metabolic disorders** and **inborn errors of metabolism**) affect the ability to convert food into energy and to remove toxic substances from the body, conditions that can lead to damage in cell development and brain function. This heterogeneous group of genetic conditions is usually caused by single-gene defects resulting in abnormal synthesis or catabolism of proteins, carbohydrates, or fats through defective enzymes or transport proteins. More than 500 different inherited metabolic disorders have been described, with the majority being rare. The estimated incidence of metabolic disorders of all kinds is approximately 1 in every 2,500 live births, or 10% of all monogenic conditions in children. It is estimated that clinical symptoms associated with damage to the CNS occur in more than 50% of individuals with IMD. Speech and other communication disorders associated with IMD are not well characterized, but evidence points to a high frequency of delayed speech and language development (Peter et al., 2022; Potter et al., 2013; Tiwari et al., 2017), developmental stuttering (Kang & Drayna, 2012), and ASD (Žigman et al., 2021).

Malocclusion (Dentofacial Disharmonies)

Malocclusion is introduced in Chapter 2. Malocclusion, dental disharmonies, and jaw disharmonies are related terms and sometimes used interchangeably. Jaw disharmonies identified after birth and that present in association with the prepubertal growth spurt are called **developmental dentofacial deformities** (Posnick & Kinard, 2020). Mandibular growth is guided by the muscles and other soft tissues of the face and oral region, as proposed in Moss' functional matrix theory (Chapter 2). Dysfunction of these tissues that can affect jaw growth include an improper swallow, prolonged thumb or pacifier habits, overactive lip and cheek muscles, mouth breathing, a resting open mouth posture, and low tongue posture. Individuals with dentofacial disharmonies and Class III malocclusion have a higher frequency of speech sound disorders than individuals without such a condition (Grudziąż-Sękowska et al., 2018; Lathrop-Marshall et al., 2022; Leavy et al., 2016; O'Gara & Wilson, 2007; Vallino & Tompson, 1993). Jacox et al. (2022) wrote that articulation problems are diagnosed in 73% to 90% of patients with dentofacial disharmonies, but the causal link is not established. Bode et al. (2023) noted that SSD occurs in about 90% of Class III patients, 83% of anterior open bite patients, and 73% to 87% of Class II patients. Class III is associated especially with difficulty in the production of the fricative /s/ (Guay et al., 1978) and a lower tongue posture (Assaf et al., 2021). Hyde et al. (2018) provide general background on dental health related to speech, and Bommangoudar et al. (2020) review the role of the pedodontist in managing speech difficulties in children with structural problems and unfavorable oral habits. Bode et al. (2023) consider patients with dentofacial disharmonies as having structural SSDs in which anatomic features of the oral cavity and vocal tract lead to speech errors and distortions.

Mouth Breathing and Long-Face Syndrome

Long-face syndrome is a contemporary term for the condition originally known as **adenoid faces**, a term introduced by Tomes (1872) to describe the dentofacial changes presumably associated with chronic nasal airway obstruction. It was suspected that such obstruction in childhood could result in a characteristic constellation of craniofacial and dental features. The term *long-face syndrome* is preferable because adenoids are not the only cause of such obstruction, which also may be caused by deviated septum, hypertrophic turbinates, and external nasal deformity (Farid & Metwalli, 2010). A large and complicated literature relates this syndrome with the behavior of **mouth breathing**, defined by Zicari et al. (2009) as "a parafunctional habit whereby air passes exclusively or partially through the mouth instead of the nose, and it is accompanied by skeletal and functional alterations in the orofacial district" (p. 60). This facial skeletal pattern is also called **hyperdivergent**, meaning that there is an excessive divergence of the skeletal planes (especially the angle between the Frankfort and mandibular planes). The commonly used craniofacial planes used in craniometrics (measurements of the cranium) are shown in Figure 2–22, and the Frankfort-mandibular angle in Figure 11–4. An increase of this angle is associated with hyperdivergence,

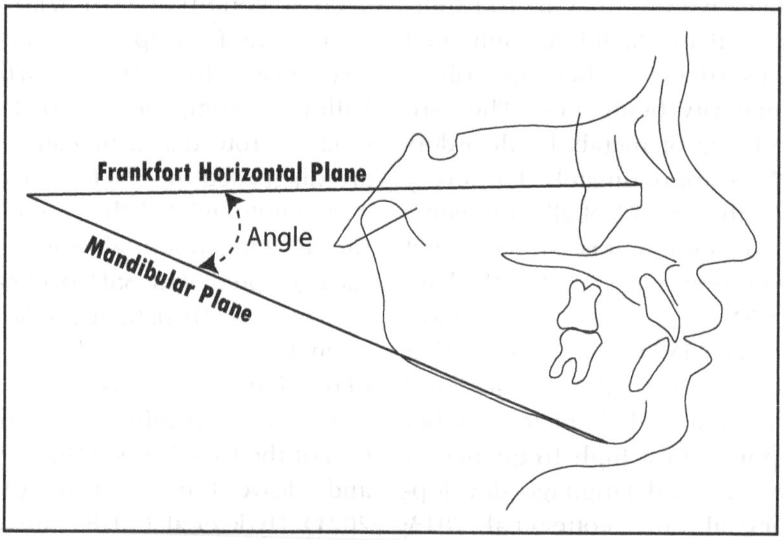

Figure 11–4. The Frankfort-mandibular angle (the angle between the Frankfort Horizontal Plane and the Mandibular Plane) is a commonly used index of facial divergence.

or separation of the cranial base and the mandible. In brief, it is proposed that the behavior of mouth breathing predisposes the craniofacial system to a particular pattern of anatomic alterations.

Evidence is accruing to support the hypothesis that mouth breathing in children can lead to alterations in craniofacial and dentofacial anatomy. In a systematic review and meta-analysis Zhao et al. (2021) identified the following anatomic features: backward and downward rotation of the mandible and maxilla, a steep occlusal plane, labial inclination of the upper anterior teeth, and airway stenosis (i.e., blockage of the airway). Table 11–2 summarizes studies on the craniofacial correlates and consequences of mouth breathing and other respiratory dysfunctions.

The consequences of mouth breathing go beyond anatomic changes, as mouth breathing has been associated with a variety of health and developmental issues including learning difficulties (Achmad & Ansar, 2021; Ribeiro et al., 2016), speech and language problems (Alhazmi, 2022; Borox et al., 2018; Lundeborg et al., 2009), asthma (Araújo et al., 2020), upper respiratory tract infections (Kukwa et al., 2018), and periodontal disease (Mummolo et al., 2020). It is difficult to know the number of children at risk for these conditions because estimates of the prevalence of mouth breathing in children range from a low of 4% to 6% (Garde et al., 2014; Kharbanda et al., 2003) to a high of 40% or 50% or greater (Abreu et al., 2008; De Menezes et al., 2006; Felcar et al., 2010; Savian et al., 2021). Breastfeeding appears to be a protective factor (Savian et al., 2021). It has been suggested that speech-language pathologists and other professionals should be involved in identifying and treating habitual mouth breathing and/or sleep-disordered breathing (Alhazmi, 2022; Bonuck et al., 2021; Mohammed et al., 2021). Alhazmi (2022) recommended that mouth-breathing children should be monitored through a multidisciplinary approach to prevent the adverse effects and improve overall development.

Oral Placement Disorder (OPD)

The main feature of this disorder is difficulty in performing the oral postures and movements for speech and other oral behaviors. Children with OPD may not respond to stimulability techniques such as imitation and instruction. The term was coined by U.S. speech-language pathologists Diane Bahr and Sara Rosenfeld-Johnson (Bahr & Rosenfeld-Johnson, 2010). Because few published studies have appeared on OPD, little is known about its prevalence or etiology.

Orofacial Myofunctional Disorders (OMDs)

Orofacial myofunctional disorders (OMDs) are "patterns involving oral and orofacial musculature that interfere with normal growth, development, or function of orofacial structures, or call attention to themselves (Mason, n.d., quoted by the American Speech-Language-Hearing Association (n.d.) https://www.asha.org/practice-portal/clinical-topics/orofacial-myofunctional-disorders/) OMDs may have direct or indirect effects on various structures and functions, including breastfeeding, facial skeletal growth

Table 11–2. Craniofacial and Oral Features Associated With Mouth Breathing, as Reported in Several Studies

Source/Feature	Facial Profile	Incisor Inclination	Lip Dysfunction	Overjet	Mandibular Rotation or Retrusion	Reduced Airway Space	Palatal Anomaly
Acharya et al. (2018)	X	X	X	X	X		X
Basheer et al. (2014)	X	X	X				
Cattoni et al. (2007)			X				X
Chambi-Rocha et al. (2018)				X			X
D'Ascanio et al. (2010)	X			X			X
Drevenek et al. (2005)	X	X					
Faria et al. (2002)					X		
Grippaudo et al. (2016)				X			
Harari et al. (2010)	X				X		
Juliano et al., (2009)		X			X	X	
Junqueira et al. (2010)			X				
Lione et al. (2015)							X
Muñoz & Orta (2014)					X	X	
Zicari et al. (2009)					X		X

and development, chewing, swallowing, speech, occlusion, temporomandibular joint movement, oral hygiene, stability of orthodontic treatment, and facial esthetics. The causes of orofacial myofunctional disorders (OMDs) are multifactorial but a common underlying factor is a low resting and functioning tongue related to genetic anomalies such as tongue tie, cleft palate, craniofacial abnormalities, and various syndromes. Factors that may cause, or are caused by, OMDs include oral habits (thumb sucking, sucking on objects), extended use of bottle or pacifier, mouth breathing, and airway constrictions (e.g., allergies, sinusitis, enlarged tonsils, or adenoids, deviated septum). There have been few studies of the prevalence of OMDs in the school-aged population of children, but a study published in 1998 on children in grades kindergarten through six (Wadsworth et al., 1998) reported relatively high prevalence of tongue thrust swallow (50.5%), open bite (24%), and abnormal resting posture of the tongue (59%). The authors concluded that SLPs in public schools are likely to find some type of OMD in about half of the children in their caseload. In a systematic review of studies of OMD and articulation disorders in children with malocclusions, Thijs et al. (2022) concluded that there is a relationship between anterior open bite and apico alveolar articulatory distortions, and between anterior open bite and atypical swallowing. Shortland et al. (2021) reviewed evidence on the use of orofacial myofunctional therapy and myofunctional devices in speech therapy and concluded that most of the studies are case reports on fewer than 10 participants, but that these techniques may yield positive outcomes, especially when used in combination with other therapies.

Conclusions

1. Speech disorders and differences in children are associated with a host of medical, educational, and social factors. The disorders and conditions considered in this chapter are by no means exhaustive, but they are ones that are likely to come to the attention of speech-language specialists. Although speech is a relatively robust human behavior, it can be compromised by numerous factors with potentially long-lasting consequences.
2. Some of the disorders and conditions discussed in this chapter are relatively rare, but others are moderately or highly prevalent. Some of those with higher prevalence are hearing loss, orofacial myopathic disorders, and malocclusions, all of which can have an impact on speech development and may contribute individually or together with other conditions to result in a speech disorder.
3. Several disorders discussed in this chapter are highly complex, affecting different aspects of speech and language, and often comorbid with other conditions such as hearing loss, intellectual disability, attention deficit and hyperactivity disorder, or ASD. Clinical services are often multidisciplinary to meet the needs of children who have these disorders.
4. Disorders in which two or more subsystems of speech production (respiratory, laryngeal, articulatory, prosodic) are affected include cerebral palsy, Down syndrome, fetal alcohol syndrome, fragile X

syndrome, and inherited metabolic disorder. Multisystem involvement poses challenges for both clinical assessment and treatment.

5. Speech disorders are generally described and classified according to salient auditory-perceptual features, but studies using instrumental methods such as kinematics and acoustics reveal features that are not always perceptually evident. For example, variability at the motor level has been reported for ASD, CAS, cerebral palsy, and developmental stuttering.
6. Advances in genetics and genomics are shedding new light on speech, language, and hearing disorders, which are associated with a variety of monogenic or multigene patterns of inheritance.
7. Disorders associated with neurological dysfunctions may be understood in the evolving field of developmental neuroscience of speech (mentioned in other chapters).

12

PREVENTION, TREATMENT, AND CLINICAL DECISION MAKING

This chapter covers the main topics of prevention and treatment of speech disorders in children and considers them in the context of clinical decision making for children's speech disorders. Therapies for these disorders have a long history and they have proliferated in recent years. Clinicians can choose from many different approaches, depending on client characteristics, therapeutic goals, available resources, levels of evidence, and other factors.

Evidence-Based Practice (EPB)

Because **evidence-based practice (EPB)** is the guideline and benchmark for clinical interventions, this chapter notes EPB concepts, illustrated in Figure 12–1. The pillars of EBP are research evidence, clinical knowledge and expertise, individual needs and personal preferences of the clients, and available resources. Research evidence pertains primarily to

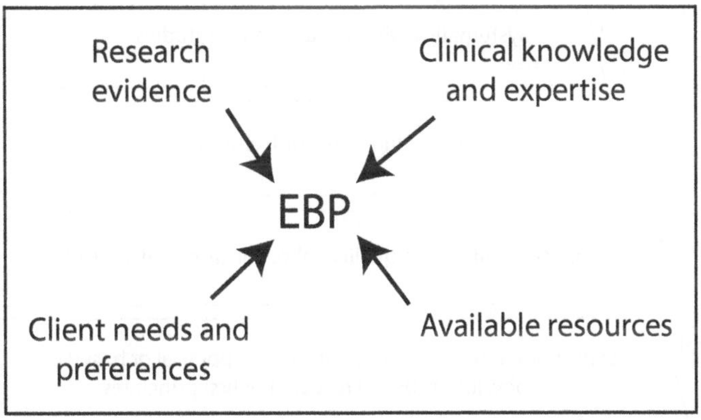

Figure 12–1. The pillars of evidence-based practice (EBP).

peer-reviewed studies relevant to a specific disorder or condition (see following discussion of levels of evidence). Clinical knowledge and expertise are based on the education and experience of an individual clinician. Client needs and personal experiences are unique to individuals, and it may not always be easy to determine these attributes for children. As noted in the Preface, clinical services often are adult centric in the sense that adults usually identify the needs and goals of treatment. Children may not be able to address these issues and must rely on the judgments of adults. Available resources are the conditions of service delivery and vary widely across settings. Even when a treatment is supported by research, conforms to a clinician's experience, and meets the goals and preferences of a client, it may not be feasible to deliver the treatment because of economic or other limitations.

Levels of evidence (LoE) is shown as the classic pyramid diagram in Figure 12–2. The different levels of the pyramid represent different LoE, with expert opinion at the base and meta-analyses and

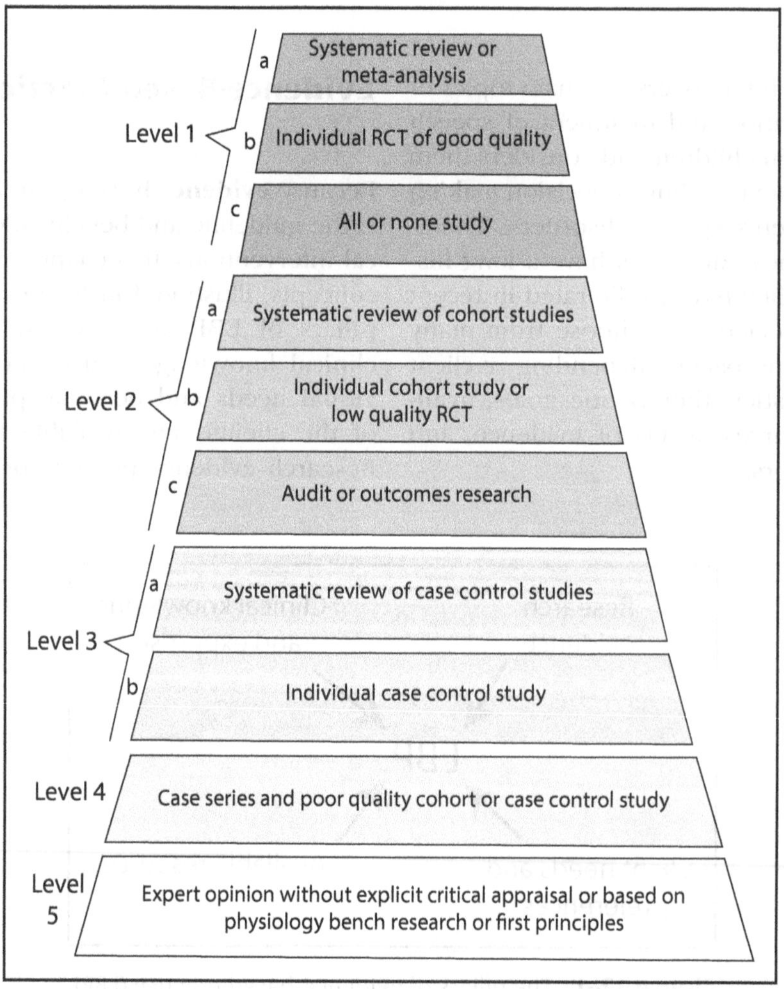

Figure 12–2. The levels of evidence (LoE) pyramid.

systematic reviews at the apex. In an ideal world, a clinician would be able to link a particular treatment with its corresponding LoE. As is the case for many clinical specialties, the evidence for speech disorders is not sufficient to provide higher levels of evidence for all treatments, but the evidence base is growing, and clinicians should be alert to newly reported data. Brief comments on LoE for different therapies are included in this chapter, but it is expected (and hoped!) that the information reported here will be quickly outdated as new data appear. Given delays in production, printed books can never be completely up to date and are, therefore, not the optimum means of disseminating current evidence. A further limitation is that the evidence base is uneven across types of speech disorders and across children's ages. DeVeney and Peterkin (2022) note that,

> Given the scarcity of empirical support available for children under the age of 3 years across all the intervention approaches reviewed, it is difficult to recommend an intervention approach for targeting speech sound productions with children in this young age group. (p. 669)

Missing from Figure 12–2 are detailed analyses of the single-subject design study (SSDS). These studies differ from one another in several ways, but they generally have the features illustrated in Figure 12–3. The dependent variable (the *y*-axis of the graph) is measured repeatedly at regular intervals over time (the *x*-axis). The study is divided into distinct phases, in which the participant is tested under one condition for each phase. The conditions are often designated by capital letters (e.g., A, B, C). Figure 12–3 shows a study called a reversal design in which the participant is tested first in condition A, then tested in condition B, and finally retested in the original condition A. As noted by Byiers et al. (2012), "The analysis of experimental control in all SSEDs is based on visual comparison between

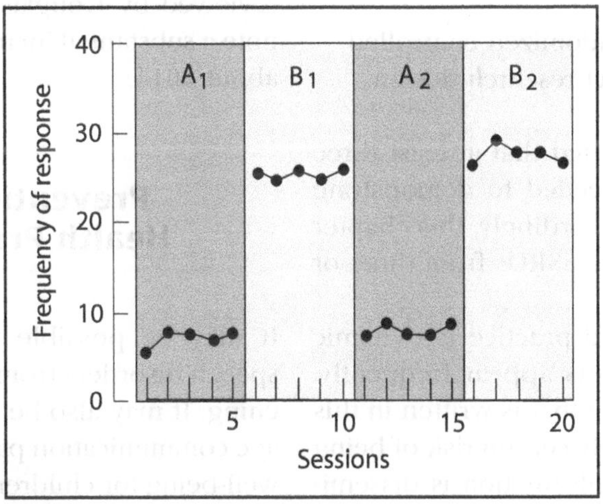

Figure 12–3. Single-subject design study called a reversal design, in which the participant is tested first in condition A, then tested in condition B, and finally retested in the original condition A.

two or more conditions. The conditions tested typically include a baseline condition, during which no intervention is in place, as well as one or more intervention conditions" (p. 398). A major attraction of SSDS is that it is applicable to clinical settings in which it is desired to measure the outcome of an intervention for an individual client. Detailed information on SSDS is available in Tate and Perdices (2019).

Levels of evidence for SSDS were proposed by Logan et al. (2008) and are summarized in the following (clear-cut results are assumed for each level).

Level 1. Randomized controlled N-of-1 (RCT), alternating treatment, and concurrent or nonconcurrent multiple baseline designs.

Level 2. Nonrandomized, controlled, concurrent multiple baseline designs.

Level 3. Nonrandomized, nonconcurrent, controlled multiple baseline designs.

Level 4. Nonrandomized, controlled SSRDs with at least three phases (ABA, ABAB, BAB, etc.).

Level 5. Nonrandomized controlled AB single-subject research design.

Logan et al. suggested that at least three participants are needed to demonstrate generalizability. Accordingly, this chapter reports results from SSRDs from three or more participants.

Evidence-based practice is dynamic because new reports appear frequently. Therefore, anything that is written in this book stands a nearly certain risk of being outdated as new information is disseminated. Fortunately, tools available to SLPs and others can help considerably to provide updated information. The American Speech-Language-Hearing Association provides two valuable resources in this regard: *The Practice Portal* and *Evidence Maps* (https://www.asha.org/practice/).

Implementation Science

As important as EBP is to clinical practice, it is not sufficient to ensure that an evidence base is incorporated in routine clinical practice and public policy. **Implementation science** is a set of strategies aimed to move evidence-based interventions into practice in clinical or community settings, thereby addressing the gap that often exists between research evidence and clinical practice. Bauer and Kirchner (2020) point out that uptake of an intervention is strongly affected by contextual factors that go beyond intervention effectiveness. A major goal of implementation science is to identify barriers and facilitators that influence the uptake of evidence-based innovation. The emerging role of implementation science in disorders of communication is reviewed by Douglas et al. (2022), who note a substantial increase in activity since about 2014.

Prevention and Health Promotion

It may be possible to prevent certain speech disorders from occurring or worsening. It may also be possible to encourage communication patterns that promote well-being for children and their families. This section considers types of prevention and the role of well-being with respect to communication disorders in children.

Types of Prevention

Prevention is complementary to treatment in that both have the goal of reducing the burden of mental, emotional, and behavioral disorders on the developing child. Prevention takes five forms, as follows.

Primordial Prevention is the most recently described preventive strategy and pertains to reducing risk factors in an entire population by focusing on social and environmental conditions that are typically implemented through laws and policies for health and education. Primordial prevention can be especially relevant to children as a means of minimizing risk exposure. Examples of primordial prevention are steps to reduce family poverty, eliminate exposure to toxic chemicals, such as lead in paint, and discourage alcohol consumption during pregnancy.

Primary Prevention is directed toward a susceptible population or individual, with the purpose of preventing the occurrence of a disease or disorder. It usually targets healthy individuals and entails activities that reduce risk exposure or increase the immunity of individuals at risk to prevent a disease or disorder from progressing in a susceptible individual. An example is advising parents on ways to promote their children's communication skills through activities such as reading aloud from age-appropriate books.

Secondary Prevention emphasizes early detection, usually targeting healthy-appearing or typically developing individuals with subclinical forms of the disorder. The subclinical disorder consists of pathologic changes or features of atypical development, but without overt symptoms leading to a diagnosis. Secondary prevention often takes the form of screenings, such as a screening for hearing loss.

Tertiary Prevention targets both the clinical and outcome stages of a disease or disorder. It does not necessarily change the disorder but can reduce the effects of the disorder and improve functional outcomes. It is implemented in affected individuals and is designed to reduce the severity of the disorder as well as of any associated sequelae. Examples are communication intervention for children with conditions such as Down syndrome, fragile X syndrome, or hearing loss.

Quaternary Prevention is an action that protects individuals from interventions that are likely to cause more harm than good. The term was coined by the Belgian family physician Marc Jamoulle, who sought to avoid or mitigate the consequences of unnecessary or excessive interventions such as over-diagnosis or over-treatment (Jamoulle, 2015). An undesirable outcome of such interventions is **iatrogeny**, an unfavorable outcome of intervention in which the patient or client is injured or harmed from the treatment. Quaternary prevention is consistent with the health care principle of *primun non nocere* (from the Latin, meaning "first do no harm") and the bioethical principle of **nonmaleficence** (meaning to avoid needless harm or injury through acts of commission or omission).

Resources on Prevention

Although prevention of communication disorders is considered a professional responsibility of speech-language pathologists (American Speech-Language-Hearing Association, 1988), there are few systematic programs that cover the different aspects of prevention. Helpful resources for such program development include the following: basic information on prevention strategies (Kisling & Das, 2022), precision or personalized prevention (August & Gewirtz, 2019), screening programs (Skarżyński & Piotrowska, 2012), language nutrition (Bang et al., 2020), and gender-related clinical services (Zanon et al., 2019).

Promotion of Health and Well-Being

According to the World Health Organization (1988), health promotion is "the process of enabling people to increase control over, and to improve their health." Well-being can be similarly defined as the process of enabling people to increase control over, and to improve their well-being. Well-being is synonymous with positive mental health, which the World Health Organization (2001) defines as "a state of well-being in which the individual realizes his or her own abilities, can cope with the normal stresses of life, can work productively and fruitfully, and is able to make a contribution to his or her community." This definition needs modification for application to children, but the basic concepts common to persons of all ages are self-realization of abilities, coping with life stresses, and satisfying family and social experiences.

Parameters of the Treatment of Speech Disorders

Treatments generally can be described with respect to five major parameters: (1) goal or target of treatment, (2) method of treatment, (3) form of service delivery, (4) support, and (5) outcome measures. Each is discussed in the following.

Goal or Target of Treatment

The goals in treatment of speech disorders range broadly, including the phonetic level (e.g., improved production on /r/), phonological patterns (e.g., correct voicing of syllable-final stops), prosody (e.g., satisfactory production of strong-weak syllables), and intelligibility or comprehensibility (e.g., being understood by unfamiliar listeners). For school-aged children, the goal often is incorporated in an Individualized Education Program (IEP). It is often the case that goals and subgoals are laid out in a sequence or hierarchy, such that progress in one goal establishes the foundation for achieving another goal. Whatever the goal may be, it is important that it is expressed clearly to guide and assess other aspects of the treatment program. Practice patterns for target selection are reviewed by McLeod and Baker (2014).

Method of Treatment

This chapter reviews many different treatments that have been designed for children's speech disorders. Therapeutic methods have been grouped in various ways, such as in the following examples.

1. ASHA (n.d.) for speech sound disorders: articulation approaches, phonological/language-based approaches.
2. Rvachew and Brosseau-Lapré, (2018) for developmental phonological disorders: input-oriented procedures, output-oriented procedures, and phonological procedures.
3. Wren et al. (2018) for speech sound disorders: environmental, auditory–perceptual, cognitive–linguistic, production, and integrated.

4. Cabbage and DeVeney (2020) for speech sound disorders: traditional motor articulatory-based approach, phonologically based approaches, and complexity.
5. Bernthal et al. (2022) for articulatory and phonological disorders: motor-based approaches, linguistically based approaches, phonological awareness, language and dialectal variations, accent modifications.

Other sources simply list interventions with little or no attempt at grouping (Bauman-Waengler & Garcia, 2019; Williams et al., 2010). A difficulty with grouping is that some treatments include more than one type of intervention, for example, a treatment may include both auditory-perceptual and motor-based approaches. Groupings can be helpful in decision making if they are based on robust and clearly identified concepts. Their utility diminishes if the boundaries between them are blurred. The approach taken here is to list the different treatments alphabetically and to comment on affinities and differences.

Forms of Service Delivery

The main forms of service delivery are individual, group, family support, telepractice, and computer assisted. These may be used in different sequences or combinations to achieve the treatment goals. There have been relatively few studies of the effectiveness of various types of service delivery, but evidence reviews are available for parent-assisted intervention (Klatte et al., 2020; Sugden et al., 2016), and remote or telehealth therapy for CAS (Bahar et al., 2022; Parnandi et al., 2015) and SSD (Coufal et al., 2018).

Support

Support means the resources available to facilitate and reinforce the treatment. Examples of support are family members, peers, and teachers. These individuals may not necessarily be directly involved in treatment, but they can help to ensure supportive environments and opportunities for monitoring.

Outcome Measures

Measures of the outcome of an intervention can take several different forms, depending on the type of intervention, client characteristics, and purpose of outcome determination. The World Health Organization defines an **outcome measure** as a "change in the health of an individual, group of people, or population that is attributable to an intervention or series of interventions." The broad definition pertains especially to health care, and typical outcome measures used by health care organizations that include mortality, readmission, patient experience, and days of hospitalization. But for speech-language services, an outcome is better defined as the effect, whether positive or negative, of an intervention delivered to an individual or a group of individuals. The Royal College of Speech and Language Therapists (RCSLT) (Gascoigne, 2015) and the Commissioning Support Programme (2011) describe three types of measures used to commission speech, language and communication services or to evaluate the outcomes of service provision: (1) the user's reported experience of services received (e.g., client-reported or parent-reported outcomes), (2) the achievement of therapy/intervention goals rated by the clinician (e.g., ratings with the ASHA

NOMS), and (3) directly measured impact of services on a client's speech, language and communication skills, attainment and well-being (e.g., documenting changes in the WHO system). The Commissioning Support Programme (2011) further suggests that a "balanced scorecard" of outcomes measures probably would consist of all three types of measures.

Tools or measures used to assess outcomes in treating children's speech disorders include the following:

1. ASHA NOMS for pediatric speech-language pathology (Mullen & Schooling, 2010)
2. Focus on the Outcomes of Communication Under Six (FOCUS; Thomas-Stonell et al., 2013).
3. Therapy Outcome Measure (TOM; John, 2011; Moyse et al., 2020).
4. ICF and ICF-children and youth (McLeod & McCormack, 2007).
5. Ratings of intelligibility along with PCC (Lousada et al., 2014), with intelligibility proposed as an end-point outcome measure and PCC used to mark change along the intervention trajectory.
6. The three dimensions of outcome: ultimate, intermediate, and instrumental (Rosen & Proctor, 1978, 1981). Ultimate outcomes are primary or long-term treatment objectives, intermediate outcomes are specific behaviors or states that are believed to be needed for progress in the intervention process, and instrumental outcomes are those effects of intervention that are expected to lead necessarily to other outcomes without further intervention. Campbell and Bain (1991) discuss these dimensions as they relate to decisions to terminate treatment in speech and language disorders. various patient-reported outcomes.

There are many opportunities for improvements in the use of outcome measures. Kearney et al. (2015) conducted a narrative review of outcome measures for studies of SSD with a motor basis. Of the 66 reports selected for analysis, the majority used perceptual methods to measure change at the impairment level of the ICF-CY and only three studies examined outcomes at the participation level. The authors emphasized the need for "accurate outcome measures that reflect the underlying deficit of the SSD as well as activity/participation level factors need to be implemented to document intervention success in this population" (p. 252). Measures at the impairment level should be sensitive to the underlying features of the disorder, and measures at the activity/participation level should be used more often. There are practical obstacles to the routine use of outcome measures in clinical practice. In a systematic review on facilitators and barriers to use of outcome measures in allied health, Duncan and Murray (2012) identified four major themes: (1) clinicians' knowledge about and perceived value for the outcome measure; (2) organization priority; (3) practical constraints including time and resources; and (4) patient considerations (such as perceived relevancy to patients care). Similar barriers may pertain to speech-language services. Kwok et al. (2022) interviewed clinicians on the use of a preschool outcome measure and identified barriers within three major domains: (1) environmental context and resources (e.g., difficulties incorporating the outcome measure into assessment sessions and intervention schedules); (2) beliefs about consequences (e.g., beliefs concerning the relevance of the measure to clinical practice); and (3) social influences (e.g., administration of the measure may interfere with rapport with families). The authors also noted the influence of facilitators in two major domains: (1) behavioral regulation (e.g., a reminder system to encourage use of the measure), and (2) environmental context and resources (e.g., availability of administrative personnel and technology support). The TOM mentioned earlier addresses the four components of: impairment (problems in body function or structure, such as deviation or loss); activity (difficulties in performing activities); participation (problems in the manner or extent of involvement in performing activities); and well-being (emotional effects resulting in upset, distress, or dissatisfaction with status).

Outcome measures for adults include patient-reported outcomes (Cohen & Hula, 2019) and universal-reporter outcome measures (Macefield et al., 2019), but such measures are not easily used for children of different ages and cognitive abilities. For that matter, attitudes of children toward communication disorders and therapy for these disorders is understudied, but some progress has been made (Lyons & Roulstone, 2018; Merrick & Roulstone, 2011). Klatte et al. (2020) report on a collaboration between parents and speech-language clinicians to determine therapy outcomes.

Treatment of Speech Disorders: Specific Methods

Treatments that have been used for children's speech disorders are summarized in the following, including a brief description of the method, typical clinical populations, and available evidence. Some of the treatments were developed for a specific clinical population, but most of the treatments are potentially applicable across disorder types. In addition, it is possible to use two or more therapies in combination to meet the therapeutic goals for an individual child. Entries are listed alphabetically.

Biofeedback

Biofeedback is a process that enables an individual to learn how to change physiological activity or behavior for the purposes of improving health and performance. The information that is fed back can be of several different types including physiological activity (e.g., brainwaves, heart function, breathing, muscle activity, and skin temperature) or sensory information (e.g., visual, auditory, tactile). The information is not necessarily subject to conscious awareness but can be displayed visually or presented auditorily to provide opportunities for monitoring or trial-and-error learning. In applications to speech-language pathology, biofeedback treatment has been used primarily with information derived from acoustic, electromyographic, and ultrasound methods. Helpful overview papers are a tutorial on visual-acoustic biofeedback (Hitchcock et al., 2023) and a clinical framework for SLPs (Allen et al., 2022).

Figure 12–4 illustrates several types of feedback that have been, or could be, used in treating speech disorders. Each type of feedback relates to a specific level of speech production. Biofeedback generally requires specialized instruments that may not be readily available to all or most SLPs. The biofeedback signals shown in Figure 12–4 are summarized as follows.

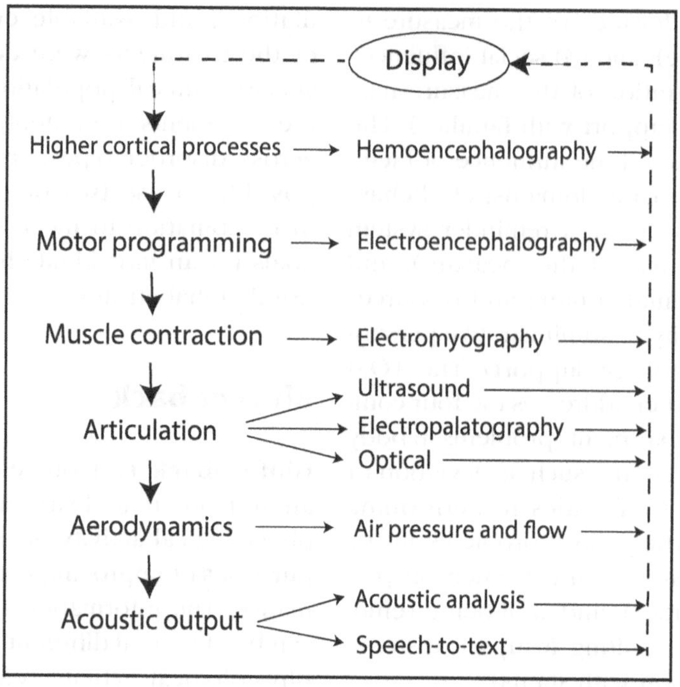

Figure 12–4. Types of biofeedback for treating speech disorders.

Hemoencephalography (HEG; Toomim, 2000) detects changes in frontal cerebral blood circulation and oxygenation using either passive infrared HEG or near infrared HEG. It is a form of **neurofeedback**, a type of biofeedback in which self-control of neural functions is achieved through feedback on brain activity. HEG has been used to accomplish self-regulation of cortical activation for treatment of ADHD, depression, and migraine. It is also much simpler to set up and monitor than electroencephalography (see the following item).

Electroencephalography (EEG) records electrical activity arising from the brain. This method has very good temporal sensitivity and is therefore well suited to study dynamic cerebral functioning. **Quantitative Electroencephalography (qEEG)** records neural activity from multiple electrodes and processes the signals with computer methods to produce displays such as color maps of brain functioning called "brain maps."

Electromyography (EMG) is a recording of electrical activity in a muscle, which is accomplished with electrodes that are inserted into, or placed over, a muscle of interest. Each electrode has two poles, and the differences in the electrical field between the poles reflects the firings of motor units. Needle electrodes are inserted into a muscle, whereas surface electrodes are attached to the skin overlying a muscle. For further discussion, see Ludlow et al. (2019).

Ultrasound and electropalatography (EPG) (both discussed in Chapter 4) are the primary means of biofeedback for articulatory positions and movements. Both require specialized instrumentation but ultrasound for speech can often be accomplished with ultrasound equipment that has general medical applications and is, therefore, available in many health care settings. EPG requires fitting and fabrication of a pseudopalate that contains embedded electrodes. Optic methods also have been used, as in the example of nasopharyngoscopy in which clients can observe their own velopharyngeal function.

The aerodynamics of speech production can be assessed with measures of air pressure, airflow, or volume. Specialized instrumentation is required but commercially available systems facilitate clinical application. Basic measures and procedures are described in Ludlow et al. (2019).

The acoustic output of speech can be analyzed with acoustic methods to display waveforms, spectra, spectrograms, or other graphic forms. Another alternative is to use speech-to-text methods in which the speech signal is processed by algorithms to yield an orthographic output. See Chapter 4 for general discussion of acoustic methods for the study of speech.

Table 12–1 summarizes selected studies reporting results from more than one child (assuming that generalization is possible when at least three participants are involved; Logan et al., 2008). Sugden et al. (2019) reported a systematic review of ultrasound visual biofeedback for treating speech sound disorders. Nearly half of the 29 studies included in the review were single-case experimental designs, and the largest number of participants was 13. Sugden et al. (2019) concluded that this therapy may be an effective adjunct to therapy for some individuals whose speech errors were not effectively treated with other therapies. A major barrier to the clinical application of biofeedback is the need for specialized equipment (Dugan et al., 2023).

Complexity

Complexity in relation to speech and language disorders has been defined in several ways, including age-of-acquisition, linguistic complexity, word frequency, and markedness (the last of these is discussed in Chapter 7). Common to these is the idea that complex forms contain or imply simpler forms, so that learning a complex form brings about improvements in simpler forms related to it. A rough analogy is the Matryoshka dolls (also called stacking dolls or nesting dolls), in which dolls of varying size are contained within one another. The largest doll contains all the other dolls, which conveys the essential idea of complexity. If one has the largest doll, all the other dolls come with it. Similarly, a complex form often contains simpler forms that compose it.

Following Rescher (1998), Gierut (2007) defines complexity from three perspectives: (1) an epistemic perspective pertaining to a description of a system (e.g., the number of descriptor terms that define the system); (2) an ontological perspective that identifies the constituent elements of a system and their hierarchical organization; and (3) a functional perspective that specifies the principles governing a system and the corresponding degrees of freedom allowed in that system. Complexity in language acquisition is often related to Pinker's (1984) writings on **language learnability**, which seeks to understand the mental operations needed for children to learn the grammar of their language based on input from adults. Pinker's solution to this problem was to propose a single framework that

Table 12–1. Selected Studies of Biofeedback Therapies for Speech Disorders in Children

Authors	Design and Participants	Type of Feedback and Treatment Goal	Results of Treatment
Byun & Hitchcock (2012)	Single-subject design; 11 children with misarticulation of /ɹ/	Acoustic for production of /ɹ/	8 children made measurable gains in the accuracy of isolated /r/ produced within treatment, with 4 showing significant generalization to untreated /r/ in words.
Cleland et al. (2019)	15 children variety of errors. We therefore employed a target selection strategy to treat the most frequent lingual error.	Visual ultrasound feedback for lingual articulation	Effect sizes for percentage of target segments correct ranged from no effect (5 children), small effect (1 child), medium effect (4 children), and large effect (5 children).
Cleland et al. (2015)	A case series of seven different children (aged 6 to 11) with persistent speech sound disorders were evaluated.	For each child, high-speed ultrasound (121 fps), audio and lip video recordings were made while probing each child's specific errors at five different time points (before, during, and after intervention).	After intervention, all the children made significant progress on targeted segments, evidenced by both perceptual measures and changes in tongue-shape.
Findley & Gasparyan (2022)	Multiple baselilne design for 3 children aged 7 to 9 years with /ɹ/ or /l/ errors	Text-to-speech feedback	All children had increased accuracy of target sound and generalized production to untrained words.
Kabakoff et al. (2022)	25 children aged 9 to14 years	Ultrasound for /ɹ/ production	A measure of tongue shape complexity predicted accuracy of /ɹ/, such that higher tongue shape complexity was associated with lower accuracy at pretreatment but higher accuracy at posttreatment.

Table 12–1. *continued*

Authors	Design and Participants	Type of Feedback and Treatment Goal	Results of Treatment
McAllister et al. (2022)	33 individuals aged 9 to 15 years with residual distortions of /ɹ/.	A course of individual intervention comprising 1 week of intensive traditional treatment and 9 weeks of ultrasound biofeedback treatment	Two major clusters were identified" (1) "low stimulability" cluster had very low accuracy at baseline, minimal response to traditional treatment, and strong response to ultrasound biofeedback; (2) "high stimulability" group was more accurate at baseline and made significant gains in both traditional and ultrasound biofeedback phases of treatment.
Neumann & Romonath (2012)	Systematic review; 6 studies using nasopharyngo-scopic biofeedback in clients with cleft lip and palate and velopharyngeal dysfunction	Optical feedback derived from nasopharyngoscopy	Low LoE showing that nasopharyngoscopy may be effective only in combination with traditional speech therapy.
Peterson et al. (2022)	4 children with misarticulation of /ɹ/	Visual-acoustic with mobile app	All participants showed a clinically significant response to the overall treatment package, with effect sizes ranging from moderate to very large. One participant showed a significant advantage for biofeedback over nonbiofeedback treatment, although the order of treatment delivery poses a potential confound for interpretation in this case.
Preston, Hitchcock, & Leece (2020)	36 children ages 8 to 16 years with /ɹ/ distortions	Ultrasound for /ɹ/ production, with or without auditory perceptual training	Similar gains in speech sound accuracy with or without auditory perceptual training
Preston et al. (2017)	Single-subject design; 6 children with CAS	Ultrasound for speech sounds	Positive outcome for visual ultrasound feedback and prosodic variation

unifies the influence of the structure of a language, the computational problems involved in language learning, and the path of child development.

The basic assumption of complexity in speech and language therapy is that treating complex targets produces changes not only in the complex targets themselves but also in simpler targets that are not targeted for treatment but are implied by the more complex targets. Figure 12–5 illustrates this idea with a simple network diagram in which three levels are represented by different shades of gray. The most basic level, shown as white circles, represents sound features that typically are acquired early in development. The next level, shown as medium gray circles, is the next developmental stage. The third level, shown as dark gray circles, is the last stage acquired in typical development. A treatment planned to follow the typical developmental pattern of speech might begin with the circles labeled 1 and 2, then proceed to the circles labeled b and c, and conclude with the circle labeled A. But from the complexity perspective, treatment would begin with circle A on the assumption that treating at this level would facilitate improvements at the other levels (circles b and C and circles 1 and 2).

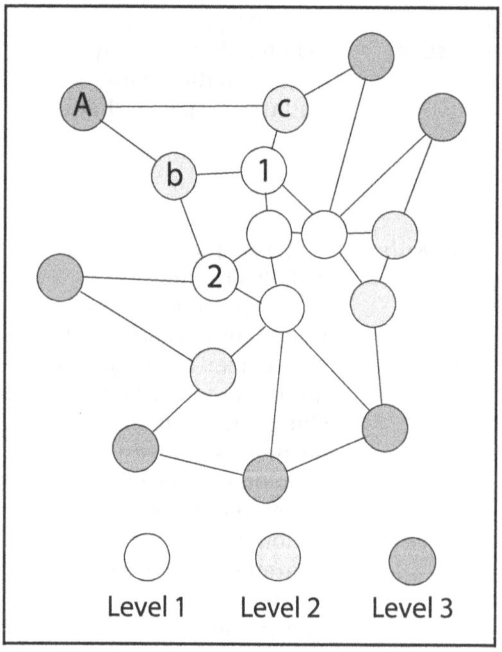

Figure 12–5. Network diagram to illustrate complexity, in which three levels are represented by different shades of gray. The most basic level, shown as white circles, represents sound features that are typically acquired early in development. The next level, shown as medium gray circles, is the next developmental stage. The third level, shown as dark gray circles, is the last stage acquired in typical development.

Complexity as an intervention has a wide spectrum of applications, including phonology, lexical-semantics, and syntax (Thompson, 2007). Gierut (2001) wrote that a strong form of the complexity hypothesis is that "complexity may be the fundamental way in which the human mind acquires, learns, processes, or retrieves information" (p. 231). Complexity offers a different perspective on target selection compared to the traditional approach of selecting targets in keeping with typical patterns of acquisition (often called the developmental approach). For example, if a child has errors on both stops and fricatives, the developmental approach typically selects stops as the first treatment target because stops are acquired before fricatives (see Chapter 4). An approach based on complexity would select fricatives as the first treatment target on the assumption that improving the production of fricatives would entail improvements for stops as well. Suggestions on implementing complexity in speech sound disorders are available in Gierut (1992, 1998, 2001, 2007) and Storkel (2018). Storkel (2018) provides a detailed discussion of target selection based on complexity, including resources for clinical implementation. She notes that treatment of targets that are late-acquired, marked, low-accuracy, or nonstimulable can facilitate system-wide change in phonology. Related discussion is under the subheadings *Contrast Therapy* and *Empty Set Therapy* in this chapter.

Although complexity has been shown to have favorable outcomes for speech sound disorders (Baker & McLeod, 2011; Kamhi, 2006; Maggu et al., 2021), this approach does not appear to be widely adopted in clinical practice, possibly because of lack of familiarity (Brumbaugh & Smit, 2013) or because it runs counter to popular (and perhaps more intuitive) approaches, such as those based on typical order of speech sound acquisition. Increased adoption may come about because of systematic descriptions of implementation (Storkel, 2018) and evidence of positive outcomes (Maggu et al., 2021). The meta-analysis of 12 studies by Maggu et al. (2021) revealed that exposure to complex input promoted production of complex sounds and facilitated production of simpler sounds that were not treated. Complexity is promoted by the following factors: greater markedness, higher word frequency, poor stimulability, articulatory difficulty, greater consistency of error, and later acquisition in typical development.

Computer-Aided Therapy

Computer-aided therapy for speech disorders in children relies primarily on the tools of speech technology, the branch of information technology pertaining to the study and practice of designing, implementing, using, and evaluating computer-based systems that allow humans and computers to interact through speech. These tools are typically a form of therapy delivery that implements specific treatments such as those described in this chapter. Therefore, computer-aided therapy is defined by both content (method of therapy) and the interaction between client and computer. Progress in this area is swift, and a variety of apps are available for clinical use. Examples of computer-aided therapy are digital games for speech therapy (Ahmed et al., 2018; Saeedi et al., 2022), automatic speech recognition (Kitzing et al., 2009), apps (Du et al., 2022; Furlong et al., 2018), and specialized systems (Attwell et al., 2023; Bílková et al., 2022; Deka et al., 2022; Saz et al., 2009). Studies of efficacy are limited, but positive outcomes have been reported for some children (Furlong et al., 2017; Jesus et al., 2019). As choices proliferate, clinicians would benefit from guidelines on the selection of therapy aids suited to individual children.

Contrast or Opposition Therapy

Contrast therapy (also known as **opposition therapy**) selects as targets speech sounds that differ in one or more features. The selected sounds are often treated in pairs. The **minimal pair approach** selects sounds that differ in a single feature, such as voicing (e.g., /t/ paired with /d/) or manner of articulation (e.g., /t/ paired with /s/). Clinicians typically select two or more exemplars for a given feature (e.g., *tea-see, tip-sip, toe-sew*, for a /t/-/s/ contrast). Elbert et al., (1991) concluded that three exemplars were sufficient for most of the phonologically impaired children in their sample to meet a generalization criterion. Lists of minimal pairs are available on several online sources. A **maximal opposition approach** (Gierut, 1989) selects sounds that differ in multiple dimensions of voice, place, and manner (e.g., /d/ paired with /tʃ/). As a child learns oppositions, the course of treatment may lead to minimal contrasts. Storkel (2022) reviewed studies on various approaches to contrast therapy and concluded that the minimal pair approach should be used with only those children who have a small number of errors, such as older children or children with mild SSD. She recommended the maximal opposition approach for children who have multiple errors across multiple sound classes. This approach targets global phoneme collapses that lead to reduced intelligibility. **Phoneme collapse** is defined as the substitution of one sound for many other different sounds, resulting in homonymy. An example is a child who produces the lateral sound /l/ for the targets /l w j ɹ/. Collapse can seriously affect intelligibility as phoneme distinctions are lost.

Core Vocabulary Therapy (CVT)

Core vocabulary therapy (CVT) typically focuses on the production of whole words rather than surface error patterns or specific sound features (Crosbie et al., 2005; Dodd et al., 2006; McIntosh & Dodd, 2008). The words are usually selected in collaboration with the child, family members, or teachers. An additional resource is the study of words that are most frequently produced by typically developing children. This information has been especially important in selecting items in AAC (Banajee et al., 2003; Beukelman et al., 1989; Laubscher & Light, 2020), but it also provides helpful guidelines for selecting a core vocabulary for other clinical populations, such as children with SSD. Core vocabulary words have communicative impact because they are used frequently in ordinary interactions, provide a framework for functional language (carrying potential for generalization outside the clinic), and do not require a well-developed phonological system. A relatively small number of words can have profound communicative value. Beukelman et al. (1989) reported that typically developing preschoolers produced 250 repeated words that accounted for 85% of their 3000-word samples.

Nouns are rare in published inventories, probably because children's use of nouns depends on context and varies considerably across children. Certain pronouns (e.g., the first person *I*), verbs (e.g., *is*), and function words (e.g., prepositions) have relatively high frequencies of occurrence and can play roles in emerging grammar. However, nouns can be important for individual children because they identify familiar people (siblings or friends), pets, toys, foods, and favorite games. Somewhat different conclusions have been reached on some aspects of CVT. For example, Crosbie et al. (2005) discouraged the use of imitation because it does not require a phonological plan but simply uses the provided model. However, Flanagan and Ttofari Eecen (2018) found that imitating words with sufficient accuracy involves phonological planning to ensure speech consistency.

Cycles

The **cycles approach** (Hodson, 2010, 2011; Hodson & Paden, 1991) has three essential principles: (1) selection of intervention targets and stimuli based on error patterns and typical development, (2) cyclical targeting of error patterns, and (3) use of focused auditory input combined with production–practice activities during treatment sessions. The basic components of this therapy, as outlined in Hodson (2010, 2011), Hodson and Paden (1991), and Prezas and Hodson (2010), are review practice, auditory bombardment (with slight amplification), stimulability practice, card coloring, production–practice activities, and metaphonology activities to promote phonological awareness. Home practice of two minutes daily is accomplished by giving parents the listening list and production-practice picture cards.

Studies of the efficacy of the cycles approach show results ranging from little or no gain (Tyler & Waterson, 1991) to some degree of benefit (Almost & Rosenbaum, 1998; Rudolph & Wendt, 2014; Rvachew et al., 1999; Tyler et al., 1987). Rvachew et al. (1999) observed an influence of stimulability and perception, with more than 50% of stimulable sounds and more than 60% of well-perceived sounds showing improvement, but with unstimulable sounds and poorly perceived sounds showing little improvement. The general indication is for positive outcome, but variations in method make it difficult to draw definitive conclusions from the published studies.

Dynamic Temporal and Tactile Cueing (DTTC)

Dynamic Temporal and Tactile Cueing (DTTC) is an integral stimulation approach to therapy for motor speech disorders such as CAS that combines motor learning principles, cues, and modeling to encourage correct production of speech targets (Strand, 2020). Articulation is shaped through multimodal cueing techniques (including tactile, visual, auditory, and proprioceptive cues) to promote accurate movements or gestures thar are practiced in words or phrases. DTTC considers issues such as the size of stimulus set, maximizing the number of practice trials per session, and using facilitators that are time efficient and maintain the child's attention to the clinician's face. Auditory, visual, and tactile cues can be added or faded to encourage independent production and automaticity. Targets are initially practiced at a slow speaking rate with progression to a more typical rate as accuracy improves. Practice is conducted across four levels: simultaneous production, direct imitation, delayed imitation, and spontaneous production. Integral stimulation therapies, including DTTC, have mostly been studied with single-case experimental designs, which have shown moderate-to-large treatment and generalization effects for most participants in rather small samples of children (Strand et al., 2006; Murray et al., 2014). A positive aspect of research on Integral Stimulation/ DTTC is that it includes studies across independent research groups (Murray et al., 2014).

Empty Set Therapy

Empty Set Therapy (or **Treatment of the Empty Set**) focuses therapy on target sounds that a child does not produce spontaneously or when imitating the clinician. In mathematics, a set can be defined as an empty set (also called a null set) if it doesn't contain any elements. As applied to speech sounds, the concept of empty set is that the set of target sounds is not in a child's productive repertoire (they are, of course, represented in the adult system). The rationale in using an empty set is that it challenges a child to learn concurrently two new sounds that are maximally different in terms of place, manner, and voice. It is expected that a child will have success in generalizing non-stimulable sounds that are linguistically complex and maximally distinct, as opposed to sounds that differ minimally. This reasoning is based on learnability theory, as discussed in this chapter under the heading of Complexity. The sounds selected in empty set therapy are complex because they involve maximal contrasts.

Integrated Therapy

See Multimodal Therapy.

Lee Silverman Voice Treatment (LSVT®)

Lee Silverman Voice Treatment (LSVT) is an intensive treatment program originally designed to improve vocal fold adduction and overall voice and speech production in individuals with Parkinson's disease (Fox, Morrison, et al., 2002). It has since been used with individuals with a variety of other neurological and neurodevelopmental disorders affecting speech production. The treatment is based on a simple set of tasks chosen to enhance phonatory and respiratory functions underlying speech production by instructing and encouraging clients to produce a loud voice with maximum effort during sustained phonation and a variety of speaking tasks. The program also encourages clients to monitor their vocal loudness and associated effort. LSVT LOUD was developed for speech pathology, and LSVT BIG is a similar program for physical therapy (C. Fox et al., 2012). With respect to children's speech disorders, this treatment has been used with children who have cerebral palsy or Down syndrome (Boliek et al., 2022; Langlois et al., 2020; Levy, 2014).

Metaphon

Metaphon therapy is a treatment for phonological disorders that focuses on metaphonological awareness, specifically, the child's awareness of phonological structure. The treatment focuses on the properties of sounds that need to be contrasted. Targets selected for intervention include processes related to speech intelligibility, processes that can be imitated, or processes not observed in typically developing children of the same age. The therapy is described in detail in Howell and Dean (1994) and Dean, Howell, Waters, and Reid (1995). Data on efficacy were reported by Dean, Howell, Grieve, et al. (1995), who concluded that this therapy has a positive effect on children's phonology. The authors emphasized the importance of improving awareness of the phonological and communicative aspects of language. Fox-Boyer (2015) pointed to a possible limitation in that Metaphon therapy requires suitable cognitive and abstraction skills so that it may not be suited to young children or those with cognitive difficulties. Siemons-Lühring et al. (2021) commented that the approach may not be suitable for certain phonological errors, such as replacement of many different initial consonants by /d/ or /h/.

Melodic Intonation Therapy (MIT)

Melodic intonation therapy (MIT) is a treatment originally developed for nonfluent aphasia resulting from left-hemisphere damage (Albert et al.,1973; Helm-Estabrooks & Albert, 2004), but is perhaps viewed more appropriately as a treatment for apraxia of speech (Zumbansen et al., 2014). MIT uses the music-like aspects of speech (melody and rhythm) to improve expressive language. The original program included the basic components of intoning (singing) simple phrases of 2 to 3 syllables, speaking phrases of 5 or more syllables across three levels of treatment. Each level consists of 20 high-probability words or social phrases presented with visual cues. Variations in procedure are described by Norton et al. (2009) and Zumbansen et al. (2014). A possible reason for its effectiveness in treating aphasia or apraxia is that it promotes use of a preserved function (singing) to engage language-capable regions in the undamaged right hemisphere.

MIT has also been used with other clinical populations including childhood apraxia of speech (Helfrich-Miller, 1984, 1994; Lagasse, 2012; Wysocka, 2019) and ASD (where it has been called Melodic Based Communication Therapy [MBCT]; Sandiford et al., 2013). Mechanisms that have been proposed to account for the therapeutic value of MIT include: neuroplastic reorganization of language function; activation of the mirror neuron system and multimodal integration; utilization of shared or specific features of music and language; and effects on motivation and mood (Merrett et al., 2014). In addition, MIT could be effective because auditory patterns provide a perceptual and cognitive scaffolding for the development of functions related to time and serial order behavior (Conway et al., 2009). That is, melodic patterns could establish an auditory reference that facilitates sequential behavior in speech production.

Motor Learning (Principles of Motor Learning)

As discussed in Chapter 9, principles of motor learning (PML) are not an intervention per se but rather a set of guidelines that reflect studies of motor skill learning. The studies of PML pertain largely to adult activities such as sports, skilled limb or finger movements, and other tasks requiring dexterity. Few studies have been done on children, and there is no assurance that results from adults can be generalized to children of different ages. PML can be integrated into treatments for speech disorders, such as rapid syllable transition treatment (ReST) or speech motor chaining (SMC), discussed later in this chapter. Some of the more frequently used principles relate to parameters of feedback, treatment intensity, and type of practice, which can be applied to several different treatments. Therefore, PML often serves as a parameter of treatment rather than a treatment itself. Decisions about type of feedback apply across a range of specific interventions.

Motor Speech Treatment Protocol

The **motor speech treatment protocol (MSTP)** is a multisensory hybrid treatment approach for children with speech sound disorders and motor difficulties (Namasivayam et al., 2015, 2019). It shares some features with other interventions, such as PROMPT and DTTC (discussed in this chapter) and incorporates PLM. The core components of MSTP are as follows: selection of speech targets based on a child's level of speech motor control, use of temporal and multisensory cueing strategies, and structuring practice opportunities in communication-based activities to facilitate acquisition and generalization of speech motor skill learning. Promising results were reported for a small number of children by Namasivayam et al. (2015, 2019), although there were large individual differences in outcomes.

Multimodal Therapy

Multimodal therapy (also called **integrated therapy** or **integrated stimulation therapy**) does not have a standardized definition in the field of speech-language pathology. The usual indication of the terms *multimodal* or *integrated* is for treatments that combine two or more modalities (e.g., manual gesture and speech production). With respect to treating aphasia, Pierce et al. (2019) proposed a broad framework to categorize multimodal treatments based in part on a common interpretation of the term *multimodal* among speech-language pathologists, specifically that the term applies to the use of nonverbal production usually combined with verbal production. A similar principle applies to the treatment of speech disorders insofar as nonverbal cues are used to facilitate correct production. Nonverbal cues include tactile cues, gestures, visual cues, drawing, singing or rhythm, symbol boards, and various devices such as bite blocks and tongue depressors. Early examples of a multimodal approach are the **moto-kinesthetic method** of Young and Hawk (1955) and the **phonetic placement method** of Van Riper (1939, 1947, 1954). More contemporary examples are Dynamic Temporal and Tactile Cueing (DTTC) and Prompts for Restructuring Oral Muscular Phonetic Targets (PROMPT), both of which are summarized in this chapter. Multimodality may be effective because it (1) leads to an overall increase in the sensory information related to speech production, (2) provides alternative sensory pathways for the regulation of movements, and (3) assists in the construction of sensorimotor maps and internal models that underlie speech.

Multiple Oppositions

Multiple oppositions therapy uses sets of multiple oppositions that are selected to induce change across a child's phonological system rather than correcting a single sound or phonetic contrast (Williams, 2000a, 2000b). This approach is suited to address the multiple absence of target sounds that can result in extensive phoneme collapses and, therefore, homonymy. The basic principle underlying multiple oppositions therapy is to consider a child's phonological system as a whole and to deliver therapy across a phonological rule or strategy. Evidence for this therapy has been reported primarily in the form of case studies (Gierut, 1990; Williams, 2000a, 2000b) and a multiple-baseline study involving both parents and speech-language pathologists (Sugden et al., 2020). Gierut proposed a scale of effectiveness for teaching distinctions, from most to least, as follows: (1) multiple and major class distinctions, (2) multiple distinctions, and (3) few distinctions. Allen (2013) reported on the effect of dose frequency for multiple oppositions therapy for preschool children with SSD. Significantly greater gains occurred with more intensive dose frequency (3 times per week for 8 weeks versus once weekly for 24 weeks).

Nonspeech Oral Movements (NSOMs)

Nonspeech oral movements are discussed in Chapters 4 and 5. Therapy based on nonspeech oral exercises is one of the most controversial approaches in speech-language pathology. Although many clinicians use NSOMs as a component of treatment for speech disorders (Kamhi, 2008; Lof & Watson, 2008), it has been concluded by several authors that evidence supporting NSOMs in treating speech sound disorders is weak or insufficient to render a judgment on efficacy (Alhairdary, 2021; Kent, 2015; A. Lee & Gibbon, 2015; McCauley et al., 2009; Vashdi et al., 2021). Questions about the suitability of nonspeech tasks in understanding speech production reach back several decades (Netsell, 1983), but the issue has come to sharper focus in recent years. Complicating factors are that NSOMs are not consistently or clearly defined across studies (Kent, 2015) and that studies vary greatly in methodology (McCauley et al., 2009; Vashdi et al., 2021). Vashdi et al. (2021) reported positive correlations between NSOMs and speech production in a large sample of children with CAS and propose that NSOMs tap basic motor skills that are relevant to speech.

Because most research has been reported on speech sound disorders in general rather than CAS, it is difficult to determine the value of NSOMs in subpopulations of speech disorders. NSOMs may hold value for children who have motor problems such as hypotonia and weakness, but relatively little research has been reported on either assessments or outcomes of treatment with NSOMs. Potter et al. (2019) reported data on tongue strength for children and adolescents with typical development, children with speech sound delay/disorders, and children with motor speech disorders. Tongue strength in all three groups increased rapidly from 3 to 6.5 years of age and then increased at a slower rate until 17 years of age. No differences were seen between typically developing children and children with speech sound delay/disorders, but children with motor speech disorders had decreased tongue strength compared to children in either of the other two groups. A survey of Australian speech-language pathologists showed that NSOMs were commonly used as part of treatment for non-progressive dysarthria (Gracia et al., 2020). Use of NSOMs is questionable without a clear rationale pertaining to aspects such as strength, endurance, or speed, which emphasizes the need for careful assessment (discussed in Chapter 5).

Nuffield Dyspraxia Program (NDP)

The **Nuffield Dyspraxia Program (NDP)** is a therapy method based on principles of motor learning and is designed primarily for children aged 3 to 7 years with CAS. Now in its third edition (NDP3; Williams & Stephens, 2004), it has been used in Australia and the United Kingdom for approximately 30 years. The treatment package includes 500 structured worksheets that address articulation, sequencing, and prosody in sounds and words in drill play activities in a psycholinguistic framework. Therapy goals are hierarchically arranged as sounds, word shapes, and phrases of increasing complexity. Positive treatment effects were reported by Murray et al. (2015). Morgan, Murray, and Liégeois (2018) noted that NDP has RCT level evidence for its effectiveness.

Orofacial Myofunctional Therapy and Myofunctional Devices

Orofacial myofunctional therapy (OMT) and **myofunctional devices (MD)** are typically used to establish an oral environment that encourages typical processes of orofacial function (Hanson & Mason, 2003). OMT methods to achieve this oral environment include isotonic exercises (in which muscle length is altered to produce the force required to move a joint) and isometric exercises (in which an effort is made to hold a stable position) (Clark, 2003). Merkel-Walsh (2020 points out that,

> OMT is a treatment modality that should be performed by a licensed professional who has this modality in their SOP [scope of practice]. To date, there is no license in the United States of America for an Orofacial Myofunctional Therapist, although the IAOM offers a formal certification process (COM®). (p. 29)

MDs are appliances that use the facial and masticatory muscles to alter the relation of teeth or arches. These are typically used to treat craniofacial muscle competence, malocclusion, atypical swallowing such as tongue thrust, obstructive sleep apnea, and sleep-disordered breathing (Shah et al., 2021; Shortland et al., 2022). Merkel-Walsh (2020) discusses OMT for young children and individuals with special needs, emphasizing the importance of an interdisciplinary team to address the needs of these populations. Shortland et al. (2021) report a systematic review of the literature on OMT and MDs, including 28 studies that met their criteria. Most were published in the last decade and targeted multiple areas of speech pathology intervention within the same study (e.g., swallowing, breathing, oral hygiene, and speech production). Although all studies reported improved function following treatment, levels of evidence were typically low and data on long-term follow-up were unavailable. Many of the studies recommended that OMT/MDs be used in a multidisciplinary or interdisciplinary team or in conjunction with other therapy.

Phonological Awareness (PA)

Phonological awareness (PA), as discussed in Chapter 7, is the ability to recognize and manipulate the elements of spoken language, usually without reference to meaning. These elements include phonemes, syllables, onsets, and rhymes. The core concept is that spoken language consists of sequences of sound units that can be independently arranged to form larger units such as words. Studies have shown that children with reduced PA can be at risk for speech disorder (Torres et al., 2020), language disorder (Vukovic et al., 2022), and dyslexia (Vander Stappen & Reybroeck, 2018). PA is, therefore, of considerable interest in clinical specialties such as speech-language pathology, reading disability, and special education.

Research on the typical and atypical development of PA has helped to define PA in relation to the development of other skills and abilities. For example, Stackhouse et al., (2002) pointed out that children's PA develops along a continuum of tacit to explicit awareness and is the cumulative result of auditory, articulatory, and reading experience. Studies have shown that PA is related to auditory skills (Bonacina et al., 2019; Jain et al., 2020), articulatory or motor factors (Cabbage et al., 2018; Erskine et al., 2020; Roepke & Brosseau-Lapré, 2023; Rvachew et al., 2007), memory (Knoop-van Campen et al., 2018), and reading (Knoop-van Campen et al., 2018). However, the picture is not entirely clear as to how PA contributes to other abilities. For example, Swanson et al. (2003) concluded from a meta-analysis that the importance of PA in accounting for reading performance has been overstated. But there is no question that PA is a matter of deep interest to specialists in several disciplines, and therapy tools are readily available to support clinical endeavors.

Therapy programs focused on PA typically address the components illustrated in Figure 7–7. Many such programs are available either free or at cost. The U.S. Department of Education (June 2012) reviewed research on PA and found that only four studies available at that time met evidence standards without reservations. Based on these studies, the report concluded that the extent of evidence of PA training on children with learning disabilities in early education settings was small for the domain communication/language competencies. More recent reports show variable evidence of efficacy and effectiveness of PA training, with outcomes being weakly or strongly positive (Al Otaiba et al., 2009; Balikci, 2020; Denne et al., 2005; Hodgins & Harrison, 2021), or neutral or negative (Krim & Lund, 2021). Because studies are heterogeneous with respect to children's characteristics, therapy setting, mode of training, and individual outcomes, it is difficult to draw an overall conclusion. In general, it appears that PA training is most beneficial when provided in early childhood and in combination with other therapies (Gillon & McNeill, 2007; Rvachew et al., 2004; Schuele & Boudreau, 2008; Taruna, 2022; van Bysterveldt et al., 2010). Hesketh et al. (2000) compared metaphonologically articulation-based therapies for 61 children, aged 3;6 to 5;0, with developmental phonological disorders. The children improved significantly in both phonological output and awareness skills, but there was no significant difference in PA between the two treatment groups.

Suggestions on treatment strategies involving PA are given by Brosseau-Lapré and Roepke (2022) and Loudermill et al. (2021). Treatments are available for computers, tablets, and mobile devices (Furlong et al., 2021; Pokorni et al., 2004). In general, positive outcomes of treatments have been reported for phonological expression and, to a lesser degree, phonological reception (Rinaldi et al., 2021). In view of the limited research on the topic, Rinaldi et al. called for methodological research on the development of software tools for the stimulation of phonological awareness. Additional research is needed to determine the role of PA in specific clinical populations such as CAS (Moriarty & Gillon, 2006), Down syndrome (van Bysterveldt et al., 2010), and co-occurring dyslexia and speech sound disorder (Cabbage et al., 2018).

The foundations of PA and other speech-related aspects of auditory processing are coming into relief through studies of speech-in-noise (SiN; Vander Ghinst et al., 2019) and various auditory processing skills (Bonacina et al., 2019; Jain et al., 2020). It is particularly important to determine how auditory maturation in preschool children contributes to PA, phonological memory, and auditory streaming. Vander Ghinst et al. (2019) found that children's difficulties in understanding speech in noise are related to an immature selective cortical tracking of the attended speech streams. Such tracking appears to be related to cortical processing of speech at its syllable rate, which may be a basic requirement of auditory speech abilities.

PhonoSens

PhonoSens is based on the **Integrated Psycholinguistic Model of Language Processing (IPMSP**; Terband, Maassen, & Maas, 2019), which combines cognitive and sensorimotor functions within a hierarchical control system. IPMSP draws on Levelt's model of speech processing (described in Chapter 3) and Guenther's neurocomputational model of speech production (described in Chapter 1). It recognizes the following processing levels: (1) selection of lexemes for the intended utterance, (2) phonological encoding that translates lexemes into sensorimotor targets, (3) motor planning that selects and sequences articulatory movements, (4) motor programming that converts motor plans into motor programs, and (5) motor execution in which motor commands are sent to the effectors. PhonoSens is unusual among treatments for speech disorders in that it takes a comprehensive view of the overall process of speech production rather than focusing on smaller parts, such as PA or articulation. An RCT showed that children treated with this method had higher PCC and a greater reduction of phonological processes after 15 therapy sessions than the wait-list control group, both with large effect sizes (Siemons-Lühring et al., 2021). The authors concluded that this therapy is effective in treating SSD in German-speaking children, and the authors believed that the treatment is adaptable for other languages.

Prompts for Restructuring Oral Muscular Phonetic Targets (PROMPT)

PROMPT is a tactile-kinesthetic method of speech therapy in which touch cues to an individual's articulators and guides them to the production of a targeted word, phrase, or sentence (Chumpelik, 1984; Hayden, 2006). It emphasizes motor control and precision of movement and is framed in terms of dynamic systems theory (discussed in Chapter 1). The control of motor speech subsystems is conceptualized in a motor speech hierarchy (MSH) that has seven levels: tone, phonatory control, mandibular control, labial/facial control, lingual control, sequenced movements, and prosody (described in Chapter 5). It can include steps to eliminate unnecessary movements of the articulators (a description is available at http://www.promptinstitute.com/).

Studies of the effectiveness of PROMPT have been mostly single-subject designs and small group studies. Kim et al. (2021) identified 16 intervention studies over the period of 1984 to 2020. PROMPT has been reported to be effective in children with several different types of speech disorder including children with motor speech disorders (Dale & Hayden, 2013; Namasivayam et al., 2021), nonverbal autism (Rogers et al., 2006), CP (Ward, et al., 2014), and cleft lip or palate (Herreras Mercadoet et al., 2019). In a case series, Fiori et al. (2021) reported neural changes induced by PROMPT in children with CAS.

Prosody Interventions

Prosody interventions use aspects of prosody, such as contrastive stress or intonation, to change speech patterns in individuals with dysarthria, apraxia of speech, ASD, hearing loss, or other conditions. These interventions can be used directly to improve prosody, or indirectly, to leverage other aspects of speech, such as articulation (e.g., using increased stress on a target syllable to enhance articulatory movements). Little information is available on effectiveness beyond case studies. The results of a review on prosody interventions for ASD showed limited evidence for treatments that directly target prosody over long durations (Holbrook & Israelsen, 2020). An important limitation is that prosodic intervention is most likely to be effective for children who are verbal and can produce utterances long enough to exhibit prosodic variations. As discussed in Chapter 6, prosody is multidimensional and some of its aspects have a long maturational course. Prosody is a treatment target in an intervention for CAS, discussed next.

Rapid Syllable Transition Treatment (ReST)

Rapid syllable transition treatment (ReST) is based on principles of motor learning for articulation or phonological disorders, especially for children with CAS (Ballard et al., 2010; Murray, McCabe, & Ballard, 2015; Thomas et al., 2014). ReST consists of (1) intensive practice in producing multisyllabic pseudowords to improve accuracy in the production of speech sounds, (2) transitioning rapidly and fluently from one sound or syllable to the next, and (3) controlling the melody by varying the stress given to each syllable in a word. The rationale for the use of pseudowords is to create a condition of novel word learning that reduces interference from previously learned patterns. Dysprosody, particularly atypical lexical stress in multisyllabic patterns, is a major focus of ReST.

Positive outcomes of ReST for treating CAS have been reported (McAllister et al., 2018; Murray, McCabe, & Ballard, 2015; Ng et al., 2022; Thomas et al., 2014). McAllister et al. (2018) concluded from a review of the literature published between 2000 and 2017 that ReST was the only method rated as having high scientific evidence for CAS. In addition to administration in person by clinician, CAS has been delivered by telehealth (Thomas et al, 2016) and combined clinician-parent involvement (Thomas, McCabe, Ballard, & Bricker-Katz, 2018; Thomas, McCabe, & Ballard, 2018).

Rate Reduction Therapy

This approach to treating speech disorders emphasizes a deliberate slowing of speaking rate. The two main methods by which a speaker can reduce speaking rate are a modification of the duration and frequency of pauses, and prolongation of phonemes (especially vowels). Presumably, reduced rate allows the speaker to have additional time for programming and execution of speech movements, as well as possibly increased opportunity to evaluate feedback. In a review of studies on speaking rate, Berry (2011) concluded that the "principal finding of research related to normal aspects of speaking rate is idiosyncrasy" (p. 15). It is likely that the same conclusion applies to disordered speech. Speakers have a preferred rate of speaking that is subject to variation within certain limits. They also differ in how they achieve different rates of speaking and the effects of speaking rate changes on articulation. The effects of reduced rate have been studied almost entirely in adult neurogenic disorders, especially apraxia of speech, ataxic dysarthria, and hypokinetic dysarthria (Blanchet & Snyder, 2010; Yorkston et al., 2007). These studies have used several different ways of controlling speaking rate, including pacing boards, alphabet board supplementation, visual and auditory feedback, cueing and pacing strategies, and delayed auditory feedback (Blanchet & Snyder, 2010). Slow speaking rate is also incorporated in some therapies for speech disorders associated with cerebral palsy (such as the systems approach described later in this chapter). A similar approach is based on the Palin Parent Child Interaction therapy (Kelman & Nichols, 2008) in which adults try to match a child's speaking rate. This approach has been used as a treatment for developmental stuttering (Millard et al., 2009; Millard et al., 2018) and stuttering in children with ASD (Preston et al., 2022). As noted in Chapter 8, speaking rate in children tends to increase with age, up to 8 years or so.

Self-Cueing and Adaptive Cueing

Self-cueing, also known as self-monitoring, has been used in therapeutic interventions to reduce the degree of therapist-driven instruction and to increase client participation. A common approach is to link production of a target sound with a tactile cue or gesture. This type of therapy is an example of an integrated or multimodal approach discussed earlier in this chapter. **Adaptive cue training** is the use of visual, auditory, or haptic cues to assist performance of a task. The usual procedure is a gradual fading of the cue as performance improves.

Cueing and monitoring techniques applied to speech disorders are described in several papers (Kawasaki-Knight et al., 2021; King et al., 2013; Klick, 1985; Xi et al., 2020). Cues can be (1) either endogenous (generated by a child) or exogenous (generated by a clinician or other person), (2) individualized to match a child's abilities and preferences, and matched to different aspects of speech (e.g., movement of a single articulator, or a series of syllables). Cues are frequently used in multimodal treatments such as PROMPT.

Speech Motor Chaining (SMC)

Speech motor chaining (Preston, Leece, & Storto, 2019) seeks to build complex speech patterns around basic core movements by incorporating several principles of motor learning, especially feedback and practice (motor learning is covered in Chapter 9). Components of SMC are as follows. Speech movement patterns are trained with feedback for both the acoustic quality of speech sounds and the articulatory actions. Training is done to address isolated speech sound errors and errors associated with symptoms of impaired transitions between sounds and syllables. The preferred speech material consists of sound sequences (syllables of the forms CV, VC, or CC) in which the target sound occupies a specific syllable position. The rationale for training sound sequences, as opposed to phonemes, is that studies of speech production indicate that the units of speech planning transcend phonemes. The concept of chaining is to move quickly from trained smaller units, such as sound sequences in syllables, to complex speech movements in words. During practice, additional movements are gradually added before the target sequence (backward chaining) or after the target sequence (forward chaining). For example, for a syllable-onset target, the training sequence might take the form of consonant cluster, syllable, monosyllabic word, multisyllabic word, short phrase, and a sentence.

Speech Systems Intelligibility Treatment (SSIT)

Speech Systems Intelligibility Treatment (SSIT) is a therapy for motor speech disorders, especially dysarthria, that targets the functions and coordination of the subsystems involved in speech production (e.g., respiration, phonation, resonance, and articulation). Treatment is conducted with the principles of motor learning, including high intensity practice, random practice of target behaviors, fading of feedback during skill acquisitions, and provision of knowledge of performance and knowledge of results. The treatment method is described by Levy (2014). Levy et al. (2021) reported on the effects of a dual-focus speech treatment targeting increased articulatory excursion and vocal intensity on the intelligibility of narrative speech, speech acoustics, and communicative participation in children with dysarthria. It was concluded that the intervention improved intelligibility and communicative participation in children with dysarthria, but the responses to treatment varied across children.

Systems Approach

The **Systems Approach** is an intervention protocol developed by Pennington et al. (2010) for children with cerebral palsy. It focuses on stabilizing respiratory and phonatory effort and control, speech rate and phrase length, or syllables per breath. These are foundations for speech production and can be important first steps in an intervention program. Therapy begins with practice that coordinates the onset of phonation with the beginning of exhalation in sustained vowels. The next step is to coordinate exhalation and phonation for producing spoken language. In the spoken language tasks, children also practice speaking slowly and maintaining breath supply across a phrase, inspiring at syntactically appropriate places. The spoken language tasks form a four-part hierarchy of exercises: (1) producing a set of 10 frequently used phrases and progressing to novel phrases consisting of (2) single words, (3) sentences, and (4) conversational speech.

A system or subsystem perspective on assessment and treatment has a long precedent in speech-language pathology, especially for dysarthrias in adults or children. Netsell (1983) comments that a component-by-component assessment may occasionally indicate adequate functions in the individual components but does not reveal difficulty in the overall coordination of the components needed to produce intelligible speech. He recommends that a solution is to use meaningful speech targets that place primary demands on one component and minimal requirements on the others. Construction of the speech sample is of primary importance to this strategy.

Traditional Speech Therapy

Traditional speech therapy is not easily defined because it is not standardized and potentially takes several different forms. However, the frequently cited source is the approach of Van Riper (1978) who prescribed a sequence of activities: (1) identify the standard sound, (2) discriminate this sound from its error sound by scanning and comparing, (3) vary and correct the different productions of this sound until it is produced correctly, and (4) strengthen and stabilize the sound in various contexts and speaking situations. Studies that compare this traditional technique with other treatment methods use some variation of the activities just listed. Traditional therapy is a gold standard or criterion standard in the sense that it is sometimes regarded as a benchmark for comparisons with other types of intervention. However, this does not mean that it is superior to all other treatments.

Transcranial Direct Current Stimulation (tDCS)

Transcranial Direct Current Stimulation (tDCS) is a noninvasive neuromodulation technique that induces prolonged brain excitability to alter and promote cerebral plasticity. Spontaneous neuronal activity is modulated by a weak direct current delivered by a stimulating electrode placed on the scalp over a target area, such as Broca's area. A reference electrode can be placed either on the scalp (bicephalic or bipolar tDCS) or some other part of the body, usually the right shoulder (monocephalic or monopolar tDCS). This treatment is not used extensively in treating SSD, but promising results have been reported for reading and phonological awareness (Mirahadi et al., 2022), language production in monozygotic twins with corpus callosum dysgenesis (Mousavi et al., 2022), and language function in girls with Rett syndrome and chronic language impairment (Fabio et al., 2018).

Practice Patterns

Surveys have been done to reveal which therapies are favored by speech-language clinicians. The results of five surveys are summarized in Table 12–2, which shows a preference for traditional articulation therapy, minimal pairs, auditory discrimination, and phonological awareness. It is interesting that traditional articulation therapy, dating back to at least 1958, retains its popularity, and that a minimal pairs approach is favored over multiple oppositions or complexity-based methods (which may have stronger evidence of efficacy). However, clinicians may favor minimal pairs when only a small number of speech sounds need treatment. In addition, clinicians may be eclectic in their approach to treatment, so that treatment methods are combined in various phases of intervention. Wren et al. (2018) discovered in their survey of speech-language therapists that the most frequently reported interventions for speech-sound disorder in preschool children were cognitive–linguistic and production approaches. They also indicated that the highest graded evidence was for studies within the auditory–perceptual and integrated categories.

Table 12–2 helps to identify general patterns of practice, but there is a risk of over-interpretation in that the results may apply to the broad classification of SSD and do not identify specific preferences for subgroups of children, such as those with CAS, for whom several treatments are available (Fish & Skinder-Meredith, 2022). Clinician preferences for therapy of CAS were reported in a survey by Gomez et al. (2022). Respondents, who were from both the U.S. and Canada, generally used an eclectic approach, and no single intervention was identified as the preferred

Table 12–2. Reports of Practice Patterns for Speech Disorders in Children

Method/Source	1	2	3	4	5	6	7
Traditional articulation	+	+	+	+	+	+	
Phonological awareness	+	+			+	+	+
Auditory discrimination	+			+	+	+	+
Minimal pairs	+	+	+	+	+	+	+
Whole language	+	+					
Core vocabulary						+	
Cued articulation				+		+	
Cycles		+	+				
Nuffield						+	

Sources: (1) Alsaad et al. (2021); (2) Brumbaugh & Smit (2013); (3) Cabbage et al. (2022); (4) Furlong et al. (2021); (5) Hegerty et al. (2018); (6) McLeod & Baker (2014); (7) Oliveira (2015).

primary treatment. Clinicians from the U.S. most often used the Kaufman Speech to Language Protocol (K-SLP) (used by 33%) and Dynamic, Temporal and Tactile Cueing (DTTC) (used by 28%). Clinicians in Canada most often used PROMPT® (31%). There is relatively strong evidence for the effectiveness of Dynamic Tactile and Temporal Cueing, Nuffield Dyspraxia Programme, and Rapid Syllable Transition. Many different factors contribute to clinician preferences in treatments for speech disorders, including available evidence, convenience and economy of application, personal experience, and potential integration in an overall program of intervention. Springle et al. (2020) concluded from a review of the evidence that motor programming treatments lead to the best speech production outcomes in CAS. These approaches include ReST, DTTC, and the Nuffield Dyspraxia Program. It is expected that eventually clinician preferences for treatments should align with the evidence base for various speech disorders.

Speech Disorders and Developmental Neuroscience

Neuroimaging opens the opportunity to examine neural features associated with speech disorders in children, thereby adding an important dimension to the developmental neuroscience of speech development. Only a few studies have been reported to date, but these offer some promising perspectives, as follows.

As mentioned in Chapter 3, already present at birth is the ventral pathway between the temporal areas to the inferior frontal gyrus and the dorsal pathway from the temporal cortex to the premotor cortex. These connections establish a basis for sensory and motor associations related to vocal development. Studies of the spatial, temporal, and spectral characteristics of gamma augmentation elicited by cooing and babbling are like those elicited by speech production in older children and adults (Cho-Hisamoto et al., 2012). Also observed was differential activation within the right inferior Rolandic region during cooing and babbling and evidence that the right superior temporal gyrus participates in an auditory feedback system during vocalization. Later maturation occurs for the dorsal pathway from the temporal cortex to the inferior frontal gyrus (IFG). The IFG is thought to be an articulatory region that accesses phonological representations that are associated with the posterior superior temporal gyrus (pSTG) (J. Wang et al., 2020). The connections between IFG and pSTG are fundamental to speech development in its phonological and motoric aspects.

Disruption to the dorsal pathway is associated with several speech and language disorders, as noted in Chapter 3. The left corticobulbar tract has been identified as a potential brain marker for developmental speech disorders (Morgan, Su, et al., 2018) and shows changes as the result of speech motor treatment for CAS (Fiori et al., 2021). It has been reported that following treatment for motor speech disorder, there is increased activation in the frontal and motor areas, followed by increased activation in the left insula (Vickie et al., 2018). Spencer et al. (in press), using fMRI to determine neural changes associated with biofeedback therapy, also observed connectivity differences near the left insula. The role of the insula in speech production is controversial. Woolnough et al. (2019) studied 27 patients implanted with penetrating intracranial electrodes for the tasks of single-word articulations, nonspeech orofacial movements, and speech listening. They concluded that the insula is not involved in pre-articulatory preparation, and that bilateral posterior insular cortices may play roles in auditory and somatosensory integration or monitoring. This interpretation of insular function may explain activation of the insula in speech treatments. Boscato et al. (2022) found that for young adults, training on a diadochokinetic oral motor task induced significant neuroplastic changes in the corticomotor pathway related to the lips, masseter, and tongue muscles. DDK rate also increased after oral motor training. As mentioned in Chapter 3, the cerebellum has a slow maturation and has been implicated in childhood onset disorders such as autism, ADHD, and developmental stuttering. The cerebellum has multiple compartments with different maturational trajectories that could provide for lifelong experience-based neuroplasticity (Romero et al., 2021). In a review of studies of speech treatment-induced neuroplasticity in adults and children with motor speech disorders, Whelan et al. (2021) noted the following brain alterations: enhanced white matter tract integrity, normalization of baseline cortical activity, right-hemisphere shifts in reorganization, perilesional activations, and cortical thinning.

Conclusions

1. Prevention of speech disorders can take any of four major forms, depending on objectives and resources. Identification of risk factors is helpful in this endeavor.
2. Several outcome measures of clinical treatment of speech disorders are available.
3. Clinicians can choose among many different types of treatment, depending on therapeutic goals, child characteristics, available resources, personal experience, and available evidence.
4. The evidence base is not uniform across treatments, but some treat-

ments have moderate to strong evidence, and it is expected that evidence is accruing for most treatments.

5. Preferred practice patterns indicate that a small number of treatments are generally favored, but it is likely that many clinicians are eclectic in their choice of treatments and that treatments are selected in due regard of child characteristics.

APPENDIX A

INTERNATIONAL PHONETIC ALPHABET (IPA)

Reproduction of the International Phonetic Alphabet (IPA).

THE INTERNATIONAL PHONETIC ALPHABET (revised to 2015)

CONSONANTS (PULMONIC)

	Bilabial	Labiodental	Dental	Alveolar	Postalveolar	Retroflex	Palatal	Velar	Uvular	Pharyngeal	Glottal
Plosive	p b			t d		ʈ ɖ	c ɟ	k ɡ	q ɢ		ʔ
Nasal	m	ɱ		n		ɳ	ɲ	ŋ	ɴ		
Trill	ʙ			r					ʀ		
Tap or Flap		ⱱ		ɾ		ɽ					
Fricative	ɸ β	f v	θ ð	s z	ʃ ʒ	ʂ ʐ	ç ʝ	x ɣ	χ ʁ	ħ ʕ	h ɦ
Lateral fricative				ɬ ɮ							
Approximant		ʋ		ɹ		ɻ	j	ɰ			
Lateral approximant				l		ɭ	ʎ	ʟ			

Symbols to the right in a cell are voiced, to the left are voiceless. Shaded areas denote articulations judged impossible.

CONSONANTS (NON-PULMONIC)

Clicks	Voiced implosives	Ejectives
ʘ Bilabial	ɓ Bilabial	ʼ Examples:
ǀ Dental	ɗ Dental/alveolar	pʼ Bilabial
ǃ (Post)alveolar	ʄ Palatal	tʼ Dental/alveolar
ǂ Palatoalveolar	ɠ Velar	kʼ Velar
ǁ Alveolar lateral	ʛ Uvular	sʼ Alveolar fricative

VOWELS

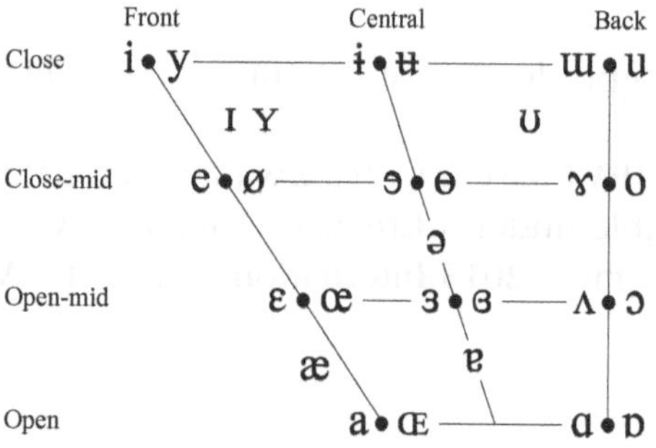

Where symbols appear in pairs, the one to the right represents a rounded vowel.

OTHER SYMBOLS

ʍ Voiceless labial-velar fricative

w Voiced labial-velar approximant

ɥ Voiced labial-palatal approximant

ʜ Voiceless epiglottal fricative

ʢ Voiced epiglottal fricative

ʡ Epiglottal plosive

ɕ ʑ Alveolo-palatal fricatives

ɺ Voiced alveolar lateral flap

ɧ Simultaneous ʃ and x

Affricates and double articulations can be represented by two symbols joined by a tie bar if necessary. t͜s k͡p

DIACRITICS Some diacritics may be placed above a symbol with a descender, e.g. ŋ̊

̥ Voiceless	n̥ d̥	̤ Breathy voiced	b̤ a̤	̪ Dental	t̪ d̪
̬ Voiced	s̬ t̬	̰ Creaky voiced	b̰ a̰	̺ Apical	t̺ d̺
ʰ Aspirated	tʰ dʰ	̼ Linguolabial	t̼ d̼	̻ Laminal	t̻ d̻
̹ More rounded	ɔ̹	ʷ Labialized	tʷ dʷ	̃ Nasalized	ẽ
̜ Less rounded	ɔ̜	ʲ Palatalized	tʲ dʲ	ⁿ Nasal release	dⁿ
̟ Advanced	u̟	ˠ Velarized	tˠ dˠ	ˡ Lateral release	dˡ
̠ Retracted	e̠	ˤ Pharyngealized	tˤ dˤ	̚ No audible release	d̚
̈ Centralized	ë	̴ Velarized or pharyngealized ɫ			
̽ Mid-centralized	e̽	̝ Raised	e̝ (ɹ̝ = voiced alveolar fricative)		
̩ Syllabic	n̩	̞ Lowered	e̞ (β̞ = voiced bilabial approximant)		
̯ Non-syllabic	e̯	̘ Advanced Tongue Root	e̘		
˞ Rhoticity	ɚ a˞	̙ Retracted Tongue Root	e̙		

SUPRASEGMENTALS

ˈ Primary stress ˌfoʊnəˈtɪʃən

ˌ Secondary stress

ː Long eː

ˑ Half-long eˑ

̆ Extra-short ĕ

| Minor (foot) group

‖ Major (intonation) group

. Syllable break ɹi.ækt

‿ Linking (absence of a break)

TONES AND WORD ACCENTS

LEVEL		CONTOUR	
e̋ or ˥	Extra high	ě or ˩˥	Rising
é ˦	High	ê ˥˩	Falling
ē ˧	Mid	e᷄ ˦˥	High rising
è ˨	Low	e᷅ ˩˨	Low rising
ȅ ˩	Extra low	e᷈ ˧˦˧	Rising-falling
ꜜ	Downstep	↗	Global rise
ꜛ	Upstep	↘	Global fall

APPENDIX B

VARIATIONS OF THE ORAL MECHANISM EXAMINATION

The following examinations pertain to specific purposes (e.g., examination of specified anatomic structures) or clinical populations (e.g., children with craniofacial anomalies or differences).

1. Pediatric feeding and swallowing (review by Heckathorn et al., 2016).
2. Oral-motor skills of preverbal children (Schedule for Oral Motor Assessment [SOMA; Skuse et al., 1995).
3. Oral movement and sensation (Marshalla Oral Sensorimotor Test [MOST; Marshalla, 2007).
4. The Movement, Articulation, Mandibular and Sensory awareness (MAMS) assessment procedure (Cook et al., 2011).
5. Verbal Motor Production Assessment for Children (VMPAC; Hayden & Square, 1999).
6. Children with craniofacial anomalies or differences (Fox, 2018; Kummer, 2009).
7. Orofacial myofunctional examination (Felício et al., 2010).
8. Lingual frenulum (Amir et al., 2006; Hazelbaker, 1993; Martinelli et al., 2012), and labial frenulum (Kotlow, 2013).
9. Oropharyngeal airway assessment (i.e., the extrapulmonary air passage, consisting of the nasal and oral cavities, pharynx, larynx, trachea, and large bronchi; Gupta et al., 2005). This assessment is performed to assess obstructive sleep apnea or to prepare for laryngoscopic tracheal intubation (Friedman et al., 2002; Mallampati, 1983; Nuckton et al., 2006), but it also can be useful in examinations of oral structure for speech and other oral functions. Mallampati and Friedman are the two most common scores. Mallampati scoring (Figure B–1) is divided into 4 classes based on the visibility of the base of the uvula, faucial pillars, and soft palate: class 1, full visibility of all three structures; class 2, visibility of hard and soft palate, upper portion of tonsils and uvula; class 3, visibility of soft and hard palate and base of the uvula; and class 4, visibility of hard palate only. Friedman classification evaluates

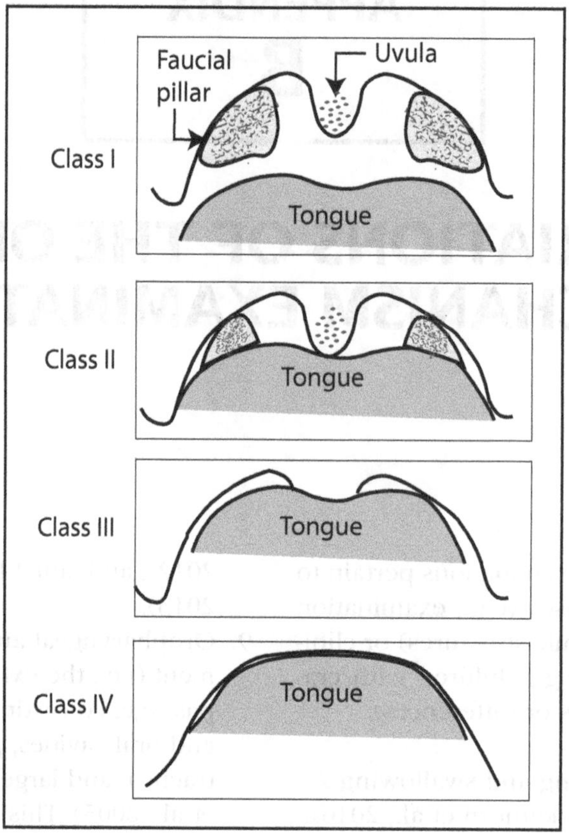

Figure B–1

tonsillar size, with scores divided into 4 classes: grade 1+, the tonsils are hidden within the tonsillar pillars; grade 2+, the tonsils extend to the tonsillar pillars; grade 3+, the tonsils extend beyond the pillars but do not reach the midline; and grade 4+, the tonsils extend to, or beyond, the midline.

10. Swansea classification for lingual tonsil (Costello et al., 2017).
11. Laryngoscopic view (Cormack & Lehane,1984)
12. Interdisciplinary examination protocol. *The Interdisciplinary Orofacial Examination Protocol for Children and Adolescents* (Grandi, 2012), was developed by four orthodontists, one ear, nose, and throat physician, and three speech-language therapists. The interdisciplinary approach has special value in the assessment of disorders in which multiple anomalies may affect diverse functions and require interactions in multispecialty clinical teams.

APPENDIX C

CRANIAL NERVE SUMMARY

Summary of Cranial Nerves: Nerve Number, Name of Nerve, Type of Nerve, and Function

Nerve Number	Name of Nerve	Nerve Type	Function of Nerve
I	Olfactory	Sensory	Olfactory (smell) information from nose
II	Optic	Sensory	Visual information from the eyes
III	Oculomotor	Motor	Eye movement, pupil constriction, lens shape
IV	Trochlear	Motor	Eye movement, turns eye downward and laterally
V	Trigeminal	Mixed	Sensory information from face and mouth, motor for chewing and other jaw movements
VI	Abducent	Motor	Eye movement, abducts the eye
VII	Facial	Mixed	Sensory information for taste, efferent for tear and salivary glands, motor control of facial muscles
XIII	Statoacoustic	Sensory	Auditory and equilibrium information from inner ear
IX	Glossopharyngeal	Mixed	Sensory information from oral cavity, sensory for baroreceptors and chemoreceptors in blood vessels, efferent for parotid gland salivary function, motor for swallowing
X	Vagus	Mixed	Sensory for parasympathetic innervation, sensory information for taste, motor for swallowing, voice, and gag reflex
XI	Spinal accessory	Sensory and motor	Controls trapezius and sternocleidomastoid muscles, controls swallowing movements
XII	Hypoglossal	Motor	Controls tongue movements

REFERENCES

Abdel-Aziz, M., El-Fouly, M., Nassar, A., & Kamel, A. (2019). The effect of hypertrophied tonsils on the velopharyngeal function in children with normal palate. *International Journal of Pediatric Otorhinolaryngology, 119*, 59–62. https://doi.org/10.1016/j.ijporl.2019.01.017

Abreu, R. R., Rocha, R. L., Lamounier, J. A., & Guerra, Â. F. M. (2008). Prevalence of mouth breathing among children. [Portuguese] *Jornal de Pediatria, 84*(5), 467–470. https://doi.org/10.2223/JPED.1806

Abur, D., Enos, N. M., & Stepp, C. E. (2019). Visual analog scale ratings and orthographic transcription measures of sentence intelligibility in Parkinson's disease with variable listener exposure. *American Journal of Speech-Language Pathology, 28*(3), 1222–1232. https://doi.org/10.1044/2019_AJSLP-18-0275

Acharya, S. S., Mali, L., Sinha, A., & Nanda, S. B. (2018). Effect of naso-respiratory obstruction with mouth breathing on dentofacial and craniofacial development. *Orthodontic Journal of Nepal, 8*(1), 22–27.

Achille, A., Rovere, M., & Soatto, S. (April 24–26, 2017). *Critical learning periods in deep neural networks* [Conference paper]. 5th International Conference on Learning Representations, ICLR 2017, Toulon, France; arXiv:1711.08856 https://doi.org/10.48550/arXiv.1711.08856

Achmad, H., & Ansar, A. W. (2021). Mouth breathing in pediatric population: A literature review. *Annals of the Romanian Society for Cell Biology, 25*(6), 4431–4455

Achmad, H., Riyanti, E., Primarti, R. S., & Imanuelly Pagal a, M. (2021). An overview of frequency malocclusion in cases of Down syndrome children: A systematic review. *European Journal of Molecular and Clinical Medicine, 8*(1), 1641–1650.

Adams, V., Mathisen, B., Baines, S., Lazarus, C., & Callister, R. (2013). A systematic review and meta-analysis of measurements of tongue and hand strength and endurance using the Iowa Oral Performance Instrument (IOPI). *Dysphagia, 28*(3), 350–369. https://doi.org/10.1007/s00455-013-9451-3

Adani, S., & Cepanec, M. (2019). Sex differences in early communication development: Behavioral and neurobiological indicators of more vulnerable communication system development in boys. *Croatian Medical Journal, 60*(2), 141–149. https://doi.org/10.3325/cmj.2019.60.141

Adolph, K. E., Cole, W. G., Komati, M., Garciaguirre, J. S., Badaly, D., Lingeman, J. M., . . . Sotsky, R. B. (2012). How do you learn to walk? Thousands of steps and dozens of falls per day. *Psychological Science, 23*(11), 1387–1394. https://doi.org/10.1177/0956797612446346

Adolph, K. E., & Franchak, J. M. (2017). The development of motor behavior. *Wiley Interdisciplinary Reviews: Cognitive Science, 8*(1–2), e1430. https://doi.org/10.1002/wcs.1430

Adolph, K. E., & Hoch, J. E. (2019). Motor development: Embodied, embedded, enculturated, and enabling. *Annual Review of Psychology, 70*, 141–164. https://doi.org/10.1146/annurev-psych-010418-102836

Adolphs, R. (2016). How should neuroscience study emotions? by distinguishing emotion states, concepts, and experiences. *Social Cognitive and Affective Neuroscience*, nsw153. https://doi.org/10.1093/scan/nsw153

Aguert, M., Laval, V., Lacroix, A., Gil, S., & Le Bigot, L. (2013). Inferring emotions from speech prosody: Not so easy at age five. *PloS ONE, 8*(12), e83657. https://doi.org/10.1371/journal.pone.0083657

Ahissar, E., Nagarajan, S., Ahissar, M., Protopapas, A., Mahncke, H., & Merzenich, M. M. (2001). Speech comprehension is correlated with temporal response patterns recorded from auditory cortex. *Proceedings of the National Academy of Science*, U.S.A., *98*, 13367–13372. https://doi.org/10.1073/pnas.201400998

Ahlsén, E. (2008). Embodiment in communication—aphasia, apraxia and the possible role of mirroring and imitation. *Clinical Linguistics & Phonetics*, *22*(4-5), 311–315. https://doi.org/10.1080/02699200801918879

Ahmed, B., Monroe, P., Hair, A., Tan, C. T., Gutierrez-Osuna, R., & Ballard, K. J. (2018). Speech-driven mobile games for speech therapy: User experiences and feasibility. *International Journal of Speech-Language Pathology*, *20*(6), 644–658. https://doi.org/10.1080/17549507.2018.1513562

Alaçam, A., Çalık Yılmaz, B. C., & Incioğlu, A. S. (2020). Assessment of orofacial dysfunction using the NOT-S method in a group of Turkish children with cerebral palsy. *European Archives of Paediatric Dentistry*, *21*, 215–221.

Albert, M. L., Sparks, R. W., & Helm, N. A. (1973). Melodic intonation therapy for aphasia. *Archives of Neurology*, *29*(2), 130–131. https://doi.org/10.1001/archneur.1973.00490260074018

Al-Dakroury, W. A. (2018). Speech and language disorders in ADHD. *Abnormal and Behavioral Psychology*, *4*(134), Article 2472–0496. https://doi.org/10.4172/2472-0496.1000134

Alderete, J., Baese-Berk, M., Leung, K., & Goldrick, M. (2021). Cascading activation in phonological planning and articulation: Evidence from spontaneous speech errors. *Cognition*, *210* 104577. https://doi.org/10.1016/j.cognition.2020.104577

Alderson-Day, B., & Fernyhough, C. (2015). Inner speech: evelopment, cognitive functions, phenomenology, and neurobiology. *Psychological Bulletin*, *141*(5), 931. https://doi.org/10.1037/bul0000021

Alexopoulos, J., Giordano, V., Janda, C., Benavides-Varela, S., Seidl, R., Doering, S., . . . Bartha-Doering, L. (2021). The duration of intrauterine development influences discrimination of speech prosody in infants. *Developmental Science*, *24*(5), e13110. https://doi.org/10.1111/desc.13110

Alhaidary, A. (2021). Treatment of speech sound disorders in children: Nonspeech oral exercises. *International Journal of Pediatrics and Adolescent Medicine*, *8*(1), 1–4. https://doi.org/10.1016/j.ijpam.2019.07.008

Alhanbali, S., Dawes, P., Millman, R. E., & Munro, K, J. (2019). Measures of listening effort are multidimensional. *Ear & Hearing*, *40*(5), 1084–1097. https://doi.org/10.1097/AUD.0000000000000697

Alhazmi, W. A. (2022). Mouth breathing and speech disorders: A multidisciplinary evaluation based on the etiology. *Journal of Pharmacy and Bioallied Sciences*, *14*(5), 911–916.

Alighieri, C., Bettens, K., Bruneel, L., D'haeseleer, E., Van Gaever, E., & Van Lierde, K. (2020). Effectiveness of speech intervention in patients with a cleft palate: Comparison of motor-phonetic versus linguistic-phonological speech approaches. *Journal of Speech, Language, and Hearing Research*, *63*(12), 3909–3933. https://doi.org/10.1044/2020_JSLHR-20-00129

Alighieri, C., Van Lierde, K., De Caesemaeker, A. S., Demuynck, K., Bruneel, L., D'haeseleer, E., & Bettens, K. (2021). Is high-intensity speech intervention better? A comparison of high-intensity intervention versus low-intensity intervention in children with a cleft palate. *Journal of Speech, Language, and Hearing Research*, *64*(9), 3398–3415. https://doi.org/10.1044/2021_JSLHR-21-00189

Allen, G. D., & Hawkins, S. (1979). Trochaic rhythm in children's speech. In H. Hollien & P. Hollien (Eds.), *Current issues in the phonetic sciences* (pp. 927–933). John Benjamins.

Allen, G. D., & Hawkins, S. (1980). Phonological rhythm: Definition and development. In G. H. Yeni-Komshian, J. F. Kavanagh, & C. A. Ferguson (Eds.), *Child phonology: Vol. 1. Production* (pp. 227–256). Academic Press.

Allen, J. E., Cleland, J., & Smith, M. (2022). An initial framework for use of ultrasound by speech and language therapists in the UK: Scope of practice, education and governance. *Ultrasound*, https://doi.org/10.1177/1742271X221122562

Allen, M. M. (2013). Intervention efficacy and intensity for children with speech sound disorder. *Journal of Speech, Language, and Hearing Research*, *56*(3), 865–877. https://doi.org/10.1044/1092-4388(2012/11-0076)

Allison, K. M. (2020). Measuring speech intelligibility in children with motor speech disorders. *Perspectives of the ASHA Special Interest Groups*, *5*(4), 809–820. https://doi.org/10.1044/2020_PERSP-19-00110

Allison, K. M., & Hustad, K. C. (2018). Acoustic predictors of pediatric dysarthria in cerebral palsy. *Journal of Speech, Language, and Hearing Research*, *61*(3), 462–478. https://doi.org/10.1044/2017_JSLHR-S-16-0414. PMID: 29466556; PMCID: PMC5963041.

Allison, K. M., Nip, I. S., & Rong, P. (2022). Use of automated kinematic diadochokinesis analysis to identify potential indicators of speech motor involvement in children with cerebral palsy. *American Journal of Speech-Language Pathology, 31*(6), 2835–2846. https://doi.org/10.1044/2022_AJSLP-21-00241

Allison, K. M., Russell, M., & Hustad, K. C. (2021). Reliability of perceptual judgments of phonetic accuracy and hypernasality among speech-language pathologists for children with dysarthria. *American Journal of Speech-Language Pathology, 30*(3S), 1558–1571. https://doi.org/10.1044/2020_AJSLP-20-00144

Almost, D. A., & Peter Rosenbaum, M. D. (1998). Effectiveness of speech intervention for phonological disorders: A randomized controlled trial. *Developmental Medicine & Child Neurology, 40*(5), 319–325. https://doi.org/10.1111/j.1469-8749.1998.tb15383.x

Al Otaiba, S., Puranik, C. S., Ziolkowski, R. A., & Montgomery, T. M. (2009). Effectiveness of early phonological awareness interventions for students with speech or language impairments. *The Journal of Special Education, 43*(2), 107–128. https://doi.org/10.1177/0022466908314869

Alsaad, M., McCabe, P., & Purcell, A. (2021). A survey of interventions used by speech-language pathologists for children with speech sound disorders in the Middle East. *Logopedics Phoniatrics Vocology, 1*, 8. https://doi.org/10.1080/14015439.2021.1991469

Alsius, A., Paré, M., & Munhall, K. G. (2018). Forty years after hearing lips and seeing voices: The McGurk effect revisited. *Multisensory Research, 31*(1-2), 111–144. https://doi.org/10.1163/22134808-00002565

Altman, K. W., Atkinson, C., & Lazarus, C. (2005). Current and emerging concepts in muscle tension dysphonia: A 30-month review. *Journal of Voice, 19*(2), 261–267. https://doi.org/10.1016/j.jvoice.2004.03.007

Alves, M. O. C., Ode, C., & Strömbergsson, S. (2020) Dealing with the unknown—addressing challenges in evaluating unintelligible speech. *Clinical Linguistics & Phonetics, 34*(1–2), 169–184. https://doi.org/10.1080/02699206.2019.1622787

American Psychiatric Association. (2013). *Diagnostic and statistical manual of mental disorders* (5th ed.). https://doi.org/10.1176/appi.books.9780890425596

American Speech-Language-Hearing Association (n.d.). *Speech sound disorders—articulation and phonology.* https://www.asha.org/practice-portal/clinical-topics/articulation-and-phonology/

American Speech-Language-Hearing Association. (1983, September). Social dialects and implications of the position on social dialects. *Asha, 25*, 23–27.

American Speech-Language-Hearing Association. (1985, June). Clinical management of communicatively handicapped minority language populations. *Asha, 27*, 29–32.

American Speech-Language-Hearing Association. (1988). *Prevention of communication disorders* [Position statement]. https://www.asha.org/policy

American Speech-Language-Hearing Association. (1998). *Provision of instruction in English as a second language by speech-language pathologists in school settings* [Technical report]. https://www.asha.org/policy

American Speech-Language-Hearing Association (2007). *Childhood apraxia of speech technical report.* https://www.asha.org/policy/tr2007-00278/

American Speech-Language-Hearing Association. (2015). *ASHA marketing solutions: Schools.* https://doi.org/10.1044/2018_PERS-SIG1-2018-0014

American Speech-Language-Hearing Association. (2021) *ASHA 2021 SLP health care survey: Caseload characteristics.* https://www.asha.org

American Speech-Language-Hearing Association (May 2022). *ASHA's National Outcomes Measurement System (NOMS) clinician user guide SLP healthcare.* https://www.asha.org/siteassets/uploadedfiles/ASHA/NOMS/NOMS-SLP-Clinician-User-Guide.pdf

Amir, L. H., James, J. P., & Donath, S. M. (2006). Reliability of the Hazelbaker Assessment Tool for lingual frenulum function. *International Breastfeeding Journal, 1*(3). https://doi.org/10.1186/1746-4358-1-3

Ananthakrishnan, S., & Narayanan, S. (2009). Unsupervised adaptation of categorical prosody models for prosody labeling and speech recognition. *IEEE Transactions on Audio, Speech & Language Processing, 17*(1), 138–149.

Anderson, D. I., Lohse, K. R., Lopes, T. C. V., & Williams, A. M. (2021). Individual differences in motor skill learning: Past, present and future. *Human Movement Science*, *78*, Article 102818. https://doi.org/10.1016/j.humov.2021.102818

Anderson, J. (1969). Syllabic or non-syllabic phonology? *Journal of Linguistics*, *5*(1), 136–142. https://www.jstor.org/stable/4175024

Andersson, H., & Sonnesen, L. (2018). Sleepiness, occlusion, dental arch and palatal dimensions in children attention deficit hyperactivity disorder (ADHD). *European Archives of Paediatric Dentistry*, *19*, 91–97.

Andrianopoulos, M. V., Darrow, K., & Chen, J. (2001). Multimodal standardization of voice among four multicultural populations formant structures. *Journal of Voice*, *2001*, *15*, 61–77. https://doi.org/10.1016/S0892-1997(01)00007-8

Anthony, J. L., & Francis, D. J. (2005). Development of phonological awareness. *Current Directions in Psychological Science*, *14*(5), 255–259. https://doi.org/10.1111/j.0963-7214.2005.00376.x

Anthony, J. L., Lonigan, C. J., Driscoll, K., Phillips, B. M., & Burgess, S. R. (2003). Phonological sensitivity: A quasi-parallel progression of word structure units and cognitive operations. *Reading Research Quarterly*, *38*, 470–487. https://doi.org/10.1598/RRQ.38.4.3

Araújo, B. C. L., de Magalhães Simões, S., de Gois-Santos, V. T., & Martins-Filho, P. R. S. (2020). Association between mouth breathing and asthma: A systematic review and meta-analysis. *Current Allergy and Asthma Reports*, *20*(7), 1–10. https://doi.org/10.1007/s11882-020-00921-9

Archibald, L. M. (2008). The promise of nonword repetition as a clinical tool. *Canadian Journal of Speech-Language Pathology and Audiology*, *32*(1), 21–28.

Archibald, L. M., & Gathercole, S. E. (2006). Nonword repetition: A comparison of tests. *Journal of Speech, Language, and Hearing Research*, *49*(5), 970–983. https://doi.org/10.1044/1092-4388(2006/070).

Arnsten, A. F., & Rubia, K. (2012). Neurobiological circuits regulating attention, cognitive control, motivation, and emotion: Disruptions in neurodevelopmental psychiatric disorders. *Journal of the American Academy of Child & Adolescent Psychiatry*, *51*(4), 356–367. https://doi.org/10.1016/j.jaac.2012.01.008

Arvaniti, A. (2012). The usefulness of metrics in the quantification of speech rhythm. *Journal of Phonetics*, *40*(3), 351–373. https://doi.org/10.1016/j.wocn.2012.02.003

Asghari, S. Z., Farashi, S., Bashirian, S., & Jenabi, E. (2021). Distinctive prosodic features of people with autism spectrum disorder: A systematic review and meta-analysis study. *Scientific Reports*, *11*(1), Article 23093. https://doi.org/10.1038/s41598-021-02487-6

Aslıer, M., Aslıer, N. G. Y., Ercan, İ., & Keskin, S. (2022). Clustering upper airway physicals, otitis media with effusion and auditory functions in children. *Auris Nasus Larynx*, *49*(2), 195–201. https://doi.org/10.1016/j.anl.2021.07.001

Assaf, D. D. C., Knorst, J. K., Busanello-Stella, A. R., Ferrazzo, V. A., Berwig, L. C., Ardenghi, T. M., & Marquezan, M. (2021). Association between malocclusion, tongue position and speech distortion in mixed-dentition schoolchildren: An epidemiological study. *Journal of Applied Oral Science*, *29*.

Astudillo-Rodriguez, C., Crespo-Martínez, E., Carvajal, F., & León-Pesantez, A. (2022). Software development of applications oriented to phonological awareness in high school children: A systematic literature review. In M. S. Islam (Ed.), *Proceedings of the 3rd Asia Pacific International Conference on Industrial Engineering and Operations Management, Johor Bahru, Malaysia, September 13–15, 2022* (pp. 2558–2569). IEOM Society International 3rd Asia Pacific Conference.

Atkinson, R. C., & Shiffrin, R. M. (1968). Human memory: A proposed system and its control processes. In K. Spence (Ed.), *The psychology of learning and motivation* (Vol. 2, pp. 115–118). Academic Press.

Attwell, G. A., Bennin, K. E., & Tekinerdogan, B. (2023). Reference architecture design for computer-based speech therapy systems. *Computer Speech & Language*, *78*, 101465. https://doi.org/10.1016/j.csl.2022.101465.

August, G. J., & Gewirtz, A. (2019). Moving toward a precision-based, personalized framework for prevention science: Introduction to the special issue. *Prevention Science*, 20, 1–9. https://doi.org/10.1007/s11121-018-0955-9

Azieb, S. (2021). The critical period hypothesis in second language acquisition: A review of the literature. *IJARS International Journal of Humanities and Social Studies*, *8*(4), 20.

Babatsouli, E. (2021). Correlation between the measure for cluster proximity (MCP) and the percentage of consonants correct (PCC). *Clinical Linguistics & Phonetics*, *35*(1), 65–83. https://doi.org/10.1080/02699206.2020.1744189

Babatsouli, E., & Sotiropoulos, D. (2018). A measure for cluster proximity (MCP) in child speech. *Clinical Linguistics & Phonetics*, *32*(12), 1071–1089. https://doi.org/10.1080/02699206.2018.1510982

Bach-y-Rita, P., Collins, C. C., Saunders, F. A., White, B. & Scadden, L. (1969). Vision substitution by tactile image projection. *Nature*, *221*, 963–964. https://doi.org/10.1038/221963a0

Baddeley, A. (1992). Working memory. *Science*, *255*(5044), 556–559. https://doi.org/10.1126/science.173635

Baddeley, A. D. (1986). *Working memory*. Clarendon Press.

Bagatto, M. (2020). Audiological considerations for managing mild bilateral or unilateral hearing loss in infants and young children. *Language, Speech, and Hearing Services in Schools*, *51*(1), 68–73. https://doi.org/10.1044/2019_LSHSS-OCHL-19-0025

Bagatto, M., DesGeorges, J., King, A., Kitterick, P., Laurnagaray, D., Lewis, D., . . .Tharpe, A. M. (2019). Consensus practice parameter: Audiological assessment and management of unilateral hearing loss in children. *International Journal of Audiology*, *58*(12), 805–815. https://doi.org/10.1080/14992027.2019.1654620

Bahar, N., Namasivayam, A. K., & van Lieshout, P. (2022). Telehealth intervention and childhood apraxia of speech: A scoping review. *Speech, Language and Hearing*, *25*(4), 450–462. https://doi.org/10.1080/2050571X.2021.1947649

Bahr, D. C., & Hillis, A. E. (2001). *Oral motor assessment and treatment: Ages and stages*. Pearson.

Bahr, D., & Rosenfeld-Johnson, S. (2010). Treatment of children with speech oral placement disorders (OPDs): A paradigm emerges. *Communication Disorders Quarterly*, *31*(3), 131–138. https://doi.org/10.1177/1525740109350217

Baigorri, M., Crowley, C., & Sommer, C. (2020). Addressing the gap in education for cleft palate: A module training series for craniofacial assessment and treatment. *Perspectives of the ASHA Special Interest Groups*, *5*(3), 662–668. https://doi.org/10.1044/2020_PERSP-19-00138

Bailey, G., & Thomas, E. (2021). Some aspects of African-American vernacular English phonology. In G. Bailey, J. Baugh, S. S. Mufwene, & Rickford, J. R. (Eds.), *African-American English: Structure, history and use* (pp. 93–118). Routledge.

Baker, A., Niles, N., Kysh, L., & Sargent, B. (2022). Effect of motor intervention for infants and toddlers with cerebral palsy: A systematic review and meta-analysis. *Pediatric Physical Therapy*, *34*(3), 297–307. https://doi.org/10.1097/PEP.0000000000000914

Baker, E., Croot, K., McLeod, S., & Paul, R. (2001). Psycholinguistic models of speech development and their application to clinical practice. *Journal of Speech, Language, and Hearing Research*, *44*(3), 685–702. https://doi.org/10.1044/1092-4388(2001/055)

Baker, E., & McLeod, S. (2011). Evidence-based practice for children with speech sound disorders: Part 1 narrative review. *Language, Speech, and Hearing Services in Schools*, *42*(2), 102–139. https://doi.org/10.1044/0161-1461(2010/09-0075)

Bakke, M., Bergendal, B., McAllister, A., Sjogreen, L., & Asten, P. (2007). Development and evaluation of a comprehensive screening for orofacial dysfunction. *Swedish Dental Journal*, *31*, 75–84.

Balas, A. (2009). Natural phonology as a functional theory. *Poznań Studies in Contemporary Linguistics*, 45(1), 43–54. https://doi.org/10.2478/v10010-009-0001-y

Balikci, O. S. (2020). Investigation of phonological awareness interventions in early childhood. *International Journal of Early Childhood Special Education*, *12*(1), 277–288.

Ball, M. J. (2015). *Principles of clinical phonology*. Routledge.

Ball, M., Müller, N., Klopfenstein, M., & Rutter, B. (2009) The importance of narrow phonetic transcription for highly unintelligible speech: Some examples. *Logopedics Phoniatrics Vocology*, *34*(2), 84–90. https://doi.org/10.1080/14015430902913535

Ballard, K. J., Robin, D. A., McCabe, P., & McDonald, J. (2010). A treatment for dysprosody in childhood apraxia of speech. *Journal of Speech, Language, and Hearing Research*, *53*(5), 1227–1245. https://doi.org/10.1044/1092-4388(2010/09-0130)

Ballard, K. J., Djaja, D., Arciuli, J., James, D. G., & van Doorn, J. (2012). Developmental trajectory for production of prosody: Lexical stress contrastivity in children ages 3 to 7 years and in adults. *Journal of Speech, Language, and Hearing Research, 55*(6), 1822–1835. https://doi.org/10.1044/1092-4388(2012/11-0257)

Baltaxe, C. A. M., & Simmons, J. Q. (1985). Prosodic development in normal and autistic children. In E. Schopler & G. B. Mesibov (Eds.), *Communication problems in autism* (pp. 95–125). Plenum.

Banai, K., Hornickel, J., Skoe, E., Nicol, T., Zecker, S., & Kraus, N. (2009). Reading and subcortical auditory function. *Cerebral Cortex, 19*(11), 2699–2707. https://doi.org/10.1093/cercor/bhp024

Banajee, M., Dicarlo, C., & Stricklin, S. B. (2003). Core vocabulary determination for toddlers. *Augmentative and Alternative Communication, 19*(2), 67–73. https://doi.org/10.1080/0743461031000112034

Bandura, A. (1986). *Social foundations of thought and action.* Prentice-Hall.

Bang, J. Y., Adiao, A. S., Marchman, V. A., & Feldman, H. M. (2020). Language nutrition for language health in children with disorders: A scoping review. *Pediatric Research, 87*(2), 300–308. https://doi.org/10.1038/s41390-019-0551-0

Bangert, K., Scott, K. S., Adams, C., Kisenwether, J. S., Giuffre, L., Reed, J., . . . Klusek, J. (2022). Cluttering in the speech of young men with Fragile X syndrome. *Journal of Speech, Language, and Hearing Research, 65*(3), 954–969. https://doi.org/10.1044/2021_JSLHR-21-00446

Bankson, N., & Bernthal, J. (1990). *Bankson-Bernthal Test of Phonology.* Riverside.

Bansal, A. K., Sharma, M., Kumar, P., Nehra, K., & Kumar, S. (2015). Long face syndrome: A literature review. *Journal of Dental Health and Oral Disorders Therapy, 2*(6), https://doi.org/10.15406/jdhodt.2015.02.00071

Barbier, G., Boë, L.-J., Captier, G., & Laboissiere, R. (2015). Human vocal tract growth: A longitudinal study of the development of various anatomical structures. *16th Annual Conference of the International Speech Communication Association (Interspeech 2015), Sep 2015, Dresden, Germany. Proceedings of Interspeech, 2015* (pp. 364–369). Curran Associates. http://www.proceedings.com/29080.html.

Barefoot, S. M., Bochner, J. H., Johnson, B. A., & Eigen, B. A. V. (1993). Rating deaf speakers' comprehensibility: An exploratory investigation. *American Journal of Speech-Language Pathology, 2*(3), 31–35. https://doi.org/10.1044/1058-0360.0203.31

Barlow, J. A., & Gierut, J. A. (1999). Optimality theory in phonological acquisition. *Journal of Speech, Language, and Hearing Research, 42*(6), 1482–1498. https://doi.org/10.1044/jslhr.4206.1482

Barnes, E. F., Roberts, J., Mirrett, P., Sideris, J., & Misenheimer, J. (2006). A comparison of oral structure and oral-motor function in young males with fragile X syndrome and Down syndrome. *Journal of Speech, Language, and Hearing Research, 49*(4), 903–917. https://doi.org/10.1044/1092-4388(2006/065)

Barnes, E., Roberts, J., Long, S. H., Martin, G. E., Berni, M. C., Mandulak, K. C., & Sideris, J. (2009). Phonological accuracy and intelligibility in connected speech of boys with Fragile X syndrome or Down syndrome. *Journal of Speech, Language, and Hearing Research, 52*(4), 1048–1061. https://doi.org/10.1044/1092-4388(2009/08-0001)

Barnes, S., & Bloch, S. (2019). Why is measuring communication difficult? A critical review of current speech pathology concepts and measures. *Clinical Linguistics & Phonetics, 33*(3), 219–236. https://doi.org/10.1080/02699206.2018.1498541

Barona-Lleo, L., & Fernandez, S. (2016). Hyperfunctional voice disorder in children with Attention Deficit Hyperactivity Disorder (ADHD). A phenotypic characteristic? *Journal of Voice, 30*(1), 114–119. https://doi.org/10.1016/j.jvoice.2015.03.002

Baron–Cohen, S., Golan, O., Wheelwright, S., Granader, Y., & Hill, J. (2010). Emotion word comprehension from 4 to 16 years old: A developmental survey. *Frontiers in Evolutionary Neuroscience, 2*, 109. https://doi.org/10.3389/fnevo.2010.00109

Barrett, C., McCabe, P., Masso, S., & Preston, J. (2020). Protocol for the connected speech transcription of children with speech disorders: An example from childhood apraxia of speech. *Folia Phoniatrica et Logopaedica, 72*(2), 152–166. https://doi.org/10.1159/000500664)

Barsties, B., & De Bodt, M. (2015). Assessment of voice quality: Current state-of-the-art. *Auris*

Nasus Larynx, *42*(3), 183–188. https://doi.org/10.1016/j.anl.2014.11.001

Basheer, B., Hegde, K. S., Bhat, S. S., Umar, D., & Baroudi, K. (2014). Influence of mouth breathing on the dentofacial growth of children: A cephalometric study. *Journal of International Oral Health*, *6*(6), 50.

Bastarache, L. (2021). Using phecodes for research with the electronic health record: From PheWAS to PheRS. *Annual Review of Biomedical Data Science*, *4*, 1–19. https://doi.org/10.1146/annurev-biodatasci-122320-112352

Bates, E., Camaioni, L., & Volterra, V. (1975). The acquisition of performatives prior to speech. *Merrill-Palmer Quarterly of Behavior and Development*, *21*(3), 205–226. https://www.jstor.org/stable/23084619

Bates, S., Titterington, J., and members of UK & Ireland's Child Speech Disorder Research Network. (2021). *Good practice guidelines for the analysis of child speech*. https://pure.ulster.ac.uk/ws/files/93134795/Good_practice_guidelines_for_the_analysis_of_child_speech_2nd_edition_2021.pdf

Bauer, M. S., & Kirchner, J. (2020). Implementation science: What is it and why should I care?. *Psychiatry Research*, *283*, 112376. https://doi.org/10.1016/j.psychres.2019.04.025

Bauman-Waengler, J, & Garcia D. (2019). *Phonological treatment of speech sound disorders in children: A practical guide*. Plural Publishing.

Baxter, R., Merkel-Walsh, R., Baxter, B. S., Lashley, A., & Rendell, N. R. (2020). Functional improvements of speech, feeding, and sleep after lingual frenectomy tongue-tie release: A prospective cohort study. *Clinical Pediatrics*, *59*(9–10), 885–892. https://doi.org/10.1177/0009922820928

Baylis, A., Chapman, K., & Whitehill, T. L. (2015). Validity and reliability of visual analog scaling for assessment of hypernasality and audible nasal emission in children with repaired cleft palate. *The Cleft Palate-Craniofacial Journal*, *52*(6), 660–670. https://doi.org/10.1597/14-040

Bearzotti, F., Tavano, A., & Fabbro, F. (2007). Development of orofacial praxis of children from 4 to 8 years of age. *Perceptual and Motor Skills*, *104*(3 Suppl.), 1355–1366. https://doi.org/10.2466/pms.104.4.1355-1

Becker, M., Oehler, K., Partsch, C. J., Ulmen, U., Schmutzler, R., Cammann, H., & Hesse, V. (2015). Hormonal 'minipuberty' influences the somatic development of boys but not of girls up to the age of 6 years. *Clinical Endocrinology*, *83*(5), 694–701.

Beking, T., Geuze, R. H., Van Faassen, M., Kema, I. P., Kreukels, B. P., & Groothuis, T. G. G. (2018). Prenatal and pubertal testosterone affect brain lateralization. *Psychoneuroendocrinology*, *88*, 78–91. https://doi.org/10.1016/j.psyneuen.2017.10.027

Belardi, K., Watson, L. R., Faldowski, R. A., Hazlett, H., Crais, E., Baranek, G. T., . . . Oller, D. K. (2017). A retrospective video analysis of canonical babbling and volubility in infants with Fragile X syndrome at 9–12 months of age. *Journal of Autism and Developmental Disorders*, *47*(4), 1193–1206. https://doi.org/10.1007/s10803-017-3033-4

Bell, R., Mouzourakis, M., & Wise, S. R. (2022). Impact of unilateral hearing loss in early development. *Current Opinion in Otolaryngology & Head and Neck Surgery*, *30*(5), 344–350. https://doi.org/10.1097/MOO.0000000000000848

Bell, V., Wilkinson, S., Greco, M., Hendrie, C., Mills. B., & Deeley, Q. (2020). What is the functional/organic distinction actually doing in psychiatry and neurology? *Wellcome Open Research*, *11*(5), 138. https://doi.org/10.12688/wellcomeopenres.16022.1.

Bellugi, U., Fischer, S., & Newkirk, C. (1988). The rate of speaking and signing. In E. S. Klima & U. Bellugi (Eds.), *The signs of language* (pp. 181–194). Harvard University Press.

Benchek, P., Igo, R. P., Voss-Hoynes, H., Wren, Y., Miller, G., Truitt, B., . . . Iyengar, S. K. (2021). Association between genes regulating neural pathways for quantitative traits of speech and language disorders. *NPJ Genomic Medicine*, *6*(1), 1–11. https://doi.org/10.1038/s41525-021-00225-5

Bérce, K. B., & Honeybone, P. (2020). Representation-based models in the current landscape of phonological theory. *Acta Linguistica Academia*, *67*(1), 3–27. https://doi.org/10.1556/2062.2020.00002

Berlucchi, G., & Buchtel, H. A. (2009). Neuronal plasticity: Historical roots and evolution of meaning. *Experimental Brain Research*, *192*(3), 307–319. https://doi.org/10.1007/s00221-008-1611-6.

Bernstein, N. (1967). *The coordination and regulation of movements*. Pergamon Press

Bernthal, J. E., Bankson, N. W., & Flipsen, P., Jr. (2022). *Articulation and phonological disorders* (7th edition). Brookes.

Berry, J. (2011). Speaking rate effects on normal aspects of articulation: Outcomes and issues. *Perspectives on Speech Science and Orofacial Disorders, 21*(1), 15–26. https://doi.org/10.1044/ssod21.1.15

Berry, M. D., & Erickson, R. L. (1973). Speaking rate: Effects on children's comprehension of normal speech. *Journal of Speech and Hearing Research, 16*(3), 367–374. https://doi.org/10.1044/jshr.1603.367

Best, C. T. (1994). The emergence of native-language phonological influences in infants: A perceptual assimilation model. In J. C. Goodman & H. C. Nusbaum (Eds.), *The development of speech perception: The transition from speech sounds to spoken words* (pp. 167–244). MIT Press.

Bettens, K., Bruneel, L., Maryn, Y., De Bodt, M., Luyten, A., & Van Lierde, K. M. (2018). Perceptual evaluation of hypernasality, audible nasal airflow and speech understandability using ordinal and visual analogue scaling and their relation with nasalance scores. *Journal of Communication Disorders, 76*, 11–20. https://doi.org/10.1016/j.jcomdis.2018.07.002

Betz, S. K., & Stoel-Gammon, C. (2005). Measuring articulatory error consistency in children with developmental apraxia of speech. *Clinical Linguistics & Phonetics, 19*(1), 53–66. https://doi.org/10.1080/02699200512331325791

Beukelman, D., Jones, R., & Rowan, M. (1989). Frequency of word usage by nondisabled peers in integrated preschool classrooms. *Augmentative Alternative Communication, 5*(4), 243–248. https://doi.org/10.1080/07434618912331275296

Bhattacharyya, N. (2015). The prevalence of pediatric voice and swallowing problems in the United States. *Laryngoscope, 125*(3), 746–750. https://doi.org/10.1002/lary.24931

Bialystok, E., & Kroll, J. F. (2018). Can the critical period be saved? A bilingual perspective. *Bilingualism: Language and Cognition, 21*(5), 908–910. https://doi.org/10.1017/S1366728918000202

Bílková, Z., Bartoš, M., Dominec, A., Greško, Š., Novozámský, A., Zitová, B., & Paroubková, M. (2022, August). ASSISLT: Computer-aided speech therapy tool. In *2022 30th European Signal Processing Conference (EUSIPCO)* (pp. 598–602). IEEE. https://doi.org/10.23919/EUSIPCO55093.2022.9909627

Binos, P., Nirgianaki, E., & Psillas, G. (2021). How effective is auditory–verbal therapy (AVT) for building language development of children with cochlear implants? A systematic review. *Life, 11*(3), 239. https://doi.org/10.3390/life11030239

Bittles, A. H., Bower, C., Hussain, R., & Glasson, E. J. (2007). The four ages of Down syndrome. *European Journal of Public Health, 17*(2), 221–225. https://doi.org/10.1093/eurpub/ckl103

Blakely, R. W. (2000). *Screening Test for Developmental Apraxia of Speech (STDAS-2)*, Second edition. Mind Resources.

Blanchet, P. G., & Snyder, G. J. (2010). Speech rate treatments for individuals with dysarthria: A tutorial. *Perceptual and Motor Skills, 110*(3), 965–982.

Blanck-Lubarsch, M., Dirksen, D., Feldmann, R., Sauerland, C., & Hohoff, A. (2019). Tooth malformations, DMFT index, speech impairment and oral habits in patients with fetal alcohol syndrome. *International Journal of Environmental Research and Public Health, 16*(22), 4401. https://doi.org/10.3390/ijerph16224401

Bland-Stewart, L. M. (2005). Difference or deficit in speakers of African American English? What every clinician should know . . . and do. *ASHA Leader, 10*(6), 6–31.

Blank, R., Barnett, A. L., Cairney, J., Green, D., Kirby, A., Polatajko, H., . . . Vinçon, S. (2019). International clinical practice recommendations on the definition, diagnosis, assessment, intervention, and psychosocial aspects of developmental coordination disorder. *Developmental Medicine & Child Neurology, 61*(3), 242–285. http://apps.who.int/classif

Blomberg, R., Danielsson, H., Rudner, M., Söderlund, G. B., & Rönnberg, J. (2019). Speech processing difficulties in attention deficit hyperactivity disorder. *Frontiers in Psychology, 10*, 1536. https://doi.org/10.3389/fpsyg.2019.01536

Bode, C., Ghaltakhchyan, N., Rezende Silva, E., Turvey, T., Blakey, G., White, R., . . . Jacox, L. (2023). Impacts of development, dentofacial disharmony, and its surgical correction on speech: A narrative review for dental professionals. *Applied Sciences, 13*(9), 5496. https://doi.org/10.3390/app13095496

Bogavac, I., Tešović, M., & Jeličić, L. (2019). Risk factors prevalence in children with speech and language disorders. *Speech and Language*, 455.

Bohannon, R. W. (2019). Considerations and practical options for measuring muscle strength: A narrative review. *BioMed Research International*, Volume 2019 | Article ID 8194537 | https://doi.org/10.1155/2019/8194537

Boliek, C. A., Halpern, A., Hernandez, K., Fox, C. M., & Ramig, L. (2022). Intensive voice treatment (Lee Silverman Voice Treatment [LSVT LOUD]) for children with Down syndrome: Phase I outcomes. *Journal of Speech, Language, and Hearing Research, 65*(4), 1228–1262. https://doi.org/10.1044/2021_JSLHR-21-00228

Boliek, C. A., Hixon, T. J., Watson, P. J., & Jones, P. B. (2009). Refinement of speech breathing in healthy 4-to 6-year-old children. *Journal of Speech, Language, and Hearing Research, 52*(4), 990–1007. https://doi.org/10.1044/1092-4388(2009/07-0214)

Bolinger, C. L., & Dembowski, J. (2019). Articulation in children with fetal alcohol syndrome. *Clinical Archives of Communication Disorders, 4*(1), 35–40. http://dx.doi.org/10.21849/cacd.2019.00010

Bolker, J. A. (2000). Modularity in development and why it matters to evo-devo. *American Zoologist, 40*(5), 770–776. https://doi.org/10.1093/icb/40.5.770

Bölte, S., Girdler, S. & Marschik, P. B. (2019). The contribution of environmental exposure to the etiology of autism spectrum disorder. *Cellular and Molecular Life Sciences, 76*, 1275–1297. https://doi.org/10.1007/s00018-018-2988-4

Bombonato, C., Casalini, C., Pecini, C., Angelucci, G., Vicari, S., Podda, I., . . . Menghini, D. (2022). Implicit learning in children with Childhood Apraxia of Speech. *Research in Developmental Disabilities, 122*, 104170. https://doi.org/10.1016/j.ridd.2021.104170

Bommangoudar, J. S., Chandrashekhar, S., Shetty, S., & Sidral, S. (2020). Pedodontist's role in managing speech impairments due to structural imperfections and oral habits: A literature review. *International Journal of Clinical Pediatric Dentistry, 13*(1), 85–90. https://doi.org/10.5005/jp-journals-10005-1745

Bonacina, S., Otto-Meyer, S., Krizman, J., White-Schwoch, T., Nicol, T., & Kraus, N. (2019). Stable auditory processing underlies phonological awareness in typically developing preschoolers. *Brain and Language, 197*, 104664. https://doi.org/10.1016/j.bandl.2019.104664

Bonneh, Y. S., Levanon, Y., Dean-Pardo, O., Lossos, L., & Adini, Y. (2011). Abnormal speech spectrum and increased pitch variability in young autistic children. *Frontiers in Human Neuroscience, 4*, 237. https://doi.org/10.3389/fnhum.2010.00237

Bono, K. E., & Bizri, R. (2014). The role of language and private speech in preschoolers' self-regulation. *Early Child Development and Care, 184*(5), 658–670. https://doi.org/10.1080/03004430.2013.813846

Bonuck, K., Battino, R., Barresi, I., & McGrath, K. (2021). Sleep problem screening of young children by speech-language pathologists: A mixed-methods feasibility study. *Autism & Developmental Language Impairments, 6*. https://doi.org/10.1177/23969415211035066

Bornstein, M. H., Hahn, C. S., & Wolke, D. (2013). Systems and cascades in cognitive development and academic achievement. *Child Development, 84*(1), 154–162. https://doi.org/10.1111/j.1467-8624.2012.01849.x

Borox, T., Leite, A. P. D., Bagarollo, M. F., Alencar, B. L. F. D., & Czlusniak, G. R. (2018). Speech production assessment of mouth breathing children with hypertrophy of palatines and/or pharyngeal tonsils. *Revista CEFAC, 20, 468–477*.

Borrie, S. A., & Delfino, C. R. (2017). Conversational entrainment of vocal fry in young adult female American English speakers. *Journal of Voice, 31*(4), 513–e525. https://doi.org/10.1016/j.jvoice.2016.12.005

Borrie, S. A., Lubold, N., & Pon-Barry, H. (2015). Disordered speech disrupts conversational entrainment: A study of acoustic-prosodic entrainment and communicative success in populations with communication challenges. *Frontiers in Psychology, 6*, 1187. https://doi.org/10.3389/fpsyg.2015.01187

Bortfeld, H., Leon, S. D., Bloom, J. E., Schober, M. F., & Brennan, S. E. (2001). Disfluency rates in conversation: Effects of age, relationship, topic, role, and gender. *Language and Speech, 44*(2), 123–147. https://doi.org/10.1177/00238309010440020101

Boscato, N., Hayakawa, H., Iida, T., Costa, Y. M., Kothari, S. F., Kothari, M., & Svensson, P. (2022). Impact of oral motor task training on corticomotor pathways and diadochokinetic rates in young healthy participants. *Journal of Oral Rehabilitation*, *49*(9), 924–934. https://doi.org/10.1111/joor.13349

Boseley, M. E., & Hartnick, C. J. (2006). Development of the human true vocal fold: Depth of cell layers and quantifying cell types within the lamina propria. *Annals of Otology, Rhinology & Laryngology*, *115*(10), 784–788. https://doi.org/10.1177/000348940611501012

Boseley, M. E., Cunningham, M. J., Volk, M. S., & Hartnick, C. J. (2006). Validation of the pediatric voice-related quality-of-life survey. *Archives of Otolaryngology-Head & Neck Surgery*, *132*(7), 717–720. https://doi.org/10.1001/archotol.132.7.717

Bosma, J. F. (1975). Anatomic and physiologic development of the speech apparatus. In D. B. Tower (Ed.), *The nervous system: Human communication and its disorders* (pp. 469–481). Raven Press.

Bottalico, P., Murgia, S., Puglisi, G. E., Astolfi, A., & Kirk, K. I. (2020). Effect of masks on speech intelligibility in auralized classrooms. *The Journal of the Acoustical Society of America*, *148*(5), 2878–2884. https://doi.org/10.1121/10.0002450

Botteron, K., Carter, C., Castellanos, F. X., Dickstein, D. P., Drevets, W., Kim, K. L., . . . Zubieta, J. K. (2012). *Consensus report of the APA work group on neuroimaging markers of psychiatric disorders*. American Psychiatric Association.

Boucher, V. J., & Lalonde, B. (2015). Effects of the growth of breath capacities on mean length of utterances: How maturing production processes influence indices of language development. *Journal of Phonetics*, *52*, 58–69. https://doi.org/10.1016/j.wocn.2015.04.005

Boutrus, M., Maybery, M. T., Alvares, G. A., Tan, D. W., Varcin, K. J., & Whitehouse, A. J. (2017). Investigating facial phenotype in autism spectrum conditions: The importance of a hypothesis driven approach. *Autism Research*, *10*, 1910–1918.

Boyce, S. E. (2015, November). The articulatory phonetics of /r/ for residual speech errors. *Seminars in Speech and Language*, *36*(4), 257–270. https://doi.org/10.1055/s-0035-1562909

Boyce, S. E., Hamilton, S. M., & Rivera-Campos, A. (2016). Acquiring rhoticity across languages: An ultrasound study of differentiating tongue movements. *Clinical Linguistics & Phonetics*, *30*(3-5), 174–201. https://doi.org/10.3109/02699206.2015.1127999

Bradford-Heit, A., & Dodd, B. (1998). Learning new words using imitation and additional cues: Differences between children with disordered speech. *Child Language Teaching and Therapy*, *14*(2), 159–179. https://doi.org/10.1177/026565909801400203

Bradlow, A. R. (1995). A comparative acoustic study of English and Spanish vowels. *The Journal of the Acoustical Society of America*, *97*, 1916–1924.

Bradlow, A. R., & Bent, T. (2008). Perceptual adaptation to non-native speech. *Cognition*, *106*(2), 707–729. https://doi.org/10.1016/j.cognition.2007.04.005

Brauer, J., Anwander, A., Perani, D., & Friederici, A. D. (2013). Dorsal and ventral pathways in language development. *Brain and Language*, *127*(2), 289–295. https://doi.org/10.1016/j.bandl.2013.03.001

Broome, K., McCabe, P., Docking, K., & Doble, M. (2017). A systematic review of speech assessments for children with autism spectrum disorder: Recommendations for best practice. *American Journal of Speech-Language Pathology*, *26*(3), 1011–1029. https://doi.org/10.1044/2017_AJSLP-16-0014

Brosseau-Lapré, F., & Roepke, E. (2019). Speech errors and phonological awareness in children ages 4 and 5 years with and without speech sound disorder. *Journal of Speech, Language, and Hearing Research*, *62*(9), 3276–3289. https://doi.org/10.1044/2019_JSLHR-S-17-0461

Brosseau-Lapré, F., & Roepke, E. (2022). Implementing speech perception and phonological awareness intervention for children with speech sound disorders. *Language, Speech, and Hearing Services in Schools*, *53*(3), 646–658. https://doi.org/10.1044/2022_LSHSS-21-00117

Browman, C. P., & Goldstein, L. (1992). Articulatory phonology: An overview. *Phonetica*, *49*(3-4), 155–180. https://doi.org/10.1159/000261913.

Brown, M. C., Sibley, D. E., Washington, J. A., Rogers, T. T., Edwards, J. R., MacDonald, M. C.,

& Seidenberg, M. S. (2015). Impact of dialect use on a basic component of learning to read. *Frontiers in Psychology*, *6*, 196. https://doi.org/10.3389/fpsyg.2015.00196

Brown, T., Murray, E., & McCabe, P. (2018). The boundaries of auditory perception for within-word syllable segregation in untrained and trained adult listeners. *Clinical Linguistics & Phonetics*, *32*(11), 979–996. https://doi.org/10.1080/02699206.2018.1463395

Brumbaugh, K. M., & Smit, A. B. (2013). Treating children ages 3–6 who have speech sound disorder: A survey. *Language, Speech, and Hearing Services in Schools*, *44*, 306–319. https://doi.org/10.1044/0161-1461(2013/12-0029)

Bruney, T. L., Scime, N. V., Madubueze, A., & Chaput, K. H. (2022). Systematic review of the evidence for resolution of common breastfeeding problems—ankyloglossia (Tongue Tie). *Acta Paediatrica*, *111*(5), 940–947. https://doi.org/10.1111/apa.16289

Brutten, G. J., & Vanryckeghem, M. (2007). *BAB: Behavior Assessment Battery for school-age children who stutter*. Plural Publishing.

Brysbaert, M. (2019). How many words do we read per minute? A review and meta-analysis of reading rate. *Journal of Memory and Language*, *109*, 104047. https://doi.org/10.1016/j.jml.2019.104047

Buder, E. H., Warlaumont, A. S., Oller, D. K., Peter, B., & MacLeod, A. (2013). An acoustic phonetic catalog of prespeech vocalizations from a developmental perspective. In B. Peter & A. A. N. MacLeod (Eds.), *Comprehensive perspectives on child speech development and disorders: Pathways from linguistic theory to clinical practice* (pp. 103–134). Nova Science Publishers.

Bunton, K. (2008, November). Speech versus nonspeech: Different tasks, different neural organization. *Seminars in Speech and Language*, *29*(4), 267–275.

Buretić-Tomljanović, A., Giacometti, J., Ostojić, S., & Kapović, M. (2007). Sex-specific differences of craniofacial traits in Croatia: The impact of environment in a small geographic area. *Annals of Human Biology*, *34*(3), 296–314. https://doi.org/10.1080/03014460701211017

Burkhardt-Reed, M. M., Long, H. L., Bowman, D. D., Bene, E. R., & Oller, D. K. (2021). The origin of language and relative roles of voice and gesture in early communication development. *Infant Behavior and Development*, *65*, 101648. https://doi.org/10.1371/journal.pone.0224956

Burrows, L., & Goldstein, B. A. (2010). Whole word measures in bilingual children with speech sound disorders. *Clinical Linguistics & Phonetics*, *24*(4-5), 357–368. https://doi.org/10.3109/02699200903581067

Buschang, P. H., & Hinton, R. J. (2005). A gradient of potential for modifying craniofacial growth. *Seminars in Orthodontics*, 11(4), 219–226. https://doi.org/10.1053/j.sodo.2005.07.006

Byiers, B. J., Reichle, J., & Symons, F. J. (2012). Single-subject experimental design for evidence-based practice. *American Journal of Speech-Language Pathology*, *21*(4), 397–414. https://doi.org/10.1044/1058-0360(2012/11-0036)

Byrd, A. S., & Brown, J. A. (2021). An interprofessional approach to dialect-shifting instruction for early elementary school students. *Language, Speech, and Hearing Services in Schools*, *52*(1), 139–148. https://doi.org/10.1044/2020_LSHSS-20-00060

Byun, T. M., & Hitchcock, E. R. (2012). Investigating the use of traditional and spectral biofeedback approaches to intervention for/r/ misarticulation. *American Journal of Speech-Language Pathology*, *21*(3), 207–222. https://doi.org/10.1044/1058-0360(2012/11-0083)

Byun, T. M., Hitchcock, E. R., & Swartz, M. T. (2014). Retroflex versus bunched in treatment for rhotic misarticulation: Evidence from ultrasound biofeedback intervention. *Journal of Speech, Language, and Hearing Research*, *57*(6), 2116–2130. https://doi.org/10.1044/2014_JSLHR-S-14-0034

Cabbage, K. L., & DeVeney, S. L. (2020). Treatment approach considerations for children with speech sound disorders in school-based settings. *Topics in Language Disorders*, *40*(4), 312–325. https://doi.org/10.1097/TLD.0000000000000229

Cabbage, K. L., Farquharson, K., Iuzzini-Seigel, J., Zuk, J., & Hogan, T. P. (2018). Exploring the overlap between dyslexia and speech sound production deficits. *Language, Speech, and Hearing Services in Schools*, *49*(4), 774–786. https://doi.org/10.1044/2018_LSHSS-DYSLC-18-0008

Cabbage, K., Farquharson, K., & DeVeney, S. (2022). Speech sound disorder treatment approaches used by school-based clinicians:

An application of the experience sampling method. *Language, Speech, and Hearing Services in Schools, 53*(3), 860–873. https://doi.org/10.1044/2022_LSHSS-21-00167

Cai, T., & McPherson, B. (2017). Hearing loss in children with otitis media with effusion: A systematic review. *International Journal of Audiology, 56*(2), 65–76. http://10.1080/14992027.2016.1250960

Callan, D. E., Kent, R. D., Guenther, F. H., & Vorperian, H. K. (2000). An auditory-feedback-based neural network model of speech production that is robust to developmental changes in the size and shape of the articulatory system. *Journal of Speech, Language, and Hearing Research, 43*(3), 721–736. https://doi.org/10.1044/jslhr.4303.721

Cámara, S., Fournier, M., Cordero, P., Melero, J., Robles, F., Esteso, B., . . . Budke, M. (2020). Neuropsychological profile in children with posterior fossa tumors with or without post-operative cerebellar mutism syndrome (CMS). *The Cerebellum, 19*(1), 78–88. https://doi.org/10.1007/s12311-019-01088-4

Campano, M., Cox, S. R., Caniano, L., & Koenig, L. L. (2021). A review of voice disorders in school-aged children. *Journal of Voice.* https://doi.org/10.1016/j.jvoice.2020.12.018

Campbell, N., & Mokhtari, P. (2003, August). Voice quality: The 4th prosodic dimension. In M.-J. Solé, D. Recasens, & J. Romero (Eds.), *Proceedings of the 15th International Congress of Phonetic Sciences.* Causal Productions.

Campbell, T. F., & Bain, B. A. (1991). How long to treat: A multiple outcome approach. *Language, Speech, and Hearing Services in Schools, 22*(4), 271–276. https://doi.org/10.1044/0161-1461.2204.271

Campbell, T. F., Dollaghan, C. A., Rockette, H. E., Paradise, J. L., Feldman, H. M., Shriberg, L. D., . . . Kurs-Lasky, M. (2003). Risk factors for speech delay of unknown origin in 3-year-old children. *Child Development, 74*(2), 346–357. https://doi.org/10.1111/1467-8624.7402002

Cantle Moore, R. (2014). The infant monitor of vocal production: Simple beginnings. *Deafness & Education International, 16*(4), 218–236. https://doi.org/10.1179/1464315414Z.00000000067

Cantle Moore R., & Colyvas, K. (2018). The Infant Monitor of vocal Production (IMP) normative study: Important foundations. *Deafness & Education International, 20*(3-4), 228–244. https://doi.org/14643154.2018.1483098

Capone, N. C., & McGregor, K. K. (2004). Gesture development. *Journal of Speech, Language, and Hearing Research, 47*(1), 173–186. https://doi.org/10.1044/1092-4388(2004/015

Carding, P. N., Roulstone, S., Northstone, K., & ALSPAC Study Team. (2006). The prevalence of childhood dysphonia: A cross-sectional study. *Journal of Voice, 20*(4), 623–630. https://doi.org/10.1016/j.jvoice.2005.07.004

Cardoso, R., Guimaraes, I., Santos, H., Loureiro, R., Domingos, J., de Abreu, D., . . . Ferreira, J. (2017). Frenchay dysarthria assessment (FDA-2) in Parkinson's disease: Cross-cultural adaptation and psychometric properties of the European Portuguese version. *Journal of Neurology, 264*, 21–31. https://https://doi.org/10.1007/s00415-016-8298-6

Carey, J. C., Cohen Jr, M. M., Curry, C. J., Devriendt, K., Holmes, L. B., & Verloes, A. (2009). Elements of morphology: standard terminology for the lips, mouth, and oral region. *American Journal of Medical Genetics Part A, 149*(1), 77–92. https://doi.org/10.1002/ajmg.a.32602

Carey, S. (2010). Beyond fast mapping. *Language Learning and Development, 6*(3), 184–205. https://doi.org/10.1080/15475441.2010.484379

Carey, S., & Bartlett, E. (1978). Acquiring a single new word. *Proceedings of the Stanford Child Language Conference, 15*, 17–29.

Carlson D. S. (2005). Growth in the postgenomic era. *Seminars in Orthodontics, 11*, 172–183.

Carpenter, M., Nagell, K., & Tomasello, M. (1998). Social cognition, joint attention, and communicative competence from 9 to 15 months of age. *Monographs of the Society for Research on Child Development, 63*, 1–143. https://doi.org/10.1037/10522-163

Cartei, V., & Reby, D. (2013). Effect of formant frequency spacing on perceived gender in pre-pubertal children's voices. *PLoS ONE, 8*(12), e81022. https://doi.org/10.1371/journal.pone.0081022

Cartei, V., Cowels, W., Banerjee, R., & Reby, D. (2014). Control of voice gender in pre-pubertal children. *British Journal of Developmental Psychology, 32*, 100–106.

Cartei, V., Cowles, H. W., & Reby, D. (2012). Spontaneous voice gender imitation abilities in adult speakers. *PloS ONE*, 7, e31353.

Cartwright, L. R., & Lass, N. J. (1975). A psychophysical study of rate of continuous speech stimuli by means of direct magnitude estimation scaling. *Language and Speech, 18*, 358–365.

Case, J., & Grigos, M. I. (2016). Articulatory control in childhood apraxia of speech in a novel word-learning task. *Journal of Speech, Language, and Hearing Research*, *59*(6), 1253–1268. https://doi.org/10.1044/2016_JSLHR-S-14-0261

Case, J., & Grigos, M. (2020). How the study of speech motor control can inform assessment and intervention in childhood apraxia of speech. *Perspectives of the ASHA Special Interest Groups, 5*(4), 784–793. https://doi.org/10.1044/2020_PERSP-19-00114

Catsman-Berrevoets C., & Patay, Z. (2018) Cerebellar mutism syndrome. *Handbook of Clinical Neurology, 155*, 273–288. https://doi.org/10.1016/B978-0-444-64189-2.00018-4

Cattoni, D. M., Fernandes, F. D., Di Francesco, R. C., & Latorre Mdo, M. R. (2007). Characteristics of the stomatognathic system of mouth breathing children: Anthroposcopic approach (original title: Características do sistema estomatognático de crianças respiradoras orais: enfoque antroposcópico). [Portuguese] *Pró-Fono Revista de Atualização Científica, 19*, 347–351. https://doi.org/10.1590/s0104-56872007000400004

Centers for Disease Control (CDC). (2020). 2020 *Annual Data Early Hearing Detection and Intervention (EHDI) Program.* https://www.cdc.gov/ncbddd/hearingloss/ehdi-data2020.html

Centers for Disease Control and Prevention. (n.d.). *CDC's developmental milestones.* https://www.cdc.gov/ncbddd/actearly/milestones/index.html

Centers for Disease Control and Prevention, Educational Center for Disease Control. (2017). *Data and statistics.* 14 Feb. 2017.

Cervin, M. (2022), Developmental signs of ADHD and autism: A prospective investigation in 3623 children. *European Child and Adolescent Psychiatry*, (2022). https://doi.org/10.1007/s00787-022-02024-4

Çetinkaya, M., Öz, F. T., Orhan, A. I., Orhan, K., Karabulut, B., Can-Karabulut, D. C., & İlk, Ö. (2011). Prevalence of oral abnormalities in a Turkish newborn population. *International Dental Journal, 61*(2), 90–100. https://doi.org/10.1111/j.1875-595X.2011.00020.x

Chai, Y., & Maxson, R. E. (2006). Recent advances in craniofacial morphogenesis. *Developmental Dynamics, 235*, 2353–2375.

Challis, J., Newnham, J., Petraglia, F., Yeganegi, M., & Bocking, A. (2013). Fetal sex and preterm birth. *Placenta, 34*(2), 95–99. https://doi.org/10.1016/j.placenta.2012.11.007

Chambi-Rocha, A., Cabrera-Domínguez, M. E., & Domínguez-Reyes, A. (2018). Breathing mode influence on craniofacial development and head posture. [Portuguese] *Jornal de Pediatria (Versão em Português), 94*(2), 123–130. https://doi.org/10.1016/j.jpedp.2017.08.022

Chan, J., Edman, J. C., & Koltai, P. J. (2004). Obstructive sleep apnea in children. *American Family Physician, 69*(5), 1147–1155.

Chang, C. B. (2012). Rapid and multifaceted effects of second-language learning on first-language speech production. *Journal of Phonetics, 40*(2), 249–268. https://doi.org/10.1016/j.wocn.2011.10.007

Chang, S. E., Garnett, E. O., Etchell, A., & Chow, H. M. (2019). Functional and neuroanatomical bases of developmental stuttering: Current insights. *The Neuroscientist, 25*(6), 566–582. https://doi.org/10.1177/1073858418803594

Charity, A. H. (2008). African American English: An overview. *Perspectives on Communication Disorders and Sciences in Culturally and Linguistically Diverse (CLD) Populations, 15*(2), 33–42.

Chauvin, R. J., Mennes, M., Llera, A., Buitelaar, J. K., & Beckmann, C. F. (2019). Disentangling common from specific processing across tasks using task potency. *NeuroImage, 184*, 632–645. https://doi.org/10.1016/j.neuroimage.2018.09.059

Chaware, S. H., Dubey, S. G., Kakatkar, V., Jankar, A., Pustake, S., & Darekar, A. (2021). The systematic review and meta-analysis of oral sensory challenges in children and adolescents with autism spectrum disorder. *Journal of International Society of Preventive & Community Dentistry, 11*(5), 469. https://doi.org/10.4103/jispcd.JISPCD_135_21

Chen, C. L., Chen, H. C., Hong, W. H., Yang, F. P. G., Yang, L. Y., & Wu, C. Y. (2010). Oromotor variability in children with mild spastic cerebral palsy: A kinematic study of speech motor control. *Journal of Neuroengineering and Rehabilitation*, *7*(1), 1–10. https://doi.org/10.1186/1743-0003-7-54

Chen, F., Cheung, C. C. H., & Peng, G. (2022). Linguistic tone and non-linguistic pitch imitation in children with autism spectrum disorders: A cross-linguistic investigation. *Journal of Autism and Developmental Disorders*, *52*(5), 2325–2343. https://doi.org/10.1007/s10803-021-05123-4

Chen, Y., Tang, E., Ding, H., & Zhang, Y. (2022). Auditory pitch perception in autism spectrum disorder: A systematic review and meta-analysis. *Journal of Speech, Language, and Hearing Research*, *65*(12), 4866–4886. https://doi.org/10.1044/2022_JSLHR-22-00254

Chenausky, K. V., & Tager-Flusberg, H. (2022). The importance of deep speech phenotyping for neurodevelopmental and genetic disorders: a conceptual review. *Journal of Neurodevelopmental Disorders*, *14*, 36. https://doi.org/10.1186/s11689-022-09443-z

Chenausky, K. V., Brignell, A., Morgan, A., Gagné, D., Norton, A., Tager-Flusberg, H., . . . Green, J. R. (2020). Factor analysis of signs of childhood apraxia of speech. *Journal of Communication Disorders*, *87*, 106033. https://doi.org/10.1016/j.jcomdis.2020.106033

Chenausky, K., Nelson III, C., & Tager-Flusberg, H. (2017). Vocalization rate and consonant production in toddlers at high and low risk for autism. *Journal of Speech, Language, and Hearing Research*, *60*(4), 865–876. https://doi.org/10.1044/2016_JSLHR-S-15-0400

Cherry, E. C. (1953). Some experiments on the recognition of speech, with one and with two ears. *The Journal of the Acoustical Society of America*, *25*(5), 975–979. https://doi.org/10.1121/1.1907229

Cheung, C., McAlonan, G. M., Fung, Y. Y., Fung, G., Yu, K. K., Tai, K. S., . . . Chua, S. E. (2011). MRI study of minor physical anomaly in childhood autism implicates aberrant neurodevelopment in infancy. *PLoS ONE*, *6*(6), e20246. https://doi.org/10.1371/journal.pone.0020246

Cheung, M. M. Y., Tsang, T. W., Watkins, R., Birman, C., Popova, S., & Elliott, E. J. (2021). Ear abnormalities among children with Fetal Alcohol Spectrum Disorder: A systematic review and meta-analysis. *The Journal of Pediatrics*, *242*, 113–120.e16. https://doi.org/10.1016/j.jpeds.2021.11.016

Chiat, S., & Polišenská, K. (2016). A framework for crosslinguistic nonword repetition tests: Effects of bilingualism and socioeconomic status on children's performance. *Journal of Speech, Language, and Hearing Research*, *59*(5), 1179–1189. https://doi.org/10.1044/2016_JSLHR-L-15-0293

Childers, D. G., & Wong, C. F. (1994). Measuring and modeling vocal source-tract interaction. *IEEE Transactions on Biomedical Engineering*, *41*(7), 663–671.

Chilosi, A. M., Podda, I., Ricca, I., Comparini, A., Franchi, B., Fiori, S., . . . Santorelli, F. M. (2022). Differences and commonalities in children with childhood apraxia of speech and comorbid neurodevelopmental disorders: A multidimensional perspective. *Journal of Personalized Medicine*, *12*(2), 313. https://doi.org/10.3390/jpm12020313

Chin. S. B., Bergeson, T. R., & Phan, J. (2012). Speech intelligibility and prosody production in children with cochlear implants. *Journal of Communication Disorders*, *45*(5), 355–366. https://doi.org/10.1016/j.jcomdis.2012.05.003

Chin, S. B., Tsai, P. L., & Gao, S. (2003). Connected speech intelligibility of children with cochlear implants and children with normal hearing. *American Journal of Speech-Language Pathology* *12*(4), 440–451. https://doi.org/10.1044/1058-0360(2003/090)

Ching, A. H., Kang, G. C. W., & Lim, G. J. S. (2021). Craniofacial measurements: A history of scientific racism, Rethinking anthropometric norms. *Journal of Craniofacial Surgery*, *32*(3), 825–827. https://doi.org/10.1097/SCS.0000000000007266

Cho-Hisamoto, Y., Kojima, K., Brown, E. C., Matsuzaki, N., & Asano, E. (2012). Cooing- and babbling-related gamma-oscillations during infancy: Intracranial recording. *Epilepsy & Behavior*, *23*(4), 494–496. https://doi.org/10.1016/j.yebeh.2012.02.012

Choi, D., Black, A. K., & Werker, J. F. (2018). Cascading and multisensory influences on speech perception development. *Mind, Brain, and Education*, *12*(4), 212–223.

Cholin, J. (2008). The mental syllabary in speech production: An integration of different approaches and domains. *Aphasiology*, *22*(11), 1127–1141. https://doi.org/10.1080/02687030701820352

Chomsky, N. (1986). *Knowledge of language: Its nature, origin and use*. Praeger.

Chomsky, N., & Halle, M. (1968). *Sound patterns of English*. Harper and Row.

Choo, A. L., Smith, S. A., & Li, H. (2022). Prevalence, severity and risk factors for speech disorders in US children: The National Survey of Children's Health. *Journal of Monolingual and Bilingual Speech*. *4* (1), 109–126. https://doi.org/10.1558/jmbs.20879.

Christopherson, E. A., Briskie, D., & Inglehart, M. R. (2009). Objective, subjective, and self-assessment of preadolescent orthodontic treatment need—A function of age, gender, and ethnic/racial background? *Journal of Public Health Dentistry*, *69*(1), 9–17. https://doi.org/10.1111/j.1752-7325.2008.00089.x

Chumpelik, D. (1984) The PROMPT system of therapy: Theoretical framework and applications for developmental apraxia of speech. In *Seminars in Speech and Language 5*(2), 139–156. Thieme Medical Publishers.

Church, M. W., & Kaltenbach, J. A. (1997). Hearing, speech, language, and vestibular disorders in the fetal alcohol syndrome: A literature review. *Alcoholism: Clinical and Experimental Research*, *21*(3), 495–512.

Çiçek, A. U., Akdag, E., & Erdivanli, O. C. (2020). Sociodemographic characteristics associated with speech and language delay and disorders. *The Journal of Nervous and Mental Disease*, *208*(2), 143–146. https://doi.org/10.1097/NMD.0000000000001120

Cielo, C. A., & Cappellari, V. M. (2008). Maximum phonation time in pre-school children. *Brazilian Journal of Otorhinolaryngology*, *74*(4), 552–560. https://doi.org/10.1016/S1808-8694(15)30602-9

Cielo, C. A., Pascotini, F. D. S., Haeffner, L. S. B., Ribeiro, V. V., & Christmann, M. K. (2016). Maximum phonation time of /e/ and voiceless /è/ and their relationship with body mass index and gender in children. *Revista CEFAC*, *18*, 491–497. https://doi.org/10.1590/1982-021620161825915

Claessen, M, & Leitão, S. (2012). Phonological representations in children with SLI. *Child Language Teaching and Therapy*, *28*(2), 211–223. https://doi.org/10.1177/0265659012436851

Claessen, M., Heath, S., Fletcher, J., Hogben, J., & Leitão, S. (2009). Quality of phonological representations: A window into the lexicon? *International Journal of Language & Communication Disorders*, *44*(2), 121–144. https://doi.org/10.1080/13682820801966317

Clark, E. V. (1982). Language change during language acquisition. In M. Lamb & A. Brown (Eds.), *Advances in developmental psychology* (Vol. 2, pp. 71–97). Erlbaum.

Clark, C., Tumanova, V., & Choi, D. (2017). Evidenced-based multifactorial assessment of preschool-age children who stutter. *Perspectives of the ASHA Special Interest Groups*, *2*(4), 4–27, https://doi.org/10.1044/persp2.SIG4.4

Clark, H. M. (2003). Neuromuscular treatments for speech and swallowing: A tutorial. *American Journal of Speech-Language Pathology*, *12*(4), 400–415. https://doi.org/10.1044/1058-0360(2003/086)

Clark, H. M., & Solomon, N. P. (2010). Submental muscle tissue compliance during relaxation, contraction, and after tone-modification interventions. *International Journal of Orofacial Myology*, *36*, 6–15.

Clark, H. M., & Solomon, N. P. (2012). Muscle tone and the speech-language pathologist: Definitions, neurophysiology, assessment, and interventions. *Perspectives on Swallowing and Swallowing Disorders (Dysphagia)*, *21*(1), 9–14. https://doi.org/10.1044/sasd21.1.9

Cleland, J., Scobbie, J. M., & Wrench, A. A. (2015). Using ultrasound visual biofeedback to treat persistent primary speech sound disorders. *Clinical Linguistics & Phonetics*, *29*(8–10), 575–597. https://doi.org/10.3109/02699206.2015.1016188

Cleland, J., Scobbie, J. M., Roxburgh, Z., Heyde, C., & Wrench, A. (2019). Enabling new articulatory gestures in children with persistent speech sound disorders using ultrasound visual biofeedback. *Journal of Speech, Language, and Hearing Research*, *62*(2), 229–246. https://doi.org/10.1044/2018_JSLHR-S-17-0360

Cler, G. J., Lee, J. C., Mittelman, T., Stepp, C. E., & Bohland, J. W. (2017). Kinematic analysis of speech sound sequencing errors induced by delayed auditory feedback. *Journal of Speech, Language, and Hearing Research*, *60*(6S), 1695–1711. https://doi.org/10.1044/2017_JSLHR–S–16–0234

Clopper, C. G., & Pisoni, D. B. (2007). Free classification of regional dialects of American English. *Journal of Phonetics*, *35*(3), 421–438. https://doi.org/10.1016/j.wocn.2006.06.001

Clopper, C. G., & Smiljanic, R. (2011). Effects of gender and regional dialect on prosodic patterns in American English. *Journal of Phonetics, 39*(2), 237–245. https://doi.org/10.1016/j.wocn.2011.02.006

Coady, J. A., & Evans, J. L. (2008). Uses and interpretations of non-word repetition tasks in children with and without specific language impairments (SLI), *International Journal of Language & Communication Disorders, 43*(1), 1–40. https://doi.org/10.1080/13682820601116485

Cobourn, K., Marayati, F., Tsering, D., Ayers, O., Myseros, J. S., Magge, S. N., . . . Keating, R. F. (2020). Cerebellar mutism syndrome: Current approaches to minimize risk for CMS. *Child's Nervous System, 36*(6), 1171–1179. https://doi.org/10.1007/s00381-019-04240-x

Cohen, M. L., & Hula, W. D. (2020). Patient-reported outcomes and evidence-based practice in speech-language pathology. *American Journal of Speech-Language Pathology, 29*(1), 357–370. https://doi.org/10.1044/2019_AJSLP-19-00076

Cohen, W., & Anderson, C. (2011). Identification of phonological processes in preschool children's single-word productions. *International Journal of Language & Communication Disorders, 46*(4), 481–488. https://doi.org/10.1111/j.1460-6984.2011.00011.x

Cohen, W., Wynne, D. M., Kubba, H., & McCartney, E. (2012). Development of a minimum protocol for assessment in the paediatric voice clinic. Part 1: Evaluating vocal function. *Logopedics Phoniatrics Vocology, 37*(1), 33–38. https://doi.org/10.3109/14015439.2011.638670

Cohn, M., Pycha, A., & Zellou, G. (2021). Intelligibility of face-masked speech depends on speaking style: Comparing casual, clear, and emotional speech. *Cognition, 210*, 104570. https://doi.org/10.1016/j.cognition.2020.104570

Cole, J. (2015). Prosody in context: a review. *Language, Cognition and Neuroscience, 30*(1–2), 1–31. https://doi.org/10.1080/23273798.2014.963130

Colonnesi, C., Stams, G. J. J., Koster, I., & Noom, M. J. (2010). The relation between pointing and language development: A meta-analysis. *Developmental Review, 30*(4), 352–366. https://doi.org/10.1016/j.dr.2010.10.001

Commissioning Support Programme. (2011). *Speech, language and communication needs Evaluating outcomes*. Available from www.commissioningsupport.org.uk

Compton, A. J. (1970). Generative studies of children's phonological disorders. *Journal of Speech and Hearing Disorders, 35*(4), 315–339. https://doi.org/10.1044/jshd.3504.315

Compton, M. T., & Walker, E. F. (2008). Physical manifestations of neurodevelopmental disruption: Are minor physical anomalies part of the syndrome of schizophrenia? *Schizophrenia Bulletin, 35, 425*–436.

Connaghan, K. P., Moore, C. A., & Higashakawa, M. (2004). Respiratory kinematics during vocalization and nonspeech respiration in children from 9 to 48 months. *Journal of Speech, Language, and Hearing Research, 47*(1), 70–84. https://doi.org/10.1044/1092-4388(2004/007)

Conway, C. M., Pisoni, D. B., & Kronenberger, W. G. (2009). The importance of sound for cognitive sequencing abilities: The auditory scaffolding hypothesis. *Current Directions in Psychological Science, 18*(5), 275–279. https://doi.org/10.1111/j.1467-8721.2009.01651.x

Cook, S., Rieger, M., Donlan, C., & Howell, P. (2011). Testing orofacial abilities of children who stutter: The Movement, Articulation, Mandibular and Sensory awareness (MAMS) assessment procedure. *Journal of Fluency Disorders, 36*(1), 27–40.

Cooper, R. P., & Aslin, R. N. (1990). Preference for infant-directed speech in the first month after birth. *Child Development, 61*(5), 1584–1595. https://doi.org/10.1111/j.1467-8624.1990.tb02885.x

Coplan, J., & Gleason, J. R. (1988). Unclear speech: Recognition and significance of unintelligible speech in preschool children. *Pediatrics, 82*(3), 447–452. https://doi.org/10.1542/peds.82.3.447

Cordaro, D. T., Keltner, D., Tshering, S., Wangchuk, D., & Flynn, L. (2016). The voice conveys emotion in ten globalized cultures and one remote village in Bhutan. *Emotion, 1*, 117–128.

Core, C., & Scarpelli, C. (2015). Phonological development in young bilinguals: Clinical implications. *Seminars in Speech and Language 36*(2), 100–108. https://doi.org/10.1055/s-0035-1549105

Cormack, R. S., & Lehane, J. (1984). Difficult tracheal intubation in obstetrics. *Anaesthesia, 39*(11), 1105–1111. https://doi.org/10.1111/j.1365-2044.1984.tb08932.x

Cortese, S. (2020). Pharmacologic treatment of attention deficit–hyperactivity disorder. *New England Journal of Medicine, 383*(11), 1050–1056. https://doi.org/10.1056/NEJMra1917069

Cortese, S., Solmi, M., Michelini, G., Bellato, A., Blanner, C., Canozzi, A., . . . Correll, C. U. (2023). Candidate diagnostic biomarkers for neurodevelopmental disorders in children and adolescents: A systematic review. *World Psychiatry, 22*(1), 129–149. https://doi.org/10.1002/wps.21037

Costello, R., Prabhu, V., & Whittet, H. (2017). Lingual tonsil: clinically applicable macroscopic anatomical classification system. *Clinical Otolaryngology, 42*(1), 144–147. https://doi.org/10.1111/coa.12715

Cote-Reschny, K. J., & Hodge, M. M. (2010). Listener effort and response time when transcribing words spoken by children with dysarthria. *Journal of Medical Speech-Language Pathology, 18*(4), 24–35.

Coufal, K., Parham, D., Jakubowitz, M., Howell, C., & Reyes, J. (2018). Comparing traditional service delivery and telepractice for speech sound production using a functional outcome measure. *American Journal of Speech-Language Pathology, 27*(1), 82–90. https://doi.org/10.1044/2017_AJSLP-16-0070

Coughlin-Woods, S., Lehman, M. E., & Cooke, P. A. (2005). Ratings of speech naturalness of children ages 8–16 years. *Perceptual and Motor Skills, 100*(2), 295–304. https://doi.org/10.2466/pms.100.2.295-304

Cowen, A. S., & Keltner, D. (2017). Self-report captures 27 distinct categories of emotion bridged by continuous gradients. *Proceedings of the National Academy of Sciences, 114*(38), E7900–E7909. https://doi.org/10.1073/pnas.1702247114

Cox, M. J., Mills-Koonce, R., Propper, C., & Gariépy, J. L. (2010). Systems theory and cascades in developmental psychopathology. *Development and Psychopathology, 22*(3), 497–506. https://doi.org/10.1017/S0954579410000234

Craig, H. K., Thompson, C. A., Washington, J. A., & Potter, S. L. (2003). Phonological features of child African American English. *Journal of Speech, Language, and Hearing Research, 46*(3), 623–635. https://doi.org/10.1044/1092-4388(2003/049)

Crais, E. R. (2011). Testing and beyond: Strategies and tools for evaluating and assessing infants and toddlers. *Language, Speech, and Hearing Services in Schools, 42*(3), 341–364. https://doi.org/10.1044/0161-1461(2010/09-0061)

Crais, E., Douglas, D., & Campbell, C. (2004). The intersection of the development of gestures and intentionality. *Journal of Speech, Language, and Hearing Research, 47*, 678–694. https://doi.org/10.1044/1092-4388(2004/052)

Cramer, S. C., Sur, M., Dobkin, B. H., O'brien, C., Sanger, T. D., Trojanowski, J. Q., . . . Vinogradov, S. (2011). Harnessing neuroplasticity for clinical applications. *Brain, 134*(6), 1591–1609. https://doi.org/10.1093/brain/awr039

Cristia, A. (2013). Input to language: The phonetics and perception of infant-directed speech. *Language and Linguistics Compass, 7*(3), 157–170. https://doi.org/10.1111/lnc3.12015

Croft, C. B., Shprintzen, R. J., & Rakoff, S. J. (1981). Patterns of velopharyngeal valving in normal and cleft palate subjects: A multi-view videofluoroscopic and nasendoscopic study. *Laryngoscope, 91*(2), 265–271. https://doi.org/10.1288/00005537-198102000-00015

Crosbie, S., Holm, A., & Dodd, B. (2005). Intervention for children with severe speech disorder: A comparison of two approaches. *International Journal of Language & Communication Disorders, 40*(4), 467–491. https://doi.org/10.1080/13682820500126049

Crowe, K., & McLeod, S. (2020). Children's English consonant acquisition in the United States: A review. *American Journal of Speech-Language Pathology, 29*(4), 2155–2169. https://doi.org/10.1044/2020_AJSLP-19-00168

Cruttenden, A. (1997). *Intonation*. Cambridge University Press.

Crystal, D. (1979). Prosodic development. In P. Fletcher & P. Garmon (Eds.), *Language acquisition* (pp. 33–48). Cambridge University Press.

Crystal, D. (1982). *Profiling linguistic disability*. Edward Arnold.

Cumming, R., Wilson, A., & Goswami, U. (2015). Basic auditory processing and sensitivity to prosodic structure in children with specific language impairments: A new look at a perceptual hypothesis. *Frontiers in Psychology, 2015, 6*, 972. https://doi.org/10.3389/fpsyg.2015.00972

Cunningham, B. J., Washington, K. N., Binns, A., Rolfe, K., Robertson, B., & Rosenbaum, P. (2017). Current methods of evaluating speech-language outcomes for preschoolers with communication disorders: A scoping review using the ICF-CY. *Journal of Speech, Language, and Hearing Research*, *60*(2), 447–464. https://doi.org/10.1044/2016_JSLHR-L-15-0329

Curtin, S., Byers-Heinlein, K., & Werker, J. F. (2011). Bilingual beginnings as a lens for theory development: PRIMIR in focus. *Journal of Phonetics*, *39*(4), 492–504. https://doi.org/10.1016/j.wocn.2010.12.002

Curtis, J. A., Borders, J. C., & Troche, M. S. (2022). Visual Analysis of Swallowing Efficiency and Safety (VASES): Establishing criterion-referenced validity and concurrent validity. *American Journal of Speech-Language Pathology*, 1–11. https://doi.org/10.1044/2021_AJSLP-21-00116

Curtis, J. F., & Hardy, J. C. (1959). A phonetic study of misarticulation of /r/. *Journal of Speech and Hearing Research*, *2*(3), 244–257. https://doi.org/10.1044/jshr.0203.244

D'Alatrri, L. U. C. I. A., & Marchese, M. R. (2014). The speech range profile (SRP): An easy and useful tool to assess vocal limits. *Acta Otorhinolaryngologica Italica*, *34*(4), 253.

D'Andrea, E., & Barbaix, E. (2006). Anatomic research on the perioral muscles, functional matrix of the maxillary and mandibular bones. *Surgical and Radiologic Anatomy*, *28*(3), 261–266. https://doi.org/10.1007/s00276-006-0095-y

D'Ascanio, L., Lancione, C., Pompa, G., Rebuffini, E., Marsi, N., & Manzini, M. (2010). Craniofacial growth in children with nasal septum deviation: A cephalometric comparative study. *International Journal of Pediatric Otorhinolaryngology*, *74*, 1180–1183.

da Costa, C. S. N., Batistão, M. V., & Rocha, N. A. C. F. (2013). Quality and structure of variability in children during motor development: A systematic review. *Research in Developmental Disabilities*, *34*(9), 2810–2830. https://doi.org/10.1016/j.ridd.2013.05.031

Dagenais, P. A., Adlington, L. M., & Evans, K. J. (2011). Intelligibility, comprehensibility, and acceptability of dysarthric speech by older and younger listeners. *Journal of Medical Speech-Language Pathology*, *19*(4), 37–49.

Dahlgren, S., Sandberg, A. D., Strömbergsson, S., Wenhov, L., Råstam, M., & Nettelbladt, U. (2018). Prosodic traits in speech produced by children with autism spectrum disorders—Perceptual and acoustic measurements. *Autism & Developmental Language Impairments*, *3*. https://doi.org/10.1177/2396941518764527

Dalbor, J. (1980). *Spanish pronunciation: Theory and practice* (2nd ed.). Holt, Rinehart & Winston.

Dale, E. W., Plumb, A. M., Sandage, M. J., & Plexico, L. W. (2020). Speech-language pathologists' knowledge and competence regarding percentage of consonants correct. *Communication Disorders Quarterly*, *41*(4), 222–230. https://doi.org/10.1177/1525740119853806

Dale, P. S., & Hayden, D. A. (2013). Treating speech subsystems in childhood apraxia of speech with tactual input: The PROMPT approach. *American Journal of Speech-Language Pathology*, *22*(4), 644–661. https://doi.org/10.1044/1058-0360(2013/12-0055)

Dallaston, K., & Docherty, G. (2020). The quantitative prevalence of creaky voice (vocal fry) in varieties of English: A systematic review of the literature. *PloS one*, *15*(3), e0229960. https://doi.org/10.1371/journal.pone.0229960

Darwin, C. (1872/1998). *The expression of the emotions in man and animals* (3rd ed.). Oxford University Press.

Davis, E., & Hodge, M. (2017). Reliability and validity of TOCS-30 for young children with severe speech and expressive language delay. *Canadian Journal of Speech-Language Pathology*, *41*(1), 92–104.

Dawson, J. I., & Tattersall, P. J. (2001). *Structured Photographic Articulation Test—II*. Janelle Publications.

Dayan, E., & Cohen, L. G. (2011). Neuroplasticity subserving motor skill learning. *Neuron*, *72*(3), 443454. https://doi.org/10.1016/j.neuron.2011.10.008

Dean, E., & Howell, J. (1986). Developing linguistic awareness: A theoretically based approach to phonological disorders. *British Journal of Disorders of Communication*, *21*, 223–238.

Dean, E.C., Howell, J., Waters, D., & Reid, J. (1995). Metaphon: A metalinguistic approach to the treatment of phonological disorder in children. *Clinical Linguistics and Phonetics*, *9*, 1–19.

Dean, E., Howell, J., Grieve, R., Donaldson, M., & Reid, J., (1995). Harnessing language awareness in a communicative context: a group study of the efficacy of Metaphon. *Interna-*

tional Journal of Language & Communication Disorders, 30(S1), 281–286. https://doi.org/10.1111/j.1460-6984.1995.tb01689.x

De Beukelaer, N., Weide, G., Huyghe, E., Vandekerckhove, I., Hanssen, B., Peeters, N., . . . Desloovere, K. (2022). Reduced cross-sectional muscle growth six months after botulinum toxin type-A injection in children with spastic cerebral palsy. *Toxins, 14*(2), 139. https://doi.org/10.3390/toxins14020139

de Boer, B. (2019). Evolution of speech: Anatomy and control. *Journal of Speech, Language, and Hearing Research, 62*(8S), 2932–2945. https://doi.org/10.1044/2019_JSLHR-S-CSMC7-18-0293

de Boer, B., & Fitch, W. T. (2010). Computer models of vocal tract evolution: An overview and critique. *Adaptive Behavior, 18*, 36–48. https://doi.org/10.1177/1059712309350972

de Bot, K., Lowie, W., & Verspoor, M. (2007). A dynamic systems theory approach to second language acquisition. *Bilingualism: Language and Cognition, 10*(1), 7–21. https://doi.org/10.1017/S1366728906002732

de Boysson-Bardies, B. (1999). *How language comes to children*. MIT Press.

de Boysson-Bardies, B., & Vihman, M. M. (1991). Adaptation to language: Evidence from babbling and first words in four languages. *Language, 67*(2), 297–319. https://doi.org/10.1353/lan.1991.0045.

de Boysson-Bardies, B., Sagart, L., & Durand, C. (1984). Discernible differences in the babbling of infants according to target language. *Journal of Child Language, 11*, 1–15. https://doi.org/10.1017/S0305000900005559

Decety, J. (1996). The neurophysiological basis of motor imagery. *Behavioural Brain Research*, 77(1-2), 45–52. https://doi.org/10.1016/0166-4328(95)00225-1

Dediu, D., & Moisik, S. R. (2019). Pushes and pulls from below: Anatomical variation, articulation and sound change. *Glossa: A Journal of General Linguistics 4*, 1–33.

De Jong, K. J. (1995). The supraglottal articulation of prominence in English: Linguistic stress as localized hyperarticulation. *The Journal of the Acoustical Society of America, 97*(1), 491–504. https://doi.org/10.1121/1.412275

de Leeuw, E., & Celata, C. (2019). Plasticity of native phonetic and phonological domains in the context of bilingualism. *Journal of Phonetics, 75*, 88–93. https://doi.org/10.1016/j.wocn.2019.05.003

de Lima Xavier, L., Hanekamp, S., & Simonyan, K. (2019). Sexual dimorphism within brain regions controlling speech production. *Frontiers in Neuroscience, 13*, 795. https://doi.org/10.3389/fnins.2019.00795

Deka, C., Shrivastava, A., Nautiyal, S., & Chauhan, P. (2022). AI-based automated speech therapy tools for persons with speech sound disorders: A systematic literature review. arXiv preprint arXiv:2204.10325. https://doi.org/10.48550/arXiv.2204.10325

Delcenserie, A., Genesee, F., Trudeau, N., & Champoux, F. (2021). The development of phonological memory and language: A multiple groups approach. *Journal of Child Language, 48*(2), 285–324. https://doi.org/10.1017/S0305000920000343

Delgado, C. E., Vagi, S. J., & Scott, K. G. (2005). Early risk factors for speech and language impairments. *Exceptionality, 13*(3), 173–191. https://doi.org/10.1207/s15327035ex1303_3

Dell, G. S. (1985). Positive feedback in hierarchical connectionist models: Applications to language production 1. *Cognitive Science, 9*(1), 3–23.

Dell, G. S. (1986). A spreading-activation theory of retrieval in sentence production. *Psychological Review, 93*(3), 283–321. https://doi.org/10.1037/0033-295X.93.3.283

De Menezes, V. A., Leal, R. B., Pessoa, R. S., & Pontes, R. M. E. S. (2006). Prevalence and factors related to mouth breathing in school children at the Santo Amaro project-Recife, 2005. *Brazilian Journal of Otorhinolaryngology, 72*(3), 394–398. https://doi.org/10.1016/S1808-8694(15)30975-7

Den Hoed, J., & Fisher, S. E. (2020). Genetic pathways involved in human speech disorders. *Current Opinion in Genetics & Development, 65*, 103–111. https://doi.org/10.1016/j.gde.2020.05.012

Denes, P. B., & Pinson, E. N. (1963). *The speech chain*. Bell Telephone Laboratories.

Denne, M., Langdown, N., Pring, T., & Roy, P. (2005). Treating children with expressive phonological disorders: Does phonological awareness therapy work in the clinic? *International Journal of Language & Communication Disorders, 40*(4), 493–504. https://doi.org/10.1080/13682820500142582

Denny, M., & McGowan, R. S. (2012a). Implications of peripheral muscular and anatomical development for the acquisition of lingual control for speech production: A review. *Folia Phoniatrica et Logopaedica*, *64*, 105–115. https://doi.org/10.1159/000338611

Denny, M., & McGowan, R. S. (2012b). Sagittal area of the vocal tract in young female children. *Folia Phoniatrica et Logopaedica*, *64*, 297–303. https://doi.10.1159/000345646

DePaolis, R. A., Vihman, M. M., & Kunnari, S. (2008). Prosody in production at the onset of word use: A cross-linguistic study. *Journal of Phonetics*, *36*, 406–422. https://doi.org/10.1016/j.wocn.2008.01.003

DePaul, R., & Kent, R. D. (2000). A longitudinal case study of ALS: Effects of listener familiarity and proficiency on intelligibility judgments. *American Journal of Speech-Language Pathology*, *9*(3), 230–240. https://doi.org/10.1044/1058-0360.0903.230

Derwing T. M., & Munro M. J. (2005). Second language accent and pronunciation teaching: A research-based approach. *TESOL Quarterly*, *39*, 379–397

DeThorne, L. S., Johnson, C. J., Walder, L., & Mahurin-Smith, J. (2009). When "Simon Says" doesn't work: Alternatives to imitation for facilitating early speech development. *American Journal of Speech-Language Pathology*, *18*(2), 133–145. https://doi.org/10.1044/1058-0360(2008/07-0090)

DeVeney, S. L., & Peterkin, K. (2022). Facing a clinical challenge: Limited empirical support for toddler speech sound production intervention approaches. *Language, Speech, and Hearing Services in Schools*, *53*(3), 659–674. https://doi.org/10.1044/2022_LSHSS-21-00104

Di Cicco, M., Kantar, A., Masini, B., Nuzzi, G., Ragazzo, V., & Peroni, D. (2021). Structural and functional development in airways throughout childhood: Children are not small adults. *Pediatric Pulmonology*, *56*(1), 240–251. https://doi.org/10.1002/ppul.25169

Dienerowitz, T., Peschel, T., Vogel, M., Poulain, T., Engel, C., Kiess, W., . . . Berger, T. (2021). Establishing normative data on singing voice parameters of children and adolescents with average singing activity using the voice range profile. *Folia Phoniatrica et Logopaedica*, *73*(6), 565-576. https://doi.org/10.1159/000513521

Di Rocco, C., Chieffo, D., Frassanito, P., Caldarelli, M., Massimi, L., & Tamburrini, G. (2011). Heralding cerebellar mutism: Evidence for presurgical language impairment as primary risk factor in posterior fossa surgery. *The Cerebellum*, *10*(3), 551–562.

Díaz-Quevedo, A. A., Castillo-Quispe, H. M. L., Atoche-Socola, K. J., & Arriola-Guillén, L. E. (2021). Evaluation of the craniofacial and oral characteristics of individuals with Down syndrome: A review of the literature. *Journal of Stomatology, Oral and Maxillofacial Surgery*, *122*(6), 583–587. https://doi.org/10.1016/j.jormas.2021.01.007

Diehl, J. J., & Paul, R. (2009). The assessment and treatment of prosodic disorders and neurological theories of prosody. *International Journal of Speech-Language Pathology*, *11*(4), 287–292. https://doi.org/10.1080/17549500902971887

Diepeveen, S., Terband, H., van Haaften, L., van de Zande, A. M., Megens-Huigh, C., de Swart, B., & Maassen, B. (2022). Process-oriented profiling of speech sound disorders. *Children*, *9*(10), 1502. https://doi.org/10.3390/children9101502

Diepeveen, S., van Haaften, L., Terband, H., De Swart, B., & Maassen, B. (2019). A standardized protocol for maximum repetition rate assessment in children. *Folia Phoniatrica et Logopaedica*, *71*(5–6), 238–250. https://doi.org/10.1159/000500305

Dietrich, S., & Hernandez (2022, August). *Language use in the United States: 2019 American community survey reports, U.S. Census.* https://www.census.gov/content/dam/Census/library/publications/2022/acs/acs-50.pdf

Diez-Itza, E., Vergara, P., Barros, M., Miranda, M., & Martínez, V. (2021). Assessing phonological profiles in children and adolescents with Down syndrome: The effect of elicitation methods. *Frontiers in Psychology*, *1610*. https://doi.org/10.3389/fpsyg.2021.662257

Dimberg, L., Lennartsson, B., Arnrup, K., & Bondemark, L. (2015). Prevalence and change of malocclusions from primary to early permanent dentition: A longitudinal study. *Angle Orthodontia*, *85*(5), 728–734. https://doi.org/10.2319/0804147542.1.

Dinç, A. E., Damar, M., Uğur, M. B., Öz, I. I., Eliçora, S. Ş., Bişkin, S., & Tutar, H. (2015). Do the angle and length of the eustachian tube influence the development of chronic otitis media? *Laryngoscope*, *125*(9), 2187–2192. https://doi.org/10.1002/lary.25231

Dodd, B. (2011). Differentiating speech delay from disorder: Does it matter? *Topics in Language Disorders*, *31*(2), 96–111. https://doi.org/10.1097/TLD.0b013e318217b66a

Dodd, B. (2014). Differential diagnosis of pediatric speech sound disorder. *Current Developmental Disorders Reports*, *1*, 189–196. https://doi.org/10.1007/s40474-014-0017-3

Dodd, B., & Gillon, G. (2001). Exploring the relationship between phonological awareness, speech impairment, and literacy. *Advances in Speech Language Pathology*, *3*(2), 139–147.

Dodd, B., & Thompson, L. (2001). Speech disorder in children with Down's syndrome. *Journal of Intellectual Disability Research*, *45*(4), 308–316. https://doi.org/10.1046/j.1365-2788.2001.00327.x

Dodd, B. J., So, L. K. H., & Wei, L. (1996). Symptoms of disorder without impairment: The written and spoken errors of bilinguals. In B. J. Dodd, R. Campbell, & L. Worall (Eds.), *Evaluating theories of language: Evidence from disordered communication* (pp. 119–136). Whurr Publishers.

Dodd, B., Holm, A., Crosbie, S., & McIntosh, B. (2006). A core vocabulary approach for management of inconsistent speech disorder. *Advances in Speech Language Pathology*, *8*(3), 220–230. https://doi.org/10.1080/14417040600738177

Dodd, B., Hua, Z., Crosbie, S., Holm, A., & Ozanne, A. (2006). *Diagnostic Evaluation of Articulation and Phonology (U.S. ed.)*. The Psychological Corporation.

Dodd, B., Leahy, J., & Hambly, G. (1989). Phonological disorders in children: Underlying cognitive deficits. *British Journal of Developmental Psychology*, 7(1), 55–71. https://doi.org/10.1111/j.2044-835X.1989.tb00788.x

Dodd, B., Reilly, S., Ttofari Eecen, K., & Morgan, A. T. (2018). Articulation or phonology? Evidence from longitudinal error data. *Clinical Linguistics & Phonetics*, *32*(11), 1027–1041.

Dollaghan, C. (1985). Child Meets Word: " Fast Mapping" in Preschool Children. *Journal of Speech, Language, and Hearing Research*, *28*(3), 449–454. https://doi.org/10.1044/jshr.2803.454

Dollaghan, C. A. (1994). Children's phonological neighborhoods: Half empty or half full? *Journal of Child Language*, *21*(2), 257–271.

Dollaghan, C., & Campbell, T. (1998). Nonword repetition and child language impairment. *Journal of Speech, Language, and Hearing Research*, *41*,1136–1146

Donegan, P. J. & Stampe, D. (1979). The study of natural phonology. In D. A. Dinnnsen (Ed.) *Current approaches to phonological theory* (pp. 126–173). Indiana University Press.

Donnelly, S., & Kidd, E. (2021). Onset neighborhood density slows lexical access in high vocabulary 30–month olds. *Cognitive Science*, *45*(9), e13022. https://doi.org/10.1111/cogs.13022

Dörnyei, Z. (2014). *The psychology of the language learner: Individual differences in second language acquisition*. Routledge. https://doi.org/10.4324/9781410613349

Doshi, R. R., & Patil, A. S. (2012). A role of genes in craniofacial growth. *The IIOAB Journal*, *3*, 19–36.

Douglas, N. F., Feuerstein, J. L., Oshita, J. Y., Schliep, M. E., & Danowski, M. L. (2022). Implementation science research in communication sciences and disorders: A scoping review. *American Journal of Speech-Language Pathology*, *31*(3), 1054–1083. https://doi.org/10.1044/2021_AJSLP-21-00126

Dowhower, S. L. (1991). Speaking of prosody: Fluency's unattended bedfellow. *Theory into Practice*, *30*, 165–175. https://doi.org/10.1080/00405849109543497

Drager, K. D., & Finke, E. H. (2012). Intelligibility of children's speech in digitized speech. *Augmentative and Alternative Communication*, *28*(3), 181–189. https://doi.org/10.3109/07434618.2012.704524

Drevenšek, M., Štefanac-Papić, J., & Farčnik, F. (2005). The influence of incompetent lip seal on the growth and development of craniofacial complex. *Collegium Antropologicum*, *29*(2), 429–434.

Drouin, J. R., Theodore, R. M., & Myers, E. B. (2016). Lexically guided perceptual tuning of internal phonetic category structure. *The Journal of the Acoustical Society of America*, *140*(4), EL307-EL313. https://doi.org/10.1121/1.4964468

Du, Y., Choe. S., Vega. J., Liu, Y., & Trujillo, A. (2022). Listening to stakeholders involved in speech-language therapy for children with communication disorders: Content analysis of Apple app store reviews. *JMIR Pediatrics and Parenting*, *5*(1), e28661. https://doi.org/10.2196/2866

Duchan, J. (n.d.). *A history of speech-language pathology—Twentieth Century*. https://www.acsu.buffalo.edu/~duchan/1965-1975.html

Duchan, J. F., & Felsenfeld, S. (2021). Cluttering framed: An historical overview. *Advances in Communication and Swallowing*, *24*(2), 75–85. https://doi.org/10.3233/ACS-210029

Duchow, H., Lindsay, A., Roth, K., Schell, S., Allen, D., & Boliek, C. A. (2019). The co-occurrence of possible developmental coordination disorder and suspected childhood apraxia of speech. *Canadian Journal of Speech-Language Pathology and Audiology*, *93*(2), 81–93.

Duffy, J. R. (2013). *Motor speech disorders: Substrates, differential diagnosis, and management*. Elsevier Health Sciences.

Duffy, J. R. (2016). Functional speech disorders: clinical manifestations, diagnosis, and management. *Handbook of Clinical Neurology*, *139*, 379–388. https://doi.org/10.1016/B978-0-12-801772-2.00033-3

Duffy, J. R. (2019). *Motor speech disorders: Substrates, differential diagnosis, and management*, 4th Edition. Elsevier.

Duffy, J. R. (2020). *Motor speech disorders* (4th ed.). Mosby.

Dugan, S., Schwab, S. M., Seward, R., Avant, J., Zhang, T., Li, S. R., . . . Boyce, S. (2023). A qualitative analysis of clinician perspectives of ultrasound biofeedback for speech sound disorders. *American Journal of Speech-Language Pathology*, *32*(3), 1252–1274. https://doi.org/10.1044/2023_AJSLP-22-00194

Dugan, S. H., Silbert, N., McAllister, T., Preston, J. L., Sotto, C., & Boyce, S. E. (2019). Modelling category goodness judgments in children with residual sound errors. *Clinical Linguistics & Phonetics*, *33*(4), 295–315. https://doi.org/10.1080/02699206.2018.1477834

Duncan, E. A., & Murray, J. (2012). The barriers and facilitators to routine outcome measurement by allied health professionals in practice: A systematic review. *BMC Health Services Research*, *12*(1), 1–9. https://doi.org/10.1186/1472-6963-12-96

Dunn, L. M., & Dunn, D. M. (2007). *Peabody Picture Vocabulary Test, Fourth Edition PPVT-4*. Pearson Assessments.

Durdiakova, J., Ostatnikova, D., & Celec, P. (2011). Testosterone and its metabolites—Modulators of brain functions. *Acta Neurobiologiae Experimentalis*, *71*(4), 434–454.

Durtschi, R. B., Chung, D., Gentry, L. R., Chung, M. K., & Vorperian, H. K. (2009). Developmental craniofacial anthropometry: Assessment of race effects. *Clinical Anatomy*, *22*, 800–808. https://doi.org/10.1002/ca.20852

Dworkin, J. P., & Culatta, R. A. (1980). *Dworkin-Culatta oral mechanism examination*. Edgewood Press.

Dyson, A. T. (1988). Phonetic inventories of 2- and 3-year-old children. *Journal of Speech and Hearing Disorders*, *53*(1), 89–93. https://doi.org/10.1044/jshd.5301.89

Dziubalska-Kołaczyk, K. (1998). Self-organization in early phonology. In S. Puppel (Ed.), *Scripta manent* (pp. 99–11). Motivex.

Eadie, P., Morgan, A., Ukoumunne, O. C., Ttofari Eecen, K., Wake, M., & Reilly, S. (2015). Speech sound disorder at 4 years: Prevalence, comorbidities, and predictors in a community cohort of children. *Developmental Medicine & Child Neurology*, *57*(6), 578–584. https://doi.org/10.1111/dmcn.12635

Eadie, T. L., & Doyle, P. C. (2002). Direct magnitude estimation and interval scaling of pleasantness and severity in dysphonic and normal speakers. *Journal of the Acoustical Society of America, 112*, 3014–3021.

Easton, C., & Verdon, S. (2021). The influence of linguistic bias upon speech-language pathologists' attitudes toward clinical scenarios involving nonstandard dialects of English. *American Journal of Speech-Language Pathology*, *30*(5), 19731989. https://doi.org/10.1044/2021_AJSLP-20-00382

Eccles, R., Van der Linde, J., le Roux, M., Holloway, J., MacCutcheon, D., Ljung, R., & Swanepoel, D. W. (2021). Is phonological awareness related to pitch, rhythm, and speech-in-noise discrimination in young children? *Language, Speech, and Hearing Services in Schools*, *52*(1), 383–395.

Eckel, F. C., & Boone, D. R. (1981). The s/z ratio as an indicator of laryngeal pathology. *Journal of Speech and Hearing Disorders, 46*(2), 147–149. https://doi.org/10.1044/jshd.4602.147

Eckman, F. (2014). Second language phonology. In S. M. Gass & A. Mackey (Eds.) *The Routledge handbook of second language acquisition* (pp. 91–105). Routledge.

Edgson, M. R., Tucker, B. V., Archibald, E. D., & A. Boliek, C. (2021). Neuromuscular and biomechanical adjustments of the speech mechanism during modulation of vocal loudness in children with cerebral palsy and dysarthria. *Neurocase, 27*(1), 30–38. https://doi.org/10.1080/13554794.2020.1862240

Edvinsson, S. E, & Lundqvist, L. O. (2016). Prevalence of orofacial dysfunction in cerebral palsy and its association with gross motor function and manual ability. *Developmental Medicine and Child Neurology, 58*, 385–394.

Edwards, M. L. (1992). In support of phonological processes. *Language, Speech, and Hearing Services in Schools, 23*(3), 233–240. http://lshss.asha.org/cgi/content/abstract/23/3/233

Eggermont, J. J., & Moore, J. K. (2012). Morphological and functional development of the auditory nervous system. In *Human auditory development* (pp. 61–105). Springer.

Ego, C., Yüksel, D., Orban de Xivry, J. J., & Lefèvre, P. (2016). Development of internal models and predictive abilities for visual tracking during childhood. *Journal of Neurophysiology, 115*(1), 301–309. https://doi.org/10.1152/jn.00534.2015

Ehrman, M. E., Leaver, B. L., & Oxford, R. L. (2003). A brief overview of individual differences in second language learning. *System, 31*(3), 313–330. https://doi.org/10.1016/S0346-251X(03)00045-9

Eikeseth, S., & Nesset, R. (2003). Behavioral treatment of children with phonological disorder: The efficacy of vocal imitation and sufficient-response-exemplar training. *Journal of Applied Behavior Analysis, 36*(3), 325–337. https://doi.org/10.1901/jaba.2003.36-325

Eilers, R. E., Oller, D. K., Levines, S., Basinger, D., Lynch, M. P., & Urbano, R. (1993). The role of prematurity and socioeconomic status in the onset of canonical babbling in infants. *Infant Behavior and Development, 16*, 297–315.

Einarsdóttir, J. T., Crowe, K., Kristinsson, S. H., & Másdóttir, T. (2020). The recovery rate of early stuttering. *Journal of Fluency Disorders, 64*, 105764. https://doi.org/10.1016/j.jfludis.2020.105764

Eisenberg, S. L., & Hitchcock, E. R. (2010). Using standardized tests to inventory consonant and vowel production: A comparison of 11 tests of articulation and phonology. *Language, Speech, and Hearing Services in Schools, 41*(4), 488–503. https://doi.org/10.1044/0161-1461(2009/08-0125)

Eising, E., Carrion-Castillo, A., Vino, A., Strand, E. A., Jakielski, K. J., Scerri, T. S., . . . Fisher, S. E. (2019). A set of regulatory genes co-expressed in embryonic human brain is implicated in disrupted speech development. *Molecular Psychiatry, 24*(7), 1065–1078. https://doi.org/10.1038/s41380-018-0020-x

Ejiri, K. (1998). Relationship between rhythmic behavior and canonical babbling in infant vocal development. *Phonetica, 55*(4), 226–237. https://doi.org/10.1159/000028434

Ekman, P. (1993). Facial expression of emotion. *American Psychologist, 48*, 384–392.

Elbert, M. & Gieret, J. A. (1986). *Handbook of clinical phonology*. College-Hill.

Elbert, M., Dinnsen, D. A., & Weismer, G. (1984). Phonological theory and the misarticulating child. *ASHA Monographs Number 22*. American Speech-Language-Hearing Association.

Elbert, M., Powell, T. W., & Swartzlander, P. (1991). Toward a technology of generalization: How many exemplars are sufficient? *Journal of Speech and Hearing Research, 34*, 81–87. https://doi.org/10.1044/jshr.3401.81

Eliasson, A. C., Krumlinde-Sundholm, L., Rösblad, B., Beckung, E., Arner, M., Öhrvall, A. M., & Rosenbaum, P. (2006). The Manual Ability Classification System (MACS) for children with cerebral palsy: Scale development and evidence of validity and reliability. *Developmental Medicine and Child Neurology, 48*(7), 549–554. https://doi.org/10.1017/S0012162206001162

Enderby, P. (1997). *Therapy Outcome Measures: Speech-language pathology user's manual*. Singular Publishing Group.

Enderby, P., & Palmer, R. (2008). *FDA-2: Frenchay Dysarthria Assessment–Second Edition*. Pro-Ed.

Engstrand, O., Williams, K., & Lacerda, F. (2003). Does babbling sound native? Listener responses to vocalizations produced by Swedish and American 12- and 18-month-olds. *Phonetica, 60*, 17–44. https://doi.org/10.1159/000070452

Eppley, B. L., van Aalst, J. A., Robey, A., Havlik, R. J., & Sadove, A. M. (2005). The spectrum of orofacial clefting. *Plastic and Reconstructive Surgery*, 115(7), 101e–114e. https://doi.org/10.1097/01.PRS.0000164494.45986.91

Eriks-Brophy, A., Gibson, S., & Tucker, S. (2013). Articulatory error patterns and phonological process use of preschool children with and without hearing loss. *The Volta Review*, *113*(2), 87–125.

Erskine, M., Munson, B., & Edwards, J. (2020). Relationship between early phonological processing and later phonological awareness: Evidence from nonword repetition. *Applied Psycholinguistics*, *41*(2), 319–346. https://doi.org/10.1017/S0142716419000547

Ertmer, D. J. (2010). Relationships between speech intelligibility and word articulation scores in children with hearing loss. *Journal of Speech, Language, and Hearing Research*, *53*(5), 1075–1086. https://doi.org/10.1044/1092-4388(2010/09-0250)

Ertmer, D. J. (2011). Assessing speech intelligibility in children with hearing loss: Toward revitalizing a valuable clinical tool. *Language, Speech, and Hearing Services in Schools*, *42*(1), 52–58. https://doi.org/10.1044/0161-1461(2010/09-0081

Esteve-Altava, B. (2020). A node-based informed modularity strategy to identify organizational modules in anatomical networks. *Biology Open*, 9(10), bio056176. https://doi.org/10.1242/bio.056176

Esteve-Altava, B., Diogo, R., Smith, C., Boughner, J. C., & Rasskin-Gutman, D. (2015). Anatomical networks reveal the musculoskeletal modularity of the human head. *Scientific Reports*, *5*, 8298.

Etchell, A., Adhikari, A., Weinberg, L. S., Choo, A. L., Garnett, E. O., Chow, H. M., & Chang, S. E. (2018). A systematic literature review of sex differences in childhood language and brain development. *Neuropsychologia*, *114*, 19–31.

Etter, N. M., Cadely, F. A., Peters, M. G., Dahm, C. R., & Neely, K. A. (2021). Speech motor control and orofacial point pressure sensation in adults with ADHD. *Neuroscience Letters*, *744*, 135592. https://doi.org/10.1016/j.neulet.2020.135592

Evans, M. A. (1985). Self-initiated speech repairs: A reflection of communicative monitoring in young children. *Developmental Psychology*, *21*(2), 365–371. https://doi.org/10.1037/0012–1649.21.2.365

Everett, C. (2017). Languages in drier climates use fewer vowels. *Frontiers in Psychology*, *8*, 1285. https://doi.org/10.3389/fpsyg.2017.01285

Everett, C., Blasi, D. E., & Roberts, S. G. (2015). Climate, vocal folds, and tonal languages: Connecting the physiological and geographic dots. *Proceedings of the National Academy of Sciences*, *112*(5), 1322–1327. https://doi.org/10.1073/pnas.1417413112

Fabio, R. A., Gangemi, A., Capri, T., Budden, S., & Falzone, A. (2018). Neurophysiological and cognitive effects of Transcranial Direct Current Stimulation in three girls with Rett syndrome with chronic language impairments. *Research in Developmental Disabilities*, *76*, 76–87. https://doi.org/10.1016/j.ridd.2018.03.008

Fabiano-Smith, L. (2019). Standardized tests and the diagnosis of speech sound disorders. *Perspectives of the ASHA Special Interest Groups*, *4*(1), 58–66. https://doi.org/10.1044/2018_PERS-SIG1-2018-0018

Fabiano-Smith, L., & Barlow, J. A. (2010). Interaction in bilingual phonological acquisition: Evidence from phonetic inventories. *International Journal of Bilingual Education and Bilinguistics*, *13*(1), 81–97. https://doi.org/10.1080/13670050902783528.

Fabiano-Smith, L., & Goldstein, B. A. (2010). Phonological acquisition in bilingual Spanish–English speaking children. *Journal of Speech, Language, and Hearing Research*, *53*(1), 160–178. https://doi.org/10.1044/1092-4388(2009/07-0064)

Fabiano-Smith, L., Oglivie, T., Maiefski, O., & Schertz, J. (2015). Acquisition of the stop-spirant alternation in bilingual Mexican Spanish–English speaking children: Theoretical and clinical implications. *Clinical Linguistics & Phonetics*, *29*(1), 1–26. https://doi.org/10.3109/02699206.2014.947540

Fagan, M. K. (2015). Why repetition? Repetitive babbling, auditory feedback, and cochlear implantation. *Journal of Experimental Child Psychology*, *137*, 125–136. https://doi.org/10.1016/j.jecp.2015.04.005

Fairs, A., Michelas, A., Dufour, S., & Strijkers, K. (2021). The same ultra-rapid parallel brain dynamics underpin the production and perception of speech. *Cerebral Cortex Communications*, *2*(3), tgab040.

Fan, S., Zhang, Y., Qin, J., Song, X., Wang, M., & Ma, J. (2021). Family environmental risk factors for developmental speech delay in children in Northern China. *Scientific Reports*, *11*, 3924. https://doi.org/10.1038/s41598-021-83554-w

Fant, G. (1995) Speech related to pure tone audiograms, In G. Plant & K. E. Spens (Eds.),

Profound deafness and speech communication (pp. 299–305). Whurr Publishers.

Farah, M. J. (1984). The neurological basis of mental imagery: A componential analysis. *Cognition, 18*(1–3), 245–272. https://doi.org/10.1016/0010-0277(84)90026-X

Faria, P. T. M., Ruellas, A. C. D. O., Matsumoto, M. A. N., Anselmo-Lima, W. T., & Pereira, F. C. (2002). Dentofacial morphology of mouth breathing children. *Brazilian Dental Journal, 13*, 129–132.

Farid, M. M., & Metwalli, N. (2010). Computed tomographic evaluation of mouth breathers among paediatric patients. *Dentomaxillofacial Radiology, 39*, 1–10.

Farkas, L. G., Katic, M. J., & Forrest, C. R. (2005). International anthropometric study of facial morphology in various ethnic groups/races. *Journal of Craniofacial Surgery, 16*, 615–646. https://https://doi.org/10.1097/01.scs.0000171847.58031.9e

Farkas, L. G., Katic, M. J., & Forrest, C. R. (2007). Comparison of craniofacial measurements of young adult African-American and North American white males and females. *Annals of Plastic Surgery, 59*, 692–698. https://doi.org/10.1097/01.sap.0000258954.55068.b4

Farnetani, E., & Recasens, D. (2010). Coarticulation and connected speech processes. In W. J. Hardcastle, J. Laver, & F. E. Gibbon (Eds.), *The handbook of phonetic sciences* (pp. 316–352). Wiley.

Farpour, H. R., Moosavi, S. A., Mohammadian, Z., & Farpour, S. (2021). Comparing the tongue and lip strength and endurance of children with Down syndrome with their typical peers using IOPI. *Dysphagia*, 1–7. https://doi.org/10.1007/s00455-021-10359-4

Farquharson, K., & Tambyraja, S. R. (2019). Describing how school-based SLPs determine eligibility for children with speech sound disorders. *Seminars in Speech and Language, 40*(2), 105–112. https://doi.org/10.1055/s-0039-1677761

Farquharson, K., Hogan, T. P., & Fox, A. B. (2021). Factors that influence non-word repetition performance in children with and without persistent speech sound disorders. *International Journal of Language & Communication Disorders, 56*(6), 1218–1234. https://doi.org/10.1111/1460-6984.12663

Fatemi, S. H., Aldinger, K. A., Ashwood, P., Bauman, M. L., Blaha, C. D., Blatt, G. J., . . . Welsh, J. P. (2012). Consensus paper: Pathological role of the cerebellum in autism. *The Cerebellum, 11*(3), 777–807. https://doi.org/10.1007/s12311-012-0355-9

Fawcett, S., Bacsfalvi, P., & Bernhardt, B. M. (2008). Ultrasound as visual feedback in speech therapy for /r/ with adults with Down Syndrome. *Down Syndrome Quarterly, 10*(1), 4–12.

Felcar, J. M., Bueno, I. R., Massan, A. C. S., Torezan, R. P., & Cardoso, J. R. (2010). Prevalence of mouth breathing in children from an elementary school. *Ciencia Saude Coletiva, 15*(2), 427–435.

Feldman, H. M. (2019). How young children learn language and speech. *Pediatrics in Review, 40*(8), 398–411. https://doi.org/10.1542/pir.2017-0325.

Felício, C. M., Folha, G. A., Ferreira, C. L. P., & Medeiros, A. P. M. (2010). Expanded protocol of orofacial myofunctional evaluation with scores: Validity and reliability. *International Journal of Pediatric Otorhinolaryngology, 74*, 1230–1239. https://doi.org/10.1016/j.ijporl.2010.07.021

Feng, Y., & Chen, F. (2022). Nonintrusive objective measurement of speech intelligibility: A review of methodology. *Biomedical Signal Processing and Control, 71*(Part B), 103204. https://doi.org/10.1016/j.bspc.2021.103204

Fernald, A. (1993). Approval and disapproval: Infant responsiveness to vocal affect in familiar and unfamiliar languages. *Child Development, 64*(3), 657–674. https://doi.org/10.1111/j.1467-8624.1993.tb02934.x

Fernyhough, C. (1996). The dialogic mind: A dialogic approach to the higher mental functions. *New Ideas in Psychology, 14*(1), 47–62. https://doi.org/10.1016/0732-118X(95)00024-B

Fernyhough, C. (2004). Alien voices and inner dialogue: Towards a developmental account of auditory verbal hallucinations. *New Ideas in Psychology, 22*(1), 49–68. https://doi.org/10.1016/j.newideapsych.2004.09.001

Fernyhough, C. (2008). Getting Vygotskian about theory of mind: Mediation, dialogue, and the development of social understanding. *Developmental Review, 28*(2), 225–262. https://doi.org/10.1016/j.dr.2007.03.001

Fernyhough, C. (2013). Inner speech. In H. Pashler (Ed.), *The encyclopedia of the mind* (Vol. 9), (pp. 418–420). Sage Publications. http://doi.org/10.4135/9781452257044.n15

Fessenden, M. (2011, December 9). 'Vocal Fry' creeping into U.S. *Science*. https://doi.org/10.1126/article.25537

Fey, M. E. (1992). Articulation and phonology: Inextricable constructs in speech pathology. *Language, Speech, and Hearing Services in Schools*, *23*(3), 225–232. https://doi.org/10.1044/0161-1461.2303.225

Field, T., & Diego, M. (2008). Vagal activity, early growth and emotional development. *Infant Behavior and Development*, *31*(3), 361–373. https://doi.org/10.1016/j.infbeh.2007.12.008.

Findley, B. R., & Gasparyan, D. (2022). Use of speech-to-text biofeedback in intervention for children with articulation disorders. *Perspectives of the ASHA Special Interest Groups*, *7*(3), 926–937. https://doi.org/10.1044/2022_PERSP-21-00276

Finestack, L. H., Richmond, E. K., & Abbeduto, L. (2009). Language development in individuals with fragile X syndrome. *Topics in Language Disorders*, *29*(2), 133. https://doi.org/10.1097/tld.0b013e3181a72016

Finnegan, D. E. (1984). Maximum phonation time for children with normal voices. *Journal of Communication Disorders*, *17*(5), 309–317. https://doi.org/10.1016/0021-9924(84)90033-9

Finneran, D. A., Heilmann, J. J., Moyle, M. J., & Chen, S. (2020). An examination of cultural-linguistic influences on PPVT-4 performance in African American and Hispanic preschoolers from low-income communities. *Clinical Linguistics & Phonetics*, *34*(3), 242–255. https://doi.org/10.1080/02699206.2019.1628811

Fior, R. (1972). Physiological maturation of auditory function between 3 and 13 years of age. *Audiology*, *11*(5-6), 317–321.

Fiori, S., Pannek, K., Podda, I., Cipriani, P., Lorenzoni, V., Franchi, B., . . . Chilosi, A. (2021). Neural changes induced by a speech motor treatment in childhood apraxia of speech: A case series. *Journal of Child Neurology*, *36*(11). https://doi.org/10.1177/08830738211015800

First, M. B. (2014). *DSM-5. Handbook of differential diagnosis*. American Psychiatric Publishing.

Fish, M., & Skinder-Meredith, A. (2022). *Here's how to treat childhood apraxia of speech*. Plural Publishing.

Fisher, H. B., & Logemann, J. A. (1971). *Fisher-Logemann Test of Articulation Competence*. Houghton Mifflin.

Fisher, S. E., Vargha-Khadem, F., Watkins, K. E., Monaco, A. P., & Pembrey, M. E. (1998). Localisation of a gene implicated in a severe speech and language disorder. *Nature Genetics*, *18*(2), 168–170. [Erratum in: *Nature Genetics*, 1998, *18*(3), 298] https://doi.org/10.1038/ng0298-168

Fishman, J. (2001). 300-plus years of heritage language education in the United States. In J. K. Peyton, D. A. Ranard, & S. McGinnis (Eds.), *Heritage languages in America: Preserving a national resource* (pp. 81–89). Center for Applied Linguistics & Delta Systems.

Fitch, W. T. (2018). The biology and evolution of speech: A comparative analysis. *Annual Review of Linguistics*, *4*(1), 255–279. https://doi.org/10.1146/annurev-linguistics-011817-045748

Fitch, W. T., & Giedd, J. (1999). Morphology and development of the human vocal tract: A study using magnetic resonance imaging. *The Journal of the Acoustical Society of America*, *106*(3), 1511–1522. https://doi.org/10.1121/1.427148

Fitts, P. M., & Posner, M. I. (1967). *Human performance*. Brooks/Cole Publishing.

Fitzpatrick, E. M., Gaboury, I., Durieux-Smith, A., Coyle, D., Whittingham, J., & Nassrallah, F. (2019). Auditory and language outcomes in children with unilateral hearing loss. *Hearing Research*, *372*, 42–51.

Fitzroy, A. B., Krizman, J., Tierney, A., Agouridou, M., & Kraus, N. (2015). Longitudinal maturation of auditory cortical function during adolescence. *Frontiers in Human Neuroscience*, *9*, 530. https://doi.org/10.3389/fnhum.2015.00530

Flanagan, K. J., & Ttofari Eecen, K. (2018). Core vocabulary therapy for the treatment of inconsistent phonological disorder: Variations in service delivery. *Child Language Teaching and Therapy*, *34*(3), 209–219. https://doi.org/10.1177/0265659018784702

Flanagan, R. M., & Symonds, J. E. (2022). Children's self-talk in naturalistic classroom settings in middle childhood: A systematic literature review. *Educational Research Review*, *100432*. https://doi.org/10.1016/j.edurev.2022.100432

Flege, J. E. (1995). Second-language speech learning: Theory, findings, and problems. In W. Strange (Ed.) *Speech perception and lin-*

guistic experience: Issue in cross-language research (pp. 229–273). York Press.

Flege, J. E. (2019). A non-critical period for second-language learning. *A sound approach to language matters: In honor of Ocke-Schwen Bohn*. Aarhus University. Open access e-book at Aurhus University Library.

Flege, J. E., & Bohn, O. S. (2021). The revised speech learning model (SLM-r). In R. Wayland (Ed.), *Second language speech learning: Theoretical and empirical progress* (pp. 3-83). Cambridge University Press.

Fleming, S., Thompson, M., Stevens, R., Heneghan, C., Plüddemann, A., Maconochie, I., . . . Mant, D. (2011). Normal ranges of heart rate and respiratory rate in children from birth to 18 years of age: a systematic review of observational studies. *The Lancet, 377*(9770), 1011–1018. https://doi.org/10.1016/S0140-6736(10)62226-X

Fletcher, A. R., Wisler, A. A., Gruver, E. R., & Borrie, S. A. (2022). Beyond speech intelligibility: Quantifying behavioral and perceived listening effort in response to dysarthric speech. *Journal of Speech, Language, and Hearing Research, 1*–11. https://doi.org/10.1044/2022_JSLHR-22-00136

Fletcher, H., & Galt, R. H. (1950). The perception of speech and its relation to telephony. *Journal of the Acoustical Society of America, 22, 89*–150. https://doi.org/10.1121/1.1906605

Fletcher, S. G. (1972). Time-by-count measurement of diadochokinetic syllable rate. *Journal of Speech and Hearing Research, 15*(4), 763–770. https://doi.org/10.1044/jshr.1504.763

Flipsen Jr., P., Shriberg, L., Weismer, G., Karlsson, H., & McSweeny, J. (1999). Acoustic characteristics of /s/ in adolescents. *Journal of Speech, Language, and Hearing Research, 42*(3), 663–677. https://doi.org/10.1044/jslhr.4203.663

Flipsen, Jr., P. (2006). Measuring the intelligibility of conversational speech in children. *Clinical Linguistics & Phonetics, 20*(4), 303–312. https://doi.org/10.1080/02699200400024863

Flipsen, P., & Lee, S. (2012). Reference data for the American English acoustic vowel space. *Clinical Linguistics and Phonetics, 26, 926*–933. https://10.3109/02699206.2012.720634

Flom, R., & Bahrick, L. E. (2007). The development of infant discrimination of affect in multimodal and unimodal stimulation: The role of intersensory redundancy. *Developmental Psychology, 43*(1), 238–252. https://doi.org/10.1037/0012-1649.43.1.238

Fluency Corporation (2020, April). *American English dialects*. https://fluencycorp.com/american-english-dialects/

Foote, J. A., & Thomson, R. I. (2021). Speech language pathologists' beliefs and knowledgebase for providing pronunciation instruction: A critical survey. *Journal of Second Language Pronunciation*, 7(2), 240–264. https://doi.org/10.1075/jslp.20031.foo

Forrest, K. (2002). Are oral-motor exercises useful in the treatment of phonological/articulatory disorders? In *Seminars in speech and language* (Vol. 23, No. 01, pp. 015–026). Thieme Medical Publishers.

Forrester, M. A. (2008). The emergence of self–repair: A case study of one child during the early preschool years. *Research on Language and Social Interaction, 41, 99*–128.

Fossa, P. (2022). Inner speech: The private area to remember, play, and dream. In P. Fossa (Ed.), *New perspectives on inner speech (Springerbriefs in psychology)* (pp. 1–5). Springer. https://doi.org/10.1007/978–3–031–06847–8_1

Fox, A. M., Reid, C. L., Anderson, M., Richardson, C., & Bishop, D. V. (2012). Maturation of rapid auditory temporal processing and subsequent nonword repetition performance in children. *Developmental Science, 15*(2), 204–211. https://doi.org/10.1111/j.1467-7687.2011.01117.x

Fox, A. V., Dodd, B., & Howard, D. (2002). Risk factors for speech disorders in children. *International Journal of Language & Communication Disorders, 37*(2), 117–131. https://doi.org/10.1080/13682820110116776

Fox, C., Ebersbach, G., Ramig, L., & Sapir, S. (2012). LSVT LOUD and LSVT BIG: behavioral treatment programs for speech and body movement in Parkinson disease. *Rehabilitation and Parkinson's Disease,* 2012, 391946. https://doi.org/10.1155/2012/391946

Fox, C. M., Morrison, C. E., Ramig, L. O., & Sapir, S. (2002). Current perspectives on the Lee Silverman Voice Treatment (LSVT) for individuals with idiopathic Parkinson disease. *American Journal of Speech-Language Pathology, 11*(2), 111–123. https://doi.org/10.1044/1058-0360(2002/012)

Fox, L. (2018). Examining the orofacial structures in patients with craniofacial differences. *Perspectives of the ASHA Special Interest Groups,*

3(5), 24–35. https://doi.org/10.1044/persp3.SIG5.24

Fox-Boyer, A. V. (2016). *Kindliche Aussprachestörungen [Speech sound disorders in children]*, (7th ed.) Schulz-Kirchner: Idstein.

Fox Tree, J. (1995). The effects of false starts and repetitions on the processing of subsequent words in spontaneous speech. *Journal of Memory and Language, 34*, 709–738.

Franchignoni, F., Salaffi, F., & Tesio, L. (2012). How should we use the visual analogue scale (VAS) in rehabilitation outcomes? I: How much of what? The seductive VAS numbers are not true measures. *Journal of Rehabilitation Medicine, 44*, 798–799.

Francis-West, P. H., Robson, L., & Evans, D. J. (2003). Craniofacial development: The tissue and molecular interactions that control development of the head. *Advances in Anatomy, Embryology and Cell Biology, 169*, III–IV, 1–138.

Fridriksson, J., Yourganov, G., Bonilha, L., Basilakos, A., Den Ouden, D. B., & Rorden, C. (2016). Revealing the dual streams of speech processing. *Proceedings of the National Academy of Sciences, 113*(52), 15108–15113. https://doi.org/10.1073/pnas.161403811

Friedman, M., Ibrahim, H., & Bass, L. (2002). Clinical staging for sleep-disordered breathing. *Otolaryngology-Head and Neck Surgery, 127*(1), 13–21. https://doi.org/10.1067/mhn.2002.126477

Friedmann, N., & Rusou, D. (2015). Critical period for first language: the crucial role of language input during the first year of life. *Current Opinion in Neurobiology, 35*, 27–34. https://doi.org/10.1016/j.conb.2015.06.003

Fromkin, V. A. (1971). The non–anomalous nature of anomalous utterances. *Language, 47*(1), 27–52. http://links.jstor.org/sici?sici=0097

Fry, D. (1977). *Homo Loquens: Man as a talking animal.* Cambridge University Press.

Fudala, J. B. (2000). *Arizona Articulation Proficiency Scale*, 3rd revision. Western Psychological Services.

Fujiki, M., Spackman, M. P., Brinton, B., & Illig, T. (2008). Ability of children with language impairment to understand emotion conveyed by prosody in a narrative passage. *International Journal of Language & Communication Disorders, 43*(3), 330–345. https://doi.org/10.1080/13682820701507377

Fujiki, R. B., & Thibeault, S. L. (2021). The relationship between auditory-perceptual rating scales and objective voice measures in children with voice disorders. *American Journal of Speech-Language Pathology, 30*(1), 228–238. https://doi.org/10.1044/2020_AJSLP-20-00188

Fujimura, J. H., & Rajagopalan, R. (2011). Different differences: The use of 'genetic ancestry' versus race in biomedical human genetic research. *Social Studies of Science, 41*(1), 5-30. https://doi.org/10.1177/0306312710379170

Furlong, L., Erickson, S., & Morris, M. E. (2017). Computer-based speech therapy for childhood speech sound disorders. *Journal of Communication Disorders, 68*, 50–69. https://doi.org/10.1016/j.jcomdis.2017.06.007

Furlong, L., Morris, M., Serry, T., & Erickson, S. (2018). Mobile apps for treatment of speech disorders in children: An evidence-based analysis of quality and efficacy. *PloS ONE, 13*(8), e0201513. https://doi.org/10.1371/journal.pone.0201513

Furlong, L. M., Morris, M. E., Serry, T. A., & Erickson, S. (2021). Treating childhood speech sound disorders: Current approaches to management by Australian speech-language pathologists. *Language, Speech, and Hearing Services in Schools, 52*(2), 581–596. https://doi.org/10.1044/2020_LSHSS-20-00092

Furrow, D. (1984). Social and private speech at two years. *Child Development, 55*(2), 355–362. https://doi.org/10.2307/1129948

Fusaroli, R., Lambrechts, A., Bang, D., Bowler, D. M., & Gaigg, S. B. (2017). Is voice a marker for autism spectrum disorder? A systematic review and meta-analysis. *Autism Research, 10*(3), 384–407. https://doi.org/10.1002/aur.1678

Fusaroli, R., Grossman, R., Bilenberg, N., Cantio, C., Jepsen, J. R. M., & Weed, E. (2022). Toward a cumulative science of vocal markers of autism: A cross-linguistic meta-analysis-based investigation of acoustic markers in American and Danish autistic children. *Autism Research, 15*(4), 653–664. https://doi.org/10.1002/aur.2661

Gabis, L. V., Shaham, M., Leon Attia, O., Shefer, S., Rosenan, R., Gabis, T., & Daloya, M. (2021). The weak link: Hypotonia in infancy and autism early identification. *Frontiers in Neurology, 12*, 612674. https://doi.org/10.3389/fneur.2021.612674

Gagné, J. P., Rochette, A. J., & Charest, M. (2002). Auditory, visual and audiovisual clear speech. *Speech Communication, 37*(3–4), 213–230. https://doi.org/10.1016/S0167-6393(01)00012-7

Galek, K. E., & Watterson, T. (2017). Perceptual anchors and the dispersion of nasality ratings. *The Cleft Palate-Craniofacial Journal, 54*(4), 423–430.2014). https://doi.org/10.1597/15-269

Gandour, J., Tong, Y., Wong, D., Talavage, T., Dzemidzic, M., Xu, Y., . . . Lowe, M. (2004). Hemispheric roles in the perception of speech prosody. *Neuroimage, 23*(1), 344–357. https://doi.org/10.1016/j.neuroimage.2004.06.004

Gangamohan, P., Kadiri, S. R., & Yegnanarayana, B. (2016). Analysis of emotional speech—A review. In A. Esposito & L. C. Jain, L. C. (Eds.), *Toward robotic socially believable behaving systems–Volume I: Modeling emotions* (Vol. 105, pp. 205–238). Springer. https://doi.org/10.1007/978-3-319-31056-5_11

Gans, C. (1988). Craniofacial growth, evolutionary questions. *Development, 103*(Suppl.), 3–15.

Garde, J. B., Suryavanshi, R. K., Jawale, B. A., Deshmukh, V., Dadhe, D. P., & Suryavanshi, M. K. (2014). An epidemiological study to know the prevalence of deleterious oral habits among 6 to12 year old children. *Journal of International Oral Health: JIOH, 6*(1), 39.

Gargano, R., Marchese, D., Oliva, S., Gerardi, S., Saraniti, C., Riggio, F., . . . Gallina, S. (2022). Swallowing, speech and orofacial disorders in children with adenotonsillar hypertrophy. *Euromediterranean Biomedical Journal, 17*. https://doi.org/10.3269/1970-5492.2022.17.8

Garmann, N. G., Hansen, P., Simonsen, H. G., & Kristoffersen, K. E. (2019). The phonology of children's early words: Trends, individual variation, and parents' accommodation in child-directed speech. *Frontiers in Communication, 4*, 10. https://doi.org/10.3389/fcomm.2019.00010

Garrido, D., Watson, L. R., Carballo, G., Garcia-Retamero, R., & Crais, E. R. (2017). Infants at-risk for autism spectrum disorder: Patterns of vocalizations at 14 months. *Autism Research, 10*(8), 1372–1383. https://doi.org/10.1002/aur.1788

Gascoigne, M. (2006). *Supporting children with speech, language and communication needs within integrated children's services*. Royal College of Speech and Language Therapists (RCSLT) [Position paper]. London. Available from the RCSLT website: www.rcslt.org

Gathercole, S. E., & Baddeley, A. D. (1996). *The children's test of nonword repetition*. Psychological Corporation.

Gathercole, S. E., Willis, C. S., Baddeley, A. D., & Emslie, H. (1994). The children's test of nonword repetition: A test of phonological working memory. *Memory, 2*(2), 103–127. https://doi.org/10.1080/09658219408258940

Gatlin, B., & Wanzek, J. (2015). Relations among children's use of dialect and literacy skills: A meta-analysis. *Journal of Speech, Language, and Hearing Research, 58*(4), 1306–1318. https://doi.org/10.1044/2015_JSLHR-L-14-0311

Gerber, R. J., Wilks, T., & Erdie-Lalena, C. (2010). Developmental milestones: Motor development. *Pediatrics in Review, 31*(7), 267–277. https://doi.org/10.1542/pir.31-7-267

Gerken, L., & McGregor, K. (1998). An overview of prosody and its role in normal and disordered child language. *American Journal of Speech-Language Pathology*, 7(2), 38–48. https://doi.org/10.1044/1058-0360.0702.38

Gervain, J. (2018). The role of prenatal experience in language development. *Current Opinion in Behavioral Sciences, 21*, 62–67. https://doi.org/10.1016/j.cobeha.2018.02.004

Gerwin, K. L., Brosseau-Lapré, F., & Weber, C. (2021). Event-related potentials elicited by phonetic errors differentiate children with speech sound disorder and typically developing peers. *Journal of Speech, Language, and Hearing Research, 64*(12), 4614–4630. https://doi.org/10.1044/2021_JSLHR-21-00203

Gerwin, K. L., Walsh, B., & Christ, S. L. (2022). Error characteristics lend specificity to nonword repetition performance in children who stutter with and without concomitant disorders. *Journal of Speech, Language, and Hearing Research, 65*(7), 2571–2585. https://doi.org/10.1044/2022_JSLHR-21-00654

Geva, S., & Fernyhough, C. (2019). A penny for your thoughts: Children's inner speech and its neuro-development. *Frontiers in Psychology, 10*, 1708. https://doi.org/10.3389/fpsyg.2019.01708

Geytenbeek J. (2019). The use of Dodd's Model for Differential Diagnosis to classify childhood speech sound disorders. *Developmen-*

tal Medicine & Child Neurology, 61(6), 626. https://doi.org/10.1111/dmcn.14022.

Gibbon, F. E., & Lee, A. (2017a). Electropalatographic (EPG) evidence of covert contrasts in disordered speech. *Clinical Linguistics & Phonetics, 31*(1), 4–20. https://doi.org/10.1080/02699206.2016.1174739

Gibbon, F. E., & Lee, A. (Eds.). (2017b). Covert contrasts [Special issue]. *Clinical Linguistics & Phonetics, 31*(1).

Gibbon, F. E., & Wood, S. E. (2002). Articulatory drift in the speech of children with articulation and phonological disorders. *Perceptual and Motor Skills, 95*(1), 295–307. https://doi.org/10.2466/pms.2002.95.1.295

Gick, B. (1999). A gesture-based account of intrusive consonants in English. *Phonology, 16*(1), 29–54. https://doi.org/10.1017/S0952675799003693

Gick, B., Kang, A., & Whalen, D. H. (2002). MRI evidence for commonality in the post-oral articulations of English vowels and liquids. *Journal of Phonetics, 30*(3), 357–371. https://doi.org/10.1006/jpho.2001.0161

Gick, B., Allen, B., Roewer-Després, F., & Stavness, I. (2017). Speaking tongues are actively braced. *Journal of Speech, Language, and Hearing Research, 60*(3), 494–506. https://doi.org/10.1044/2016_JSLHR-S-15-0141

Gick, B., Wilson, I., Koch, K., & Cook, C. (2004). Language-specific articulatory settings: Evidence from inter-utterance rest position. *Phonetica, 61*(4), 220–233. https://doi.org/10.1159/000084159

Gierut, J. A. (1989). Maximal opposition approach to phonological treatment. *Journal of Speech and Hearing Disorders, 54*(1), 9–19. https://doi.org/10.1044/jshd.5401.09

Gierut, J., A. (1990). Differential learning of phonological oppositions. *Journal of Speech, Language, and Hearing Research, 33*, 540–549. https://doi.org/10.1044/jshr.3303.540

Gierut, J. A. (1992). The conditions and course of clinically induced phonological change. *Journal of Speech, Language, and Hearing Research, 35*, 1049–1063. https://doi.org/10.1044/jshr.3505.1049

Gierut, J. A. (1998). Treatment efficacy: Functional phonological disorders in children. *Journal of Speech, Language, and Hearing Research, 41*(1), 85–100. https://doi.org/10.1044/jslhr.4101.s85

Gierut, J. A. (2001). Complexity in phonological treatment: Clinical factors. *Language, Speech, and Hearing Services in Schools. 32*(4), 229–241. https://doi.org/10.1044/0161-1461(2001/021)

Gierut, J. A. (2007). Phonological complexity and language learnability. *American Journal of Speech-Language Pathology, 16*(1), 6–17. https://doi.org/10.1044/1058-0360(2007/003)

Gildersleeve-Neumann, C. E., Kester, E. S., Davis, B. L., & Peña, E. D. (2008). English speech sound development in preschool-aged children from bilingual English–Spanish environments. *Language, Speech, & Hearing Services in Schools, 39*(3), 314–328 https://doi.org/10.1044/0161-1461(2008/030)

Gill, C., Mehta, J., Fredenburg, K., & Bartlett, K. (2011). Imitation therapy for non-verbal toddlers. *Child Language Teaching and Therapy, 27*(1), 97–108. https://doi.org/10.1177/0265659010375179

Gillam, R. B., Logan, K. J., & Pearson, N. A. (2009). *TOCS: Test of Childhood Stuttering*. Pro-Ed.

Gillon, G. T., & McNeill, B. C. (2007). *Integrated phonological awareness. An intervention program for preschool children with speech-language impairment*. University of Canterbury.

Gillon, G., Hyter, Y., Fernandes, F. D., Ferman, S., Hus, Y., Petinou, K., . . . Westerveld, M. (2017). International survey of speech-language pathologists' practices in working with children with autism spectrum disorder. *Folia Phoniatrica et Logopaedica, 69*(1-2), 8–19. https://doi.org/10.1159/000479063

Giovannoli, J., Martella, D., Federico, F., Pirchio, S., & Casagrande, M. (2020). The impact of bilingualism on executive functions in children and adolescents: A systematic review based on the PRISMA method. *Frontiers in Psychology, 11*, 574789. https://doi.org/10.3389/fpsyg.2020.574789

Gironda, F., Fabus, R., & Musayeva, (2011). Assessment of the oral-peripheral speech mechanism. In R. Fabus & C. Stein-Rubin (Eds.), *Guide to clinical assessment and professional report writing in speech-language pathology* (pp. 116–134). Plural Publishing.

Glaspey, A. M., & MacLeod, A. A. (2010). A multidimensional approach to gradient change in phonological acquisition: A case study of disordered speech development. *Clinical Lin-*

guistics & Phonetics, 24(4–5), 283–299. https://doi.org/10.3109/02699200903581091

Gleason, J. B. (2019). *The Wug Test.* Larchwood Press.

Gleitman, L., Gleitman, H., Landau, B., & Wanner, E. (1988). Where learning begins: Initial representations for language learning. In F. Newmeyer (Ed.), *Linguistics: The Cambridge survey III. Language: Psychological and biological aspects* (pp. 150–193). Cambridge University Press.

Godde, E., Bosse, M. L., & Bailly, G. (2020). A review of reading prosody acquisition and development. *Reading and Writing, 33*(2), 399–426. https://doi.org/10.1007/s11145-019-09968-1

Goetz, M., Vesela, M., & Ptacek, R. (2014). Notes on the role of the cerebellum in ADHD. *Austin Journal of Psychiatry and Behavioral Science, 1*(3), 1013.

Goffman, L. (2004). Kinematic differentiation of prosodic categories in normal and disordered language development. *Journal of Speech, Language, and Hearing Research, 47*(5), 1088–1102. https://doi.org/10.1044/1092-4388(2004/081)

Goffman, L., Gerken, L., & Lucchesi, J. (2007). Relations between segmental and motor variability in prosodically complex nonword sequences. *Journal of Speech, Language, and Hearing Research, 50*(2), 444–458. https://doi.org/10.1044/1092-4388(2007/031)

Goldin-Meadow, S. (2015). Gesture as a window onto communicative abilities: Implications for diagnosis and intervention. *Perspectives on Language Learning and Education, 22*(2), 50–60. https://doi.org/10.1044/lle22.2.50

Goldman, R., & Fristoe, M. (2000). *Goldman-Fristoe Test of Articulation* (2nd ed.). AGS.

Goldrick, M., & Chu, K. (2014). Gradient coactivation and speech error articulation: Comment on Pouplier and Goldstein (2010). *Language, Cognition and Neuroscience, 29*(4), 452–458. https://doi.org/10.1080/01690965.2013.807347

Goldsack, J. C., Coravos, A., Bakker, J. P., Bent, B., Dowling, A. V., Fitzer-Attas, C., . . . Dunn, J. (2020). Verification, analytical validation, and clinical validation (V3): The foundation of determining fit-for-purpose for Biometric Monitoring Technologies (BioMeTs). *npj Digital Medicine, 3*(1), 55. https://doi.org/10.1038/s41746-020-0260-4

Goldsmith, J. A. (1976). *Autosegmental phonology* [Doctoral dissertation]. Massachusetts Institute of Technology.

Goldsmith, J. A. (2001). An overview of autosegmental phonology. In C. W. Kreidler (Ed.), *Phonology: Critical concepts in linguistics* (Vol. 3, pp. 382–425). Routledge.

Goldstein, B. (2001). Transcription of Spanish and Spanish-influenced English. *Communication Disorders Quarterly, 23*(1), 54–60. https://doi.org/10.1177/152574010102300108

Goldstein, B. A., & Iglesias, A. (2001). The effect of dialect on phonological analysis: Evidence from Spanish speaking children. *American Journal of Speech-Language Pathology, 10*(4), 394–406. https://doi.org/10.1044/1058-0360(2001/034)

Goldstein, B., & Iglesias, A. (2006). *CPACS: Contextual probes of articulation competence: Spanish.* Super Duper.

Goldstone, R. L. (1998). Perceptual learning. *Annual review of psychology, 49*(1), 585–612. https://doi.org/10.1146/annurev.psych.49.1.585

Gomez, M., McCabe, P., & Purcell, A. (2022). A survey of the clinical management of childhood apraxia of speech in the United States and Canada. *Journal of Communication Disorders, 96*, 106193.

Goo, M., Tucker, K., & Johnston, L. M. (2018). Muscle tone assessments for children aged 0 to 12 years: a systematic review. *Developmental Medicine & Child Neurology, 60*(7), 660–671. https://doi.org/10.1111/dmcn.13668

Goodrich, L. V., & Kanold, P. O. (2020). Functional circuit development in the auditory system. In J. Rubenstein, B. Chen, P. Rakic, & K. Y. Kwann (Eds.), *Neural circuit and cognitive development* (pp. 27–55). Academic Press.

Goodwin, C., & Lillo-Martin, D. (2019). Morphological accuracy in the speech of bimodal bilingual children with CIs. *The Journal of Deaf Studies and Deaf Education, 24*(4), 435–447. https://doi.org/10.1093/deafed/enz019

Goodwyn, S. W., Acredolo, L. P., & Brown, C. A. (2000). Impact of symbolic gesturing on early language development. *Journal of Nonverbal Behavior, 24*, 81–103. https://doi.org/10.1023/A:1006653828895

Gordon-Brannan, & Hodson, B. W. (2000). Intelligibility/severity measurements of prekindergarten children's speech. *American Journal of Speech-Language Pathology*, *9*(2), 141–150. https://doi.org/10.1044/1058-0360.0902.141

Gracia, N., Rumbach, A., & Finch, E. (2020). A survey of speech-language pathology treatment for non-progressive dysarthria in Australia. *Brain Impairment*, *21*(2), 173–190. https://doi.org/10.1017/BrImp.2020.3

Graf Estes, K., Evans, J. L., & Else-Quest, N. E. (2007). Differences in the nonword repetition performance of children with and without specific language impairment: A meta-analysis. *Journal of Speech, Language, and Hearing Research*, *50*(1), 177–195. https://doi.org/10.1044/1092-4388(2007/015)

Grandchamp, R., Rapin, L., Perrone-Bertolotti, M., Pichat, C., Haldin, C., Cousin, E., . . . Lœvenbruck, H. (2019). The ConDialInt model: Condensation, dialogality, and intentionality dimensions of inner speech within a hierarchical predictive control framework. *Frontiers in Psychology*, *10*. https://doi.org/10.3389/fpsyg.2019.02019

Grandi, D. (2012). Interdisciplinary Orofacial Examination Protocol for Children and Adolescents": A resource for the interdisciplinary assessment of the stomatognatic system. *International Journal of Orofacial Myology*, *38*, 15–26.

Grandjean, D. (2021). Brain networks of emotional prosody processing. *Emotion Review*, *13*(1), 34–43. https://doi.org/10.1177/1754073919898522

Granocchio, E., Gazzola, S., Scopelliti, M. R., Criscuoli, L., Airaghi, G., Sarti, D., & Magazù, S. (2021). Evaluation of oro-phonatory development and articulatory diadochokinesis in a sample of Italian children using the protocol of Robbins & Klee. *Journal of Communication Disorders*, *91*, 106101. https://doi.org/10.1016/j.jcomdis.2021.106101

Green, M. (Fall 2021). Speech acts. In E. N. Zalta (Ed.), *The Stanford encyclopedia of philosophy*. https://plato.stanford.edu/archives/fall2021/entries/speech-acts/>

Green, J. R., Moore, C. A., & Reilly, K. J. (2002). The sequential development of jaw and lip control for speech. *Journal of Speech, Language, and Hearing Research*, *45*(1), 66–79. https://doi.org/10.1044/1092-4388(2002/005)

Grigos, M. I., & Patel, R. (2007). Articulator movement associated with the development of prosodic control in children. *Journal of Speech, Language, and Hearing Research*, *50*(1), 119–130. https://doi.org/10.1044/1092-4388(2007/010)

Grimley, S. J., Ko, C. M., Morrell, H. E., Grace, F., Bañuelos, M. S., Bautista, B. R., . . . Olson, L. E. (2018). The need for a neutral speaking period in psychosocial stress testing. *Journal of Psychophysiology*, *33*(4). https://doi.org/10.1027/0269-8803/a000228

Grimm, R., Cassani, G., Gillis, S., & Daelemans, W. (2019). Children probably store short rather than frequent or predictable chunks: Quantitative evidence from a corpus study. *Frontiers in Psychology*, *10*, 80. https://doi.org/10.3389/fpsyg.2019.00080

Grimme, B., Fuchs, S., Perrier, P., & Schöner, G. (2011). Limb versus speech motor control: A conceptual review. *Motor Control, Human Kinetics*, *15*(1), 5–33. https://doi.org/10.1123/mcj.15.1.5.

Grippaudo, C., Paolantonio, E. G., Antonini, G., Saulle, R., La Torre, G., & Deli, R. (2016). Association between oral habits, mouth breathing and malocclusion. *Acta Otorhinolaryngologica Italica*, *36*(5), 386.

Grisso, T. (2000). What we know about youths' capacities as trial defendants. In T. Grisso & R. G. Schwartz (Eds.), *Youth on trial: A developmental perspective on juvenile justice* (pp. 139–171). University of Chicago Press.

Grosbras, M. H., Ross, P. D. & Belin, P. (2018). Categorical emotion recognition from voice improves during childhood and adolescence. *Scientific Reports*, *8*, 14791. https://doi.org/10.1038/s41598-018-32868-3

Gross, M. C., & Kaushanskaya, M. (2022). Language control and code-switching in bilingual children with developmental language disorder. *Journal of Speech, Language, and Hearing Research*, *65*(3), 1104–1127. https://doi.org/10.1044/2021_JSLHR-21-00332

Grossman, R. C., Hattis, B. F., & Ringel, R. L. (1965). Oral tactile experience. *Archives of Oral Biology*, *10*(4), 691-IN36. https://doi.org/10.1016/0003-9969(65)90014-2

Grossman. R. B., Edelson, L. R., & Tager-Flusberg, H. (2013). Emotional facial and vocal expressions during story retelling by children and adolescents with high-functioning autism. *Journal of Speech, Language, and Hearing Research*, *56*(3), 1035–1044. https://doi.org/10.1044/1092–4388(2012/12–0067)

Grossmann, T., Striano, T., & Friederici, A. D. (2005). Infants' electric brain responses to emotional prosody. *Neuroreport, 16*(16), 1825–1828. https://doi.org/10.1097/01.wnr.0000185964.34336.b1

Grover, V., Namasivayam, A., & Mahendra, N. (2022). A viewpoint on accent services: Framing and terminology matter. *American Journal of Speech-Language Pathology, 31*(2), 639–648. https://doi.org/10.1044/2021_AJSLP-20-00376

Grudziąż-Sękowska, J, Olczak-Kowalczyk, D., & Zadurska, M. (2018). Correlation between functional disorders of the masticatory system and speech sound disorders in children aged 7–10 years. *Dental and Medical Problems, 55*(2), 161–165. https://doi.org/10.17219/dmp/86006.

Grundy, J. G., Anderson, J. A., & Bialystok, E. (2017). Neural correlates of cognitive processing in monolinguals and bilinguals. *Annals of the New York Academy of Sciences, 1396*(1), 183–201. https://https://doi.org/10.1111/nyas.13333

Grünheid, T., Langenbach, G. E. J., Korfage, J. A. M., Zentner, A., & van Eijden, T. M. (2009). The adaptive response of jaw muscles to varying functional demands. *European Journal of Orthodontics, 31*(6), 596–612. https://doi.org/10.1093/ejo/cjp093

Grunwell, P., (1985). *Phonological assessment of child speech (PACS)*. NFER-Nelson.

Grunwell, P. (1987). *Clinical phonology* (2nd ed.). Blackwell.

Guay, A. H., Maxwell, D. L., & Beecher, R. (1978). A radiographic study of tongue posture at rest and during the phonation of /s/ in class III malocclusion. *The Angle Orthodontist, 48*(1), 10–22. https://doi.org/10.1043/0003-3219(1978)048<0010:arsotp>2.0.co;2

Guenther, F. H. (1994). A neural network model of speech acquisition and motor equivalent speech production. *Biological Cybernetics, 72*(1), 43–53. https://doi.org/10.1007/BF00206237

Guenther, F. H. (2006). Cortical interactions underlying the production of speech sounds. *Journal of Communication Disorders, 39*(5), 350–365. https://doi.org/10.1016/j.jcomdis.2006.06.013

Guerra, J., & Cacabelos, R. (2019). Genomics of speech and language disorders. *Journal of Translational Genetics and Genomics, 3*(9). https://doi.org/10.20517/jtgg.2018.03

Guidali, G., Pisoni, A., Bolognini, N., & Papagno, C. (2019). Keeping order in the brain: The supramarginal gyrus and serial order in short-term memory. *Cortex, 119*, 89–99. https://doi.org/10.1016/j.cortex.2019.04.009

Guilleminault, C., Huang, Y. S., & Quo, S. (2019). Apraxia in children and adults with obstructive sleep apnea syndrome. *Sleep, 42*(12), zsz168.

Guiraud, H., Bedoin, N., Krifi-Papoz, S., Herbillon, V., Caillot-Bascoul, A., Gonzalez-Monge, S., & Boulenger, V. (2018). Don't speak too fast! Processing of fast rate speech in children with specific language impairment. *PloS ONE, 13*(1), e0191808. https://doi.org/10.1371/journal.pone.0191808

Gunnerud, H. L., ten Braak, D., Reikerås, E. K. L., Donolato, E., & Melby-Lervåg, M. (2020). Is bilingualism related to a cognitive advantage in children? A systematic review and meta-analysis. *Psychological Bulletin, 146*(12), 1059–1083. https://doi.org/10.1037/bul0000301

Gupta, S., Sharma, R., & Jain, D. (2005). Airway assessment: Predictors of difficult airway. *Indian Journal of Anesthesiology, 49*(4), 257–262.

Guttentag, O. E. (1949). On the clinical entity. *Annals of Internal Medicine, 31*(3), 484–496. https://doi.org/10.7326/0003-4819-31-3-484

Haake, M., Hansson, K., Gulz, A., Schötz, S., & Sahlén, B. (2014). The slower the better? Does the speaker's speech rate influence children's performance on a language comprehension test? *International Journal of Speech and Language Pathology, 16*(2), 181–190. https://doi.org/10.3109/17549507.2013.845690.

Haas, E., Ziegler, W., & Schölderle, T. (2021). Developmental courses in childhood dysarthria: Longitudinal analyses of auditory-perceptual parameters. *Journal of Speech, Language, and Hearing Research, 64*(5), 1421–1435. https://doi.org/10.1044/2020_JSLHR-20-00492

Haas, E., Ziegler, W., & Schölderle, T. (2022). Intelligibility, speech rate, and communication efficiency in children with neurological conditions: A longitudinal study of childhood dysarthria. *American Journal of Speech-Language Pathology, 31*(4), 1817–1835. https://doi.org/10.1044/2022_AJSLP-21-00354d

Haelsig, P. C., & Madison, C. L. (1986). A study of phonological processes exhibited by 3-, 4-, and 5-year-old children. *Language, Speech, and Hearing Services in Schools, 17*(2), 107–114. https://doi.org/10.1044/0161-1461.1702.107

Hall, M. L., Hall, W. C., & Caselli, N. K. (2019). Deaf children need language, not (just) speech. *First Language, 39*(4), 367–395. https://doi.org/10.1177/0142723719834102

Hall, J. A., Horgan, T. G., & Murphy, N. A. (2019). Nonverbal communication. *Annual Review of Psychology, 70*, 271–294. https://doi.org/10.1146/annurev-psych-010418103145

Hallé, P. A., De Boysson-Bardies, B., & Vihman, M. M. (1991). Beginnings of prosodic organization: Intonation and duration patterns of disyllables produced by Japanese and French infants. *Language and Speech, 34*(4), 299–318. https://doi.org/10.1177/002383099103400401

Hambly, H., Wren, Y., McLeod, S., & Roulstone, S. (2013). The influence of bilingualism on speech production: A systematic review. *International Journal of Language & Communication Disorders, 48*(1), 1–24. https://doi.org/10.1111/j.1460-6984.2012.00178.x

Hammer, J., & Eber, E. (2005). The peculiarities of infant respiratory physiology. In J. Hammer & E. Eber (Eds.), *Paediatric pulmonary function testing* (Vol. 33, pp. 2–7). Karger Publishers.

Hanley, L., Ballard, K. J., Dickson, A., & Purcell, A. (2022). Speech intervention for children with cleft palate using principles of motor learning. *American Journal of Speech-Language Pathology*, 1–21. https://doi.org/10.1044/2022_AJSLP-22-00007

Hanley, L., Ballard, K. J., Dickson, A., & Purcell, A. (2023). Speech intervention for children with cleft palate using principles of motor learning. *Journal of Speech-Language Pathology, 32*(1),169–189.

Hannahs, S. J., & Bosch, A. R. K. (2022). *The Routledge handbook of phonological theory*. Routledge Handbooks Online.

Hanson, M. L., & Mason, R. M. (2003). *Orofacial myology: International perspectives* (2nd ed.). Charles C Thomas.

Harari, D., Redlich, M., Miri, S., Hamud, T., & Gross, M. (2010). The effect of mouth breathing versus nasal breathing on dentofacial and craniofacial development in orthodontic patients. *The Laryngoscope, 120*, 2089–2093. https://doi.org/10.1002/lary.20991

Harley, T. A. (1984). A critique of top–down independent levels models of speech production: Evidence from non-plan-internal speech errors. *Cognitive Science, 8*(3), 191–219. https://doi.org/10.1016/S0364–0213(84)80001–4

Harris, M. (2013). *Language experience and early language development: From input to uptake*. Psychology Press.

Harris, S. R. (2008). Congenital hypotonia: Clinical and developmental assessment. *Developmental Medicine & Child Neurology, 50*(12), 889–892. https://doi.org/10.1111/j.1469-8749.2008.03097.x

Harrison, L. J., & McLeod, S. (2010). Risk and protective factors associated with speech and language impairment in a nationally representative sample of 4-to 5-year-old children. *Journal of Speech, Language, and Hearing Research, 53*(2), 508–529. https://doi.org/10.1044/1092-4388(2009/08-0086)

Hartnick, C. J. (2002). Validation of a pediatric voice quality-of-life instrument: The pediatric voice outcome survey. *Archives of Otolaryngology-Head & Neck Surgery, 128*(8), 919–922. https://doi.org/10.1001/archotol.128.8.919

Hartnick, C. J., Rehbar, R., & Prasad, V. (2005). Development and maturation of the pediatric human vocal fold lamina propria. *Laryngoscope, 115*(1), 4–15. https://doi.org/10.1097/01.mlg.0000150685.54893.e9

Hartshorne, J. K., Tenenbaum, J. B., & Pinker, S. (2018). A critical period for second language acquisition: Evidence from 2/3 million English speakers. *Cognition, 177*, 263–277. https://doi.org/10.1016/j.cognition.2018.04.007

Haselager, G. J. T., Slis, I. H., & Rietveld, A, C, M. (1991) An alternative method of studying the development of speech rate, *Clinical Linguistics & Phonetics, 5*(1), 53–63. https://doi.org/10.3109/02699209108985502

Hawthorne, K., & Fischer, S. (2020). Speech-language pathologists and prosody: Clinical practices and barriers. *Journal of Communication Disorders, 87*, 106024. https://doi.org/10.1016/j.jcomdis.2020.106024.

Hayden, D. (2006). The PROMPT model: Use and application for children with mixed phonological-motor impairment. *Advances in Speech Language Pathology, 8*(3), 265–281. https://doi.org/10.1080/14417040600861094

Hayden, D., & Square, P. (1994). Motor speech treatment hierarchy: A systems approach. *Clinics in Communication Disorders, 4*(3), 162–174.

Hayden, D., & Square-Storer, P. (1999). *VMPAC: Verbal Motor Production Assessment for Children*. Psychological Corporation.

Hayden, D., Eigen, J., Walker, A., & Olsen, L. (2010). PROMPT: A tactually grounded model. In L. Williams, S. McLeod, & R. McCauley (Eds.), *Interventions for speech sound disorders in children* (pp. 453–474). Brookes.

Hazan, V., & Markham, D. (2004). Acoustic-phonetic correlates of talker intelligibility for adults and children. *The Journal of the Acoustical Society of America, 116*(5), 3108–3118. https://doi.org/10.1121/1.1806826

Hazelbaker, A. K. (1993). *The Assessment Tool for Lingual Frenulum Function (ATLFF): Use in a lactation consultant private practice*. Pacific Oaks College.

Healey, E. C., & Reid, R. (2003). ADHD and stuttering: A tutorial. *Journal of Fluency Disorders, 28*(2), 79–93. https://doi.org/10.1016/S0094-730X(03)00021-4

Hearnshaw, S., Baker, E., & Munro, N. (2019). Speech perception skills of children with speech sound disorders: A systematic review and meta-analysis. *Journal of Speech, Language, and Hearing Research, 62*(10), 3771–3789. https://doi.org/10.1044/2019_JSLHR-S-18-0519

Heavey, C. L., & Hurlburt, R. T. (2008). The phenomena of inner experience. *Consciousness and Cognition*, 17(3), 798-810. https://doi.org/10.1016/j.concog.2007.12.006

Heckathorn, D.-E., Speyer, R., Taylor, J., & Cordier, R. (2016). Systematic review: Non-instrumental swallowing and feeding assessments in pediatrics. *Dysphagia, 31*, 1–23. https://doi.org/10.1007/s00455-015-9667-5

Hegarty, N., Titterington, J., McLeod, S., & Taggart, L. (2018). Intervention for children with phonological impairment: Knowledge, practices and intervention intensity in the UK. *International Journal of Language & Communication Disorders, 53*(5), 995–1006. https://doi.org/10.1111/1460-6984.12416

Hegde, M. N. (2021). A critical review of phonological theories. *Journal of All India Institute of Speech and Hearing, 40*(1), 3–17.

Heidlmayr, K., Ferragne, E., & Isel, F. (2021). Neuroplasticity in the phonological system: The PMN and the N400 as markers for the perception of non-native phonemic contrasts by late second language learners. *Neuropsychologia, 156*, 107831. https://doi.org/10.1016/j.neuropsychologia.2021.107831

Helfrich-Miller, K. R. (1984, May). Melodic intonation therapy with developmentally apraxic children. *Seminars in Speech and Language, 2*(5), 119–126.

Helfrich-Miller, K. R. (1994). A clinical perspective: Melodic intonation therapy for developmental apraxia. *Clinics In Communication Disorders, 4*(3), 175–182.

Helm-Estabrooks, N., & Albert, M. L. (2004). Melodic intonation therapy. In N. Helm-Estabrooks & M. L. Albert (Eds.), *Manual of aphasia and aphasia therapy* (2nd ed., pp. 221–233). Pro-Ed.

Hendricks, A. E., Watson-Wales, M., & Reed, P. E. (2021). Perceptions of African American English by students in speech-language pathology programs. *American Journal of Speech-Language Pathology, 30*(5), 1962–1972. https://doi.org/10.1044/2021_AJSLP-20-00339

Hendricks, G., Malcolm-Smith, S., Adnams, C., Stein, D., & Donald, K. (2019). Effects of prenatal alcohol exposure on language, speech and communication outcomes: A review longitudinal studies. *Acta Neuropsychiatrica, 31*(2), 74–83. https://doi.org/10.1017/neu.2018.28

Henningsson, G., Kuehn, D. P., Sell, D., Sweeney, T., Trost-Cardamone, J. E., & Whitehill, T. L. (2008). Universal parameters for reporting speech outcomes in individuals with cleft palate. *The Cleft Palate-Craniofacial Journal, 45*(1), 1–17. https://doi.org/10.1597/06-086.1

Hensch, T. K. (2004). Critical period regulation. *Annual Review of Neuroscience.*, 27, 549–579. https://doi.org/10.1146/annurev.neuro.27.070203.144327

Herreras Mercado, R., Simpson, K., & Bellom-Rohrbacher, K. H. (2019). Effect of prompts for restructuring oral muscular phonetic targets (PROMPT) on compensatory articulation in children with cleft palate/lip. *Global Pediatric Health, 6*. https://doi.org/10.1177/2333794X19851417

Hesketh, C. A., Nightingale, C., & Hall, R. A. (2000). Phonological awareness therapy and articulatory training approaches for children with phonological disorders: A comparative outcome study. *International Journal of Lan-*

guage & Communication Disorders, 35(3), 337–354. 10.1080/136828200410618

Hesling, I., Clément, S., Bordessoules, M., & Allard (2005). Cerebral mechanisms of prosodic integration: Evidence from connected speech. *Neuroimage, 24*(4), 937–947. https://doi.org/10.1016/j.neuroimage.2004.11.003

Heyes, C., & Catmur, C. (2022). What happened to mirror neurons? *Perspectives on Psychological Science, 17*(1), 153–168. https://doi.org/10.1177/1745691621990638

Heylen, L., Wuyts, F. L., Mertens, F., Bodt, M. D., Pattyn, J., Croux, C., & Heyning, P. H. V. D. (1998). Evaluation of the vocal performance of children using a voice range profile index. *Journal of Speech, Language, and Hearing Research, 41*(2), 232–238. https://doi.org/10.1044/jslhr.4102.232

Hickman, L. A. (1997). *Apraxia Profile: A Descriptive Assessment Tool for Children*. Communication Skill Builders.

Hickok, G. (2012). Computational neuroanatomy of speech production. *Nature Reviews Neuroscience, 13, 135*–145. https://doi.org/10.1038/nrn3158

Hickok, G. (2014). *The myth of mirror neurons: The real neuroscience of communication and cognition*. W. W. Norton & Company.

Hickok, G., & Poeppel, D. (2004). Dorsal and ventral streams: A framework for understanding aspects of the functional anatomy of language. *Cognition, 92*(1–2), 67–99. https://doi.org/10.1016/j.cognition.2003.10.011

Hidecker, M. J. C., Paneth, N., Rosenbaum, P. L., Kent, R. D., Lillie, J., Eulenberg, J. B., . . . Taylor, K. (2011). Developing and validating the Communication Function Classification System for individuals with cerebral palsy. *Developmental Medicine & Child Neurology, 53*(8), 704–710. https://doi.org/10.1111/j.1469-8749.2011.03996.x

Hildebrand, M. S., Jackson, V. E., Scerri, T. S., Van Reyk, O., Coleman, M., Braden, R. O., . . . Morgan, A. T. (2020). Severe childhood speech disorder: Gene discovery highlights transcriptional dysregulation. *Neurology, 94*(20), e2148–e2167. https://doi.org/10.1212/WNL.0000000000009441

Hill, R. R., Lee, C. S., & Pados, B. F. (2021). The prevalence of ankyloglossia in children aged <1 year: A systematic review and meta-analysis. *Pediatric Research, 90*(2), 259–266. https://doi.org/10.1038/s41390-020-01239-y

Hirano, M. (1974). Morphological structure of the vocal cord as a vibrator and its variations. *Folia Phoniatrica (Basel), 26*(2), 89–94.

Hirano, M. (1981). *Clinical examination of voice*. Springer.

Hirano, M., Kurita, S., & Nakashima, T. (1983). Growth development and aging of vocal folds. In D. M. Bless & J. H. Abbs (Eds.), *Vocal fold physiology: Contemporary research and clinical issues* (pp. 22–43). College-Hill Press.

Hiremath, C. S., Sagar, K. J. V., Yamini, B. K., Girimaji, A. S., Kumar, R., Sravanti, S. L., & Kumar, M. (2021). Emerging behavioral and neuroimaging biomarkers for early and accurate characterization of autism spectrum disorders: A systematic review. *Translational Psychiatry, 11*(1), 42. https://doi.org/10.1038/s41398-020-01178-6

Hirsch, M. E., Thompson, A., Kim, Y., & Lansford, K. L. (2022). The reliability and validity of speech-language pathologists' estimations of intelligibility in dysarthria. *Brain Sciences, 12*(8), 1011. https://doi.org/10.3390/brainsci12081011

Hitchcock, E. R., Ochs, L. C., Swartz, M. T., Leece, M. C., Preston, J. L., & McAllister, T. (2023). Tutorial: Using visual–acoustic biofeedback for speech sound training. *American Journal of Speech-Language Pathology, 1*–19. https://doi.org/10.1044/2022_AJSLP-22-00142

Hixon, T. J., Hawley, J. L., & Wilson, K. J. (1982). An around-the-house device for the clinical determination of respiratory driving pressure: A note on making simple even simpler. *Journal of Speech and Hearing Disorders, 47*(4), 413–415. https://doi.org/10.1044/jshd.4704.413

Ho, A. K., & Wilmut, K. (2010). Speech and oromotor function in children with Developmental Coordination Disorder: A pilot study. *Human Movement Science, 29*(4), 605–614. https://doi.org/10.1016/j.humov.2010.01.007

Hodge, M. M. (1998). Developmental coordination disorder: A diagnosis with theoretical and clinical implications for developmental apraxia of speech. *Perspectives on Language Learning and Education, 5*(2), 8–12. https://doi.org/10.1044/lle5.2.8

Hodge, M. (2003). *TOCS-30 Probe*. University of Alberta.

Hodge, M., & Daniels, J. (2007). *TOCS+ Intelligibility Measures*. University of Alberta.

Hodge, M., & Gotzke, C. L. (2014). Criterion-related validity of the Test of Children's

Speech sentence intelligibility measure for children with cerebral palsy and dysarthria. *International Journal of Speech-Language Pathology*, *16*(4), 417–426. https://doi.org/10.3109/17549507.2014.930174

Hodgins, H., & Harrison, G. L. (2021). Improving phonological awareness with Talking Tables in at-risk kindergarten readers. *Research in Developmental Disabilities*, *115*, 103996. https://doi.org/10.1016/j.ridd.2021.103996

Hodson, B. W. (2004). *Hodson Assessment of Phonological Patterns* (3rd ed.). Pro-Ed.

Hodson, B. W. (2010). *Evaluation & enhancing children's phonological systems*. PhonoComb Publishing.

Hodson, B. W. (2011). Enhancing phonological patterns of young children with highly unintelligible speech. *The ASHA Leader*, *16*(4), 16–19. https://doi.org/10.1044/leader.FTR2.16042011.16

Hodson, B. W., & Paden, E. P. (1981). Phonological processes which characterize unintelligible and intelligible speech in early childhood. *Journal of Speech and Hearing Disorders*, *46*(4), 369–373. https://doi.org/10.1044/jshd.4604.369

Hodson, B. W., & Paden, E. P. (1991). *A phonological approach to remediation: Targeting intelligible speech* (2nd ed.). Pro-Ed.

Hoemann, K., Xu, F., & Barrett, L. F. (2019). Emotion words, emotion concepts, and emotional development in children: A constructionist hypothesis. *Developmental Psychology*, *55*(9), 1830–1849. https://doi.org/10.1037/dev0000686

Hoffman, P. R., Schuckers, G. H., & Ratusnik, D. L. (1977). Contextual-coarticulatory inconsistency of /r/ misarticulation. *Journal of Speech and Hearing Research*, *20*(4), 631–643. https://doi.org/10.1044/jshr.2004.631

Hogikyan, N. D., & Sethuraman, G. (1999). Validation of an instrument to measure voice-related quality of life (V-RQOL). *Journal of Voice*, *13*(4), 557–569. https://doi.org/10.1016/S0892-1997(99)80010-1

Hoit, J. D., & Hixon, T. J. (1992). Age and laryngeal resistance during vowel production in women. *Journal of Speech and Hearing Research*, *35*, 309–313. https://doi.org/10.1044/jshr.3502.309

Hoit, J. D., Hixon, T. J., Watson, P. J., & Morgan, W. J. (1990). Speech breathing in children and adolescents. *Journal of Speech, Language, and Hearing Research*, *33*(1), 51–69. https://doi.org/10.1044/jshr.3301.51

Holbrook, S., & Israelsen, M. (2020). Speech prosody interventions for persons with autism spectrum disorders: A systematic review. *American Journal of Speech-Language Pathology*, *29*(4), 2189–2205. https://doi.org/10.1044/2020_AJSLP-19-00127

Holbrook, S., & Israelsen, M. (2020). Speech prosody interventions for persons with autism spectrum disorders: A systematic review. *American Journal of Speech-Language Pathology*, *29*(4), 2189–2205. https://doi.org/10.1044/2020_AJSLP-19-00127

Holm, A., Crosbie, S., & Dodd, B. (2007). Differentiating normal variability from inconsistency in children's speech: Normative data. *International Journal of Language & Communication Disorders*, *42*(4), 467–486. https://doi.org/10.1080/13682820600988967

Holm, A., Farrier, F., & Dodd, B. (2008). Phonological awareness, reading accuracy and spelling ability of children with inconsistent phonological disorder. *International Journal of Language & Communication Disorders*, *43*(3), 300–322. https://doi.org/10.1080/13682820701445032

Holm, A., van Reyk, O., Crosbie, S., De Bono, S., Morgan, A., & Dodd, B. (2022). Preschool children's consistency of word production. *Clinical Linguistics & Phonetics*, 119. https://doi.org/10.1080/02699206.2022.2041099

Holt, L., & Lotto, A. (2014). The alluring but misleading analogy between mirror neurons and the motor theory of speech. *Behavioral and Brain Sciences*, *37*(2), 204–205. https://doi.org/10.1017/S0140525X13002331

Homøe, P., Heidemann, C. H., Damoiseaux, R. A., Lailach, S., Lieu, J. E., Phillips, J. S., & Venekamp, R. P. (2020). Panel 5: Impact of otitis media on quality of life and development. *International Journal of Pediatric Otorhinolaryngology*, *130* (Suppl. 1), 109837. https://doi.org/10.1016/j.ijporl.2019.109837

Honikman, B. (1964). Articulatory settings. In D. Abercrombie, D. B. Fry, P. A. D. MacCarthy, N. C. Scott, & J. L. M. Trim (Eds.), *In Honour of Daniel Jones* (pp. 73–84). Longman.

Hoque, F., Akhter, S., & Mannan, M. (2021). Risk factors identification of speech and language delay in children in a tertiary level hospital: A pilot study. *World Journal of Advanced Research and Reviews*, *11*(01), 103–112.

https://doi.org/10.30574/wjarr.2021.11.1.0323

Hosseinabad, H. H., Washington, K. N., Boyce, S. E., Silbert, N., & Kummer, A. W. (2022). Assessment of intelligibility in children with velopharyngeal insufficiency: The relationship between Intelligibility in Context Scale and experimental measures. *Folia Phoniatrica et Logopaedica*, *74*(1), 17–28. https://doi.org/10.1159/000516537

Howard, S. (2004). Compensatory articulatory behaviours in adolescents with cleft palate: Comparing the perceptual and instrumental evidence. *Clinical Linguistics & Phonetics*, *18*(4-5), 313–340. https://doi.org/10.1080/02699200410001701314

Howell, J., & Dean, E. (1994). *Treating phonological disorders in children: Metaphon theory to practice*. Whurr.

Howson, P. J., & Monahan, P. J. (2019). Perceptual motivation for rhotics as a class. *Speech Communication*, *115*, 15–28. https://doi.org/10.1016/j.specom.2019.10.002

Howson, P. J., & Redford, M. A. (2021). The acquisition of articulatory timing for liquids: Evidence from child and adult speech. *Journal of Speech, Language, and Hearing Research*, *64*(3), 734–753. https://doi.org/10.1044/2020_JSLHR-20-00391

Huber, J. E., Chandrasekaran, B., & Wolstencroft, J. J. (2005). Changes to respiratory mechanisms during speech as a result of different cues to increase loudness. *Journal of Applied Physiology*, *98*(6), 2177–2184. https://doi.org/10.1152/japplphysiol.01239.2004

Huensch, A., & Tremblay, A. (2015). Effects of perceptual phonetic training on the perception and production of second language syllable structure. *Journal of Phonetics*, *52*, 105–120. https://doi.org/10.1016/j.wocn.2015.06.007

Hughes, C., & de Rosnay, M. (2006). The role of conversations in children's social, emotional and cognitive development—Introduction. *British Journal of Developmental Psychology*, *24*, 1–5.

Hulme, C., & Snowling, M. J. (2009). *Developmental disorders of language learning and cognition*. Wiley-Blackwell.

Hunter, E. J., Cantor-Cutiva, L. C., van Leer, E., van Mersbergen, M., Nanjundeswaran, C. D., Bottalico, P., . . . Whitling, S. (2020). Toward a consensus description of vocal effort, vocal load, vocal loading, and vocal fatigue. *Journal of Speech, Language, and Hearing Research*, 63(2), 509–532. https://doi.org/10.1044/2019_JSLHR-19-00057

Hunter, P. (2019). The riddle of speech. *EMBO Reports*, *20*:e47618. https://doi.org/10.15252/embr.201847618

Hurlburt, R. T., & Heavey, C. L. (2001). Telling what we know: Describing inner experience. *Trends in Cognitive Sciences*, *5*(9), 400–403. https://doi.org/10.1016/j.concog.2007.12.006

Hustad, K. C., & Borrie, S. A. (2021). Intelligibility impairment. In J. S. Damico, N. Müller, & M. J. Ball (Eds.) *The handbook of language and speech disorders* (pp. 81–94). Wiley/Blackwell.

Hustad, K. C., Mahr, T. J., Natzke, P., & Rathouz, P. J. (2021). Speech development between 30 and 119 months in typical children I: Intelligibility growth curves for single-word and multiword productions. *Journal of Speech, Language, and Hearing Research*, *64*(10), 3707–3719. https://doi.org/10.1044/2021_JSLHR-21-00142

Hyde, A. C., Moriarty, L., Morgan, A. G., Elsharkasi, L., & Deery, C. (2018). Speech and the dental interface. *Dental Update*, *45*(9), 795–803. https://doi.org/10.12968/denu.2018.45.9.795

Icht, M., & Ben-David, B. M. (2021). Evaluating rate and accuracy of real word vs. nonword diadochokinetic productions from childhood to early adulthood in Hebrew speakers. *Journal of Communication Disorders*, *92*, 106112. https://doi.org/10.1016/j.jcomdis.2021.106112

Inada, E., Saitoh, I., Kaihara, Y., & Yamasaki, Y. (2021). Factors related to mouth-breathing syndrome and the influence of an incompetent lip seal on facial soft tissue form in children. *Pediatric Dental Journal*, *31*(1), 1–10. https://doi.org/10.1016/j.pdj.2020.10.002

Ingram, D. (2002). The measurement of whole-word productions. *Journal of Child Language*, *29*, 713–733. https://doi.org/10.1017/S0305000902005275

International Cluttering Association (ICA). (n.d.). https://sites.google.com/view/icacluttering/home

Ireland, M., McLeod, S., Farquharson, K., & Crowe, K. (2020). Evaluating children in U.S.public schools with speech sound disorders: Considering federal and state laws, guidance, and research. *Topics in Language Disorders*, *40*(4), 326–340. https://doi.org/10.1097/TLD.0000000000000226

Irwin, R. B., West, J. F., & Trombetta, M. A. (1966). Effectiveness of speech therapy for second grade children with misarticulations—Predictive factors. *Exceptional Children*, *32*(7), 471–479. https://doi.org/10.1177/001440296603200705

Isel, F. (2021). Neuroplasticity of second language vocabulary acquisition: The role of linguistic experience in individual learning. *Language, Interaction and Acquisition*, *12*(1), 54–81. https://doi.org/10.1075/lia.20023.ise

Iskarous, K., & Pouplier, M. (2022). Advancements of phonetics in the 21st century: A critical appraisal of time and space in Articulatory Phonology. *Journal of Phonetics*, *95*, 101195. https://doi.org/10.1016/j.wocn.2022.101195

Iuzzini-Seigel, J. (2021). Procedural learning, grammar, and motor skills in children with childhood apraxia of speech, speech sound disorder, and typically developing speech. *Journal of Speech, Language, and Hearing Research*, *64*(4), 1081–1103. https://doi.org/10.1044/2020_JSLHR-20-00581

Iuzzuni-Seigel, J., Allison, K. M., & Stoeckel, R. (2022). A tool for differential diagnosis of childhood apraxia of speech and dysarthria in children: A tutorial. *Language, Speech, and Hearing Services in Schools*, *53*, 926–946. https://doi.org/10.1044/2022_LSHSS-21-00164

Iuzzini-Seigel, J., Hogan, T. P., & Green, J. R. (2017). Speech inconsistency in children with childhood apraxia of speech, language impairment, and speech delay: Depends on the stimuli. *Journal of Speech, Language, and Hearing Research*, *60*(5), 1194–1210. https://doi.org/10.1044/2016_JSLHR-S-15-0184

Iuzzini-Seigel, J., Moorer, L., & Tamplain, P. (2022). An investigation of developmental coordination disorder characteristics in children with childhood apraxia of speech. *Language, Speech, and Hearing Services in Schools*, *53*(4), 1006–1021. https://doi.org/10.1044/2022_LSHSS-21-00163

Iuzzini-Seigel, J., Hogan, T. P., Rong, P., & Green, J. R. (2015). Longitudinal development of speech motor control: Motor and linguistic factors. *Journal of Motor Learning and Development*, *3*(1), 53–68.

Iverson, J. M. (2021). Developmental variability and developmental cascades: Lessons from motor and language development in infancy. *Current directions in Psychological Science*, *30*(3), 228–235. https://doi.org/10.1177/0963721421993822

Izard, C. (2010). The many meaningsaAspects of emotion: Definitions, functions, activation, and regulation. *Emotion Review*, *2*(4). https://doi.org/10.1177/1754073910374661

Jack, R. E., Garrod, O. G., & Schyns, P. G. (2014). Dynamic facial expressions of emotion transmit an evolving hierarchy of signals over time. *Current Biology*, *24*(2), 187–192. https://doi.org/10.1016/j.cub.2013.11.064

Jackson, E., Leitao, S., Claessen, M., & Boyes, M. (2019). Fast mapping short and long words: Examining the influence of phonological short-term memory and receptive vocabulary in children with developmental language disorder. *Journal of Communication Disorders*, *79*, 11–23. https://doi.org/10.1016/j.jcomdis.2019.02.001

Jacobs, R., Serhal, C. & van Steenberghe, D. (1998). Oral stereognosis: a review of the literature. *Clinical Oral Investigations, 2*, 3–10. https://doi.org/10.1007/s007840050035

Jacobson, B. H., Johnson, A., Grywalski, C., Silbergleit, A., Jacobson, G., Benninger, M. S., & Newman, C. W. (1997). The voice handicap index (VHI) development and validation. *American Journal of Speech-Language Pathology*, *6*(3), 66–70. https://doi.org/10.1044/1058-0360.0603.66

Jacox, L. A., Turvey, T. A., Mielke, J., Zajac, D. A., & Blakey, G. H. (2022). Impacts of jaw disproportions on speech of dentofacial disharmony patients. *Journal of Oral and Maxillofacial Surgery*, *80*(9), S26. https://doi.org/10.1016/j.joms.2022.07.039

Jaeger, J. (1992). 'Not by the chair of my hinny hin hin': Some general properties of slips of the tongue in young children. *Journal of Child Language*, *199*(2), 335–366. https://doi.org/10.1017/S0305000900011442

Jaeger, J. (2004). *Kids' slips: What young children's slips of the tongue reveal about language development*. Psychology Press. https://doi.org/10.4324/9781410611550

Jafari, Z., Malayeri, S., & Rostami, R. (2015). Subcortical encoding of speech cues in children with attention deficit hyperactivity disorder. *Clinical Neurophysiology*, *126*(2), 325–332. https://doi.org/10.1016/j.clinph.2014.06.007

Jain, C., Priya, M. B., & Joshi, K. (2020). Relationship between temporal processing and phonological awareness in children with speech sound disorders. *Clinical Linguistics & Phonetics, 34*(6), 566–575. https://doi.org/10.1080/02699206.2019.1671902

Jakobson, R. (1941). *Kindersprache, aphasie, und allgemeine lautgesetze*. Almqvist & Wiksell.

Jakobson, R. (1968). *Child language: Aphasia and phonological universals* (No. 72). Walter de Gruyter.

Jakobson, R., Fant, G. M., & Halle, M. (1963). *Preliminaties to speech analysis: The distinctive features and their correlates.* MIT Press.

James, D., van Doorn, J., & McLeod, S. (2001). Vowel production in mono-, di- and polysyllabic words in children 3:0 to 7:11 years. In L. Wilson & S. Hewat (Eds.), *Proceedings of the speech pathology conference* (pp. 127–136). Speech Pathology Australia.

Jamoulle, M. (2015). Quaternary prevention, an answer of family doctors to overmedicalization. *International Journal of Health Policy and Management*, *4*(2), 61–64. https://doi.org/10.15171/ijhpm.2015.24

Jasmin, K., Dick, F., & Tierney, A. T. (2020). The multidimensional battery of prosody perception (MBOPP). *Wellcome Open Research, 5*. https://doi.org/10.12688/wellcomeopenres.15607.2

Jaw, T. S., Sheu, R. S., Liu, G. C., & Lin, W. C. (1999). Development of adenoids: A study by measurement with MR images. *The Kaohsiung Journal of Medical Sciences, 15*(1), 12–18.

Jeans, W. D., Fernando, D. C. J., Maw, A. R., & Leighton, B. C. (1981). A longitudinal study of the growth of the nasopharynx and its contents in normal children. *The British Journal of Radiology*, *54*(638), 117–121.

Jelm, J. (2001). *Verbal dyspraxia profile.* Janelle Publications.

Jensen, J. K., & Neff, D. L. (1993). Development of basic auditory discrimination in preschool children. *Psychological Science*, *4*(2), 104–107. https://doi.org/10.1111/j.1467-9280.1993.tb00469.x

Jesney, K. (2004). The use of global foreign accent rating in studies of L2 acquisition. *Calgary, AB: University of Calgary Language Research Centre Reports*, 1–44.

Jesus, L. M., Martinez, J., Santos, J., Hall, A., & Joffe, V. (2019). Comparing traditional and tablet-based intervention for children with speech sound disorders: A randomized controlled trial. *Journal of Speech, Language, and Hearing Research*, *62*(11), 4045–4061. https://doi.org/10.1044/2019_JSLHR-S-18-0301

Jing, L., & Grigos, M. I. (2022). Speech-language pathologists' ratings of speech accuracy in children with speech sound disorders. *American Journal of Speech-language Pathology*, *31*(1), 419–430. https://doi.org/10.1044/2021_AJSLP-20-00381

Jobson, K. R., Hoffman, L. J., Metoki, A., Popal, H., Dick, A. S., Reilly, J., & Olson, I. R. (2022). Language and the cerebellum: Structural connectivity to the eloquent brain. *Neurobiology of Language*. https//doi.org/10.1162/nol_a_00085

Joffe, V., & Pring, T., 2008, Children with phonological problems: A survey of clinical practice. *International Journal of Language and Communication Disorders*, *43*, 154–164.

Johannisson, T. B., Lohmander, A., & Persson, C. (2014). Assessing intelligibility by single words, sentences and spontaneous speech: A methodological study of the speech production of 10-year-olds. *Logopedics Phoniatrics Vocology*, *39*(4), 159–168. https://doi.org/10.3109/14015439.2013.820487

John, A. (2011) Therapy outcome measures: Where are we now? *International Journal of Speech-Language Pathology*, *13*(1), 36–42. https://doi.org/10.3109/17549507.2010.497562

Johnson, K. N., Walden, T. A., Conture. E. G., & Karrass, J. (2010). Spontaneous regulation of emotions in preschool children who stutter: Preliminary findings. *Journal of Speech, Language, and Hearing Research*, *53*(6), 1478–1495. https://doi.org/10.1044/1092–4388(2010/08–0150).

Johnson-Root, B. A. (2015). *Oral-facial examination for speech-language pathologists.* Plural Publishing.

Jones, H. E. (1955). The vital capacity of children. *Archives of Disease in Childhood, 30*(153), 445–448. https://doi.org/10.1136/adc.30.153.445

Jones, H. N., Crisp, K. D., Kuchibhatla, M., Mahler, L., Risoli, T., Jr., Jones, C. W., & Kishnani, P. (2019). Auditory-perceptual speech features in children with Down syndrome. *American Journal on Intellectual and Developmental Disabilities*, *124*(4), 324–338. https://doi.org/10.1352/1944-7558-124.4.324

Jones, M., Castile, R., Davis, S., Kisling, J., Filbrun, D., Flucke, R., & Tepper, R. S. (2000). Forced expiratory flows and volumes in infants: Normative data and lung growth. *American Journal of Respiratory and Critical Care Medicine*, *161*(2), 353–359. https://doi.org/10.1164/ajrccm.161.2.9903026

Jongman, A., Wayland, R., & Wong, S. (2000). Acoustic characteristics of English fricatives. *The Journal of the Acoustical Society of America*, *108*, 1252–1263. https://doi.org/10.1121/1.1288413

Joshi, S., & Kotecha, S. (2007). Lung growth and development. *Early Human Development*, *83*(12), 789–794. https://doi.org/10.1016/j.earlhumdev.2007.09.007

Juliano, M. L., Machado, M. A. C., Carvalho, L. B. C. D., Prado, L. B. F. D., & Prado, G. F. D. (2009). Mouth breathing children have cephalometric patterns similar to those of adult patients with obstructive sleep apnea syndrome. *Arquivos de neuro-psiquiatria*, *67*(3B), 860–865. https://doi.org/10.1590/S0004-282X2009000500015

Junqueira, P., Marchesan, I. Q., de Oliveira, L. R., Ciccone, E., Haddad, L., & Rizzo, M. C. (2010). Speech-language pathology findings in patients with mouth breathing: multidisciplinary diagnosis according to etiology. *International Journal of Orofacial Myology*, *36*.

Juslin, P. N., & Laukka, P. (2003). Communication of emotions in vocal expression and music performance: Different channels, same code? *Psychological Bulletin*, *129*(5), 770–814.

Kabakoff, H., Harel, D., Tiede, M., Whalen, D. H., & McAllister, T. (2021). Extending ultrasound tongue shape complexity measures to speech development and disorders. *Journal of Speech, Language, and Hearing Research*, *64*(7), 2557–2574.

Kabakoff, H., Gritsyk, O., Harel, D., Tiede, M., Preston, J. L., Whalen, D. H., & McAllister, T. (2022). Characterizing sensorimotor profiles in children with residual speech sound disorder: A pilot study. *Journal of Communication Disorders*, *99*, 106230. https://doi.org/10.1016/j.jcomdis.2022.106230

Kaczorowska, N., Kaczorowski, K., Laskowska, J., & Mikulewicz, M. (2019). Down syndrome as a cause of abnormalities in the craniofacial region: A systematic literature review. *Advances in Clinical and Experimental Medicine*, *28*(11), 1587–1592. https://doi.org/10.17219/acem/112785

Kafri, M., & Atun-Einy, O. (2019). From motor learning theory to practice: A scoping review of conceptual frameworks for applying knowledge in motor learning to physical therapist practice. *Physical Therapy*, *99*(12), 1628–1643. https://doi.org/10.1093/ptj/pzz118

Kaipa, R., & Peterson, A. M. (2016). A systematic review of treatment intensity in speech disorders. *International Journal of Speech-Language Pathology*, *18*(6), 507–520. https://doi.org/10.3109/17549507.2015.1126640

Kalathottukaren, R. T., Purdy, S. C., & Ballard, E. (2015). Behavioral measures to evaluate prosodic skills: A review of assessment tools for children and adults. *Issues in Communication Science and Disorders*, *42*, 138–154. https://pubs.asha.org 70.226.170.179

Kamhi, A. G. (2006). Treatment decisions for children with speech sound disorders. *Language, Speech, and Hearing Services in Schools*, *37*(4), 271–279. https://doi.org/10.1044/0161-1461(2006/031)

Kamhi, A. (2008). A meme's-eye view of nonspeech oral motor exercises. *Seminars in Speech and Language*, *29*(4), 331–339. https://doi.org/10.1055/s-0028-1103397

Kang, C., & Drayna, D. (2012). A role for inherited metabolic deficits in persistent developmental stuttering. *Molecular Genetics and Metabolism*, *107*(3), 276–280. https://doi.org/10.1016/j.ymgme.2012.07.020

Kanold, P. O. (2022). Listening to mom: How the early auditory experience sculpts the auditory cortex of the brain. *Acoustics Today*, *18*(1), 32–40. https://doi.org/org/10.1121/AT.2022.181.132.

Kara, M., Calis, M., Kara, I., Incebay, O., Kayikci, M. E. K., Gunaydin, R. O., & Ozgur, F. (2020). Does early cleft palate repair make difference? Comparative evaluation of the speech outcomes using objective parameters. *Journal of Cranio-Maxillofacial Surgery*, *48*(11), 1057–1065. https://doi.org/10.1016/j.jcms.2020.09.003

Karlsson, H. B., Shriberg, L. D., Flipsen Jr, P. F., & McSweeny, J. L. (2002). Acoustic phenotypes for speech-genetics studies: Toward an acoustic marker for residual /s/ distortions. *Clinical Linguistics & Phonetics*, *16*(6), 403–424. https://doi.org/10.1080/02699200210128954

Kaspi, A., Hildebrand, M. S., Jackson, V. E., Braden, R., van Reyk, O., Howell, T., . . . Morgan, A. T. (2022). Genetic aetiologies for childhood speech disorder: Novel pathways co-expressed during brain development. *Molecular Psychiatry*. https://doi.org/10.1038/s41380-022-01764-8

Katz, R. V., Dearing, B. A., Ryan, J. M., Ryan, L. K., Zubi, M. K., & Sokhal, G. K. (2020). Development of a tongue-tie case definition in newborns using a Delphi survey: The NYU-Tongue-Tie Case Definition. *Oral Surgery, Oral Medicine, Oral Pathology and Oral Radiology, 129*(1), 21–26. https://doi.org/10.1016/j.oooo.2019.01.012

Kaufman, N. (1995). *Kaufman Speech Praxis Test for Children*. Wayne State University Press.

Kawasaki-Knight, L., Wolgemuth, K. S., & Becerra, B. J. (2021). Integrated approach on the acquisition of phonological targets in 4-to-6-year-old children. *Journal of Child Language Acquisition and Development-JCLAD*, 249–283.

Kearney, E., & Guenther, F. H. (2019). Articulating: The neural mechanisms of speech production. *Language, Cognition and Neuroscience, 34*(9), 1214–1229. https://doi.org/10.1080/23273798.2019.1589541

Kearney, E., Granata, F., Yunusova, Y., Van Lieshout, P., Hayden, D., & Namasivayam, A. (2015). Outcome measures in developmental speech sound disorders with a motor basis. *Current Developmental Disorders Reports, 2*(3), 253–272. https://doi.org/10.1007/s40474-015-0058-2

Keating, D., Turrell, G., & Ozanne, A. (2001). Childhood speech disorders: Reported prevalence, comorbidity and socioeconomic profile. *Journal of Paediatrics and Child Health, 37*(5), 431–436. https://doi.org/10.1046/j.1440-1754.2001.00697.x

Keating, P. (2003). Phonetic encoding of prosodic structure. In S. Palethorpe & M. Tabain (Eds.), *Proceedings of the Sixth International Seminar on Speech Production* (pp. 119–124). Macquarie Centre for Cognitive Science.

Kehoe, M., & Stoel-Gammon, C. (1997). The acquisition of prosodic structure: An investigation of current accounts of children's prosodic development. *Language*, 113–144. https://doi.org/10.2307/416597

Kelchner, L. N., Brehm, S. B., de Alarcon, A., & Weinrich, B. (2012). Update on pediatric voice and airway disorders: Assessment and care. *Current Opinion in Otolaryngology & Head and Neck Surgery, 20*(3), 160–164. https://doi.org/10.1097/MOO.0b013e3283530ecb

Keller, E. (2004, September). The analysis of voice quality in speech processing. In *International School on Neural Networks*, Initiated by IIASS and EMFCSC (pp. 54–73). Springer.

Kelly, M. P., Vorperian, H. K., Wang, Y., Tillman, K. K., Werner, H. M., Chung, M. K. & Gentry, L. R. (2017). Characterizing mandibular growth using three-dimensional imaging techniques and anatomic landmarks. *Archives of Oral Biology, 77*(1), 27–38. https://doi.org/10.1016/j.archoralbio.2017.01.018

Kelman, E., & Nicholas, A. (2008). *Practical intervention for early childhood* stammering: *Palin PCI Approach*. Speechmark.

Kelso, J. A., & Tuller, B. (1984). Converging evidence in support of common dynamical principles for speech and movement coordination. *American Journal of Physiology-Regulatory, Integrative and Comparative Physiology, 246*(6), R928–R935. https://doi.org/10.1152/ajpregu.1984.246.6.R928

Keltner, D., Sauter, D., Tracy, J., & Cowen, A. (2019). Emotional expression: Advances in basic emotion theory. *Journal of Nonverbal Behavior, 43*(2), 133–160. https://doi.org/10.1007/s10919-019-00293-3

Kempster, G., Gerratt, B., Abbott, K., Barkmeier-Kraemer, J., & Hillman, R. (2009). Consensus auditory-perceptual evaluation of voice: Development of a standardized clinical protocol. *American Journal of Speech-Language Pathology, 18*(2), 124–132. https://doi.org/10.1044/1058-0360(2008/08-0017)

Kent, R. D. (1982). Contextual facilitation of correct sound production. *Language, Speech, and Hearing Services in Schools, 13*(2), 66–76. https://doi.org/10.1044/0161-1461.1302.66

Kent, R. D. (1992). The biology of phonological development. In C. A. Ferguson, L. Menn & C. Stoel-Gammon (Eds.), *Phonological development: Models, research, implications* (pp. 65–90). York Press.

Kent, R. D. (2000). Research on speech motor control and its disorders: A review and prospective. *Journal of Communication Disorders, 33*, 391–428. https://doi.org/10.1016/S0021–9924(00)00023–X

Kent, R. D. (2004). The uniqueness of speech among motor systems. *Clinical linguistics & phonetics, 18(*6-8), 495–505. https://doi.org/10.1080/02699200410001703600

Kent, R. D. (2015). Nonspeech oral movements and oral motor disorders: A narrative review.

American Journal of Speech-Language Pathology, 24, 763–789. https://doi.org/10.1044/2015_AJSLP14-0179

Kent, R. D. (2021). Developmental functional modules in infant vocalizations. *Journal of Speech, Language, and Hearing Research, 64*(5), 1581–1604. https://doi.org/10.1044/2021_JSLHR-20-00703

Kent, R. D. (2022). The maturational gradient of infant vocalizations: Developmental stages and functional modules. *Infant Behavior and Development, 66*, 101682. https://doi.org/10.1016/j.infbeh.2021.101682

Kent, R. D., & Moll, K. L. (1972). Cinefluorographic analyses of selected lingual consonants. *Journal of Speech and Hearing Research, 15*(3), 453–473. https://doi.org/10.1044/jshr.1503.453

Kent, R. D., & Netsell, R. (1978). Articulatory abnormalities in athetoid cerebral palsy. *Journal of Speech and Hearing Disorders, 43*, 353–373. https://doi.org/10.1044/jshd.4303.353

Kent, R. D., & Rountrey, C. (2020). What acoustic studies tell us about vowels in developing and disordered speech. *American Journal of Speech-Language Pathology, 29*(3), 1749–1778. https://doi.org/10.1044/2020_AJSLP-19-00178

Kent, R. D., & Vorperian, H. K. (1995). Anatomic development of the craniofacial-oral-laryngeal systems: A review. *Journal of Medical Speech-Language Pathology, 3*, 145–190.

Kent, R. D., & Vorperian, H. K. (2013). Speech impairments in Down syndrome: A review. *Journal of Speech, Language, and Hearing Research, 56*, 1044–1092. https://doi.org/10.1044/1092-4388(2012/12-0148)

Kent, R. D., & Vorperian. H. K. (2018). Static measurements of vowel formant frequencies and bandwidths: A review. *Journal of Communication Disorders, 74*, 74–97. https://doi.org/10.1016/j.jcomdis.2018.05.004

Kent, R. D., Eichhorn, J. T., & Vorperian, H. K. (2021). Acoustic parameters of voice in typically developing children ages 4–19 years. *International Journal of Pediatric Otorhinolaryngology, 142*, 110614. https://doi.org/10.1016/j.ijporl.2021.110614

Kent, R. D., Kent, J. F., & Rosenbek, J. C. (1987). Maximum performance tests of speech production. *Journal of Speech and Hearing Disorders, 52*, 367–387. https://doi.org/10.1044/jshd.5204.367

Kent, R. D., Kim, Y., & Chen, L. M. (2022). Oral and laryngeal diadochokinesis across the life span: A scoping review of methods, reference data, and clinical applications. *Journal of Speech, Language, and Hearing Research, 65*(2), 574–623. https://doi.org/10.1044/2021_JSLHR-21-00396

Kent, R. D., Martin, R. E. & Suffit, R. L. (1990) Oral sensation: A review and clinical prospective. In H. Winitz (Ed.) *Human communication and its disorders: A review* (pp. 135–191). Ablex Press.

Kent, R. D., Miolo, G., & Bloedel, S. (1994). The intelligibility of children's speech: A review of evaluation procedures. *American Journal of Speech-Language Pathology, 3*(2), 81–95. https://doi.org/10.1044/1058-0360.0302.81

Kent, R. D., Wiley, T. L., & Strennen, M. L. (1979). Consonant discrimination as a function of presentation level. *Audiology, 18*(3), 212–224. https://doi.org/10.3109/00206097909081524

Kent, R. D., Eichhorn, J., Wilson, E. M., Suk, Y., Bolt, D. M., & Vorperian, H. K. (2021). Auditory-perceptual features of speech in children and adults with Down syndrome: A speech profile analysis. *Journal of Speech, Language, and Hearing Research, 64*(4), 1157–1175. https://doi.org/10.1044/2021_JSLHR-20-00617

Kester, E. S. (2014). *Difference or disorder: Understanding speech and language patterns in culturally and linguistically diverse students.* Bilinguistics.

Khan, L. M., & Lewis, N. (2002). *Khan-Lewis Phonological Analysis* (2nd ed.). AGS.

Kharbanda, O. P., Sidhu, S. S., Sundaram, K., & Shukla, D. K. (2003). Oral habits in school going children of Delhi: A prevalence study. *Journal of the Indian Society of Pedodontics and Preventive Dentistry, 21*(3), 120–124.

Khavarghazalani, B., Hosseini Dastgerdi, Z., Gohari, N., & Khakzand, S. (2022). Auditory temporal processing in children with history of recurrent otitis media with effusion. *Hearing, Balance, and Communication, 20*(1), 46–51. https://doi.org/10.1080/21695717.2022.2029091

Kidd, E., Bidgood, A., Donnelly, S., Durrant, S., Peter, M. S., & Rowland, C. F. (2020). Individual differences in first language acquisition and their theoretical implications. *Trends in Language Acquisition Research, 27*, 189–219.

Kidd, G. R., Watson, C. S., & Gygi, B. (2007). Individual differences in auditory abilities. *The*

Journal of the Acoustical Society of America, 122(1), 418–435.

Kier, W. M., & Smith, K. K. (1985). Tongues, tentacles and trunks: The biomechanics of movement in muscular-hydrostats. *Zoological Journal of the Linnean Society, 83*(4), 307–324. https://doi.org/10.1111/j.1096-3642.1985.tb01178.x

Kilner, J. M., & Lemon, R. N. (2013). What we know currently about mirror neurons. *Current Biology, 2*(23), R1057–R1062. https://doi.org/10.1016/j.cub.2013.10.051.

Klick, S. L. (1985). Adapted cuing technique for use in treatment of dyspraxia. *Language, Speech, and Hearing Services in Schools*, 16(4), 256–259. https://doi.org/10.1044/0161-1461.1604.256

Kim, J., Toutios, A., Lee, S., & Narayanan, S. S. (2015). A kinematic study of critical and noncritical articulators in emotional speech production. *The Journal of the Acoustical Society of America, 137*(3), 1411–1429. http://doi.org/10.1121/1.4908284

Kim, W. S., Lee, R., & Lee, J. W. (2021). Literature analysis on PROMPT treatment (1984–2020). *Journal of Digital Convergence, 19*(2), 447–456. https://doi.org/10.14400/JDC.2021.19.2.447

Kim, Y., & Thompson, A. (2022). An acoustic-phonetic approach to effects of face masks on speech intelligibility. *Journal of Speech, Language, and Hearing Research*, 1–11. https://doi.org/10.1044/2022_JSLHR-22-00245

King, A. M., Hengst, J. A., & DeThorne, L. S. (2013). Severe speech sound disorders: An integrated multimodal intervention. *Language, Speech, and Hearing Services in Schools, 44*(2), 195–210. https://doi.org/10.1044/0161-1461(2012/12-0023)

King, E., Remington, M., & Berger, H. (2022). Family perspectives on gaps in health care for people with Down syndrome. *American Journal of Medical Genetics Part A, 188*(4), 1160–1169. https://doi.org/10.1002/ajmg.a.62635

Kisling, L. A., & Das, J. M. (2022). Prevention strategies. *StatPearls* [Internet]. StatPearls Publishing. https://www.ncbi.nlm.nih.gov/books/NBK537222/

Kitago, T. & Krakauer, J. W. (2013). Motor learning principles for neurorehabilitation. In M. P. Barnes & D. C. Good (Eds.), *Handbook of clinical neurology* (Vol. 110, 3rd series, pp. 93–103). Elsevier.

Kitzing, P., Maier, A., & Åhlander, V. L. (2009). Automatic speech recognition (ASR) and its use as a tool for assessment or therapy of voice, speech, and language disorders. *Logopedics Phoniatrics Vocology, 34*(2), 91–96. https://doi.org/10.1080/14015430802657216

Kjellmer, L., Raud Westberg, L., & Lohmander, A. (2021). Treatment of active nasal fricatives substituting /s/ in young children with normal palatal function using motor-based intervention. *International Journal of Speech-Language Pathology, 23*(6), 593–603. https://doi.org/10.1080/17549507.2021.1891285

Klatte, I. S., Lyons, R., Davies, K., Harding, S., Marshall, J., McKean, C., & Roulstone, S. (2020). Collaboration between parents and SLTs produces optimal outcomes for children attending speech and language therapy: Gathering the evidence. *International Journal of Language & Communication Disorders, 55*(4), 618–628. https://doi.org/10.1111/1460-6984.12538

Klein, E. S. (1996). *Clinical phonology*. Singular Publishing.

Kleynen, M., Braun, S. M., Bleijlevens, M. H., Lexis, M. A., Rasquin, S. M., Halfens, J., . . . Masters, R. S. (2014). Using a Delphi technique to seek consensus regarding definitions, descriptions and classification of terms related to implicit and explicit forms of motor learning. *PLoS ONE, 9*(6), e100227. https://doi.org/10.1371/journal.pone.0100227

Klopfenstein, M. (2009). Interaction between prosody and intelligibility. *International Journal of Speech-Language Pathology, 11*(4), 326–331. https://doi.org/10.1080/17549500903003094

Klopfenstein, M., Bernard, K. & Heyman, C. (2019). The study of speech naturalness in communication disorders: A systematic review of the literature, *Clinical Linguistics & Phonetics*. https://doi.org/10.1080/02699206.2019.1652692

Knight, R. A., Bandali , C., Woodhead, C., & Vansadia, P. (2018). Clinicians' views of the training, use and maintenance of phonetic transcription in speech and language therapy. *International Journal of Language & Communication Disorders, 53*(4), 776–787.

Knoop-van Campen, C. A., Segers, E., & Verhoeven, L. (2018). How phonological awareness mediates the relation between working memory and word reading efficiency in children with dyslexia. *Dyslexia, 24*(2), 156–169. https://doi.org/10.1002/dys.1583

Koegel, L. K., Koegel, R. L., & Ingham, J. C. (1986). Programming rapid generalization of correct articulation through self-monitoring procedures. *Journal of Speech and Hearing Disorders, 51*(1), 24–32. https://doi.org/10.1044/jshd.5101.24

Koegel, R. L., Koegel, L. K., Ingham, J. C., & Van Voy, K. (1988). Within clinic versus outside-of-clinic self-monitoring of articulation to promote generalization. *Journal of Speech and Hearing Disorders, 53*(4), 392–399. https://jshd.pubs.asha.org/article.aspx?articleid=1775200

Koenig, L. L., Lucero, J. C., & Perlman, E. (2008). Speech production variability in fricatives of children and adults: Results of functional data analysis. *The Journal of the Acoustical Society of America, 124*(5), 3158–3170. https://doi.org/10.1121/1.2981639

Kohler, K. J. (1966). Is the syllable a phonological universal? *Journal of Linguistics, 2*, 207–208.

Kollara, L., Perry, J. L., & Hudson, S. (2016). Racial variations in velopharyngeal and craniometrics morphology in children: An imaging study. *Journal of Speech, Language, and Hearing Research, 59*, 27–38. https://doi.org/10.1044/2015_JSLHR-S-14-0236

Kondraciuk, A., Manias, S., Misiuk, E., Kraszewska, A., Kosztyła-Hojna, B., Szczepański, M., & Cybulski, M. (2014). Impact of the orofacial area reflexes on infant's speech development. *Progress in Health Sciences, 4*(1), 188–194.

Kooi-van Es, M., Erasmus, C. E., de Swart, B. J., Voet, N., van der Wees, P. J., de Groot, I. J., & Van den Engel-Hoek, L. (2020). Dysphagia and dysarthria in children with neuromuscular diseases, a prevalence study. *Journal of Neuromuscular Diseases, 7*(3), 287–295. https://doi.org/10.3233/JND-190436

Kools, J. A., & Tweedie, D. (1975). Development of praxis in children. *Perceptual and Motor Skills, 40*(1), 11–19.

Koopmans-van Beinum, F. J., & van der Stelt, J. M. (1986). Early stages in the development of speech movements. In B. Lindblom & R. Zetterström (Eds.), *Precursors of early speech* (pp. 37–50). Palgrave Macmillan.

Kopera, H. C., & Grigos, M. I. (2020). Lexical stress in childhood apraxia of speech: Acoustic and kinematic findings. *International Journal of Speech-Language Pathology, 22*(1), 12–23. https://doi.org/10.1080/17549507.2019.1568571

Korkalainen, J., McCabe, P., Smidt, A., & Morgan, C. (2023). Motor speech interventions for children with cerebral palsy: A systematic review. *Journal of Speech, Language, and Hearing Research, 66*(1), 110–125. https://doi.org/10.1044/2022_JSLHR-22-00375

Kotlow, L. A. (2013). Diagnosing and understanding the maxillary lip-tie (superior labial, the maxillary labial frenum) as it relates to breastfeeding. *Journal of Human Lactation, 29*, 458–464.

Kover, S. T, & Abbeduto, L. (2010). Expressive language in male adolescents with fragile X syndrome with and without comorbid autism. *Journal of Intellectual Disabilities Research, 54*(3), 246–265. https://doi.org/10.1111/j.1365-2788. 2010.01255.x

Kowal, S., O'Connell, D., & Sabin, E. (1975). Development of temporal patterning and vocal hesitations in spontaneous narratives. *Journal of Psycholinguistic Research, 4*, 195–207. https://doi.org/10.1007/BF01066926

Kozhevnikov, V. A. & Chistovich, L.A. (1965). *Rech: Artikulyatsiya i Vospriyatiye* (Moscow Leningrad, 1965). Trans. *Speech: Articulation and perception*. Joint Publication Research Service, No. 30, 543.

Krakauer, J. W., Hadjiosif, A. M., Xu, J., Wong, A. L., & Haith, A. M. (2019). Motor learning. *Comprehensive Physiology, 9*(2), 613–663. https://doi.org/10.1002/cphy.c170043

Kral, A., & O'Donoghue, G. M. (2010). Profound deafness in childhood. *New England Journal of Medicine, 363*(15), 1438–1450. https://doi.org/10.1056/NEJMra0911225.

Kraus, N., & Nicol, T. (2014). The cognitive auditory system: The role of learning in shaping the biology of the auditory system. In A. Popper & R. Fay, R. (Eds.), *Perspectives on auditory research. Springer handbook of auditory research* (Vol. 50, pp. 299–319). Springer. https://doi.org/10.1007/978-1-4614-9102-6_17

Kreiman, J., Gerratt, B. R., Kempster, G. B., Erman, A., & Berke, G. S. (1993). Perceptual evaluation of voice quality: Review, tutorial, and a framework for future research. *Journal of Speech, Language, and Hearing Research, 36*(1), 21–40. https://doi.org/10.1044/jshr.3601.21

Krimm, H., & Lund, E. (2021). Efficacy of online learning modules for teaching dialogic reading strategies and phonemic awareness. *Language, Speech, and Hearing Services in Schools, 52*(4), 1020–1030. https://doi.org/10.1044/2021_LSHSS-21-00011

Kronfeld-Duenias, V., Amir, O., Ezrati-Vinacour, R., Civier, O., & Ben-Shachar, M. (2016). Dorsal and ventral language pathways in persistent developmental stuttering. *Cortex, 81*, 79–92. https://doi.org/10.1016/j.cortex.2016.04.001

Kronrod, Y., Coppess, E., & Feldman, N. H. (2016). A unified account of categorical effects in phonetic perception. *Psychonomic Bulletin Review, 23*, 1681–1712. https://doi.org/10.3758/s13423-016-1049-y

Krustev, M. B., Krustev, B. P., & Mileva, S. A. (2000). Neonatal muscle hypotonia–an early manifestation of cerebral palsy. *Folia Medica, 42*(3), 37–40.

Kruyt, J., & Beňuš, Š. (2021). Prosodic entrainment in individuals with autism spectrum disorder. *Topics in Linguistics, 22*(2), 47–61. https://doi.org/10.2478/topling-2021-0010

Kuberski, S. R., & Gafos, A. I. (2021). Fitts' law in tongue movements of repetitive speech. *Phonetica, 78*(1), 3–27. https://doi.org/10.1159/000501644

Kuhl, P. K., & Meltzoff, A. N. (1996). Infant vocalizations in response to speech: Vocal imitation and developmental change. *The Journal of the Acoustical Society of America, 100*(4), 2425–2438. https://doi.org/10.1121/1.417951

Kuhl, P. K., Conboy, B. T., Padden, D., Nelson, T., & Pruitt, J. (2005). Early speech perception and later language development: Implications for the" critical period." *Language Learning and Development, 1*(3–4), 237–264. https://doi.org/10.1080/15475441.2005.9671948

Kuhl, P., Williams, K., Lacerda, F., Stevens, K., & Lindblom, B. (1992). Linguistic experience alters phonetic perception in infants by 6 months of age. *Science, 255*, 606–608. https://doi.org/10.1126/science.1736364

Kuhl, P. K., Conboy, B. T., Coffey-Corina, S., Padden, D., Rivera-Gaxiola, M., & Nelson, T. (2008). Phonetic learning as a pathway to language: New data and Native Language Magnet theory expanded (NLM-e). *Philosophical Transactions of the Royal Society B: Biological Sciences, 363*, 979–1000. https://doi.org/10.1098/rstb.2007.2154

Kukwa, W., Guilleminault, C., Tomaszewska, M., Kukwa, A., Krzeski, A., & Migacz, E. (2018). Prevalence of upper respiratory tract infections in habitually snoring and mouth breathing children. *International Journal of Pediatric Otorhinolaryngology, 107*, 37–41. https://doi.org/10.1016/j.ijporl.2018.01.022

Kumar A, Zubair M, & Gulraiz A. (2022, September 26) An assessment of risk factors of delayed speech and language in children: A cross-sectional study. *Cureus 14*(9), e29623. https://doi.org/10.7759/cureus.29623

Kumin, L. (1994). Intelligibility of speech in children with Down syndrome in natural settings: Parents' perspective. *Perceptual and Motor Skills, 78*, 307–313. https://doi.org/10.2466/pms.1994.78.1.307

Kumin, L. (2006). Speech intelligibility and childhood verbal apraxia in children with Down syndrome. *Down Syndrome Research and Practice, 10*(1), 10–22. https://doi.org/10.3104/reports.301

Kumin, L. B., Saltysiak, E. B., Bell, K., Forget, K., Goodman, M. S., Goytisolo, M., . . . Thomas, S. (1984). Relationships of oral stereognostic ability to age and sex of children. *Perceptual and Motor Skills, 59*(1), 123–126.

Kummer, A. W. (2009). Evaluation of speech and resonance for children with craniofacial anomalies. *Facial Plastic Surgery Clinics of North America, 24*, 445–451.

Kwiatkowski, J., & Shriberg, L. D. (1992). Intelligibility assessment in developmental phonological disorders: Accuracy of caregiver gloss. *Journal of Speech, Language, and Hearing Research, 35*(5), 1095–1104. https://doi.org/10.1044/jshr.3505.1095

Kwok, E. Y., Rosenbaum, P., & Cunningham, B. J. (2022). Speech-language pathologists' treatment goals for preschool language disorders: An ICF analysis. *International Journal of Speech-Language Pathology*, 1–8. https://doi.org/10.1080/17549507.2022.2142665

Kwok, E. Y., Moodie, S. T., Cunningham, B. J., & Cardy, J. O. (2022). Barriers and facilitators to implementation of a preschool outcome measure: An interview study with speech-language pathologists. *Journal of Communication Disorders, 95*, 106166. https://doi.org/10.1016/j.jcomdis.2021.106166

Laakso, M. (2006). Kaksivuotiaiden lasten oman puheen korjaukset keskustelussa [Self-repair of speech by two-year-old children in conversation]. *Puhe ja Kieli, 26*, 123–136.

Labov, W., Ash, S., & Boberg, C. (2006). *The atlas of North American English*. Mouton de Gruyter.

Ladányi, E., Persici, V., Fiveash, A., Tillmann, B., & Gordon, R. L. (2020). Is atypical rhythm a risk factor for developmental speech and language disorders? *Wiley Interdisciplinary Reviews: Cognitive Science*, *11*(5), e1528. https://doi.org/10.1002/wcs.1528

Lagan, N., Huggard, D., Mc Grane, F., Leahy, T. R., Franklin, O., Roche, E., . . . Molloy, E. J. (2020). Multiorgan involvement and management in children with Down syndrome. *Acta Paediatrica*, *109*(6), 1096–1111. https://doi.org/10.1111/apa.15153

Lagasse, B. (2012). Evaluation of melodic intonation therapy for developmental apraxia of speech. *Music Therapy Perspectives*, *30*(1), 49–55. https://doi.org/10.1093/mtp/30.1.49

Lagerberg, T. B., Anrep-Nordin, E., Emanuelsson, H., & Strömbergsson, S. (2021). Parent rating of intelligibility: A discussion of the construct validity of the Intelligibility in Context Scale (ICS) and normative data of the Swedish version of the ICS. *International Journal of Language & Communication Disorders*, (4), 873–886. https://doi.org/10.1111/1460-6984.12634

Lagerberg, T. B., Åsberg, J., Hartelius, L., & Persson, C. (2014). Assessment of intelligibility using children's spontaneous speech: Methodological aspects. *International Journal of Language & Communication Disorders*, *49*, 228–239. https://doi.org/10.1111/1460-6984.12067

Lagerberg, T. B., Holm, K., McAllister, A., & Strömbergsson, S. (2021). Measuring intelligibility in spontaneous speech using syllables perceived as understood. *Journal of Communication Disorders*, *92*, 106108. https://doi.org/10.1016/j.jcomdis.2021.106108

Lagerberg, T. B., Johnels, J. Å., Hartelius, L., & Persson, C. (2015). Effect of the number of presentations on listener transcriptions and reliability in the assessment of speech intelligibility in children. *International Journal of Language & Communication Disorders*, *50*(4), 476–487. https://doi.org/10.1111/1460-6984.12149

Lai, C. S., Fisher, S. E., Hurst, J. A., Vargha-Khadem, F., & Monaco, A. P. (2001). A forkhead-domain gene is mutated in a severe speech and language disorder. *Nature*, *413*(6855), 519–523. https://doi.org/10.1038/35097076

Lalonde, K., Buss, E., Miller, M. K., & Leibold, L. J. (2022). Face masks impact auditory and audiovisual consonant recognition in children with and without hearing loss. *Frontiers in Psychology*, *13*, 874345. https://doi.org/10.3389/fpsyg.2022.874345

Land, W. M., Volchenkov, D., Bläsing, B. E., & Schack, T. (2013). From action representation to action execution: exploring the links between cognitive and biomechanical levels of motor control. *Frontiers in Computational Neuroscience*, *7*, 127. https://doi.org/10.3389/fncom.2013.00127

Landa, S., Pennington, L., Miller, N., Robson, S., Thompson, V., & Steen, N. (2014). Association between objective measurement of the speech intelligibility of young people with dysarthria and listener ratings of ease of understanding. *International Journal of Speech-Language Pathology*, *16*(4), 408–416. https://doi.org/10.3109/17549507.2014.927922

Lang, S., Bartl-Pokorny, K. D., Pokorny, F. B., Garrido, D., Mani, N., Fox-Boyer, A. V., . . . Marschik, P. B. (2019). Canonical babbling: A marker for earlier identification of late detected developmental disorders. *Current Developmental Disorders Reports*, *6*(3), 111–118. https://doi.org/10.1007/s40474-019-00166-w

Lange, B., Euler, H., & Zaretsky, E. (2016). Sex differences in language competence of 3- to 6-year-old children. *Applied Psycholinguistics*, *37*(6), 1417–1438. https://doi.org/10.1017/S0142716415000624

Langlois, C., Tucker, B. V., Sawatzky, A. N., Reed, A., & Boliek, C. A. (2020). Effects of an intensive voice treatment on articulatory function and speech intelligibility in children with motor speech disorders: A phase one study. *Journal of Communication Disorders*, *86*, 106003. https://doi.org/10.1016/j.jcomdis.2020.106003

Lashley, K. S. (1951). The problem of serial order in behavior. In L. A. Jeffress (Ed.), *Cerebral mechanisms in behavior: The Hixon symposium* (pp. 112–136). Wiley.

Latash, M. L. (2012). The bliss (not the problem) of motor abundance (not redundancy). *Experimental Brain Research*, *217*(1), 1–5. https://doi.org/10.1007/s00221-012-3000-4.

Latash, M., Wood, L., & Ulrich, D. (2008). What is currently known about hypotonia, motor skill development, and physical activity in Down syndrome. *Down Syndrome Research and Practice*, 1–21.

Lathrop-Marshall, H., Keyser, M. M. B., Jhingree, S., Giduz, N., Bocklage, C., Couldwell, S., . . . Jacox, L. A. (2022). Orthognathic speech pathology: Impacts of Class III malocclusion on speech. *European Journal of Orthodontics, 44*(3), 340–351. https://doi.org/10.1016/j.rasd.2023.102118

Lau, J. C., Losh, M., & Speights, M. (2023). Differences in speech articulatory timing and associations with pragmatic language ability in autism. *Research in Autism Spectrum Disorders, 102*, 102118. https://doi.org/10.1093/ejo/cjab067

Lau, J. C., Patel, S., Kang, X., Nayar, K., Martin, G. E., Choy, J., . . . Losh, M. (2022). Cross-linguistic patterns of speech prosodic differences in autism: A machine learning study. *PloS ONE, 17*(6), e0269637. https://doi.org/10.1371/journal.pone.0269637

Laubscher, E., & Light, J. (2020). Core vocabulary lists for young children and considerations for early language development: A narrative review. *Augmentative and Alternative Communication, 36*(1), 43–53. https://doi.org/10.1080/07434618.2020.1737964

Lausen, A., & Hammerschmidt, K. (2020). Emotion recognition and confidence ratings predicted by vocal stimulus type and prosodic parameters. *Humanities and Social Sciences Communications*, 7(1), 1–17. https://doi.org/10.1057/s41599-020-0499-z

Laver, John (1980). *The phonetic description of voice quality*. Cambridge University Press.

Laws, G., & Gunn, D. (2004). Phonological memory as a predictor of language development in children with Down syndrome: A five year follow up study. *Journal of Child Psychology and Psychiatry, 45*, 326–337. https://doi.org/10.1111/j.1469-7610.2004.00224.x

Leavy, K. M., Cisneros, G. J., & LeBlanc, E. M. (2016). Malocclusion and its relationship to speech sound production: Redefining the effect of malocclusal traits on sound production. *American Journal of Orthodontics and Dentofacial Orthopedics, 150*, 116–123.

Lee, A. S.-Y., & Gibbon, F. E. (2015). Non-speech oral motor treatment for children with developmental speech sound disorders. *Cochrane Database of Systematic Reviews* 2015, Issue 3. Art. No. CD009383. https://doi.org/10.1002/14651858.CD009383.pub2

Lee, J., Russell, C. G., Mohebbi, M., & Keast, R. (2022). Grating orientation task: A screening tool for determination of oral tactile acuity in children. *Food Quality and Preference, 95*, 104365. https://doi.org/10.1016/j.foodqual.2021.104365

Lee, Y. C., Chen, V. C., Yang, Y.H., Kuo, T. Y., Hung, T. H., Cheng, Y. F., & Huang, K.Y. (2020). Association between emotional disorders and speech and language impairments: A national population–based study. *Child Psychiatry and Human Development, 51*(3), 355–365. https://doi.org/10.1007/s10578-019-00947-9

Lehnert-LeHouillier, H., Terrazas, S., & Sandoval, S. (2020). Prosodic entrainment in conversations of verbal children and teens on the autism spectrum. *Frontiers in Psychology, 11*,2718. https://doi.org/10.3389/fpsyg.2020.582221

Lenneberg, E. H. (1964). Speech as a motor skill with special reference to nonaphasic disorders. *Monographs of the Society for Research in Child Development, 29*(1), 115–127. https://www.jstor.org/stable/1165759

Lenneberg, E. (1967). *Biological foundations of language*. Wiley.

Lenneberg, E. H. (1969). On explaining language: The development of language in children can best be understood in the context of developmental biology. *Science, 164*(3880), 635–643. https://doi.org/10.1126/science.164.3880.635

Leong, V., & Goswami, U. (2015). Acoustic-emergent phonology in the amplitude envelope of child-directed Speech. *PLoS ONE, 10*(12), e0144411-e0144411. 1307. http://doi.org/10.1371/journal.pone.0144411

Levelt, W. J. M. (1993). *Speaking: From intention to articulation*. MIT Press.

Levin, K. (1999). Babbling in infants with cerebral palsy. *Clinical Linguistics & Phonetics, 13*(4), 249–267. https://doi.org/10.1080/026992099299077

Levy, E. S. (2014) Implementing two treatment approaches to childhood dysarthria, *International Journal of Speech-Language Pathology, 16*(4), 344–354. https://doi.org/10.3109/17549507.2014.894123

Levy, E. S., & Crowley, C. J. (2012). Policies and practices regarding students with accents in speech-language pathology training programs.

Communication Disorders Quarterly, 34, 59–68. http://doi.org/10.1177/152574011140 9567

Levy, E. S., Chang, Y. M., Hwang, K., & McAuliffe, M. J. (2021). Perceptual and acoustic effects of dual-focus speech treatment in children with dysarthria. *Journal of Speech, Language, and Hearing Research, 64*(6S), 2301–2316. https://doi.org/10.1044/2020_JSLHR-20-00301

Lewis, B. A., Short, E. J., Iyengar, S. K., Taylor, H. G., Freebairn, M. L., Tag, M. J., . . . Stein, C. M. (2012). Speech-sound disorders and attention-deficit/hyperactivity disorder symptoms. *Topics in Language Disorders, 32*(3), 247. https://doi.org/10.1097/tld.0b013e318261f086

Lewis, K., Casteel, R., & McMahon, J. (1982). Duration of sustained/a/related to the number of trials. *Folia Phoniatrica et Logopaedica, 34*(1), 41–48. https://doi.org/10.1159/000265626

Li, P., Legault, J., & Litcofsky, K. A. (2014). Neuroplasticity as a function of second language learning: anatomical changes in the human brain. *Cortex, 58, 301*-324. https://doi.org/10.1016/j.cortex.2014.05.001

Liberman, I. Y., Shankweiler, D. & Liberman, A. M. (1989). The alphabetic principle and learning to read. In D. Shankweiler & I. Y. Liberman (Eds.), *Phonology and reading disability: Solving the reading puzzle* (pp. 1–33). University of Michigan Press.

Libertus, K., & Violi, D. A. (2016). Sit to talk: Relation between motor skills and language development in infancy. *Frontiers in Psychology*, 7, 475. https://doi.org/10.3389/fpsyg.2016.00475

Licari, M. K., Alvares, G. A., Bernie, C., Elliott, C., Evans, K. L., McIntyre, S., . . . Williams, J. (2021). The unmet clinical needs of children with developmental coordination disorder. *Pediatric Research, 90*(4), 826–831. https://doi.org/10.1038/s41390-021-01373-1

Liebenthal, E., Silbersweig, D. A., & Stern E. (2016). The language, tone and prosody of emotions: Neural substrates and dynamics of spoken-word emotion perception. *Frontiers in Neuroscience, 10*, 506. https://www.frontiersin.org/article/10.3389/fnins.2016.00506

Lieberman, D. E. (2011). Epigenetic integration, complexity, and evolvability of the head. In B. Hallgrímsson & B. K. Hall (Eds.), *Epigenetics: Linking genotype and phenotype in development and evolution* (pp. 271–289). University of California Press.

Lieberman, D. E., & McCarthy, R. C. (1999). The ontogeny of cranial base angulation in humans and chimpanzees and its implications for reconstructing pharyngeal dimensions. *Journal of Human Evolution, 36*, 487–517. https://doi.org/10.1006/jhev.1998.0287

Lieberman, D. E., McCarthy, R. D., Hiiemae, K. M., & Palmer, J. B. (2001). Ontogeny of postnatal hyoid and larynx descent in humans. *Archives of Oral Biology, 46*, 117–128. https://doi.org/10.1016/S0003-9969(00)00108-4

Lieberman, P., Crelin, E. S., & Klatt, D. H. (1972). Phonetic ability and related anatomy of the newborn and adult human, Neanderthal man, and the chimpanzee. *American Anthropologist, 74*(3), 287–307. https://doi.org/10.1525/aa.1972.74.3.02a00020

Liberman, I. Y., Shankweiler, D., & Liberman, A. M. (1989). In D. Shankweiler & I. Y. Liberman (eds), *The alphabetic principle and learning to read* (pp. 1–33). University of Michigan Press

Liégeois, F. J., & Morgan, A. T. (2012). Neural bases of childhood speech disorders: Lateralization and plasticity for speech functions during development. *Neuroscience & Biobehavioral Reviews, 36*(1), 439–458. https://doi.org/10.1016/j.neubiorev.2011.07.011

Liégeois, F. J., Turner, S. J., Mayes, A., Bonthrone, A. F., Boys, A., Smith, L., . . . Morgan, A. T. (2019). Dorsal language stream anomalies in an inherited speech disorder. *Brain, 142*(4), 966–977. https://doi.org/10.1093/brain/awz018

Lieu, J. E. C. (2004). Speech-language and educational consequences of unilateral hearing loss in children. *Archives of Otolaryngology-Head & Neck Surgery, 130*(5), 524–530. https://doi.org/10.1001/archotol.130.5.524

Lieu, J. E., Kenna, M., Anne, S., & Davidson, L. (2020). Hearing loss in children: A review. *JAMA, 324*(21), 2195–2205. https://doi.org/10.1001/jama.2020.17647.

Lillo-Martin, D., & Henner, J. (2021). Acquisition of sign languages *Annual Review of Linguistics*, 7(1), 395–419. https://doi.org/10.1146/annurev-linguistics-043020-092357

Lin, A. (2013). Classroom code-switching: Three decades of research. *Applied Linguistics Review, 4*(1), 195–218. http://hdl.handle.net/10722/184270)

Lind, A., & Hartsuiker, R. J. (2020). Self-monitoring in speech production: Comprehending the conflict between conflict- and comprehension-based accounts. *Journal of Cognition*, *3*(1),16. https://doi.org/10.5334/joc.118.

Lindblom, B. (1990). On the notion of "possible speech sound". *Journal of Phonetics*, *18*(2), 135–152.

Lindquist, K. A., MacCormack, J. K., & Shablack, H. (2015). The role of language in emotion: Predictions from psychological constructionism. *Frontiers in Psychology*, *6*, 444. https://doi.org/10.3389/fpsyg.2015.00444

Lione, R., Franchi, L., Ghislanzoni, L. T. H., Primozic, J., Buongiorno, M., & Cozza, P. (2015). Palatal surface and volume in mouth-breathing subjects evaluated with three-dimensional analysis of digital dental casts—A controlled study. *The European Journal of Orthodontics*, *37* (1), 101–104.

Lippke, B. A., Dickey, S. E., Selmar, J. W., & Soder, A. L. (1997). *Photo-Articulation Test* (3rd ed.). Pro-Ed.

Lisi, E. C., & Cohn, R. D. (2011). Genetic evaluation of the pediatric patient with hypotonia: Perspective from a hypotonia specialty clinic and review of the literature. *Developmental Medicine & Child Neurology*, *53*(7), 586–599. https://doi.org/10.1111/j.1469-8749.2011.03918.x

Liss, J. M., White, L., Mattys, S. L., Lansford, K., Lotto, A. J., Spitzer, S. M., & Caviness, J. N. (2009). Quantifying speech rhythm abnormalities in the dysarthrias. *Journal of Speech, Language, and Hearing Research*, *52*(5),1334–1352. https://doi.org/10.1044/10924388(2009/08-0208).

Litovsky, R. (2015). Development of the auditory system. *Handbook of Clinical Neurology*, *129*, 55–72. https://doi.org/10.1016/B978-0-444-62630-1.00003-2

Liu, Y., Lee, S. A. S., & Chen, W. (2022). The correlation between perceptual ratings and nasalance scores in resonance disorders: A systematic review. *Journal of Speech, Language, and Hearing Research*, *65*(6), 1–20. https://doi.org/10.1044/2022_JSLHR-21-00588

Locke, J. L. (1983). Clinical phonology: the explanation and treatment of speech sound disorders. *Journal of Speech and Hearing Disorders*, *48*(4), 339–341. https://doi.org/10.1044/jshd.4804.339.

Lof, G. L. (1996). Factors associated with speech-sound stimulability. *Journal of Communication Disorders*, *29*(4), 255–278. https://doi.org/10.1016/0021-9924(96)00013-5

Lof, G. L., & Watson, M. M. (2008). A nationwide survey of nonspeech oral motor exercise use: Implications for evidence-based practice. *Language, Speech, and Hearing Services in Schools*, *39*, 392–407. https://doi.org/10.1044/0161-1461(2008/037)

Lof, G., & Watson, M. (2010). Five reasons why nonspeech oral-motor exercises do not work. *Perspectives on School Based Issues, American Speech-Language-Hearing Association*, *11*, 109–117.

Logan, K. J., Byrd, C. T., Mazzocchi, E. M., & Gillam, R. B. (2011). Speaking rate characteristics of elementary-school-aged children who do and do not stutter. *Journal of Communication Disorders*, *44*(1), 130–147. https://doi.org/10.1016/j.jcomdis.2010.08.001

Logan, L. R., Hickman, R. R., Harris, S. R., & Heriza, C. B. (2008). Single-subject research design: recommendations for levels of evidence and quality rating. *Developmental Medicine & Child Neurology*, *50*(2), 99–103. https://doi.org/10.1111/j.1469-8749.2007.02005.x

Lohmander, A., Westberg, L. R., Olsson, S., Tengroth, B. I., & Flynn, T. (2021). Canonical babbling and early consonant development related to hearing in children with otitis media with effusion with or without cleft palate. *The Cleft Palate-Craniofacial Journal*, *58*(7), 894–905. https://doi.org/10.1177/1055665620966198

Long, H. L., & Hustad, K. C. (2023). Marginal and canonical babbling in 10 infants at risk for cerebral palsy. *American Journal of Speech-Language Pathology*, 1–15. https://doi.org/10.1044/2022_AJSLP-22-00165

Long, H. L., Bowman, D. D., Yoo, H., Burkhardt-Reed, M. M., Bene, E. R., & Oller, D. K. (2020). Social and endogenous infant vocalizations. *PLoS ONE*, *15*(8), e0224956. https://doi.org/10.1371/journal.pone.0224956

Long, H. L., Mahr, T. J., Natzke, P., Rathouz, P. J., & Hustad, K. C. (2022). Longitudinal change in speech classification between 4 and 10 years in children with cerebral palsy. *Developmental Medicine & Child Neurology*, *64*(9), 1096–1105. https://doi.org/10.1111/dmcn.15198

Long, H., Ramsay, G., Bowman, D. D., Burkhardt-Reed, M. M., & Oller, D. K. (2021). Social and endogenous motivations in the emergence of canonical babbling in infants at low and high risk for autism. *Research Square*. https://doi.org/10.21203/rs.3.rs-528843/v1

Loudermill, C., Greenwell, T., & Brosseau-Lapré, F. (2021, March). A comprehensive treatment approach to address speech production and literacy skills in school-age children with speech sound disorders. *Seminars in Speech and Language 42*(2) 136–146.

Lousada, M., Jesus, L. M., Hall, A., & Joffe, V. (2014). Intelligibility as a clinical outcome measure following intervention with children with phonologically based speech–sound disorders. *International Journal of Language & Communication Disorders, 49*(5), 584–601. https://doi.org/10.1111/1460-6984.12095

Lowit, A., Kent, R. D., & Kuschmann, A. (2022). Management of dysarthria. In I. Papathanasiou & P. Coppens (Eds.), *Aphasia* (3rd ed., pp. 641–671). Jones & Bartlett Learning.

Luchini, P. L. (2017). Measurements for accentedness, pause and nuclear stress placement in the EFL context. *Ilha Desterro, 70*(3), 185–200. https://doi.org/10.5007/2175-8026.2017v70n3p185

Ludlow, C. L., Kent, R. S., & Gray, L. C. (2019). *Measuring voice, speech, and swallowing in the clinic and laboratory*. Plural Publishing.

Ludlow, C. L., Hoit, J., Kent, R., Ramig, L. O., Shrivastav, R., Strand, E., . . . Sapienza, C. M. (2008). Translating principles of neural plasticity into research on speech motor control recovery and rehabilitation. *Journal of Speech, Language, and Hearing Research, 51*(1), S240–S258. https://doi.org/10.1044/1092-4388(2008/019)

Lundeborg, I., Ericsson, E., Hultcrantz, E., & McAllister, A. M. (2011). Influence of adenotonsillar hypertrophy on/s/-articulation in children—effects of surgery. *Logopedics Phoniatrics Vocology, 36*(3), 100–108. https://doi.org/10.3109/14015439.2010.531047

Lundeborg, I., McAllister, A., Samuelsson, C., & Ericsson, E. (2009). Phonological development in children with obstructive sleep-disordered breathing. *Clinical Linguistics & Phonetics, 23*, 751–761. https://doi.org/10.3109/02699200903144770

Lust, J. M., Spruijt, S., Wilson, P. H., & Steenbergen, B. (2018) Motor planning in children with cerebral palsy: A longitudinal perspective. *Journal of Clinical and Experimental Neuropsychology, 40*(6), 559–566. https://doi.org/10.1080/13803395.2017.1387645

Lyakso, E., Frolova, O., & Nikolaev, A. (2021). Voice and speech features as a diagnostic symptom. In C. Pracana & M. Wang (Eds.) *Psychological applications and trends* (pp. 259–263). InScience Press.

Lyons, R., & Roulstone, S. (2018). Listening to the voice of children with developmental speech and language disorders using narrative inquiry: Methodological considerations. *Journal of Communication Disorders, 72*, 16–25. https://doi.org/10.1016/j.jcomdis.2018.02.006

Ma, E.P.-M., & Yiu, E. M.-L. (2007). Scaling voice activity limitation and participation restriction in dysphonic individuals. *Folia Phoniatrica Logopaedica, 59*, 74–82.

Maas, E., & Mailend, M. L. (2017). Fricative contrast and coarticulation in children with and without speech sound disorders. *American Journal of Speech-language Pathology, 26*(2S), 649–663. https://doi.org/10.1044/2017_AJSLP-16-0110

Maas, E., Gildersleeve-Neumann, C. E., Jakielski, K. J., & Stoeckel, R. (2014). Motor-based intervention protocols in treatment of childhood apraxia of speech (CAS). *Current Developmental Disorders Reports, 1*(3), 197–206. https://doi.org/10.1007/s40474-014-0016-4

Maas, E., Robin, D. A., Hula, S. N. A., Freedman, S. E., Wulf, G., Ballard, K. J., & Schmidt, R. A. (2008). Principles of motor learning in treatment of motor speech disorders. *American Journal of Speech-Language Pathology, 17*(3), 277–298. https://doi.org/10.1044/1058-0360(2008/025)

Maassen, B., Nijland, L., & Van Der Meulen, S. (2001). Coarticulation within and between syllables by children with developmental apraxia of speech. *Clinical Linguistics & Phonetics, 15*(1–2), 145–150. https://doi.org/10.3109/02699200109167647

Macefield, R., Brookes, S., Blazeby, J., & Avery, K. (2019). Development of a 'universal-reporter' outcome measure (UROM) for patient and healthcare professional completion: A mixed methods study demonstrating a novel concept for optimal questionnaire design. *BMJ Open, 9*(8), e029741. https://doi.org/10.1136/bmjopen-2019-029741

Macken, M. A., & Barton, D. (1980). The acquisition of the voicing contrast in English: A study of voice onset time in word-initial stop consonants. *Journal of Child Language*, *7*(1), 41–74. https://doi.org/10.1017/S0305000900007029

MacNeilage, P. F. (1998). The frame/content theory of evolution of speech production. *Behavioral and Brain Sciences*, *21*(4), 499–511. https://doi.org/10.1017/S0140525X98001265

Maddieson, I. (1984). *Patterns of sounds*. Cambridge University Press. https://doi.org/10.1017/CBO9780511753459

Madell, J. (2013, April 23). Can children understand fast speech? *Hearing Health and Technology Matters*.

Maenner, M. J., Shaw, K. A., Baio, J., Washington, A., Patrick, M., DiRienzo, M., . . . Dietz, P. M. (2020). Prevalence of autism spectrum disorder among children aged 8 years—Autism and developmental disabilities monitoring network, 11 sites, United States, 2016. *MMWR Surveillance Summaries*, *69*(4), 1. https://doi.org/10.15585/mmwr.ss6904a1

Maggu, A. R., Kager, R., To, C. K., Kwan, J. S., & Wong, P. C. (2021). Effect of complexity on speech sound development: Evidence from meta-analysis review of treatment-based studies. *Frontiers in Psychology*, *12*, 651900. https://doi.org/10.3389/fpsyg.2021.651900

Maguire, G. A., Nguyen, D. L., Simonson, K. C., & Kurz, T. L. (2020). The pharmacologic treatment of stuttering and its neuropharmacologic basis. *Frontiers in Neuroscience*, *14*, 158. https://doi.org/10.3389/fnins.2020.00158

Mahler, L. A., & Jones, H. N. (2012). Intensive treatment of dysarthria in two adults with Down syndrome. *Developmental Neurorehabilitation*, *15*(1), 44–53. https://doi.org/10.3109/17518423.2011.632784

Mahr, T. J., Soriano, J. U., Rathouz, P. J., & Hustad, K. C. (2021). Speech development between 30 and 119 months in typical children II: Articulation rate growth curves. *Journal of Speech, Language, and Hearing Research*, *64*(11), 4057–4070. https://doi.org/10.1044/2021_JSLHR-21-00206

Maier, M., Ballester, B. R., & Verschure, P. F. (2019). Principles of neurorehabilitation after stroke based on motor learning and brain plasticity mechanisms. *Frontiers in Systems Neuroscience*, *13*, 74. https://doi.org/10.3389/fnsys.2019.00074

Majorano, M., Bastianello, T., Morelli, M., Lavelli, M., & Vihman, M. M. (2019). Vocal production and novel word learning in the first year. *Journal of Child Language*, *46*(3), 606–616.

Malik, F., & Marwaha, R. (2022). *Developmental stages of social emotional development in children*. [Updated 2022 Feb 7]. In StatPearls [Internet]. StatPearls Publishing. https://www.ncbi.nlm.nih.gov/books/NBK534819/

Malisz, Z., Brandt, E., Möbius, B., Oh, Y. M., & Andreeva, B. (2018). Dimensions of segmental variability: Interaction of prosody and surprisal in six languages. *Frontiers of Communication*. https://doi.org/10.3389/fcomm.2018.00025

Mallampati, S. R. (1983). Clinical sign to predict difficult tracheal intubation (hypothesis). *Canadian Anaesthetists' Society Journal*, *30*(3), 316–317. https://doi.org/10.1007/BF03013818

Malmenholt, A., Lohmander, A., & McAllister, A. (2017). Childhood apraxia of speech: A survey of praxis and typical speech characteristics. *Logopedics Phoniatrics Vocology*, *42*(2), 84–92.

Maniwa, K., Jongman, A., & Wade, T. (2009). Acoustic characteristics of clearly spoken English fricatives. *The Journal of the Acoustical Society of America*, *125*(6), 3962–3973. https://doi.org/10.1121/1.2990715

Manouilenko, I., Eriksson, J. M., Humble, M. B., & Bejerot, S. (2014). Minor physical anomalies in adults with autism spectrum disorder and healthy controls. *Autism Research and Treatment*. Article ID 743482, 9 pages. http://dx.doi.org/10.1155/2014/743482.

Marecka, M., Wrembel, M., Otwinowska, A., Szewczyk, J., Banasik-Jemielniak, N., & Wodniecka, Z. (2020). Bilingual children's phonology shows evidence of transfer, but not deceleration in their L1. *Studies in Second Language Acquisition*, *42*(1), 89–114. https://doi.org/10.1017/S0272263119000408

Mariën, P., & Borgatti, R. (2018). Language and the cerebellum. *Handbook of Clinical Neurology*, *154*, 181–202. https://doi.org/10.1016/B978-0-444-63956-1.00011-4

Marshalla, P. (2007). *Marshalla Oral Sensorimotor Test (MOST)*. Super Duper Publications.

Marslen-Wilson, W. D. (1984). Function and process in spoken word recognition. In H. Bouma & D. Bouwhuis (Eds.), *Attention and performance X: Control of language processes* (pp. 125–150). Erlbaum.

Martikainen, A. L., Savinainen-Makkonen, T., & Kunnari, S. (2021). Speech inconsistency and its association with speech production, phonological awareness and nonword repetition skills. *Clinical Linguistics & Phonetics*, *35*(8), 743–760. https://doi.org/10.1080/02699206.2020.1827296

Martin, G. E., Roberts, J. E., Helm-Estabrooks, N., Sideris, J., Vanderbilt, J., & Moskowitz, L. (2012). Perseveration in the connected speech of boys with fragile X syndrome with and without autism spectrum disorder. *American Journal on Intellectual and Developmental Disabilities*, *117*(5), 384–399. https://doi.org/10.1352/1944-7558-117.5.384

Martin, R. R., Haroldson, S. K., & Triden, K. A. (1984). Stuttering and speech naturalness. *Journal of Speech and Hearing Disorders*, *49*(1), 53–58. https://doi.org/10.1044/jshd.4901.53

Martinelli, R. L., Marchesan, I. Q., & Berretin-Felix, G. (2012). Lingual frenulum protocol with scores for infants. *International Journal of Orofacial Myology*, *38*, 104–112.

Martino, J., Brogna, C., Robles, S. G., Vergani, F., & Duffau, H. (2010). Anatomic dissection of the inferior fronto-occipital fasciculus revisited in the lights of brain stimulation data. *Cortex*, *46*(5), 691–699. https://doi.org/10.1016/j.cortex.2009.07.015

Marvel, C. L., & Desmond, J. E. (2012). From storage to manipulation: How the neural correlates of verbal working memory reflect varying demands on inner speech. *Brain and Language*, *120*(1), 42–51. https://doi.org/10.1016/j.bandl.2011.08.005

Maryn, Y., Van Lierde, K., De Bodt, M., & Van Cauwenberge, P. (2004). The effects of adenoidectomy and tonsillectomy on speech and nasal resonance. *Folia Phoniatrica et Logopaedica*, *56*(3), 182–191.

Mason, K. M., Marsh, R. L., Pelton, S. I., & Harvill, E. T. (2022). Otitis media. *Frontiers in Cellular and Infection Microbiology*, *12*, 1736. https://doi.org/10.3389/fcimb.2022.1063153

Masterson, J. J., Bernhardt, B. H., & Hofheinz, M. K. (2005). A comparison of single words and conversational speech in phonological evaluation. *American Journal of Speech-Language Pathology*, *14*(3), 229–241. https://doi.org/10.1044/1058-0360(2005/023)

Matthews, H. S., Penington, A. J., Hardiman, R., Fan, Y., Clement, J. G., Kilpatrick, N. M., & Claes, P. D. (2018). Modelling 3D craniofacial growth trajectories for population comparison and classification illustrated using sex-differences. *Scientific Reports*, *8*(1), 1–11. https://doi.org/10.1038/s41598-018-22752-5

Maurer, C. W., Duffy, J. R. (2022). Functional speech and voice disorders. In K. LaFaver, C. W. Maurer, T. R. Nicholson, & D. L. Perez (Eds.), *Functional movement disorder. Current clinical neurology*. Humana. https://doi.org/10.1007/978-3-030-86495-8_13

May, T., Adesina, I., McGillivray, J., & Rinehart, N. J. (2019). Sex differences in neurodevelopmental disorders. *Current Opinion in Neurology*, *32*(4), 622–626. https://doi.org/10.1097/WCO.0000000000000714

Mayo, R., & Grant, W. (1995). Fundamental frequency, perturbation, and vocal tract resonance characteristics of African-American and White American males. *Echo*, *17*, 32–38.

Mayo, R., & Manning, W. (1994). Vocal tract characteristics of African-American and Caucasian-American adult males. *Tejas: Texas Journal of Audiology and Speech Pathology*, *20*, 33–36.

McAllister, A., & Sjölander, P. (2013). Children's voice and voice disorders. *Seminars in Speech and Language 34*(2), 071–079.

McAllister, A., Brodén, M., Gonzalez Lindh, M., Krüssenberg, C., Ristic, I., Rubensson, A., & Sjögreen, L. (2018). Oral sensory-motor intervention for children and adolescents (3–18 years) with developmental or early acquired speech disorders: A review of the literature 2000–2017. *Annals of Otolaryngology and Rhinology*, *5*(5), 1221.

McAllister Byun, T., Buchwald, A., & Mizoguchi, A. (2016). Covert contrast in velar fronting: An acoustic and ultrasound study. *Clinical Linguistics & Phonetics*, *30*(3–5), 249–276. https://doi.org/10.3109/02699206.2015.1056884

McAllister, T., Eads, A., Kabakoff, H., Scott, M., Boyce, S., Whalen, D. H., & Preston, J. L. (2022). Baseline stimulability predicts patterns of response to traditional and ultrasound biofeedback treatment for residual speech sound disorder. *Journal of Speech, Language, and Hearing Research*, *65*(8), 2860–2880. https://doi.org/10.1044/2022_JSLHR-22-00161

McAuliffe, M. J., & Cornwell, P. L. (2008). Intervention for lateral /s/ using electropalatography (EPG) biofeedback and an intensive motor learning approach: A case report. *International Journal of Language & Communication Disorders*, *43*(2), 219–229. https://doi.org/10.1080/13682820701344078

McAuliffe, M. J., Lin E., Robb M. P., & Murdoch B. E (2008). Influence of a standard electropalatography artificial palate upon articulation. *Folia Phoniatrica et Logopaedica*. *60*, 45–53. https://doi.org/10.1159/000112216

McCabe, D. J., & Altman, K. W. (2017). Prosody: An overview and applications to voice therapy. *Global Journal of Otolaryngology*, *7*, 1–8. https://doi.org/10.19080/GJO.2017.07.555719

McCann, J., & Peppé, S. (2003). Prosody in autism spectrum disorders: A critical review. *International Journal of Language & Communication Disorders*, *38*(4), 325–350. https://10.1080/1368282031000154204

McCauley, R. J., & Skenes, L. L. (1987). Contrastive stress, phonetic context, and misarticulation of /r/ in young speakers. *Journal of Speech, Language, and Hearing Research*, *30*(1), 114–121. https://doi.org/10.1044/jshr.3001.114

McCauley, R. J., & Strand, E. A. (2008). A review of standardized tests of nonverbal oral and speech motor performance in children. *American Journal of Speech-Language Pathology*, *17*, 81–91.

McCauley, R. J., Strand, E., Lof, G. L., Schooling, T., & Frymark, T. (2009). Evidence-based systematic review: Effects of nonspeech oral motor exercises on speech. *American Journal of Speech-Language Pathology*, *18*(4), 343–360. https://doi.org/10.1044/1058-0360(2009/09-0006)

McCauley, S. M., Bannard, C., Theakston, A., Davis, M., Cameron-Faulkner, T., & Ambridge, B. (2021). Multiword units lead to errors of commission in children's spontaneous production: "What corpus data can tell us?" *Developmental Science*, *24*(6), e13125. https://doi.org/10.1111/desc.13125

McCormack, J., McLeod, S., Harrison, L. J., & McAllister, L. (2010). The impact of speech impairment in early childhood: Investigating parents' and speech-language pathologists' perspectives using the ICF-CY. *Journal of Communication Disorders*, *43*(5), 378–396.

McCormack, J., McLeod, S., McAllister, L., & Harrison, L. J. (2009). A systematic review of the association between childhood speech impairment and participation across the lifespan. *International Journal of Speech-Language Pathology*, *11*(2), 155–170.

McCune, L., & Vihman, M. (1987). Vocal motor schemes. *Papers and Reports on Child Language Development*, *26*, 72–79.

McCune, L., & Vihman, M. M. (2001). Early phonetic and lexical development: A productivity approach. *Journal of Speech, Language, and Hearing Research*, *44*(3), 670–684. https://doi.org/10.1044/1092-4388(2001/054)

McDaniel, J., Woynaroski, T., Keceli-Kaysili, B., Watson, L. R., & Yoder, P. (2019). Vocal communication with canonical syllables predicts later expressive language skills in preschool-aged children with autism spectrum disorder. *Journal of Speech, Language, and Hearing Research*, *62*(10), 3826–3833. https://doi.org/10.1044/2019_JSLHR-L-19-0162

McGillion, M. L., Herbert, J. S., Pine, J., Vihman, M. M., Depaolis, R., Keren-Portnoy, T., & Matthews, D. (2016). What paves the way to conventional language? The predictive value of babble, pointing and SES. *Child Development*, *88*(1), 156–166.

McGowan, R. S., & Nittrouer, S. (1988). Differences in fricative production between children and adults: Evidence from an acoustic analysis of /ʃ/ and /s/. *The Journal of the Acoustical Society of America*, *83*(1), 229–236. https://doi.org/10.1121/1.396425

McGrath, L. M., Hutaff-Lee, C., Scott, A., Boada, R., Shriberg, L. D., & Pennington, B. F. (2008). Children with comorbid speech sound disorder and specific language impairment are at increased risk for attention-deficit/hyperactivity disorder. *Journal of Abnormal Child Psychology*, *36*, 151–163. https://doi.org/10.1007/s10802-007-9166-8

McGregor, K. K., Williams, D., Hearst, S., & Johnson, A. C. (1997). The use of contrastive analysis in distinguishing difference from disorder: A tutorial. *American Journal of Speech-Language Pathology*, *6*(3), 45–56. https://doi.org/10.1044/1058-0360.0603.45

McGurk, H., & MacDonald, J. (1976). Hearing lips and seeing voices. *Nature*. 264, 746–748. https://doi.org/10.1038/264746a0

Mchugh, R. K., & Friedman, R. A. (2006). Genetics of hearing loss: Allelism and modifier genes produce a phenotypic continuum. *The Anatomical Record Part A: Discoveries in Molec-*

ular, Cellular, and Evolutionary Biology, *288*(4), 370–381. https://doi.org/10.1002/ar.a.20297

McIntosh, B., & Dodd, B. (2008). Evaluation of Core Vocabulary intervention for treatment of inconsistent phonological disorder: Three treatment case studies. *Child Language Teaching and Therapy*, *24*(3), 307–327. https://doi.org/10.1177/0265659007096295

McKay, R., Smart, S., & Cocks, N. (2020). Investigating tongue strength and endurance in children aged 6 to 11 years. *Dysphagia*, *35*(5), 762–772. https://doi.org/10.1007/s00455-019-10081-2

McKechnie, J., Shahin, M., Ahmed, B., McCabe, P., Arciuli, J., & Ballard, K. J. (2021). An automated lexical stress classification tool for assessing dysprosody in childhood apraxia of speech. *Brain Sciences*, *11*(11), 1408. https://doi.org/10.3390/brainsci11111408

McLaughlin, S. A., Thorne, J. C., Jirikowic, T., Waddington, T., Lee, A. K., & Astley Hemingway, S. J. (2019). Listening difficulties in children with fetal alcohol spectrum disorders: More than a problem of audibility. *Journal of Speech, Language, and Hearing Research*, *62*(5), 1532–1548. https://doi.org/10.1044/2018_JSLHR-H-18-0359

McLeod, S. (2015). Intelligibility in Context Scale: A parent-report screening tool translated into 60 languages. *Journal of Clinical Practice in Speech-Language Pathology*, *17*(1), 9–14.

McLeod, S. (2020). Intelligibility in Context Scale: Cross-linguistic use, validity, and reliability. *Speech, Language and Hearing*, *23*(1), 9–16. https://doi.org/10.1080/2050571X.2020.1718837

McLeod, S., & Baker, E. (2014). Speech-language pathologists' practices regarding assessment, analysis, target selection, intervention, and service delivery for children with speech sound disorders. *Clinical Linguistics & Phonetics*, *28*(7-8), 508–531. https://doi.org/10.3109/02699206.2014.926994

McLeod, S., & Bleile, K. (2004). The ICF: a framework for setting goals for children with speech impairment. *Child Language Teaching and Therapy*, *20*(3), 199–219.

McLeod, S., & McCormack, J. (2007). Application of the ICF and ICF-children and youth in children with speech impairment. *Seminars in Speech and Language 28*(4), 254–264).

McLeod, S., & Searl, J. (2006). Adaptation to an electropalatography palate: Acoustic, impressionist, and perceptual data. *American Journal of Speech-Language Pathology*, *15*, 192–206. https://doi.org/10.1044/1058-0360(2006/018)

McLeod, S., & Verdon, S. (2014). A review of 30 speech assessments in 19 languages other than English. *American Journal of Speech-Language Pathology*, *23*(4), 708–723.

McLeod, S., Crowe, K., & Shahaeian, A. (2015). Intelligibility in Context Scale: Normative and validation data for English-speaking preschoolers. *Language, Speech, and Hearing Services in Schools*, *46*(3), 266–276. https://doi.org/10.1044/2015_LSHSS-14-0120

McLeod, S., Harrison, L. J., & McCormack, J. (2012). *Intelligibility in Context Scale*. Charles Sturt University. https://doi.org/10.1037/t35980-000

McLeod, S., Roberts, A., & Sita, J. (2006). Tongue/palate contact for the production of /s/ and /z/. *Clinical Linguistics & Phonetics*, *20*(1), 51–66. https://doi.org/10.1080/02699200400021331

McMillan, C. T., & Corley, M. (2010). Cascading influences on the production of speech: Evidence from articulation. *Cognition*, *117*(3), 243–260. https://doi.org/10.1016/j.cognition.2010.08.019

McMurray, B., Danelz, A., Rigler, H., & Seedorff, M. (2018). Speech categorization develops slowly through adolescence. *Developmental Psychology*, *54*(8), 1472–1491. https://doi.org/10.1037/dev0000542

McNeill, B. C., Gillon, G. T., & Dodd, B. (2009). Phonological awareness and early reading development in childhood apraxia of speech (CAS). *International Journal of Language & Communication Disorders*, *44*(2), 175–192. https://doi.org/10.1080/13682820801997353

McQueen, J. M. (2007). Eight questions about spoken-word recognition. In M. G. Gaskell & G. Altmann (Eds.), *The Oxford handbook of psycholinguistics* (pp. 37–53). Oxford University Press.

McReynolds, L. V., & Elbert, M. (1981). Criteria for phonological process analysis. *Journal of Speech and Hearing Disorders*, *46*(2), 197–204. https://doi.org/10.1044/jshd.4602.197

Meditch, A. (1975). The development of sex-specific speech patterns in young children. *Anthropological Linguistics*, *17*, 421–433.

Medline Plus. (n.d.). *Speech disorders—children*. National Library of Medicine. https://medlineplus.gov/ency/article/001430.htm#:~:text=A%20speech%20disorder%20is%20a,Phonological%20disorders

Medwetsky, L. (2011). Spoken language processing model: Bridging auditory and language processing to guide assessment and intervention. *Language, Speech, and Hearing Services in Schools, 42*(3), 286–296. https://doi.org/10.1044/0161-1461(2011/10-0036)

Mehl, M. R., Vazire, S., Ramirez-Esparza, N., Slatcher, R. B., & Pennebaker, J. W. (2007). Are women really more talkative than men? *Science, 317*, 82.

Mehrabian, A., & Ferris, S. (1967). Inference of attitudes from nonverbal communication in two channels. *Journal of Consulting Psychology, 13*, 248–252. https://doi.org/10.1037/h0024532

Mehrabian A., & Wiener, M. (1967). Decoding of inconsistent communications. *Journal of Personality and Social Psychology, 6*, 109–114. https://doi.org/10.1037/h0024648

Mehrdad, A. G., & Ahghar, M. R. (2015). Markedness and syllabus design in SLA. *Procedia—Social and Behavioral Sciences, 177*, 104–108.

Mei, C., Reilly, S., Bickerton, M., Mensah, F., Turner, S., Kumaranayagam, D., . . . Morgan, A. T. (2020). Speech in children with cerebral palsy. *Developmental Medicine & Child Neurology, 62*(12), 1374–1382. https://doi.org/10.1111/dmcn.14592

Mennen, I., Scobbie, J. M., de Leeuw, E., Schaeffler, S., & Schaeffler, F. (2010). Measuring language-specific phonetic settings. *Second Language Research, 26*(1), 13–41. https://doi.org/10.1177/0267658309337617

Merel, J., Botvinick, M. & Wayne, G. (2019). Hierarchical motor control in mammals and machines. *Nature Communications, 10*, 5489. https://doi.org/10.1038/s41467-019-13239-6

Merkel-Walsh, R. (2020). Orofacial myofunctional therapy with children ages 0-4 and individuals with special needs. *International Journal of Orofacial Myology and Myofunctional Therapy, 46* (1), 22–36.

Merrett, D. L., Peretz, I., & Wilson, S. J. (2014). Neurobiological, cognitive, and emotional mechanisms in melodic intonation therapy. *Frontiers in Human Neuroscience, 8*, 401. https://doi.org/10.3389/fnhum.2014.00401

Merrick, R., & Roulstone, S. (2011). Children's views of communication and speech-language pathology. *International Journal of Speech-Language Pathology, 13*(4), 281–290. https://doi.org/10.3109/17549507.2011.577809

Merritt, B., & Bent, T. (2020). Perceptual evaluation of speech naturalness in speakers of varying gender identities. *Journal of Speech, Language, and Hearing Research, 63*(7), 2054–2069. https://doi.org/10.1044/2020_JSLHR-19-00337

Mesquita, B. (2022). *Between us: How cultures create emotions*. W. W. Norton & Co.

Messner, A. H., & Lalakea, M. L. (2002). The effect of ankyloglossia on speech in children. *Otolaryngology-Head and Neck Surgery, 127*(6), 539–545. https://doi.org/10.1067/mhn.2002.129731

Messner, A. H., Walsh, J., Rosenfeld, R. M., Schwartz, S. R., Ishman, S. L., Baldassari, C., . . . Satterfield, L. (2020). Clinical consensus statement: Ankyloglossia in children. *Otolaryngology-Head and Neck Surgery, 162*(5), 597–611. https://doi.org/10.1177/0194599820915457

Mesulam, M. M. (1990). Large-scale neurocognitive networks and distributed processing for attention, language, and memory. *Annals of Neurology, 28*(5), 597–613. https://doi.org/10.1002/ana.410280502

Mesulam, M. M. (Editor) (2000). *Principles of behavioral and cognitive neurology* (2nd ed.). Oxford University Press.

Metsala, J. L. & Walley, A. C. (1998). Spoken vocabulary growth and the segmental restructuring of lexical representations: Precursors to phonemic awareness and early reading ability. In J. L. Metsala & L. C. Ehri (Eds.), *Word recognition in beginning literacy* (pp. 89–120). Erlbaum.

Meyer, A. S. (1992). Investigation of phonological encoding through speech error analyses: Achievements, limitations, and alternatives. *Cognition, 42*(1–3), 181–211. https://doi.org/10.1016/0010–0277(92)90043–H

Miccio, A. W., & Scarpino, S. E. (2008). Phonological analysis, phonological processes. In M. J. Ball, M. R. Perkins, N. Müller & S. Howard (Eds.), *The handbook of clinical linguistics* (pp. 412–421). Blackwell Publishing.

Miles, B. L., Van Simaeys, K., Whitecotton, M., & Simons, C. T. (2018). Comparative tactile sensitivity of the fingertip and apical tongue using complex and pure tactile tasks. *Physiology & Behavior, 194*, 515–521.

Millard, S. K., Edwards, S., & Cook, F. M. (2009). Parent-child interaction therapy: Adding to the evidence. *International Journal of Speech-Language Pathology, 11*(1), 61–76. https://doi.org/10.1080/17549500802603895

Millard, S. K., Zebrowski, P., & Kelman, E. (2018). Palin parent–child interaction therapy: The bigger picture. *American Journal of Speech-Language Pathology, 27*(3S), 1211–1223. https://doi.org/10.1044/2018_AJSLP-ODC11-17-0199

Miller, G. A. (1956). The magical number seven, plus or minus two: Some limits on our capacity for processing information. *Psychological Review, 63*, 81–97.

Miller, G. (1977). *Spontaneous apprentices: Children and language*. Seabury Press.

Miller, J. L. (1994). On the internal structure of phonetic categories: A progress report. *Cognition, 50*(1-3), 271–285. https://doi.org/10.1016/0010-0277(94)90031-0

Miller N. (2013). Measuring up to speech intelligibility. *International Journal of Language & Communication Disorders, 48*(6), 601–612. https://doi.org/10.1111/1460-6984.12061

Mills, N., Geddes, D. T., Amirapu, S., & Mirjalili, S. A. (2020). Understanding the lingual frenulum: Histological structure, tissue composition, and implications for tongue tie surgery. *International Journal of Otolaryngology*, 1820978. https://doi.org/10.1155/2020/1820978

Mills, N., Pransky, S. M., Geddes, D. T., & Mirjalili, S. A. (2019). What is a tongue tie? Defining the anatomy of the in-situ lingual frenulum. *Clinical Anatomy, 32*(6), 749–761. https://doi.org/10.1002/ca.23343

Mirahadi, S. S., Nitsche, M. A., Pahlavanzadeh, B., Mohamadi, R., Ashayeri, H., & Abolghasemi, J. (2022). Reading and phonological awareness improvement accomplished by transcranial direct current stimulation combined with phonological awareness training: A randomized controlled trial. *Applied Neuropsychology: Child, 12*(2) 137–149.

Mishra, A., Ceballos, V., Himmelwright, K., McCabe, S., & Scott, L. (2021). Gesture production in toddlers with autism spectrum disorder. *Journal of Autism and Developmental Disorders, 51*, 1658–1667. https://doi.org/10.1007/s10803-020-04647-5

Missiuna, C., Gaines, B. R., & Pollock, N. (2002). Recognizing and referring children at risk for developmental coordination disorder: Role of the speech-language pathologist. *Journal of Speech-Language Pathology and Audiology, 26*(4), 172–179.

Mitchell, R. B., Call, E., & Kelly, J. (2003). Diagnosis and therapy for airway obstruction in children With Down syndrome. *Archives of Otolaryngology-Head and Neck Surgery, 129*(6), 642–645. https://doi.org/10.1001/archotol.129.6.642

Mo, Y., Cole, J., & Hasegawa-Johnson, M. (2009). Prosodic effects on vowel production: Evidence from formant structure. In H. Terband, F. V. Brenk, P. V. Lieshout, L. Nijland, & B. A, Maassen (Eds.), *Proceedings of the 10th Annual Conference of the International Speech Communication Association, Interspeech 2009*, 2483–2486. ISCA, printed by Curran Associates.

Moayedi, Y., Michlig, S., Park, M., Koch, A., & Lumpkin, E. A. (2021). Somatosensory innervation of healthy human oral tissues. *Journal of Comparative Neurology, 529*(11), 3046–3061. https://doi.org/10.1002/cne.25148

Mody, M., & Belliveau, J. W. (2013). Speech and language impairments in autism: Insights from behavior and neuroimaging. *North American Journal of Medicine & Science, 5*(3), 157. https://doi.org/10.7156/v5i3p157

Moeller, M. P., Thomas, A. E., Oleson, J., & Ambrose, S. E. (2019). Validation of a parent report tool for monitoring early vocal stages in infants. *Journal of Speech, Language, and Hearing Research, 62*(7), 2245–2257. https://doi.org/10.1044/2019_JSLHR-S-18-0485

Moffitt, J. M., Ahn, Y. A., Custode, S., Tao, Y., Mathew, E., Parlade, M., . . . Messinger, D. S. (2022). Objective measurement of vocalizations in the assessment of autism spectrum disorder symptoms in preschool age children. *Autism Research, 15*(9), 1665–1674. https://doi.org/10.1002/aur.2731

Mogren, Å., McAllister, A., & Sjögreen, L. (2022). Range of motion (ROM) in the lips and jaw during vowels assessed with 3D motion analysis in Swedish children with typical speech development and children with speech sound disorders. *Logopedics Phoniatrics Vocology, 47*(4), 219–229. https://doi.org/10.1080/14015439.2021.1890207

Mogren, Å., Sjögreen, L., Barr Agholme, M., & McAllister, A. (2020). Orofacial function in children with Speech Sound Disorders persisting after the age of six years. *International Journal of Speech-Language Pathology,*

22(5), 526–536. https://doi.org/10.1080/17549507.2019.1701081

Mohammed, D., Park, V., Bogaardt, H., & Docking, K. (2021). The impact of childhood obstructive sleep apnea on speech and oral language development: A systematic review. *Sleep Medicine, 81*, 144–153. https://doi.org/10.1016/j.sleep.2021.02.015

Molemans, I., van den Berg, R., Van Severen, L., & Gillis, S. (2012). How to measure the onset of babbling reliably? *Journal of Child Language, 39*(3), 523–552, 10.1017/s0305000911000171\

Molini-Avejonas, D. R., Ferreira, L. V., & de La Higuera Amato, C. A. (2017). Risk factors for speech-language pathologies in children. In F. D. M. Fernandes (Ed.), *Advances in speech-language pathology*. IntechOpen. https://doi.org/10.5772/intechopen.70107

Mondal, N., Bhat, B. V., Plakkal, N., Thulasingam, M., Ajayan, P., & Poorna, D. R. (2016). Prevalence and risk factors of speech and language delay in children less than three years of age. *Journal of Comprehensive Pediatrics*, *7*(2), e33173. https://doi.org/10.17795/compreped-33173

Monk, C. (2008). The development of emotion–related neural circuitry in health and psychopathology. *Development and Psychopathology*, *20*(4), 1231–1250. https://doi.org/10.1017/S095457940800059X

Monnier, P. (2011). Applied surgical anatomy of the larynx and trachea. In P. Monnier (Ed.), *Pediatric airway surgery* (pp. 7–29). Springer. https://doi.org/10.1007/978-3-642-13535-4_2

Montgomery, J. W. (2004). Sentence comprehension in children with specific language impairment: Effects of input rate and phonological working memory. *International Journal of Language and Communication Disorders, 39*(1) 115–133. https://doi.org/10.1080/13682820310001616985

Moore, D. R., Zobay, O., & Ferguson, M. A. (2020). Minimal and mild hearing loss in children: Association with auditory perception, cognition, and communication problems. *Ear and Hearing, 41*(4), 720. https://doi.org/10.1097/AUD.0000000000000802

Moore, D. R., Cowan, J. A., Riley, A., Edmondson-Jones, A. M., & Ferguson, M. A. (2011). Development of auditory processing in 6-to 11-yr-old children. *Ear and Hearing*, *32*(3), 269–285. https://doi.org/10.1097/AUD.0b013e318201c468

Moore, J. K., & Linthicum Jr, F. H. (2007). The human auditory system: A timeline of development. *International Journal of Audiology*, *46*(9), 460–478. https://doi.org/10.1080/14992020701383019

Moore, M. W., Tompkins, C. A., & Dollaghan, C. A. (2010). Manipulating articulatory demands in non-word repetition: A 'late-8' non-word repetition task. *Clinical Linguistics & Phonetics*, *24*(12), 997–1008. https://doi.org/10.3109/02699206.2010.510917

Morgan, A. T., & Liégeois, F. (2010). Re-thinking diagnostic classification of the dysarthrias: A developmental perspective. *Folia Phoniatrica et Logopaedica, 62*(3), 120–126. https://doi.org/10.1159/000287210

Morgan, A. T., & Vogel, A. P. (2008). Intervention for dysarthria associated with acquired brain injury in children and adolescents. *Cochrane Database of Systematic Reviews*, (3). https://doi.org/10.1002/14651858.CD006279.pub2

Morgan, A. T., Murray, E., & Liégeois, F. J. (2018). Interventions for childhood apraxia of speech. *Cochrane Database of Systematic Reviews, 5*(5).

Morgan, A. T., Su, M., Reilly, S., Conti-Ramsden, G., Connelly, A., & Liégeois, F. J. (2018). A brain marker for developmental speech disorders. *The Journal of Pediatrics*, *198*, 234–239. https://doi.org/10.1016/j.jpeds.2018.02.043

Morgan, L., & Wren, Y. E. (2018). A systematic review of the literature on early vocalizations and babbling patterns in young children. *Communication Disorders Quarterly*, *40*(1), 3–14. https://doi.org/10.1177/1525740118760215

Moriarty, B. C., & Gillon, G. T. (2006). Phonological awareness intervention for children with childhood apraxia of speech. *International Journal of Language & Communication Disorders*, *41*(6), 713–734. https://doi.org/10.1080/13682820600623960

Morin, A., & Racy, F. (2022). Frequency, content, and functions of self–reported inner speech in young adults: A synthesis. In *Inner speech, culture & education* (pp. 147–170). Springer. https://doi.org/10.1007/978–3–031–14212–3_9

Moritz Jr., J., Turk, P., Williams, J. D., & Stone-Roy, L. M. (2017). Perceived intensity and discrimination ability for lingual electrotactile stimulation depends on location and orientation of electrodes. *Frontiers in Human Neuroscience, 11*, 186.

Morningstar, M., Garcia, D., Dirks, M. A., & Bagner, D. M. (2019). Changes in parental prosody mediate effect of parent-training intervention on infant language production. *Journal of Consulting and Clinical Psychology, 87*(3), 313. https://doi.org/10.1037/ccp0000375

Morris, S. R. (2010). Clinical application of the mean babbling level and syllable structure level. *Language, Speech, and Hearing Services in Schools, 41*(2), 223–230. https://doi.org/10.1044/0161-1461(2009/08-0076)

Morris, S. R., & Wilcox, K. A. (1999). *The Children's Speech Intelligibility Measure*. Psychological Corp.

Morris, S. R., Wilcox, K. A., & Schooling, T. L. (1995). The preschool speech intelligibility measure. *American Journal of Speech-Language Pathology, 4*(4), 22–28. https://doi.org/10.1044/1058-0360.0404.22

Morrison, J. A., & Shriberg, L. D. (1992). Articulation testing versus conversational speech sampling. *Journal of Speech, Language, and Hearing Research, 35*(2), 259–273. https://doi.org/10.1044/jshr.3502.259

Morrow, E. L., & Duff, M. C. (2020). Sleep supports memory and learning: Implications for clinical practice in speech-language pathology. *American Journal of Speech-Language Pathology, 29*(2), 577–585. https://doi.org/10.1044/2019_AJSLP-19-00125

Morton, S. U., Christodoulou, J., Costain, G., Muntoni, F., Wakeling, E., Wojcik, M. H., . . . Agrawal, P. B. (2022). Multicenter consensus approach to evaluation of neonatal hypotonia in the genomic era: A review. *JAMA Neurology, 79*(4), 405–413. https://doi.org/10.1001/jamaneurol.2022.0067

Moss, M. L. (1962). The functional matrix. In B. Kraus & R. Reidel (Eds.), *Vistas in orthodontics* (pp. 85–98). Lea and Febiger.

Moss, M. L. (1963). The primacy of functional matrices on orofacial growth. *Dental Practice, 19*, 65–73.

Moss, M. (1968). A theoretical analysis of the functional matrix. *Acta Biotheoretica, 18*, 195–202.

Moss, M. L. (1997a). The functional matrix hypothesis revisited. 1. The role of mechanotransduction. *American Journal of Orthodontics and Dentofacial Orthopedics, 112*, 8–11.

Moss, M. L. (1997b). The functional matrix hypothesis revisited. 2. The role of an osseous connected cellular network. *American Journal of Orthodontics and Dentofacial Orthopedics, 112*, 221–226.

Moss, M. L. (1997c). The functional matrix hypothesis revisited. 3. The genomic thesis. *American Journal of Orthodontics and Dentofacial Orthopedics, 112*, 338–342.

Moss, M. L. (1997d). The functional matrix hypothesis revisited. 4. The epigenetic antithesis and the resolving synthesis. *American Journal of Orthodontics and Dentofacial Orthopedics, 112*, 410–417.

Most, T., & Aviner, C. (2009). Auditory, visual, and auditory–visual perception of emotions by individuals with cochlear implants, hearing aids, and normal hearing. *Journal of Deaf Studies and Deaf Education, 14*(4), 449–464. https://doi.org/10.1093/deafed/enp007

Mou, Z., Teng, W., Ouyang, H., Chen, Y., Liu, Y., Jiang, C., . . . Chen, Z. (2019). Quantitative analysis of vowel production in cerebral palsy children with dysarthria. *Journal of Clinical Neuroscience, 66*, 77–82. https://doi.org/10.1016/j.jocn.2019.05.020

Mountford, H. S., Braden, R., Newbury, D. F., & Morgan, A. T. (2022). The genetic and molecular basis of developmental language disorder: A review. *Children, 9*(5), 586. https://doi.org/10.3390/children9050586

Mousavi, N., Nitsche, M. A., Jahan, A., Nazari, M. A., & Hassanpour, H. (2022). Efficacy of transcranial Direct Current Stimulation (tDCS) combined with intensive speech therapy for language production in monozygotic twins with corpus callosum dysgenesis (CCD): A sham-controlled single subject study. *Neurocase, 28*(2), 218–225.

Mowrey, R. & MacKay, I. (1990). Phonological primitives: electro–myographic speech error evidence. *Journal of the Acoustical Society of America, 88*(3), 1299–1312. https://doi.org/10.1121/1.399706

Moyse, K., Enderby, P., Chadd, K., Gadhok, K., Bedwell, M., & Guest, P. (2020). Outcome measurement in speech and language therapy: A digital journey. *BMJ Health & Care Informatics, 27*(1) e100085. https://doi.org/10.1136/bmjhci-2019-100085

Mulder, T. (2007). Motor imagery and action observation: Cognitive tools for rehabilitation.

Journal of Neural Transmission, *114*, 1265–1278. https://doi.org/10.1007/s00702-007-0763-z

Mullen, R., & Schooling, T. (2010) The National Outcomes Measurement System for pediatric speech-language pathology. *Language, Speech, and Hearing Services in Schools*, *41*(1), 44–60. https://doi.org/10.1044/0161-1461(2009/08-0051)

Müller, N. (2017). Different sources of delay and acceleration in early child bilingualism. *Zeitschrift für Sprachwissenschaft*, *36*(1), 7–30. https://doi.org/10.1515/zfs-2017-0002

Multani, I., Manji, J., Hastings-Ison, T., Khot, A., & Graham, K. (2019). Botulinum toxin in the management of children with cerebral palsy. *Pediatric Drugs*, *21*(4), 261–281. https://doi.org/10.1007/s40272-019-00358-2

Mulvihill, A., Carroll, A., Dux, P. E., & Matthews, N. (2020). Self-directed speech and self-regulation in childhood neurodevelopmental disorders: current findings and future directions. *Development and Psychopathology*, *32*(1), 205–217. https://doi.org/10.1017/S0954579418001670

Mummolo, S., Quinzi, V., Dedola, A., Albani, F., Marzo, G., & Campanella, V. (2020). Oral microbiota in mouth-breathing patients. *Journal of Oral Hygiene & Health*, *8*(2), 2–6, 1000259.

Muñoz, I. C. L., & Orta, P. B. (2014). Comparison of cephalometric patterns in mouth breathing and nose breathing children. *International Journal of Pediatric Otorhinolaryngology*, *78*(7), 1167–1172. https://doi.org/10.1016/j.ijporl.2014.04.046

Munro, M. J. & Derwing, T. M. (1995). Foreign accent, comprehensibility and intelligibility in the speech of second language learners. *Language Learning*, *45*, 73–97. https://doi.org/10.1111/j.1467-1770.1995.tb00963.x

Munson, B., Edwards, J., & Beckman, M. E. (2005). Relationships between nonword repetition accuracy and other measures of linguistic development in children with phonological disorders. *Journal of Speech, Language, and Hearing Research*, *48*(1), 61–78. https://doi.org/10.1044/1092-4388(2005/006)

Munson, B., Schellinger, S. K., & Carlson, K. U. (2012). Measuring speech-sound learning using visual analog scaling. *Perspectives on Language Learning and Education*, *19*(1), 19–30. https://doi.org/10.1044/lle19.1.19

Munson, B., Edwards, J., Schellinger, S. K., Beckman, M. E., & Meyer, M. K. (2010). Deconstructing phonetic transcription: Covert contrast, perceptual bias, and an extraterrestrial view of Vox Humana. *Clinical Linguistics & Phonetics*, *24*(4-5), 245–260. https://doi.org/10.3109/02699200903532524

Munzert, J., Lorey, B., & Zentgraf, K. (2009). Cognitive motor processes: the role of motor imagery in the study of motor representations. *Brain Research Reviews*, *60*(2), 306–326. https://doi.org/10.1016/j.brainresrev.2008.12.024

Murillo-Rincón. A. P., & Kaucka, M. (2020). Insights into the complexity of craniofacial development from a cellular perspective. *Frontiers in Cell and Developmental Biology*, *8*, 620735. https://www.frontiersin.org/articles/10.3389/fcell.2020.620735

Murray, E. S. H., & Chao, A. (2021). The relationships among vocal variability, vocal-articulatory coordination, and dysphonia in children. *Journal of Voice*. https://doi.org/10.1016/j.jvoice.2021.06.008

Murray, E., McCabe, P., & Ballard, K. J. (2014). A systematic review of treatment outcomes for children with childhood apraxia of speech. *American Journal of Speech-Language Pathology*, *23*(3), 486–504. https://doi.org/10.1044/2014_AJSLP-13-0035

Murray, E., McCabe, P., & Ballard, K. J. (2015). A randomized controlled trial for children with childhood apraxia of speech comparing rapid syllable transition treatment and the Nuffield Dyspraxia Programme–Third Edition. *Journal of Speech, Language, and Hearing Research*, *58*(3), 669–686. https://doi.org/10.1044/2015_JSLHR-S-13-0179

Murray, E., McCabe, P., Heard, R., & Ballard, K. J. (2015). Differential diagnosis of children with suspected childhood apraxia of speech. *Journal of Speech, Language, and Hearing Research*, *58*(1), 43–60. https:/doi.org/10.1044/2014_JSLHR-S-12-0358

Murray, E., Iuzzini-Seigel, J., Maas, E., Terband, H., & Ballard, K. J. (2021). Differential diagnosis of childhood apraxia of speech compared to other speech sound disorders: A systematic review. *American Journal of Speech-Language Pathology*, *30*(1), 279–300. https://doi.org/10.1044/2020_AJSLP-20-00063

Murray, E., Velleman, S., Preston, J., Heard, R., Shibu, A., & McCabe, P. (in press). The reliability of expert diagnosis of Childhood Apraxia of Speech. *Journal of Speech, Language, and Hearing Research*.

Myers, B. R., Lense, M. D., & Gordon, R. L. (2019). Pushing the envelope: Developments in neural entrainment to speech and the biological underpinnings of prosody perception. *Brain Sciences*, *9*(3), 70. https://doi.org/10.3390/brainsci9030070

Nagle, C. L., & Huensch, A. (2020). Expanding the scope of L2 intelligibility research: Intelligibility, comprehensibility, and accentedness in L2 Spanish. *Journal of Second Language Pronunciation*, *6*(3), 329–351. https://doi.org/10.1075/jslp.20009.nag

Nagle, K. F., & Eadie, T. L. (2018). Perceived listener effort as an outcome measure for disordered speech. *Journal of Communication Disorders*, *73*, 34–49. https://doi.org/10.1016/j.jcomdis.2018.03.003

Naidu, P., Yao, C. A., Chong, D. K., & Magee III, W. P. (2022). Cleft palate repair: A history of techniques and variations. *Plastic and Reconstructive Surgery Global Open*, *10*(3). https://doi.org/10.1097/GOX.0000000000004019

Nair, V. K., Farah, W., & Cushing, I. (2023). A critical analysis of standardized testing in speech and language therapy. *Language, Speech, and Hearing Services in Schools*, 1–13. Advance online publication. https://doi.org/10.1044/2023_LSHSS-22-00141

Nakai, Y., Takashima, R., Takiguchi, T., & Takada, S. (2014). Speech intonation in children with autism spectrum disorder. *Brain and Development*, *36*(6), 516–522. https://doi.org/10.1016/j.braindev.2013.07.006

Nam, H. W., Ahn, J. B., & Kwon, D. H. (2006). Diadochokinetic characteristics in the subjects with spastic cerebral palsy by severity: In terms of rate, regularity, accuracy and consistency. *MALSORI–Journal of the Phonetic Society of Korea*, 58, 1–18.

Namasivayam, A. K., & Van Lieshout, P. (2011). Speech motor skill and stuttering. *Journal of Motor Behavior*, *43*(6), 477–489. https://doi.org/10.1080/00222895.2011.628347

Namasivayam, A. K., Coleman, D., O'Dwyer, A., & Van Lieshout, P. (2020). Speech sound disorders in children: An articulatory phonology perspective. *Frontiers in Psychology*, *10*, 2998. https://doi.org/10.3389/fpsyg.2019.02998

Namasivayam, A. K., Huynh, A., Granata, F., Law, V., & van Lieshout, P. (2021). PROMPT intervention for children with severe speech motor delay: a randomized control trial. *Pediatric Research*, *89*, 613–621. https://doi.org/10.1038/s41390-020-0924-4

Namasivayam, A. K., Pukonen, M., Goshulak, D., Granata, F., Le, D. J., Kroll, R., & van Lieshout, P. (2019). Investigating intervention dose frequency for children with speech sound disorders and motor speech involvement. *International Journal of Language & Communication Disorders*, *54*(4), 673–686.

Namasivayam, A., Pukonen, M., Hard, J., Jahnke, R., Kearney, E., Kroll, R., & van Lieshout, P. (2015). Motor speech treatment protocol for developmental motor speech disorders. *Developmental Neurorehabilitation*, *18*(5), 296–303. https://doi.org/10.3109/17518423.2013.832431

Namasivayam, A. K., Huynh, A., Bali, R., Granata, F., Law, V., Rampersaud, D., . . . Hayden, D. (2021). Development and validation of a probe word list to assess speech motor skills in children. *American Journal of Speech-Language Pathology*, *30*(2), 622–648. https://doi.org/10.1044/2020_AJSLP-20-00139

Namasivayam, A. K., Pukonen, M., Goshulak, D., Vickie, Y. Y., Kadis, D. S., Kroll, R., . . . Luc, F. (2013). Relationship between speech motor control and speech intelligibility in children with speech sound disorders. *Journal of Communication Disorders*, *46*(3), 264–280. https://doi.org/10.1016/j.jcomdis.2013.02.003

Närhi, V., Ahonen, T., Aro, M., Leppäsaari, T., Korhonen, T. T., Tolvanen, A., & Lyytinen, H. (2005). Rapid serial naming: Relations between different stimuli and neuropsychological factors. *Brain and Language*, *92*(1), 45–57. https://doi.org/10.1016/j.bandl.2004.05.004

Nathani, S., Ertmer, D. J., & Stark, R. E. (2006). Assessing vocal development in infants and toddlers. *Clinical Linguistics & Phonetics*, *20*(5), 351–369. https://doi.org/10.1080/02699200500211451

Nathani, S., Oller, D. K., & Cobo-Lewis, A. (2003). Final syllable lengthening (FSL) in infant vocalizations. *Journal of Child Language*, *30*, 3–25. https://doi.org/10.1017/S0305000902005433

National Organization for Rare Disorders. (NORD). *Functional neurological disorder*. https://rarediseases.org/rare-diseases/fnd/

Neil, N., & Jones, E. A. (2018). Communication intervention for individuals with Down syndrome: Systematic review and meta-analysis. *Developmental Neurorehabilitation*, *21*(1), 1–12. https://doi.org/10.1080/17518423.2016.1212947

Neilson, P. D., & O'Dwyer, N. J. (1981). Pathophysiology of dysarthria in cerebral palsy. *Journal of Neurology, Neurosurgery & Psychiatry*, *44*(11), 1013–1019.

Neilson, P. D., & O'Dwyer, N. J. (1984). Reproducibility and variability of speech muscle activity in athetoid dysarthria of cerebral palsy. *Journal of Speech, Language, and Hearing Research*, *27*(4), 502–517. https://doi.org/10.1044/jshr.2704.502

Nelson III, C. A., & Gabard-Durnam, L. J. (2020). Early adversity and critical periods: Neurodevelopmental consequences of violating the expectable environment. *Trends in Neurosciences*, *43*(3), 133–143. https://doi.org/10.1016/j.tins.2020.01.002

Nelson, N. W. (1976). Comprehension of spoken language by normal children as a function of speaking rate, sentence difficulty, and listener age and sex. *Child Development*, *47*(1), 299–303. https://doi.org/10.2307/1128319

Nespor, M. & I. Vogel (1986). *Prosodic phonology*. Foris.

Netsell, R. (1982). Speech motor control and selected neurologic disorders. In S. Grillner, B. Lindblom, J. Lubker, & A. Persson (Eds.), *Speech motor control* (pp. 247–261). Pergamon Press.

Netsell, R. (1983). Speech motor control: Theoretical issues with clinical impact. In W. Barry (Ed.), *Clinical dysarthria* (pp. 1–19). College-Hill.

Netsell, R., & Hixon, T. J. (1978). A noninvasive method for clinically estimating subglottal air pressure. *Journal of Speech and Hearing Disorders*, *43*, 326–330. https://doi.org/10.1044/jshd.4303.326

Netsell, R., Lotz, W., Peters, J. E., & Schulte, L. (1994). Developmental patterns of laryngeal and respiratory function for speech production. *Journal of Voice*, *8*, 123–131. https://doi.org/10.1016/S0892-1997(05)80304-2

Neumann, K., Euler, H. A., Bosshardt, H. G., Cook, S., Sandrieser, P., & Sommer, M. (2017). The pathogenesis, assessment and treatment of speech fluency disorders. *Deutsches Ärzteblatt International*, *114*(22–23), 383. https://doi.org/10.3238/arztebl.2017.0383

Neumann, S., & Romonath, R. (2012). Effectiveness of nasopharyngoscopic biofeedback in clients with cleft palate speech—A systematic review. *Logopedics Phoniatrics Vocology*, *37*(3), 95–106.

Neves, L., Martins, M., Correia, A. I., Castro, S. L., & Lima, C. F. (2021). Associations between vocal emotion recognition and socio-emotional adjustment in children. *Royal Society Open Science*, *8*(11), 211412. https://doi.org/10.1098/rsos.211412

Newbury, D. F., & Monaco, A. P. (2010). Genetic advances in the study of speech and language disorders. *Neuron*, *68*(2), 309–320. https://doi.org/10.1016/j.neuron.2010.10.001

Ng, W. L., McCabe, P., Heard, R., Park, V., Murray, E., & Thomas, D. (2022). Predicting treatment outcomes in Rapid Syllable Transition Treatment: An individual participant data meta-analysis. *Journal of Speech, Language, and Hearing Research*, *65*(5), 1784–1799. https://doi.org/10.1044/2022_JSLHR-21-00617

Ngerncham, S., Laohapensang, M., Wongvisutdhi, T., Ritjaroen, Y., Painpichan, N., Hakularb, P., . . . Chaturapitphothong, P. (2013). Lingual frenulum and effect on breastfeeding in Thai newborn infants. *Paediatrics and International Child Health*, *33*(2), 86–90. https://doi.org/10.1179/2046905512Y.0000000023

Nguyen, T. V., McCracken, J., Ducharme, S., Botteron, K. N., Mahabir, M., Johnson, W., . . . Brain Development Cooperative Group. (2013). Testosterone-related cortical maturation across childhood and adolescence. *Cerebral Cortex*, *23*(6), 1424–1432. https://doi.org/10.1093/cercor/bhs125

Nickel, J. C., Iwasaki, L. R., Gonzalez, Y. M., Gallo, L. M., & Yao, H. (2018). Mechanobehavior and ontogenesis of the temporomandibular joint. *Journal of Dental Research*, *97*(11), 1185–1192. https://doi.org/10.1177/0022034518786469

Nightingale, E., Yoon, P., Wolter-Warmerdam, K., Daniels, D., & Hickey, F. (2017). Understanding hearing and hearing loss in children with Down syndrome. *American Journal of Audiology*, *26*(3), 301–308. https://doi.org/10.1044/2017_AJA-17-0010

Nijland, L., Maassen, B., Meulen, S. V. D., Gabreëls, F., Kraaimaat, F. W., & Schreuder, R. (2002). Coarticulation patterns in children with developmental apraxia of speech. *Clinical Linguistics & Phonetics*, *16*(6), 461–483. https://doi.org/10.1080/02699200210159103

Nip, I. S. B. (2013). Kinematic characteristics of speaking rate in individuals with cerebral palsy: A preliminary study. *Journal of Medical Speech-Language Pathology, 20*(4), 88–94.

Nip, I. S., & Garellek, M. (2021). Voice quality of children with cerebral palsy. *Journal of Speech, Language, and Hearing Research, 64*(8), 3051–3059. https://doi.org/10.1044/2021_JSLHR-20-00633

Nissen, S. L., & Fox, R. A. (2005). Acoustic and spectral characteristics of young children's fricative productions: A developmental perspective. *The Journal of the Acoustical Society of America, 118*, 2570–2578. https://doi.org/10.1044/1092-4388(2005/052)

Nita, L. M., Battlehner, C. N., Ferreira, M. A., Imamura, R., Sennes, L. U., Caldini, E. G., & Tsuji, D. H. (2009). The presence of a vocal ligament in fetuses: A histochemical and ultrastructural study. *Journal of Anatomy, 215*, 692–697.

Nittrouer, S. (1995). Children learn separate aspects of speech production at different rates: Evidence from spectral moments. *The Journal of the Acoustical Society of America, 97*(1), 520–530. https://doi.org/10.1121/1.2010407

Noel, A., Manikandan, M., & Kumar, P. (2023). Efficacy of auditory verbal therapy in children with cochlear implantation based on auditory performance—A systematic review. *Cochlear Implants International, 24*(1), 43–53. https://doi.org/10.1080/14670100.2022.2141418

Nogami, Y., Saitoh, I., Inada, E., Murakami, D., Iwase, Y., Kubota, N., . . . Kaihara, Y. (2021). Prevalence of an incompetent lip seal during growth periods throughout Japan: A large-scale, survey-based, cross-sectional study. *Environmental Health and Preventive Medicine, 26*(1), 1–9. https://doi.org/10.1186/s12199-021-00933-5

Noiray, A., Abakarova, D., Rubertus, E., Krüger S. & Tiede M. (2018). How do children organize their speech in the first years of life? Insight from ultrasound imaging. *Journal of Speech, Language, and Hearing Research, 61*(6), 1355–1368. https://doi.org/10.1044/2018_JSLHR-S-17-0148

Noris, A., Zicca, A., Lenge, M., Picetti, E., Zanaboni, C., Rossi, S., & Giordano, F. (2021). The medical therapy for cerebellar mutism syndrome: A case report and literature review. *Child's Nervous System, 37*(9), 2727–2734. https://doi.org/10.1007/s00381-021-05233-5

Norton, A., Zipse, L., Marchina, S., & Schlaug, G. (2009). Melodic intonation therapy: Shared insights on how it is done and why it might help. *Annals of the New York Academy of Sciences, 1169*, 431–436. https://doi.org/10.1111/j.1749-6632.2009.04859.x

Norton, E. S., & Wolf, M. (2012). Rapid automatized naming (RAN) and reading fluency: Implications for understanding and treatment of reading disabilities. *Annual Review of Psychology, 63, 427*–452. https://doi.org/10.1146/annurev-psych-120710-100431

Novak, A. (1972). The voice of children with Down's syndrome. *Folia Phoniatrica (Basel), 24*, 182–194. https://doi.org/10.1159/000263566

Nuckton, T. J., Glidden, D. V., Browner, W. S., & Claman, D. M. (2006). Physical examination: Mallampati score as an independent predictor of obstructive sleep apnea. *Sleep, 29*(7), 903–908. https://doi.org/10.1093/sleep/29.7.903

Nyman, A., Strömbergsson, S., & Lohmander, A. (2021). Canonical babbling ratio–Concurrent and predictive evaluation of the 0.15 criterion. *Journal of Communication Disorders, 94*, 106164. https://doi.org/10.1016/j.jcomdis.2021.106164

Oberklaid, F., & Drever, K. (2011). Is my child normal? Milestones and red flags for referral. *Australian Family Physician, 40*(9), 666–670.

O'Brien, A. M., Perrachione, T. K., Weil, L. W., Araujo, Y. S., Halverson, K., Harris, A., . . . Qi, Z. (2022). Altered engagement of the speech motor network is associated with reduced phonological working memory in autism. *NeuroImage: Clinical*, 103299. https://doi.org/10.1016/j.nicl.2022.103299

Oetting, J. B., Gregory, K. D., & Rivière, A. M. (2016). Changing how speech-language pathologists think and talk about dialect variation. *Perspectives of the ASHA Special Interest Groups, 1*(16), 28–37. https://doi.org/10.1044/persp1.SIG16.28

O'Farrell, C., McCabe, P., Purcell, A., & Heard, R. (2022). The adult perceptual limen of syllable segregation in typically developing paediatric speech. *Frontiers in Communication*, 7, 61. https://doi.org/10.3389/fcomm.2022.839415

Oganian, Y., & Chang, E. F. (2019). A speech envelope landmark for syllable encoding in human superior temporal gyrus. *Science Advances, 5*(11). https://doi.org/10.1126/sciadv.aay6279

O'Gara, M., & Wilson, K. (2007). The effects of maxillofacial surgery on speech and velopharyngeal function. *Clinics in Plastic Surgery*, *34*(3), 395–402. https://doi.org/10.1016/j.cps.2007.04.001

Ohala, J. J. (1990). There is no interface between phonology and phonetics: A personal view. *Journal of Phonetics*, *18*(2), 153–171.

Ojakangas, C. L. (2013). What brain research can tell us about accent modification. *Perspectives on Communication Disorders and Sciences in Culturally and Linguistically Diverse (CLD) Populations*, *20*(3), 101–108.

Oliveira, C., Lousada, M., & Jesus, L. (2015). The clinical practice of speech and language therapists with children with phonologically based speech sound disorders. *Child Language Teaching and Therapy*, *31*, 173–194. https://doi.org/10.1177/0265659014550420

Oller, D. K. (2000). *The emergence of the speech capacity*. Erlbaum. https://doi.org/10.4324/9781410602565

Oller, D. K., Eilers, R. E., Neal, A. R., & Schwartz, H. K. (1999). Precursors to speech in infancy: The prediction of speech and language disorders. *Journal of Communication Disorders*, *32*, 223–245.

Oller, D. K., Wieman, L. A., Doyle, W. J., & Ross, C. (1976). Infant babbling and speech. *Journal of Child Language*, *3*(1), 1–11. https://doi.org/10.1017/S0305000900001276

Oller, D. K., Buder, E. H., Ramsdell, H. L., Warlaumont, A. S., Chorna, L., & Bakeman, R. (2013). Functional flexibility of infant vocalization and the emergence of language. *Proceedings of the National Academy of Sciences*, *110*(16), 6318–6323. https://doi.org/10.1073/pnas.1300337110

Oller, D. K., Griebel, U., Iyer, S. N., Jhang, Y., Warlaumont, A. S., Dale, R., & Call, J. (2019). Language origins viewed in spontaneous and interactive vocal rates of human and bonobo infants. *Frontiers in Psychology*, *10*, 729. https://doi.org/10.3389/fpsyg.2019.00729

Oren, L., Kummer, A., & Boyce, S. (2020). Understanding nasal emission during speech production: A review of types, terminology, and causality. *The Cleft Palate-Craniofacial Journal*, *57*(1), 123–126.

Ortiz, J. A. (2021). Using nonword repetition to identify language impairment in bilingual children: A meta-analysis of diagnostic accuracy. *American Journal of Speech-Language Pathology*, *30*(5), 2275–2295. https://doi.org/10.1044/2021_AJSLP-20-00237

Osberger, M. J. (1994). Speech intelligibility of children with cochlear implants. *Volta Review*, *96*(5), 169–80.

O'Shea, J. E., Foster, J. P., O'Donnell, C. P. F., Breathnach, D., Jacobs, S. E., Todd, D. A., & Davis, P. G. (2017). Frenotomy for tongue-tie in newborn infants. *Cochrane Database of Systematic Reviews*, Issue 3. Art. No. CD011065. https://doi.org/10.1002/14651858.CD011065.pub2

Öster Cattu Alves, M., Ode, C., & Strömbergsson, S. (2020). Dealing with the unknown–addressing challenges in evaluating unintelligible speech. *Clinical Linguistics & Phonetics*, *34*(1-2), 169–184. https://doi.org/10.1080/02699206.2019.1622787

Overby, M., Belardi, K., & Schreiber, J. (2020). A retrospective video analysis of canonical babbling and volubility in infants later diagnosed with childhood apraxia of speech. *Clinical Linguistics & Phonetics*, *34*(7), 634–651. https://doi.org/10.1080/02699206.2019.1683231

Overby, M. S., Caspari, S. S., & Schreiber, J. (2019). Volubility, consonant emergence, and syllabic structure in infants and toddlers later diagnosed with childhood apraxia of speech, speech sound disorder, and typical development: A retrospective video analysis. *Journal of Speech, Language, and Hearing Research*, *62*(6), 1657–1675. https://doi.org/10.1044/2019_JSLHR-S-18-0046

Ozawa, Y., Shiromoto, O., Ishizaki, F., & Watamori, T. (2001). Symptomatic differences in decreased alternating motion rates between individuals with spastic and with ataxic dysarthria: An acoustic analysis. *Folia Phoniatrica et Logopaedica*, *53*(2), 67–72. https://doi.org/10.1159/000052656

Özçalışkan, Ş., Adamson, L. B., & Dimitrova, N. (2016). Early deictic but not other gestures predict later vocabulary in both typical development and autism. *Autism*, *20*(6), 754–763. https://doi.org/10.1177/1362361315605

Özçalışkan, Ş., Adamson, L. B., Dimitrova, N., & Baumann, S. (2017). Early gesture provides a helping hand to spoken vocabulary development for children with autism, Down syndrome, and typical development. *Journal of Cognition and Development*, *18*(3), 325–337. https://doi.org/10.1080/15248372.2017.1329735

Ozgen, H. M., Hop, J. W., Hox, J. J., Beemer, F. A., & Van Engeland, H. (2010). Minor physical anomalies in autism: a meta-analysis. *Molecular Psychiatry, 15*, 300–307.

Page, C. G., & Johnson, K. (2021). Electropalatographic therapy and speech production for children with down syndrome. *Perspectives of the American Speech-Language-Hearing Association, 6*(2), 485–493. https://doi.org/10.1044/2021_PERSP-20-00175

Pamir, Z., Canoluk, M. U., Jung, J. H., & Peli, E. (2020). Poor resolution at the back of the tongue is the bottleneck for spatial pattern recognition. *Scientific Reports, 10*(1), 1–13. https://doi.org/10.1038/s41598-020-59102-3

Pandian, G. S. B., Jain, A., Raza, Q., & Sahu, K. K. (2021). Digital health interventions (DHI) for the treatment of attention deficit hyperactivity disorder (ADHD) in children-a comparative review of literature among various treatment and DHI. *Psychiatry Research, 297*, 113742. https://doi.org/10.1016/j.psychres.2021.113742

Pang, E. W., Valica, T., MacDonald, M. J., Taylor, M. J., Brian, J., Lerch, J. P., & Anagnostou, E. (2016). Abnormal brain dynamics underlie speech production in children with autism spectrum disorder. *Autism Research, 9*(2), 249–261. https://doi.org/10.1002/aur.1526

Papaeliou, C., Minadakis, G., & Cavouras, D. (2002). Acoustic patterns of infant vocalizations expressing emotions and communicative functions. *Journal of Speech, Language, and Hearing Research, 45*(2), 311–317. https://doi.org/10.1044/1092-4388(2002/024)

Papoušek, M., Bornstein, M. H., Nuzzo, C., Papoušek, H., & Symmes, D. (1990). Infant responses to prototypical melodic contours in parental speech. *Infant Behavior and Development, 13*(4), 539–545. https://doi.org/10.1016/0163-6383(90)90022-Z

Paquier, P. F., Walsh, K. S., Docking, K. M., Hartley, H., Kumar, R., & Catsman-Berrevoets, C. E. (2020). Post-operative cerebellar mutism syndrome: Rehabilitation issues. *Child's Nervous System, 36*(6), 1215–1222. https://doi.org/10.1007/s00381-019-04229-6

Paradis, J., & Genesee, F. (1996). Syntactic acquisition in bilingual children: Autonomous or interdependent? *Studies in Second Language Acquisition, 18*(1), 1–25. https://doi.org/10.1017/S0272263100014662

Parlato-Oliveira, E., Saint-Georges, C., Cohen, D., Pellerin, H., Pereira, I. M., Fouillet, C., . . . Viaux-Savelon, S. (2021). "Motherese" prosody in fetal-directed speech: An exploratory study using automatic social signal processing. *Frontiers in Psychology, 12*, 649. https://doi.org/10.3389/fpsyg.2021.646170

Parnandi, A., Karappa, V.,Lan, T., & Shahin, M. A.(2015). Development of a remote therapy tool for childhood apraxia of speech. *ACM Transactions on Accessible Computing (TACCESS), 7*(3), 1–23. https://doi.org/10.1145/2776895

Parrell, B., Lammert, A. C., Ciccarelli, G., & Quatieri, T. F. (2019). Current models of speech motor control: A control-theoretic overview of architectures and properties. *The Journal of the Acoustical Society of America, 145*(3), 1456–1481. https://doi.org/10.1121/1.5092807

Pasman, J. W., Rotteveel, J. J., Maassen, B., & Visco, Y. M. (1999). The maturation of auditory cortical evoked responses between (preterm) birth and 14 years of age. *European Journal of Paediatric Neurology, 3*(2), 79–82.

Patel, R. R. (2018). Pediatric laryngeal endoscopic imaging: Current research and clinical implications. *Perspectives of the ASHA Special Interest Groups SIG 3*, Vol. 3(2), 34–39. https://doi.org/10.1044/persp3.SIG3.34

Patel, R., & Brayton, J. T. (2009). Identifying prosodic contrasts in utterances produced by 4-, 7-, and 11-year-old children. *Journal of Speech, Language, and Hearing Research, 52*(3), 790–801. https://doi.org/10.1044/1092-4388(2008/07-0137)

Patel, R., Connaghan, K., Franco, D., Edsall, E., Forgit, D., Olsen, L., . . . Russell, S. (2013). "The Caterpillar": A novel reading passage for assessment of motor speech disorders. *American Journal of Speech-Language Pathology, 22*(1), 1–9. https://doi.org/10.1044/1058-0360(2012/11-0134)

Patel, S. P., Kim, J. H., Larson, C. R., & Losh, M. (2019). Mechanisms of voice control related to prosody in autism spectrum disorder and first-degree relatives. *Autism Research, 12*(8), 1192–1210. https://doi.org/10.1002/aur.2156

Patel, S. P., Cole, J., Lau, J. C., Fragnito, G., & Losh, M. (2022). Verbal entrainment in autism spectrum disorder and first-degree relatives. *Scientific Reports, 12*(1), 11496. https://doi.org/10.1038/s41598-022-12945-4

Patel, S. P., Nayar, K., Martin, G. E., Franich, K., Crawford, S., Diehl, J. J., & Losh, M. (2020). An acoustic characterization of prosodic differences in autism spectrum disorder and first-degree relatives. *Journal of Autism and Developmental Disorders*, *50*(8), 3032–3045. https://doi.org/10.1007/s10803-020-04392-9.

Patil, S., Rao, R. S., & Majumdar, B. (2014). Chromosomal and multifactorial genetic disorders with oral manifestations. *Journal of International Oral Health: JIOH*, *6*(5), 118.

Patkee, P. A., Baburamani, A. A., Kyriakopoulou, V., Davidson, A., Avini, E., Dimitrova, R., . . . Rutherford, M. A. (2020). Early alterations in cortical and cerebellar regional brain growth in Down Syndrome: An in vivo fetal and neonatal MRI assessment. *NeuroImage: Clinical*, *25*, 102139. https://doi.org/10.1016/j.nicl.2019.102139

Patkowski, M. (1980). The sensitive period for the acquisition of syntax in a second language. *Language Learning*, *30*, 449–472.

Patkowski, M. (1990). Age and accent in a second language: A reply to James Emil Flege, *Applied Linguistics*, *11*, 73–89.

Patten, E., Belardi, K., Baranek, G. T., Watson, L. R., Labban, J. D., & Oller, D. K. (2014). Vocal patterns in infants with autism spectrum disorder: Canonical babbling status and vocalization frequency. *Journal of Autism and Developmental Disorders*, *44*(10), 2413–2428. https://doi.org/10.1007/s10803-014-2047-4

Patton, M. H., Blundon, J. A., & Zakharenko, S. S. (2019). Rejuvenation of plasticity in the brain: opening the critical period. *Current Opinion in Neurobiology*, *54*, 83–89. https://doi.org/10.1016/j.conb.2018.09.003

Paul, R., & Jennings, P. (1992). Phonological behavior in toddlers with slow expressive language development. *Journal of Speech and Hearing Research*, *35*, 99–107. https://doi.org/10.1044/jshr.3501.99

Paul, R., Augustyn, A., Klin, A., & Volkmar, F. R. (2005). Perception and production of prosody by speakers with autism spectrum disorders. *Journal of Autism and Developmental Disorders*, *35*(2), 205–220. https://doi.org/10.1007/s10803-004-1999-1

Paus, T., Wong, A. P. Y., Syme, C., & Pausova, Z. (2017). Sex differences in the adolescent brain and body: Findings from the saguenay youth study. *Journal of Neuroscience Research*, *95*(1-2), 362–370. https://doi.org/10.1002/jnr.23825

Pawlak, M. (2021). Investigating language learning strategies: Prospects, pitfalls and challenges. *Language Teaching Research*, *25*(5), 817–835. https://doi.org/10.1177/1362168819876156

Pearson, B. Z., Velleman, S. L., Bryant, T. J., & Charko, T. (2009). Phonological milestones for African American English-speaking children learning Mainstream American English as a second dialect. *Language, Speech, and Hearing Services in Schools*, *40*(3), 229–244. https://doi.org/10.1044/0161-1461(2008/08-0064

Pebbili, G. K., Kashyap, R., Rashmi, J., Karike, A., & Navya, A. (2019). Laryngeal aerodynamic analysis of glottal valving in children with Down syndrome. *Journal of Voice*, *35*(1), 156.e15–156.e21. https://doi.org/10.1016/j.jvoice.2019.05.011

Peelle, J. E. (2018). Listening effort: How the cognitive consequences of acoustic challenge are reflected in brain and behavior. *Ear & Hearing*, *39*(2), 204–214. https://doi.org/10.1097/AUD.0000000000000494.

Peeters, C., Prescher, A., & Angerstein, W. (2019). Anatomy of the orbicularis oris muscle: A historical review. *History of Otorhinolaryngology*, *1*, 239–252.

Peña, E. D., Gutiérrez-Clellen, V. F., Iglesias, A., Goldstein, B. A., & Bedore, L. M. (2014). *BESA: Bilingual English-Spanish Assessment*. AR-Clinical Publications.

Penfield, W., & Roberts, L. (1959). *Speech and brain mechanisms*. Athenaeum.

Pennington L., & McConachie H. (1999). Mother-child interaction revisited: Communication with non-speaking physically disabled children. *International Journal of Language & Communication Disorders*, *34*, 391–416. https://doi.org/10.1080/136828299247351

Pennington L., & McConachie H (2001). Predicting patterns of interaction between children with cerebral palsy and their mothers. *Developmental Medicine and Child Neurology*, *43*, 83–90.

Pennington, L., Miller, N., Robson, S., & Steen, N. (2010). Intensive speech and language therapy for older children with cerebral palsy: A systems approach. *Developmental Medicine & Child Neurology*, *52*(4), 337–344.

Pennington, L., Rauch, R., Smith, J., & Brittain, K. (2020). Views of children with cerebral palsy and their parents on the effectiveness and acceptability of intensive speech therapy. *Disability and Rehabilitation*, *42*(20), 2935–2943. https://doi.org/10.1080/09638288.2019.1577504

Penuelas-Calvo, I., Jiang-Lin, L. K., Girela-Serrano, B., Delgado-Gomez, D., Navarro-Jimenez, R., Baca-Garcia, E., & Porras-Segovia, A. (2020). Video games for the assessment and treatment of attention-deficit/hyperactivity disorder: A systematic review. *European Child & Adolescent Psychiatry*, 1–16. https://doi.org/10.1016/j.psychres.2021.113742

Peppé, S. J. (2009). Why is prosody in speech-language pathology so difficult? *International Journal of Speech-Language Pathology, 11*(4), 258–271. https://doi.org/10.1080/17549500902906339

Peppé, S. (2015). *PEPS-C 2015*. http://www.peps-c.com/

Peppé, S., & McCann, J. (2003). Assessing intonation and prosody in children with atypical language development: The PEPS–C test and the revised version. *Clinical Linguistics & Phonetics, 17*, 345–354. https://doi.org/10.1080/0269920031000079994

Peppé, S., Cleland, J., Gibbon, F., O'Hare, A., & Castilla, P. M. (2011). Expressive prosody in children with autism spectrum conditions. *Journal of Neurolinguistics, 24*(1), 41–53. https://doi.org/10.1016/j.jneuroling.2010.07.005

Peredo, D. E., & Hannibal, M. C. (2009). The floppy infant: evaluation of hypotonia. *Pediatrics in Review, 30*(9), e66–e76. https://doi.org/10.1542/pir.30-9-e66

Perkell, J. S. (2012). Movement goals and feedback and feedforward control mechanisms in speech production. *Journal of Neurolinguistics, 25*(5), 382–407. https://doi.org/10.1016/j.jneuroling.2010.02.011

Perkell, J. S., Boyce, S. E., & Stevens, K. N. (1979). Articulatory and acoustic correlates of the [s-sh] distinction. *The Journal of the Acoustical Society of America, 65*(S1), S24. https://doi.org/10.1121/1.2017169

Perkell, J. S., Matthies, M. L., Tiede, M., Lane, H., Zandipour, M., Marrone, N., . . . Guenther, F. H. (2004). The distinctness of speakers' (s)-(sh) contrast is related to their auditory discrimination and use of an articulatory saturation effect. *Journal of Speech, Language, and Hearing Research, 47*, 1259–1269. https://doi.org/10.1044/1092-4388(2004/095)

Perkins, K., & Zhang, L. J. (2022). The effect of first language transfer on second language acquisition and learning: From contrastive analysis to contemporary neuroimaging. *RELC Journal, 0*(0). https://doi.org/10.1177/00336882221081894

Perone, S., & Simmering, V. R. (2017). Applications of dynamic systems theory to cognition and development: New frontiers. *Advances in Child Development and Behavior, 52*, 43–80. https://doi.org/10.1016/bs.acdb.2016.10.002

Perrachione, T. K., Lee, J., Ha, L. Y., & Wong, P. C. (2011). Learning a novel phonological contrast depends on interactions between individual differences and training paradigm design. *The Journal of the Acoustical Society of America, 130*(1), 461–472. https://doi.org/10.1121/1.3593366

Perrachione, T. K., Ghosh, S. S., Ostrovskaya, I., Gabrieli, J. D., & Kovelman, I. (2017). Phonological working memory for words and nonwords in cerebral cortex. *Journal of Speech, Language, and Hearing Research, 60*(7), 1959–1979. https://doi.org/10.1044/2017_JSLHR-L-15-0446.

Perry, J. L., Haenssler, A. E., Kotlarek, K. J., Fang, X., Middleton, S., Mason, R., & Kuehn, D. P. (2022). A midsagittal-view magnetic resonance imaging study of the growth and involution of the adenoid mass and related changes in selected velopharyngeal structures. *Journal of Speech, Language, and Hearing Research, 65*(4), 1282–1293. https://doi.org/10.1044/2021_JSLHR-21-00514

Peter, B., Lancaster, H., Vose, C., Middleton, K., & Stoel-Gammon, C. (2018). Sequential processing deficit as a shared persisting biomarker in dyslexia and childhood apraxia of speech. *Clinical Linguistics & Phonetics, 32*(4), 316–346. https://doi.org/10.1080/02699206.2017.1375560

Peter, B., Davis, J., Finestack, L., Stoel-Gammon, C., VanDam, M., Bruce, L., . . . Potter, N. (2022). Translating principles of precision medicine into speech-language pathology: Clinical trial of a proactive speech and language intervention for infants with classic galactosemia. *Human Genetics and Genomics Advances*, 100119. https://doi.org/10.1016/j.xhgg.2022.10011

Peterson, G. E., & Barney, H. E. (1952). Control methods used in a study of vowels. *The Journal of the Acoustical Society of America, 24*(2), 175–184. https://doi.org/10.1121/1.1906875

Peterson, L., Savarese, C., Campbell, T., Ma, Z., Simpson, K. O., & McAllister, T. (2022). telepractice treatment of residual rhotic errors using app-based biofeedback: A pilot study. *Language, Speech, and Hearing Services in*

Schools, 53(2), 256–274. https://doi.org/10.1044/2021_LSHSS-21-00084

Pettersson, S. D., Kitlinski, M., Miękisiak, G., Ali, S., Krakowiak, M., & Szmuda, T. (2021). Risk factors for postoperative cerebellar mutism syndrome in pediatric patients: a systematic review and meta-analysis. *Journal of Neurosurgery: Pediatrics, 29*(4), 467–475. https://doi.org/10.3171/2021.11.PEDS21445

Piaget, J. (1926). *The language and thought of the child.* Routledge & Kegan Paul.

Piek, J. P., & Carman, R. (1994). Developmental profiles of spontaneous movements in infants. *Early Human Development, 39*(2), 109–126. https://doi.org/10.1016/0378-3782(94)90160

Pierce, J. E., O'Halloran, R., Togher, L., & Rose, M. L. (2019). What is meant by "Multimodal Therapy" for Aphasia? *American Journal of Speech-Language Pathology, 28*(2), 706–716. https://doi.org/10.1044/2018_AJSLP-18-0157

Pigdon, L., Willmott, C., Reilly, S., Conti-Ramsden, G., Liegeois, F., Connelly, A., & Morgan, A.T. (2020). The neural basis of nonword repetition in children with developmental speech or language disorder: An fMRI study. *Neuropsychologia*, S0028–3932(19)30355. https://doi.org/https://doi.org/10.1016/j.neuropsychologia.2019.107312.

Pigdon, L., Willmott, C., Reilly, S., Conti-Ramsden, G., & Morgan, A. T. (2020). What predicts nonword repetition performance? *Child Neuropsychology, 26*(4), 518–533. https://doi.org/10.1080/09297049.2019.1674799

Pinborough-Zimmerman, J., Satterfield, R., Miller, J., Bilder, D., Hossain, S., & McMahon, W. (2007). Communication disorders: Prevalence and comorbid intellectual disability, autism, and emotional/behavioral disorders. *American Journal of Speech-Language Pathology, 16*(4), 359–367. https://doi.org/10.1044/1058-0360(2007/039)

Pinker, S. (1984). *Language learnability and language development.* Harvard University Press.

Pisanski, K., Fraccaro, P. J., Tigue, C. O'Connor, J. J. M., Röder, S., Andrews, P. W., . . . Feinberg, D. R. (2014). Vocal indicators of body size in men and women: A meta-analysis. *Animal Behavior, 95*, 89–99.

Plante, E., Holland, S. K., & Schmithorst, V. J. (2006). Prosodic processing by children: an fMRI study. *Brain & Language, 97*(3), 332–342. https://doi.org/10.1016/j.bandl.2005.12.004.

Plate, S., Yankowitz, L., Resorla, L., Swanson, M. R., Meera, S. S., Estes, A., . . . IBIS Network. (2022). Infant vocalizing and phenotypic outcomes in autism: Evidence from the first 2 years. *Child Development, 93*(2), 468–483. https://doi.org/10.1111/cdev.13697

Pleger, B., & Timmann, D. (2018). The role of the human cerebellum in linguistic prediction, word generation and verbal working memory: Evidence from brain imaging, non-invasive cerebellar stimulation and lesion studies. *Neuropsychologia, 115*, 204–210. https://doi.org/10.1016/j.neuropsychologia.2018.03.012

Plutchik, R. (1980). A general psychoevolutionary theory of emotion. In R. Plutchik & H. Kellerman (Eds.), *Emotion: Theory, research and experience, Theories of emotion, Vol. 1* (pp. 3–33). Academic Press.

Poeppel, D., & Assaneo, M. F. (2020). Speech rhythms and their neural foundations. *Nature Reviews Neuroscience*, 21(6), 322–334. https://doi.org/10.1038/s41583-020-0304-4

Pointer, N. F., van Mersbergen, M., & Nanjundeswaran, C. D. (2022). Listeners' attitudes towards young women with glottal fry. *Journal of Voice.* https://doi.org/10.1016/j.jvoice.2022.09.007

Pokorni, J. L., Worthington, C. K., & Jamison, P. J. (2004). Phonological awareness intervention: comparison of Fast ForWord, Earobics, and LiPS. *The Journal of Educational Research, 97*(3), 147–158. https://doi.org/10.3200/JOER.97.3.147-158

Polikowsky, H. G., Shaw, D. M., Petty, L. E., Chen, H. H., Pruett, D. G., Linklater, J. P., . . . Kraft, S. J. (2022). Population-based genetic effects for developmental stuttering. *Human Genetics and Genomics Advances, 3*(1), 100073. https://doi.org/10.1016/j.xhgg.2021.100073

Poljak, L. (2019). Trends in accentedness and comprehensibility research, with respect of L2 speech ratings: A literature review. *SFU Educational Review, 12*(2), 36–63. https://doi.org/10.21810/sfuer.v12i2.929

Polka, L., & Bohn, O. S. (2011). Natural Referent Vowel (NRV) framework: An emerging view of early phonetic development. *Journal of Phonetics, 39*, 467–478. https://doi.org/10.1016/j.wocn.2010.08.007

Pollock, K. E. (1991). The identification of vowel errors using traditional articulation or phonological process test stimuli. *Language, Speech, and Hearing Services in Schools*, *22*(2), 39–50. https://doi.org/10.1044/0161-1461.2202.39

Pommée, T., Balaguer, M., Mauclair, J., Pinquier, J., & Woisard, V. (2022). Intelligibility and comprehensibility: A Delphi consensus study. *International Journal of Language & Communication Disorders*, *57*. 21–41. https://doi.org/10.1111/1460-6984.12672

Pommée, T., Balaguer, M., Pinquier, J., Mauclair, J., Woisard, V., & Speyer, R. (2021). Relationship between phoneme-level spectral acoustics and speech intelligibility in healthy speech: A systematic review. *Speech, Language and Hearing*, *24*(2), 105–132. https://doi.org/10.1080/2050571X.2021.1913300

Pontecorvo, E., Higgins, M., Mora, J., Lieberman, A. M., Pyers, J., & Caselli, N. K. (2023). Learning a sign language does not hinder acquisition of a spoken language. *Journal of Speech, Language, and Hearing Research*, 66(4), 1291–1308. https://doi.org/10.1044/2022_JSLHR-22-00505

Porges, S. W. (2001). The polyvagal theory: Phylogenetic substrates of a social nervous system. *International Journal of Psychophysiology*, *42*(2), 123–146. https://doi.org/10.1016/S0167-8760(01)00162-3

Porges, S. W. (2009). The polyvagal theory: new insights into adaptive reactions of the autonomic nervous system. *Cleveland Clinic Journal of Medicine*, *76* (Suppl 2), S86–S90. https://doi.org/10.3949/ccjm.76.s2.17.

Porges, S. W., & Lewis, G. F. (2010). In S. M. Brudzynski, *The polyvagal hypothesis: Common mechanisms mediating autonomic regulation, vocalizations and listening*.

Posnick, J. C, & Kinard, B. E. (2020). Common patterns of developmental dentofacial deformities: A biologic classification system. *FACE*, *1*(2), 131–139. https://doi.org/10.1177/2732501620973032

Post, B., & Payne, E. (2018). Speech rhythm in development: What is the child acquiring? In N. Esteve-Gibert & P. Prieto (Eds.), *Prosodic development in first language acquisition* (pp. 125–144). John Benjamins. https://doi.org/10.1075/tilar.23.07pos

Postma, A. (2000). Detection of errors during speech production: A review of speech monitoring models. *Cognition*, *77*(2), 97–132. https://doi.org/10.1016/S0010-0277(00)00090-1

Potter, N. L., Kent, R. D., & Lazarus, J. C. (2009). Oral and manual force control in preschool-aged children: Is there evidence for common control? *Journal of Motor Behavior*, *41*(1), 66–82. https://doi.org/10.1080/00222895.2009.10125919.

Potter, N. L., Nievergelt, Y., & Shriberg, L. D. (2013). Motor and speech disorders in classic galactosemia. *JIMD Reports*, *11*, 31–41. https://doi.org/10.1007/8904_2013_219

Potter, N. L., Nievergelt, Y., & VanDam, M. (2019). Tongue strength in children with and without speech sound disorders. *American Journal of Speech-Language Pathology*, *28*(2), 612–622. 10.1044/2018_AJSLP-18-0023

Potter, N., & Short, R. (2009). Maximal tongue strength in typically developing children and adolescents. *Dysphagia*, *24*(4), 391–397. https://doi.org/10.1007/s00455-009-9215-2

Pouplier, M., & Hardcastle, W. (2005). A re-evaluation of the nature of speech errors in normal and disordered speakers. *Phonetica*, *62*(2–4), 227–243. https://doi.org/10.1159/000090100

Powell, T. W. (2006). A comparison of English reading passages for elicitation of speech samples from clinical populations. *Clinical Linguistics & Phonetics*, *20*, 91–97. https://doi.org/10.1080/02699200400026488

Powell, T. W., & Miccio, A. W. (1996). Stimulability: A useful clinical tool. *Journal of Communication Disorders*, *29*(4), 237–253. https://doi.org/10.1016/0021-9924(96)00012-3

Prath, S. (2016). Red flags for speech-language impairment in bilingual children: Differentiate disability from disorder by understanding common developmental milestones. *The ASHA Leader*, *21*(11), 32–33. https://doi.org/10.1044/leader.SCM.21112016.32

Prelock, P. A., Hutchins, T., & Glascoe, F. P. (2008). Speech-language impairment: How to identify the most common and least diagnosed disability of childhood. *The Medscape Journal of Medicine*, *10*(6), 136.

Preston, J. L., & Edwards, M. L. (2009). Speed and accuracy of rapid speech output by adolescents with residual speech sound errors including rhotics. *Clinical Linguistics & Phonetics*, *23*(4), 301–318. https://doi.org/10.1080/02699200802680833

Preston, J., & Edwards, M. L. (2010). Phonological awareness and types of sound errors in preschoolers with speech sound disorders.

Journal of Speech, Language, and Hearing Research, *53*(1), 44–60. https://doi.org/10.1044/1092-4388(2009/09-0021)

Preston, J. L., Hitchcock, E. R., & Leece, M. C. (2020). Auditory perception and ultrasound biofeedback treatment outcomes for children with residual /ɹ/ distortions: A randomized controlled trial. *Journal of Speech, Language, and Hearing Research*, *63*(2), 444–455. https://doi.org/10.1044/2019_JSLHR-19-00060

Preston, J. L., Hull, M., & Edwards, M. L. (2013). Preschool speech error patterns predict articulation and phonological awareness outcomes in children with histories of speech sound disorders. *American Journal of Speech-Language Pathology*, *22*(2), 173–184. https://doi.org/10.1044/1058-0360(2012/12-0022)

Preston, J. L., Leece, M. C., & Storto, J. (2019). Tutorial: Speech motor chaining treatment for school-age children with speech sound disorders. *Language, Speech, and Hearing Services in Schools*, *50*(3), 343–355. 10.1044/2018_LSHSS-18-0081

Preston, J. L., Benway, N. R., Leece, M. C., & Caballero, N. F. (2021). Concurrent validity between two sound sequencing tasks used to identify childhood apraxia of speech in school-age children. *American Journal of Speech-Language Pathology*, *30*(3S), 1580–1588. https://doi.org/10.1044/2020_AJSLP-20-00108

Preston, R., Halpin, M., Clarke, G., & Millard, S. (2022). Palin parent-child interaction therapy with children with autism spectrum disorder and stuttering. *Journal of Communication Disorders*, *97*, 106217. https://doi.org/10.1016/j.jcomdis.2022.106217

Preston, J. L., Leece, M. C., McNamara, K., & Maas, E. (2017). Variable practice to enhance speech learning in ultrasound biofeedback treatment for childhood apraxia of speech: A single case experimental study. *American Journal of Speech-Language Pathology*, *26*(3), 840–852. https://doi.org/10.1044/2017_AJSLP-16-0155

Preston, J. L., McCabe, P., Tiede, M., & Whalen, D. H. (2019). Tongue shapes for rhotics in school-age children with and without residual speech errors. *Clinical Linguistics & Phonetics*, *33*(4), 334–348. https://doi.org/10.1080/02699206.2018.1517190

Preston, J. L., Benway, N. R., Leece, M. C., Hitchcock, E. R., & McAllister, T. (2020). Tutorial: Motor-based treatment strategies for /r/ distortions. *Language, Speech, and Hearing Services in Schools*, *51*(4), 966–980. https://doi.org/10.1044/2020_LSHSS-20-00012.

Preston, J. L., Ramsdell, H. L., Oller, D. K., Edwards, M. L., & Tobin, S. J. (2011). Developing a weighted measure of speech sound accuracy. *Journal of Speech, Language, and Hearing Research*, *54*(1), 1–18. https://doi.org/10.1044/1092-4388(2010/10-0030)

Prezas, R. F., & Hodson, B. W. (2010). The cycles phonological remediation approach: Enhancing children's phonological systems. In L. Williams, S. McLeod, & R. McCauley R, (Eds.), *Interventions for speech sound disorders in children* (pp. 137–158). Brookes Publishing Company.

Price, C. N., & Moncrieff, D. (2021). Defining the role of attention in hierarchical auditory processing. *Audiology Research*, *11*(1), 112–128. https://doi.org/10.3390/audiolres11010012

Prieto, P., & Esteve-Gibert, N. (2018). *The development of prosody in first language acquisition*. John Benjamins.

Prince, A., & Smolensky, P. (2008). *Optimality theory: Constraint interaction in generative grammar*. Wiley.

Proctor, M. (2011). Towards a gestural characterization of liquids: Evidence from Spanish and Russian. *Laboratory Phonology*, *2*, 451–485.

Pruett, D. G., Shaw, D. M., Chen, H. H., Petty, L. E., Polikowsky, H. G., Kraft, S. J., . . . Below, J. E. (2021). Identifying developmental stuttering and associated comorbidities in electronic health records and creating a phenome risk classifier. *Journal of Fluency Disorders*, *68*, 105847. https://doi.org/10.1016/j.jfludis.2021.105847

Pulgram, E. (1970). *Homo Loquens*: An ecological view. *Lingua*, *24*, 309–342.

Raghavan, R., Camarata, S., White, K., Barbaresi, W., Parish, S., & Krahn, G. (2018). Population health in pediatric speech and language disorders: Available data sources and a research agenda for the field. *Journal of Speech, Language, and Hearing Research*, *61*(5), 1279–1291. https://doi.org/10.1044/2018_JSLHR-L-16-0459

Ramanarayanan, V., Lammert, A., Goldstein, L., & Narayanan, S. (2014). Are articulatory settings mechanically advantageous for speech motor control? *PLoS ONE*, *9*(8), e104168. https://doi.org/10.1371/journal.pone.0104168

Ramanarayanan, V., Lammert, A. C., Rowe, H. P., Quatieri, T. F., & Green, J. R. (2022). Speech as a biomarker: Opportunities, interpretability, and challenges. *Perspectives of the ASHA Special Interest Groups*, *7*(1), 276–283. https://doi.org/10.1044/2021_PERSP-21-00174

Ramírez-Esparza, N., García-Sierra, A., & Kuhl, P. K. (2014). Look who's talking: Speech style and social context in language input to infants are linked to concurrent and future speech development. *Developmental Science*, *17*(6), 880–891. https://doi.org/10.1111/desc.12172

Ramos, L. de A., Souza, B. O., & Gama, A. C. C. (2017). Vocal analysis in children: An integrative review. *Distúrbios da Comunicação, São Paulo*, *29*(1), 20–32. https://doi.org/10.23925/2176-2724.2017v29i1p20-32

Ramus, F., Nespor, M., & Mehler, J. (1999). Correlates of linguistic rhythm in the speech signal. *Cognition*, *73*(3), 265–292. https://doi.org/10.1016/S0010-0277(00)00101-3

Ranieri, D., Von Holzen, K., Newman, R., & Bernstein Ratner, N. (2020). Change in maternal speech rate to preverbal infants over the first two years of life. *Journal of Child Language*, *47*(6), 1263–1275. https://doi.org/10.1017/S030500091900093X

Rapin, I., and Dunn, M. (2003). Update on the language disorders of individuals on the autistic spectrum. *Brain Development*, *25*, *166*–172. https://doi.org/10.1016/S0387-7604(02)00191-2

Ratcliff, A., Coughlin, S., & Lehman, M. (2002). Factors influencing ratings of speech naturalness in augmentative and alternative communication, *Augmentative and Alternative Communication*, *18*(1), 11–19. https://doi.org/10.1080/aac.18.1.11.19

Rauschecker, J. P., & Tian, B. (2000). Mechanisms and streams for processing of "what" and "where" in auditory cortex. *Proceedings of the National Academy of Sciences*, *97*(22), 11800–11806. https://doi.org/10.1073/pnas.97.22.11800

Redford, M. A. (2014). The perceived clarity of children's speech varies as a function of their default articulation rate. *The Journal of the Acoustical Society of America*, *135*(5), 2952–2963. https://doi.org/10.1121/1.4869820

Redford, M. A. (2019). Speech production from a developmental perspective. *Journal of Speech, Language, and Hearing Research*, *62*(8S), 2946–2962. https://doi.org/10.1044/2019_JSLHR-S-CSMC7-18-0130

Redford, M., & Gildersleeve-Neumann, C. E. (2009). The development of distinct speaking styles in preschool children. *Journal of Speech, Language, and Hearing Research*, *52*(6), 1434–1448. https://doi.org/10.1044/1092-4388(2009/07-0223)

Redmond, S. (1992). The critical period hypothesis for language acquisition and it's implication for the management of communication disorders. *NSSLHA Journal*, (20), 25–31.

Reh, R. K., Dias, B. G., Nelson III, C. A., Kaufer, D., Werker, J. F., Kolb, B., . . . Hensch, T. K. (2020). Critical period regulation across multiple timescales. *Proceedings of the National Academy of Sciences*, *117*(38), 23242–23251. https://doi.org/10.1073/pnas.1820836117

Reilly, K. J., & Moore, C. A. (2009). Respiratory movement patterns during vocalizations at 7 and 11 months of age. *Journal of Speech, Language, and Hearing Research*, *52*(1), 223–239. https://doi.org/10.1044/1092-4388(2008/06-0215)

Reiter, R., Brosch, S., Wefel, H., Schlömer, G., & Haase, S. (2011). The submucous cleft palate: diagnosis and therapy. *International Journal of Pediatric Otorhinolaryngology*, *75*(1), 85–88. https://doi.org/10.1016/j.ijporl.2010.10.015

Rendall, D., Kollias, S., Ney, C., & Lloyd, P. (1995). Pitch (F0) and formant profiles of human vowels and vowel-like baboon grunts: The role of vocalizer body size. *The Journal of the Acoustical Society of America*, *117*, 944–955. https://doi.org/10.1121/1.1848011

Rescher N. (1998). *Complexity: A philosophical overview*. Transaction.

Ribeiro, G. C. A., Santos, I. D. D., Santos, A. C. N., Paranhos, L. R., & César, C. P. H. A. R. (2016). Influence of the breathing pattern on the learning process: A systematic review of literature. *Brazilian Journal of Otorhinolaryngology*, *82*(4), 466–478.

Richardson, U., Thomson, J. M., Scott, S. K., & Goswami, U. (2004). Auditory processing skills and phonological representation in dyslexic children. *Dyslexia*, *10*(3), 215–233. https://doi.org/10.1002/dys.276

Rickford, J. R. (1996). *What is Ebonics? (African American Vernacular English)*. https://www.linguisticsociety.org/content/what-ebonics-african-american-english

Riley, G. D. (1994). *Stuttering severity instrument for children and adults* (3rd ed.). Pro-Ed.

Rinaldi, S., Caselli, M. C., Cofelice, V., D'Amico, S., De Cagno, A. G., Della Corte, G., . . . Zoccolotti,

P. (2021). Efficacy of the treatment of developmental language disorder: A systematic review. *Brain Sciences*, *11*(3), 407. https://doi.org/10.3390/brainsci11030407

Robb, M. P., & Bleile, K. M. (1994). Consonant inventories of young children from 8 to 25 months. *Clinical Linguistics and Phonetics*, *8*(4), 295–320. https://doi.org/10.3109/02699209408985314. PMID: 22320895.

Robbins, J., & Klee, T. (1987). Clinical assessment of oropharyngeal motor development in young children. *Journal of Speech and Hearing Disorders*, *52*(3), 271–277. https://doi.org/10.1044/jshd.5203.271

Roberts, J. E., Burchinal, M., & Footo, M. M. (1990). Phonological process decline from 2½ to 8 years. *Journal of Communication Disorders*, *23*(3), 205–217.

Roberts, J. E., Rosenfeld, R. M., & Zeisel, S. A. (2004). Otitis media and speech and language: A meta-analysis of prospective studies. *Pediatrics*, *113*(3), e238–e248. http: //www.pediatrics.org/cgi/content/full/113/3/e238

Robin, J., Harrison, J. E., Kaufman, L. D., Rudzicz, F., Simpson, W., & Yancheva, M. (2020). Evaluation of speech-based digital biomarkers: review and recommendations. *Digital Biomarkers*, *4*(3), 99–108. https://doi.org/10.1159/000510820

Robles-Bykbaev, V. E., López-Nores, M., Pazos-Arias, J. J., & Arévalo-Lucero, D. (2015). SPELTA: An expert system to generate therapy plans for speech and language disorders. *Expert Systems with Applications*, *42*(21), 7641–7651. https://doi.org/10.1016/j.eswa.2015.06.011

Roche, L., Zhang, D., Bartl-Pokorny, K. D., Pokorny, F. B., Schuller, B. W., Esposito, G., . . . Marschik, P. B. (2018). Early vocal development in autism spectrum disorder, Rett syndrome, and fragile X syndrome: Insights from studies using retrospective video analysis. *Advances in Neurodevelopmental Disorders*, *2*(1), 49–61. https://doi.org/10.1007/s41252-017-0051-3

Rochet-Capellan, A., Richer, L., & Ostry, D. J. (2012). Nonhomogeneous transfer reveals specificity in speech motor learning. *Journal of Neurophysiology*, *107*(6), 1711–1717. https://doi.org/10.1152/jn.00773.2011

Roelofs, A. (1997). The WEAVER model of word–form encoding in speech production. *Cognition*, *64*, *249*–284. https://doi.org/10.1016/S0010–0277(97)00027–9

Roelofs, A. (2000). WEAVER++ and other computational models of lemma retrieval and word–form encoding. In L. Wheeldon (Ed.), *Aspects of language production* (pp. 71–114). Psychology Press.

Roepke, E., & Brosseau-Lapré, F. (2021). Vowel errors produced by preschool-age children on a single-word test of articulation. *Clinical Linguistics & Phonetics*, 1–23. https://doi.org/10.1080/02699206.2020.1869834

Roepke, E., & Brosseau-Lapré, F. (2023). Speech error variability and phonological awareness in preschoolers. *American Journal of Speech-Language Pathology*, *32*(1), 246–263. https://doi.org/10.1044/2022_AJSLP-22-00031

Rogers, R. (1978). Self–initiated corrections in the speech of infant–school children. *Journal of Child Language* 5, 365–371.

Rogers, S. J., Hayden, D., Hepburn, S., Charlifue-Smith, R., Hall, T., & Hayes, A. (2006). Teaching young nonverbal children with autism useful speech: A pilot study of the Denver model and PROMPT interventions. *Journal of Autism and Developmental Disorders*, *36*(8), 1007–1024. https://doi.org/10.1007/s10803-006-0142-x

Rohlfs, A. K., Friedhoff, J., Bohnert, A., Breitfuss, A., Hess, M., Müller, F., . . . Wiesner, T. (2017). Unilateral hearing loss in children: A retrospective study and a review of the current literature. *European Journal of Pediatrics*, *176*, 475–486. https://doi.org/10.1007/s00431-016-2827-2

Roizen, N. J. (2003). Nongenetic causes of hearing loss. *Mental retardation and Developmental Disabilities Research Reviews*, *9*(2), 120–127. https://doi.org/10.1002/mrdd.10068

Roizen, N. J. (2010). Overview of health issues among persons with Down syndrome. In *International Review of Research in Mental Retardation 39*, 2–33. https://doi.org/10.1016/S0074-7750(10)39001-X

Rolf, M., Steil, J. J., and Gienger, M. (2010). Goal babbling permits direct learning of inverse kinematics. *IEEE Transactions on Autonomous Mental Development*, *2*(3), 216–229. https://doi.org/10.1109/TAMD.2010.2062511

Romero, J. E., Coupe, P., Lanuza, E., Catheline, G., Manjón, J. V., & Alzheimer's Disease Neuroimaging Initiative. (2021). Toward a unified analysis of cerebellum maturation and aging across the entire lifespan: A MRI analysis.

Human Brain Mapping, *42*(5), 1287–1303. https://doi.org/10.1002/hbm.25293

Roosenboom, J., Hens, G., Mattern, B. C., Shriver, M. D., & Claes, P. (2016). Exploring the underlying genetics of craniofacial morphology through various sources of knowledge. *BioMed Research International*, Article ID 3054578. | https://doi.org/10.1155/2016/3054578.

Rosa-Lugo, L. I., Mihai, F. M., & Nutta, J. W. (2017). Preparation of speech-language pathologists to work with English learners (ELs): Incorporating interprofessional education (IPE) and interprofessional collaborative practice (IPP) competencies. *Perspectives of the ASHA Special Interest Groups*, *2*(14), 103–121. https://doi.org/10.1044/persp2.SIG14.103

Rosen, A., & Proctor, E. (1978). Specifying the treatment process: The basis for effectiveness research. *Journal of Social Service Research*, *2*, 25–43.

Rosen, A., & Proctor, E. K. (1981). Distinctions between treatment outcomes and their implications for treatment evaluation. *Journal of Consulting and Clinical Psychology*, *49*(3), 418–425

Rosen, C. A., Lee, A. S., Osborne, J., Zullo, T., & Murry, T. (2004). Development and validation of the voice handicap index-10. *Laryngoscope*, *114*(9), 1549–1556. https://doi.org/10.1097/00005537-200409000-00009

Rosenbaum, P. L., Palisano, R. J., Bartlett, D. J., Galuppi, B. E., & Russell, D. J. (2008). Development of the gross motor function classification system for cerebral palsy. *Developmental Medicine & Child Neurology*, *50*(4), 249–253. https://doi.org/10.1111/j.1469-8749.2008.02045.x

Rosenbaum, P., Paneth, N., Leviton, A., Goldstein, M., & Bax, M. (2007). A report: The definition and classification of cerebral palsy April 2006. *Developmental Medicine and Child Neurology. Supplement*, *109*(SUPPL. 2), 8–14. https://doi.org/10.1111/j.14698749.2007.tb12610.x

Rosenberg, T. L., & Schweinfurth, J. M. (2009). Cell density of the lamina propria of neonatal vocal folds. *Annals of Otology, Rhinology & Laryngology*, *118*(2), 87–90. https://doi.org/10.1177/000348940911800202

Ross, A. H., & Williams, S. E. (2021). Ancestry studies in forensic anthropology: Back on the frontier of racism. *Biology*, *10*(7), 602. https://doi.org/10.3390/biology10070602

Rosso, M., Fremion, E., Santoro, S. L., Oreskovic, N. M., Chitnis, T., Skotko, B. G., & Santoro, J. D. (2020). Down syndrome disintegrative disorder: a clinical regression syndrome of increasing importance. *Pediatrics*, *145*(6). https://doi.org/10.1542/peds.2019-2939

Roug, L., Landberg, I., & Lundberg, L. J. (1989). Phonetic development in early infancy: A study of four Swedish children during the first eighteen months of life. *Journal of Child Language*, *16*(1), 19–40. https://doi.org/10.1017/S0305000900013416

Roy, P., & Chiat, S. (2004). A prosodically controlled word and nonword repetition task for 2- to 4- year-olds: Evidence from typically developing children. *Journal of Speech, Language, and Hearing Research*, *47*(1), 223–234. https://doi.org/10.1044/1092-4388(2004/019)

Rozen-Blay, O., Novogrodsky, R., & Degani, T. (2022). Talking while signing: The influence of simultaneous communication on the spoken language of bimodal bilinguals. *Journal of Speech, Language, and Hearing Research*, *65*(2), 785–796. https://doi.org/10.1044/2021_JSLHR-21-00326

Rozin, P., & Gleitman, L.R. (1977). The structure and acquisition of reading: II. The reading process and the acquisition of the alphabetic principle. In A. S. Reber & D. L. Scarborough (Eds.), *Toward a psychology of reading* (pp. 44–141). Erlbaum.

Rudolph, J. M., & Wendt, O. (2014). The efficacy of the cycles approach: A multiple baseline design. *Journal of Communication Disorders*, *47*, 1–16. https://doi.org/10.1016/j.jcomdis.2013.12.003

Ruessink, M., van den Engel-Hoek, L., van Gerven, M., Spek, B., de Swart, B., & Kalf, J. (2021). Validation of the pediatric Radboud dysarthria assessment. *Journal of Pediatric Rehabilitation Medicine*, (Preprint), 1–12. https://doi.org/10.3233/PRM-190671

Runnqvist, E., Chanoine, V., Strijkers, K., Pattamadilok, C., Bonnard, M., Nazarian, B., . . . Alario, F. X. (2021). Cerebellar and cortical correlates of internal and external speech error monitoring. *Cerebral Cortex Communications*, *2*(2), tgab038. https://doi.org/10.1093/texcom/tgab038

Rupela, V., & Manjula, R. (2010). Diadochokinetic assessment in persons with Down syndrome. *Asia Pacific Journal of Speech, Language and Hearing*, *13*(2), 109–120. http://doi.org/10.1179/136132810805335092

Rupela, V., Velleman, S. L., & Andrianopoulos, M. V. (2016). Motor speech skills in children with Down syndrome: A descriptive study. *International Journal of Speech-Language Pathology, 18*(5), 483–492. https://doi.org/10.3109/17549507.2015.1112836

Ruscello, D. M. (2000). A summary of commercial tests and protocols for examining the speech mechanism. *Perspectives on Speech Science and Orofacial Disorders, 10*(2), 9–12. https://doi.org/10.1044/ssod10.2.9

Ruscello, D. M., & Shelton, R. L. (1979). Planning and self-assessment in articulatory training. *Journal of Speech and Hearing Disorders, 44*, 504–512. https://doi.org/10.1044/jshd.4404.504

Ruscello, D., & Vallino, L. (2014). The application of motor learning concepts to the treatment of children with compensatory speech sound errors. *Perspectives on Speech Science and Orofacial Disorders, 24*(2), 39–47. https://doi.org/10.1044/ssod24.2.39

Rvachew, S. (2005). Stimulability and treatment success. *Topics in Language Disorders. 25*(3), 207–219.

Rvachew, S., & Brosseau-Lapré, F. (2018). *Developmental phonological disorders: Foundations of clinical practice* (2nd ed.). Plural Publishing.

Rvachew, S., & Matthews, T. (2017). Using the Syllable Repetition Task to reveal underlying speech processes in childhood apraxia of speech: A Tutorial. *Canadian Journal of Speech-Language Pathology & Audiology, 41*, 106–126.

Rvachew, S., Chiang, P. Y., & Evans, N. (2007). Characteristics of speech errors produced by children with and without delayed phonological awareness skills. *Language, Speech, and Hearing Services in Schools, 38*(1), 60–71. https://doi.org/10.1044/0161-1461(2007/006)

Rvachew, S., Hodge, M., & Ohberg, A. (2005). Obtaining and interpreting m0aximum performance tasks from children: A tutorial. *Journal of Speech-Language Pathology and Audiology, 29*(4), 146–157.

Rvachew, S., Nowak, M., & Cloutier, G. (2004). Effect of phonemic perception training on the speech production and phonological awareness skills of children with expressive phonological delay. *American Journal of Speech-Language Pathology, 13*, 250–263. https://doi.org/10.1044/1058-0360(2004/026)

Rvachew, S., Rafaat, S., & Martin, M. (1999). Stimulability, speech perception skills, and the treatment of phonological disorders. *American Journal of Speech-Language Pathology, 8*(1), 33–43. https://doi.org/10.1044/1058-0360.0801.33

Saarni, C., Campos, J. J., Camras, L. A., & Witherington, D. (2006). Emotional development: Action, communication, and understanding. In N. Eisenberg, W. Damon, & R. M. Lerner (Eds.), *Handbook of child psychology: Social, emotional, and personality development* (pp. 226–299). John Wiley & Sons.

Sachs, J., Lieberman, P., & Erickson, D. (1973). Anatomical and cultural determinants of male and female speech. In R. W. Shuy & R. W. Fasold (Eds.), *Language attitudes* (pp. 74–83). Georgetown University Press.

Sadagopan, N., & Smith, A. (2008). Developmental changes in the effects of utterance length and complexity on speech movement variability. *Journal of Speech, Language, and Hearing Research, 51*(5), 1138–1151. https://doi.org/10.1044/1092-4388(2008/06-0222)

Sadowska, M., Sarecka-Hujar, B., & Kopyta, I. (2020). Cerebral palsy: Current opinions on definition, epidemiology, risk factors, classification and treatment options. *Neuropsychiatric Disease and Treatment, 16*, 1505–1518. https://doi.org/10.2147/NDT.S235165

Saeedi, S., Bouraghi, H., Seifpanahi, M. S., & Ghazisaeedi, M. (2022). Application of digital games for speech therapy in children: A systematic review of features and challenges. *Journal of Healthcare Engineering*, Article ID 4814945. https://doi.org/10.1155/2022/4814945

Sagr, A. A., & Sagr, N. A. (2021). The effect of Otitis media on the language acquisition among children: Findings from a systematic review. *Journal of Health Informatics in Developing Countries, 15*(1). https://jhidc.org/index.php/jhidc/article/view/317

Saibene, A., Assale, M., & Giltri, M. (2021). Expert systems: Definitions, advantages and issues in medical field applications. *Expert Systems with Applications, 177*, 114900. https://doi.org/10.1016/j.eswa.2021.114900

Sakash, A., Mahr, T. J., & Hustad, K. C. (2023). Perceptual measurement of articulatory goodness in young children: Relationships with age, speech sound acquisition, and intelligibility, *Clinical Linguistics & Phonetics.*

https://doi.org/10.1080/02699206.2022.2150893

Salari, N., Darvishi, N., Heydari, M., Bokaee, S., Darvishi, F., & Mohammadi, M. (2021). Global prevalence of cleft palate, cleft lip and cleft palate and lip: A comprehensive systematic review and meta-analysis. *Journal of Stomatology, Oral and Maxillofacial Surgery. 123*(2), 110–120. https://doi.org/10.1016/j.jormas.2021.05.008

Salt, H., Claessen, M., Johnston, T., & Smart, S. (2020). Speech production in young children with tongue-tie. *International Journal of Pediatric Otorhinolaryngology, 134*, 110035. https://doi.org/10.1016/j.ijporl.2020.110035

Samuel, A. G., & Kraljic, T. (2009). Perceptual learning for speech. *Attention, Perception, & Psychophysics, 71* (6), 1207–1218. https://doi.org/10.3758/APP.71.6.1207

Sanders, I., Mu, L., Amirali, A., Su, H., & Sobotka, S. (2013). The human tongue slows down to speak: Muscle fibers of the human tongue. *Anatomical Record, 296*(10), 1615–1627. https://doi.org/10.1002/ar.22755

Sandiford, G. A., Mainess, K. J., & Daher, N. S. (2013). A pilot study on the efficacy of melodic based communication therapy for eliciting speech in nonverbal children with autism. *Journal of Autism and Developmental Disorders, 43*, 1298–1307. https://doi.org/10.1007/s10803-012-1672-z

Sanli, E. A., Patterson, J. T., Bray, S. R., & Lee, T. D. (2013). Understanding self-controlled motor learning protocols through the self-determination theory. *Frontiers in Psychology, 11*. https://doi.org/10.3389/fpsyg.2012.00611

Santa Maria, C., Aby, J., Truong, M. T., Thakur, Y., Rea, S, & Messner, A. (2018). The superior labial frenulum in newborns: What is normal? *Global Pediatric Health, 4*, 1–6. https://doi.org/10.1177/2333794X17718896

Sato, K., Nakashima, T., Nonaka, S., & Harabuchi, Y. (2008). Histopathologic investigations of the unphonated human vocal fold mucosa. *Acta Oto-Laryngologica, 128*(6), 694–701. https://doi.org/10.1080/00016480701675643

Saur, D., Kreher, B. W., Schnell, S., Kümmerer, D., Kellmeyer, P., Vry, M. S., . . . Weiller, C. (2008). Ventral and dorsal pathways for language. *Proceedings of the National Academy of Sciences, 105*(46), 18035–18040. https://doi.org/10.1073/pnas.0805234105

Savian, C. M., Bolsson, G. B., Botton, G., Antoniazzi, R. P., de Oliveira Rocha, R., Zanatta, F. B., & Santos, B. Z. (2021). Do breastfed children have a lower chance of developing mouth breathing? A systematic review and meta-analysis. *Clinical Oral Investigations*, 1–14. https://doi.org/10.1007/s00784-021-03791-1

Savill, N. J., Cornelissen, P., Pahor, A., & Jefferies, E. (2019). rTMS evidence for a dissociation in short-term memory for spoken words and nonwords. *Cortex, 112*, 5–22. https://doi.org/10.1016/j.cortex.2018.07.021

Sayahi, F., & Jalaie, S. (2016). Diagnosis of childhood apraxia of speech: A systematic review. *Journal of Diagnostics, 3*(1), 21–26. https://doi.org/10.18488/journal.98/2016.3.1/98.1.21.26

Saz, O., Yin, S. C., Lleida, E., Rose, R., Vaquero, C., & Rodríguez, W. R. (2009). Tools and technologies for computer-aided speech and language therapy. *Speech Communication, 51*(10), 948–967. https://doi.org/10.1016/j.specom.2009.04.006

Scammon, R. E. (1930). The measurement of the body in childhood. In J. A. Harris, C. M. Jackson, D. G. Patterson & R. E. Scammon (Eds.), *The measurement of man* (pp. 173–215). University of Minnesota Press.

Scarborough, H. S., & Brady, S. A. (2002). Toward a common terminology for talking about speech and reading: A glossary of the "phon" words and some related terms. *Journal of Literacy Research, 34*(3), 299–336.

Scharff Rethfeldt, W., McNeilly, L., Abutbul-Oz, H., Blumenthal, M., Salameh, E. K., Smolander, S., . . . Thordardottir, E. (2020). *Common questions by speech and language therapists/speech-language pathologists about bilingual/multilingual children and informed, evidence-based answers*. International Association of Communication Sciences and Disorders. https://ialpasoc.info/committees/multilingual-and-multicultural-affairs-committee/

Scheerer, N. E., Jacobson, D. S., & Jones, J. A. (2020). Sensorimotor control of vocal production in early childhood. *Journal of Experimental Psychology: General, 149*(6), 1071–1077. https://doi.org/10.1037/xge0000706

Schiavetti, N. (1992). Scaling procedures for the measurement of speech intelligibility. In R. D. Kent (Ed.), *Intelligibility in speech disorders: Theory, measurement and management* (pp. 11–34). John Benjamins.

Schiavetti, N., Metz, D. E., & Sitler, R. W. (1981). Construct validity of direct magnitude estimation and interval scaling of speech intelligibility. Evidence from a study of the hearing impaired. *Journal of Speech, Language, and Hearing Research*, *24*, 441–445.

Schiavetti, N., Sacco, P. R., Metz, D. E., & Sitler, R. W. (1983). Direct magnitude estimation and interval scaling of stuttering severity. *Journal of Speech, Language, and Hearing Research*, *26*, 568–573.

Schiller, I. S., Morsomme, D., Kob, M., & Remacle, A. (2020). Noise and a speaker's impaired voice quality disrupt spoken language processing in school-aged children: Evidence from performance and response time measures. *Journal of Speech, Language, and Hearing Research*, *63*(7), 2115–2131.

Schiller, N. O., Meyer, A. S., Baayen, R. H., & Levelt, W. J. M. (1996). A comparison of lexeme and speech syllables in Dutch. *Journal of Quantitative Linguistics*, *3*, 8–28.

Schilling-Estes, N. (2002). American English social dialect variation and gender. *Journal of English Linguistics*, *30*(2), 122H137. https://doi.org/10.1177/007242030002003

Schmahmann, J. D. (2020). Pediatric post-operative cerebellar mutism syndrome, cerebellar cognitive affective syndrome, and posterior fossa syndrome: Historical review and proposed resolution to guide future study. *Child's Nervous System*, *36*(6), 1205–1214. https://doi.org/10.1007/s00381-019-04253-6

Schmidt, A. M., & Sullivan, S. (2003). Clinical training in foreign accent modification: A national survey. *Contemporary Issues in Communication Science and Disorders*, *30*(Fall), 127–135.

Schmitt, L. M., Wang, J., Pedapati, E. V., Thurman, A. J., Abbeduto, L., Erickson, C. A., & Sweeney, J. A. (2020). A neurophysiological model of speech production deficits in fragile X syndrome. *Brain Communications*, *2*(1), fcz042. https://doi.org/10.1093/braincomms/fcz042

Schmidt, R. A. (1975). A schema theory of discrete motor skill learning. *Psychological Review*, *82*(4), 225–260. https://doi.org/10.1037/h0076770

Schmidt, R. A. (1976). The schema as a solution to some persistent problems in motor learning theory. In G. E. Stelmach (Ed.), *Motor control issues and trends* (pp. 41–65). Academic Press.

Schoen, E., Paul, R., & Chawarska, K. (2011). Phonology and vocal behavior in toddlers with autism spectrum disorders. *Autism Research*, *4*(3), 177–188. https://doi.org/10.1002/aur.183

Schölderle, T., Haas, E., & Ziegler, W. (2020). Age norms for auditory-perceptual neurophonetic parameters: A prerequisite for the assessment of childhood dysarthria. *Journal of Speech, Language, and Hearing Research*, *63*(4), 1071–1082. https://doi.org/10.1044/2020_JSLHR-19-00114

Schölderle, T., Haas, E., & Ziegler, W. (2021). Dysarthria syndromes in children with cerebral palsy. *Developmental Medicine & Child Neurology*, *63*(4), 444–449. https://doi.org/10.1111/dmcn.14679

Schölderle, T., Haas, E., & Ziegler, W. (2022). Childhood dysarthria: Auditory-perceptual profiles against the background of typical speech motor development. *Journal of Speech, Language, and Hearing Research*, *65*(6). 2114–2127. https://doi.org/10.1044/2022_JSLHR-21-00608

Schölderle, T., Haas, E., Baumeister, S., & Ziegler, W. (2021). Intelligibility, articulation rate, fluency, and communicative efficiency in typically developing children. *Journal of Speech, Language, and Hearing Research*, *64*(7), 2575–2585. https://doi.org/10.1044/2021_JSLHR-20-00640

Schuele, C. M., & Boudreau, D. (2008). Phonological awareness intervention: Beyond the basics. *Language, Speech, and Hearing Services in Schools*, *39*(1), 3–20. https://doi.org/10.1044/0161-1461(2008/002)

Schwob, S., Eddé, L., Jacquin, L., Leboulanger, M., Picard, M., Oliveira, P. R., & Skoruppa, K. (2021). Using nonword repetition to identify developmental language disorder in monolingual and bilingual children: A systematic review and meta-analysis. *Journal of Speech, Language, and Hearing Research*, *64*(9), 3578–3593. https://doi.org/10.1044/2021_JSLHR-20-00552

Scobbie, J., Gibbon, F., Hardcastle, W., & Fletcher, P. (2000). Covert contrast as a stage in the acquisition of phonetics and phonology. In M. B. Broe & J. B. Pierrehumbert (Eds.), *Papers in Laboratory Phonology V: Acquisition and the lexicon* (pp. 194–207). Cambridge University Press.

Scovel, T. (1988). *A time to speak. A psycholinguistic inquiry into the critical period for human speech*. Newbury House Publishers.

Secord, W. A., & Donohoe, J. S. (2002). *Clinical Assessment of Articulation and Phonology*. Super Duper Publications.

Segal, L. M., Stephenson, R., Dawes, M., & Feldman, P. (2007). Prevalence, diagnosis, and treatment of ankyloglossia: Methodologic review. *Canadian Family Physician*, *53*(6), 1027–1033.

Seidenberg, M. (2017). *Language at the speed of sight: How we read, why so many can't, and what can be done about it*. Hachette Book Group: Basic Books.

Seifert, M., Davies, A., Harding, S., McLeod, S., & Wren, Y. (2021). Intelligibility in 3-year-olds with cleft lip and/or palate using the intelligibility in context scale: Findings from the Cleft Collective Cohort Study. *The Cleft Palate-Craniofacial Journal*, *58*(9), 1178–1189. https://doi.org/10.1177/105566562098574

Sekścińska, I. (2021). The role of inner speech in the speech production process. *Studia Linguistica*, *40*, 93–111. https://doi.org/10.19195/0137–1169.40.7

Selby, J. C., Robb, M. P., & Gilbert, H. R. (2000). Normal vowel articulations between 15 and 36 months of age. *Clinical Linguistics & Phonetics*, *14*, 255256. https://doi.org/10.1080/02699200050023976

Selkirk, E. O. (1980). Prosodic domains in phonology. Sanskrit revisited. In M. Aronoff & M. L. Kean (Eds.), *Juncture. A collection of original papers* (pp. 107–129). Anma Libri.

Selkirk, E. O. (1995). The prosodic structure of function words. In J. N. Beckman, L. W. Dickey, & Urbanczyk (Eds.), *Papers in optimality theory* (pp. 439–469). GSLA.

Service, E. (2013). Working memory in second language acquisition: Phonological short-term. In C. A. Chapelle (Ed.), *The encyclopedia of applied linguistics*. Wiley Blackwell. https://doi.org/10.1002/9781405198431.wbeal1287

Sforza, C., Dellavia, C., Allievi, C., Tommasi, D. G., & Ferrario, V. F. (2012). Anthropometric indices of facial features in Down's syndrome subjects. In V. R. Preedy (Ed.), *Handbook of anthropometry: Physical measures of human form in health and disease* (pp. 1603–1618). Springer.

Shablack, H., & Lindquist, K.A. (2019). The role of language in emotional development. In V. LoBue, K. Pérez-Edgar, & K. A. Buss (Eds.), *Handbook of emotional development* (pp. 451–478). Springer. https://doi.org/10.1007/978-3-030-17332-6_18

Shah, S. S., Nankar, M. Y., Bendgude, V. D., & Shetty, B. R. (2021). Orofacial myofunctional therapy in tongue thrust habit: A narrative review. *International Journal of Clinical Pediatric Dentistry*, *14*(2), 298. https://doi.org/10.5005/jp-journals-10005-1926

Sharda, M., Subhadra, T. P., Sahay, S., Nagaraja, C., Singh, L., Mishra, R., . . . Singh, N. C. (2010). Sounds of melody—Pitch patterns of speech in autism. *Neuroscience Letters*, *478*(1), 42–45. https://doi.org/10.1016/j.neulet.2010.04.066

Sharma, A., & Couture, J. (2014). A review of the pathophysiology, etiology, and treatment of attention-deficit hyperactivity disorder (ADHD). *Annals of Pharmacotherapy*, *48*(2), 209–225. https://doi.org/10.1177/1060028013510699

Sharma, S. D., Cushing, S. L., Papsin, B. C., & Gordon, K. A. (2020). Hearing and speech benefits of cochlear implantation in children: A review of the literature. *International Journal of Pediatric Otorhinolaryngology*, *133*, 109984. https://doi.org/10.1016/j.ijporl.2020.109984

Shattuck–Hufnagel, S. (1983). Sublexical units and suprasegmental structure in speech production planning. In P. F. MacNeilage (Ed.) *The production of speech*. (pp. 109–136). Springer. https://doi.org/10.1007/978–1–4613–8202–7_6

Shattuck-Hufnagel, S., & Turk, A. E. (1996). A prosody tutorial for investigators of auditory sentence processing. *Journal of Psycholinguistic Research*, *25*(2), 193–247. https://doi.org/10.1007/BF01708572

Shea, C. H., & Kohl, R. M. (1990). Specificity and variability of practice. *Research Quarterly for Exercise and Sport*, *61*(2), 169–177. https://doi.org/10.1080/02701367.1990.10608671.

Sheffield, A. M., & Smith, R. J. (2019). The epidemiology of deafness. *Cold Spring Harbor Perspectives in Medicine*, *9*(9), a033258.

Sherman, S. L., Allen, E. G., Bean, L. H., & Freeman, S. B. (2007). Epidemiology of Down syndrome. *Mental Retardation and Developmental Disabilities Research Reviews*, *13*(3), 221–227. https://doi.org/10.1002/mrdd.20157

Shields, C., Willis, H., Nichani, J., Slade, M., & Kluk-de Kort, K. (2022) Listening effort: WHAT is it, HOW is it measured and WHY is it important? *Cochlear Implants International, 23*(2), 114–117, https://doi.org/10.1080/14670100.2021.1992941

Shiller, D. M., & Rochon, M.-L. (2014). Auditory-perceptual learning improves speech motor adaptation in children. *Journal of Experimental Psychology: Human Perception and Performance, 40*(4), 1308–1315. https://doi.org/10.1037/a0036660

Shiohama, T., Levman, J., Baumer, N., & Takahashi, E. (2019). Structural magnetic resonance imaging-based brain morphology study in infants and toddlers with Down syndrome: The effect of comorbidities. *Pediatric Neurology, 100*, 67–73. https://doi.org/10.1016/j.pediatrneurol.2019.03.015

Shirali-Shahreza, S., & Penn, G. (2018, December). MOS Naturalness and the quest for human-like speech. *2018 IEEE Spoken Language Technology Workshop (SLT)* (pp. 346–352). IEEE. https://doi.org/10.1109/SLT.2018.8639599

Shortland, H. A. L., Hewat, S., Vertigan, A., & Webb, G. (2021). Orofacial myofunctional therapy and myofunctional devices used in speech pathology treatment: A systematic quantitative review of the literature. *American Journal of Speech-Language Pathology, 30*(1), 301–317. https://doi.org/10.1044/2020_AJSLP-20-00245

Shortland, H. A. L., Webb, G., Vertigan, A. E., & Hewat, S. (2022). Speech-language pathologists' use of myofunctional devices in therapy programs. *Perspectives of the ASHA Special Interest Groups, 7*(6), 2012–2026. https://pubs.asha.org/doi/10.1044/2022_PERSP-22-00145

Shriberg, L. D. (1993). Four new speech and prosody-voice measures for genetics research and other studies in developmental phonological disorders. *Journal of Speech and Hearing Research, 36*(1), 105–140. https://doi.org/10.1044/jshr.3601.105-

Shriberg, L. D., & Kwiatkowski, J. (1982). Phonological disorders III: A procedure for assessing severity of involvement. *Journal of Speech and Hearing Disorders, 47*(3), 256–270. https://doi.org/10.1044/jshd.4703.256

Shriberg, L. D., & Kwiatkowski, J. (1990). Self–monitoring and generalization in preschool speech–delayed children. *Language, Speech, and Hearing Services in Schools, 21*, 157–170. https://doi.org/10.1044/0161-1461.2103.157

Shriberg, L. D., Kwiatkowski, J., & Rasmussen, C. (1990). *The Prosody-Voice Screening Profile*. Communication Skill Builders.

Shriberg, L. D., Campbell, T. F., Mabie, H. L., & McGlothlin, J. H. (2019). Initial studies of the phenotype and persistence of Speech Motor Delay (SMD). *Clinical Linguistics & Phonetics 33*(8), 737–756. https://doi.org/10.1080/02699206.2019.1595733

Shriberg, L. D., Kent, R. D., McAllister, T., & Preston, J. L. (2019). *Clinical phonetics* (5th ed.). Pearson.

Shriberg, L. D., Austin, D., Lewis, B. A., McSweeny, J. L., & Wilson, D. L. (1997a). The percentage of consonants correct (PCC) metric: Extensions and reliability data. *Journal of Speech, Language, and Hearing Research, 40*(4), 708–722. https://doi.org/10.1044/jslhr.4004.708

Shriberg, L. D., Austin, D., Lewis, B. A., McSweeny, J. L., & Wilson, D. L. (1997b). The Speech Disorders Classification System (SDCS) extensions and lifespan reference data. *Journal of Speech, Language, and Hearing Research, 40*(4), 723–740. https://doi.org/10.1044/jslhr.4004.723

Shriberg, L. D., Campbell, T. F., Karlsson, H. B., Brown, R. L., McSweeny, J. L., & Nadler, C. J. (2003). A diagnostic marker for childhood apraxia of speech: The lexical stress ratio. *Clinical Linguistics & Phonetics, 17*(7), 549–574. https://doi.org/10.1080/0269920031000138123

Shriberg, L. D., Lohmeier, H. L., Campbell, T. F., Dollaghan, C. A., Green, J. R., & Moore, C. A. (2009). A nonword repetition task for speakers with misarticulations: The Syllable Repetition Task (SRT). *Journal of Speech, Language, and Hearing Research, 52*(5), 1189–1212. https://doi.org/10.1044/1092-4388(2009/08-0047)

Shriberg, L. D., Paul, R., McSweeny, J. L., Klin, A. M., Cohen, D. J., & Volkmar, F. R. (2001). Speech and prosody characteristics of adolescents and adults with high-functioning autism and Asperger syndrome. *Journal of Speech, Language, and Hearing Research, 44*, 1097–1115. https://doi.org/10.1044/1092-4388(2001/087)

Shriberg, L. D., Strand, E. A., Fourakis, M., Jakielski, K. J., Hall, S. D., Karlsson, H. B., . . . Wilson, D. L. (2017). A diagnostic marker to discriminate childhood apraxia of speech from speech delay: I. Development and description of the pause marker. *Journal of Speech, Language, and Hearing Research, 60*(4), S1096–S1117. https://doi.org/10.1044/2016_JSLHR-S-15-0296

Shriberg, L. D., Fourakis, M., Hall, S. D., Karlsson, H. B., Lohmeier, H. L., McSweeny, J. L . . . Wilson, D. L. (2010). Extensions to the speech disorders classification system (SDCS). *Clinical Linguistics & Phonetics, 24*(10), 795–824. https://doi.org/10.3109/02699206.2010.503006

Sidtis, D. V. L., & Yang, S. Y. (2020). Pathological prosody: Overview, assessment, and treatment. In C. Gussenhoven & A. Chen (Eds.), *The Oxford Handbook of Language Prosody.* https://doi.org/10.1093/oxfordhb/9780198832232.013.48

Siemons-Lühring, D. I., Euler, H. A., Mathmann, P., Suchan, B., & Neumann, K. (2021). The effectiveness of an integrated treatment for functional speech sound disorders—A randomized controlled trial. *Children, 8*(12), 1190. https://doi.org/10.3390/children8121190

Sigafoos, J., Roche, L., O'Reilly, M. F., & Lancioni, G. (2021). Persistence of primitive reflexes in developmental disorders. *Current Developmental Disorders Reports. 8*, 98–105. https://doi.org/10.1007/s40474-021-00232-2

Silva, G. M. D., Couto, M. I. V., & Molini-Avejonas, D. R. (2013). Risk factors identification in children with speech disorders: Pilot study. *CoDAS, 25*, 456–462. Sociedade Brasileira de Fonoaudiologia. https://doi.org/10.1590/S2317-17822013000500010

Silverman, K., Beckman, M., Pitrelli, J., Ostendorf, M., Wightman, C., Price, P., . . . Hirschberg, J. 1992. ToBI: A standard for labelling English prosody. *Proceedings ICSLP92, 2*, 867–870, Banff, Canada. http://www.ling.ohio-state.edu/~tobi/

Simpson, E. A., Murray, L., Paukner, A., & Ferrari, P. F. (2014). The mirror neuron system as revealed through neonatal imitation: presence from birth, predictive power and evidence of plasticity. *Philosophical Transactions of the Royal Society B: Biological Sciences, 369*(1644), 20130289. https://doi.org/10.1098/rstb.2013.0289

Sinagra, C., & Wiener, S. (2022). The perception of intonational and emotional speech prosody produced with and without a face mask: An exploratory individual differences study. *Cognitive Research, 7*, 89. https://doi.org/10.1186/s41235-022-00439-w

Singer, C. M., Hessling, A., Kelly, E. M., Singer, L., & Jones, R. M. (2020). Clinical characteristics associated with stuttering persistence: A meta-analysis. *Journal of Speech, Language, and Hearing Research, 63*(9), 2995–3018. https://doi.org/10.1044/2020_JSLHR-20-00096

Sivapathasundharam, B., & Biswas, P. G. (2020). Oral stereognosis-A literature review. *European Journal of Molecular & Clinical Medicine*, 7(9), 1053–1063. 10.31838/ejmcm.07.09.108

Skahan, S. M., Watson, M., & Lof, G. L. (2007). Speech-language pathologists' assessment practices for children with suspected speech sound disorders: Results of a national survey. *American Journal of Speech-Language Pathology, 16*(3), 246–259. https://doi.org/10.1044/1058-0360(2007/029)

Skarżyński, H., & Piotrowska, A. (2012). Prevention of communication disorders—screening pre-school and school-age children for problems with hearing, vision and speech: European Consensus Statement. *Medical Science Monitor: International Medical Journal of Experimental and Clinical Research, 18*(4), SR17–SR21. https://doi.org/10.12659/MSM.882603

Skelton, S. L., & Richard, J. T. (2016). Application of a motor learning treatment for speech sound disorders in small groups. *Perceptual and Motor Skills*, 122(3), 840–854. https://doi.org/10.1177/0031512516647693

Skuse, D., Stevenson, J., Reilly, S., & Mathisen, B. (1995). Schedule for oral-motor assessment (SOMA): Methods of validation. *Dysphagia, 10*, 192–202. https://doi.org/10.1007/BF00260976

Small, S. L., Buccino, G., & Solodkin, A. (2012). The mirror neuron system and treatment of stroke. *Developmental Psychobiology, 54*(3), 293–310. https://doi.org/10.1002/dev.20504

Smartt Jr, J. M., Low, D. W., & Bartlett, S. P. (2005). The pediatric mandible: I. A primer on growth and development. *Plastic and Reconstructive Surgery, 116*(1), 14e–23e. https://doi.org/10.1097/01.PRS.0000169940.69315.9C

Smit, A. B., & Hand, L. (1992). *Smit-Hand Articulation and Phonology Evaluation.* Eastern Psychological Services.

Smith, A., & Weber, C. (2017). How stuttering develops: The Multifactorial Dynamic Pathways

Theory. *Journal of Speech, Language, and Hearing Research, 60*(9), 2483–2505. htpps://doi.org/10.1044/2017_JSLHR-S-16-0343.

Smith, A., Goffman, L., Sasisekaran, J., & Weber-Fox, C. (2012). Language and motor abilities of preschool children who stutter: Evidence from behavioral and kinematic indices of nonword repetition performance. *Journal of Fluency Disorders, 37*(4), 44–58. https://doi.org/10.1016/j.jfludis.2012.06.001.

Smith, A., Goffman, L., Zelaznik, H. N., Ying, G., & McGillem, C. (1995). Spatiotemporal stability and patterning of speech movement sequences. *Experimental Brain Research, 104*(3), 493–501. https://doi.org/10.1007/BF00231983

Smith, K. E., Plumb, A. M., & Sandage, M. J. (2022). Speech-language pathologists' knowledge of Spanish-Influenced English and dialectical differences: A survey. *Communication Disorders Quarterly, 43*(2), 128–132.

Snow, D. (1994). Phrase-final syllable lengthening and intonation in early child speech. *Journal of Speech, Language, and Hearing Research, 37*(4), 831–840. https://doi.org/10.1044/jshr.3704.831

Snyder, H. M., Bain, L. J., Brickman, A. M., Carrillo, M. C., Esbensen, A. J., Espinosa, J. M., . . . Rafii, M. S. (2020). Further understanding the connection between Alzheimer's disease and Down syndrome. *Alzheimer's & Dementia, 16*(7), 1065–1077. https://doi.org/10.1002/alz.12112

Soderstrom, M., Reimchen, M., Sauter, D., & Morgan, J. L. (2017). Do infants discriminate non-linguistic vocal expressions of positive emotions? *Cognition and Emotion, 31*(2), 298–311. http://dx.doi.org/10.1080/02699931.2015.1108904

Sodoro, J., Allinder, R. M., & Rankin-Erickson, J. L. (2002). Assessment of phonological awareness: Review of methods and tools. *Educational Psychology Review, 14*(3), 223–260. https://doi.org/10.1023/A:1016050412323

Solomon, N. P., & Clark, H. M. (2010). Quantifying orofacial muscle stiffness using damped oscillation. *Journal of Medical Speech-Language Pathology, 18*(4), 120–124.

Solomon, N. P., Garlitz, S. J., & Milbrath, R. L. (2000). Respiratory and laryngeal contributions to maximum phonation duration. *Journal of Voice, 14*(3), 331–340. https://doi.org/10.1016/S0892-1997(00)80079-X

Soriano, J. U., & Hustad, K. C. (2021). Speech-language profile groups in school aged children with cerebral palsy: Nonverbal cognition, receptive language, speech intelligibility, and motor function. *Developmental Neurorehabilitation, 24*(2), 118–129. https://doi.org/10.1080/17518423.2020.1858360

Soriano, J. U., Olivieri, A., & Hustad, K. C. (2021). Utility of the Intelligibility in Context Scale for predicting speech intelligibility of children with cerebral palsy. *Brain Sciences, 11*(11), 1540. https://doi.org/10.3390/brainsci11111540

Sosa, A. V. (2015). Intraword variability in typical speech development. *American Journal of Speech-Language Pathology, 24*(1), 24–35. https://doi.org/10.1044/2014_AJSLP-13-0148

Southwood, M. H., & Flege, J. E. (1999). Scaling foreign accent: Direct magnitude estimation versus interval scaling. *Clinical Linguistics & Phonetics, 13*, 335–349.

Speer, S. R., & Ito, K. (2009). Prosody in first language acquisition–Acquiring intonation as a tool to organize information in conversation. *Language and Linguistics Compass, 3*(1), 90–110. https://doi.org/10.1111/j.1749-818X.2008.00103.x

Spencer, C., Vannest, J., Preston, J. L., Maas, E., Sizemore, E. R., McAllister, T., . . . Boyce, S. (in press). Neural changes in children with residual speech sound disorder after ultrasound biofeedback speech therapy. *Journal of Speech, Language, and Hearing Research.*

Spinelli, M., Fasolo, M., & Mesman, J. (2017). Does prosody make the difference? A meta-analysis on relations between prosodic aspects of infant-directed speech and infant outcomes. *Developmental Review, 44*, 1–18. https://doi.org/10.1016/j.dr.2016.12.001

Spinelli, M., Rocha, A. C. D. O., Giacheti, C. M., & Richieri-Costa, A. (1995). Word-finding difficulties, verbal paraphasias, and verbal dyspraxia in ten individuals with fragile x syndrome. *American Journal of Medical Genetics, 60*(1), 39–43. https://doi.org/10.1002/ajmg.1320600108

Spinu, L. E., Hwang, J., & Lohmann, R. (2018). Is there a bilingual advantage in phonetic and phonological acquisition? The initial learning of word-final coronal stop realization in a novel accent of English. *International Journal of Bilingualism, 22*(3), 350–370. https://doi.org/org/10.1177/1367006916681080

Springle, A. P., Breeden, A., & Raymer, A. M. (2020). Speech intervention effects for childhood apraxia of speech: Quality appraisal of systematic reviews. *Perspectives of the ASHA Special Interest Groups*, *5*(3), 646–653. https://doi.org/10.1044/2020_PERSP-19-00019

Sproat, R., & Fujimura, O. (1993). Allophonic variation in English /l/ and its implications for phonetic implementation. *Journal of Phonetics*, *2*(3), 291–311. https://doi.org/10.1016/S0095-4470(19)31340-3

St. Louis, K. O., & Ruscello, D. (2000). *Oral Speech Mechanism Screening Examination, Third Edition*. Pro-Ed.

St. Louis, K. O., Hansen, G. R., Buch, J. L., & Oliver, T. L. (1992). Voice deviations and coexisting communication disorders. *Language, Speech, and Hearing Services in Schools*, *23*, 82–87. https://doi.org/10.1044/0161-1461.2301.82

Stackhouse, J., & Wells, B. (1997). *Children's speech and literacy difficulties: A psycholinguistic framework*. Wiley.

Stackhouse, J., Wells, B., Pascoe, M., & Rees, R. (2002). From phonological therapy to phonological awareness. *Seminars in Speech and Language 23*(1), 27–42.

Stamenov, M. I., & Gallese, V. (Eds.) (2002). *Mirror neurons and the evolution of brain and language*. John Benjamins.

Stampe, D. (1969). The acquisition of phonetic representation. In R. Binnick et al. (Eds.), *Papers from the Fifth Regional Meeting of the Chicago Linguistic Society* (pp. 443–454). Chicago Linguistic Society. Reprinted in 2003 in B. Lust & C. Foley (Eds.), *First language acquisition: The essential readings* (pp. 307–315.). Blackwell.

Stathopoulos, E. T., & Sapienza, C. (1993). Respiratory and laryngeal measures of children during vocal intensity variation. *The Journal of the Acoustical Society of America*, *94*(5), 2531–2543. https://doi.org/10.1121/1.407365

Steels, L., & De Boer, B. (2008). Embodiment and self-organization of human categories: A case study for speech. In T. Ziemke, J. Zlatev, & R. M. Frank (Eds.), *Body, language and mind, Vol. 1: Embodiment* (pp. 411–430). Mouton de Gruyter.

Stein, C. M., Benchek, P., Miller, G., Hall, N. B., Menon, D., Freebairn, L., . . . Lyengar, S. K. (2020). Feature-driven classification reveals potential comorbid subtypes within childhood apraxia of speech. *BMC Pediatrics*, *20*(1), 519. https://doi.org/10.1186/s12887-020-02421-1

Stemberger, J. P. (1989). Speech errors in early child language production. *Journal of Memory and Language*, *28*(2), 164–188. https://doi.org/10.1016/0749-596X(89)90042-9

Stephan, F., Saalbach, H., & Rossi, S. (2020). Inner versus overt speech production: Does this make a difference in the developing brain? *Brain Sciences*, *10*(12), 939. https://doi.org/10.3390/brainsci10120939

Stepp, C. E., & Vojtech, J. M. (2019). Speech naturalness. In J. S. Damico & M. J. Ball (Eds.), *The SAGE encyclopedia of human communication sciences and disorders* (p. 1777). Sage Publications. https://doi.org/10.4135/9781483380810.n577

Stevens, S. S. (1946). On the theory of scales of measurement. *Science, 103*, 677–680.

Stewart, K. J., Ahmad, T., Razzell, R. E., & Watson, A. C. (2002). Altered speech following adenoidectomy: A 20 year experience. *British Journal of Plastic Surgery*. 55(6), 469–473. https://doi.org/10.1054/bjps.2002.3886

Stilp, C. (2020). Acoustic context effects in speech perception. *Wiley Interdisciplinary Reviews: Cognitive Science*, *11*(1), e1517. https://doi.org/10.1002/wcs.1517

Stipancic, K. L., Tjaden K., & Wilding G. (2016). Comparison of intelligibility measures for adults with Parkinson's disease, adults with multiple sclerosis, and healthy controls. *Journal of Speech, Language, and Hearing Research*, *59*(2), 230–238. https://doi.org/10.1044/2015_JSLHR-S-15-0271

Stockman, I. J. (2010). A review of developmental and applied language research on African American children: From a deficit to difference perspective on dialect differences. *Language, Speech, and Hearing Services in Schools*, *41*(1), 23–38. https://doi.org/10.1044/0161-1461(2009/08-0086

Stoel-Gammon C. (1985). Phonetic inventories, 15-24 months: A longitudinal study. *Journal of Speech and Hearing Research*, *28*(4), 505–512. https://doi.org/10.1044/jshr.2804.505

Stoel-Gammon, C. (1987). Language production scale. In L. Olswang, C. Stoel-Gammon, T. Coggins, & R. Carpenter (Eds.), *Assessing prelinguistic and early linguistic behaviors in developmentally young children* (pp. 120–150). University of Washington Press.

Stoel-Gammon, C. (1991). Normal and disordered phonology in two-year olds. *Topics in Language Disorders, 11*, 21–32.

Stoel-Gammon, C. (2001). Down syndrome phonology: Development patterns and intervention strategies. *Down Syndrome Research and Practice, 7*, 93–100. https://doi.org/10.3104/reviews.118

Stoel-Gammon, C., & Stone, J. R. (1991). Assessing phonology in young children. *Clinics in Communication Disorders, 1*(2), 25–39.

Stokes, S. F. (2014). The impact of phonological neighborhood density on typical and atypical emerging lexicons. *Journal of Child Language, 41*(3), 634–657. https://doi.org/10.1017/S030500091300010X

Stollman, M. H. P., van Velzen, E. C. W., Simkens, H. M. F., Snik, A. F. M., & van den Broek, P. (2004). Development of auditory processing in 6–12-year-old children: A longitudinal study, *International Journal of Audiology, 43*(1), 34–44. https://doi.org/10.1080/14992020400050006

Stone, M., Faber, A., Raphael, L. J., & Shawker, T. H. (1992). Cross-sectional tongue shape and linguopalatal contact patterns in [s], [ʃ], [f], and [l]. *Journal of Phonetics, 20*(2), 253–270.

Storkel, H. L. (2018). The complexity approach to phonological treatment: How to select treatment targets. *Language, Speech, and Hearing Services in Schools, 49*(3), 463–481. https://doi.org/10.1044/2017_LSHSS-17-0082

Storkel, H. L. (2022). Minimal, maximal, or multiple: Which contrastive intervention approach to use with children with speech sound disorders? *Language, Speech, and Hearing Services in Schools,* 1–14. https://doi.org/10.1044/2021_LSHSS-21-00105

Størvold, G. V., Aarethun, K., & Bratberg, G. H. (2013). Age for onset of walking and prewalking strategies. *Early Human Development, 89*(9), 655–659. https://doi.org/10.1016/j.earlhumdev.2013.04.010

Strand, E. A. (1995, May). Treatment of motor speech disorders in children. In *Seminars in speech and language* (Vol. 16, No. 02, pp. 126–139). Thieme Medical Publishers.

Strand, E. A. (2020). Dynamic temporal and tactile cueing: A treatment strategy for childhood apraxia of speech. *American Journal of Speech-Language Pathology, 29*(1), 30–48. https://doi.org/10.1044/2019_AJSLP-19-0005

Strand, E. A., Stoeckel, R., & Baas, B. (2006). Treatment of severe childhood apraxia of speech: A treatment efficacy study. *Journal of Medical Speech-Language Pathology, 14*(4), 297–308.

Strand, E. A., McCauley, R. J., Weigand, S. D., Stoeckel, R. E., & Baas, B. S. (2013). A motor speech assessment for children with severe speech disorders: Reliability and validity evidence. *Journal of Speech, Language, and Hearing Research, 56*(2), 505–520. https://doi.org/10.1044/1092-4388(2012/12-0094)

Strange, W. (2011). Automatic selective perception (ASP) of first and second language speech: A working model. *Journal of Phonetics, 39*(4), 456–466. https://doi.org/10.1016/j.wocn.2010.09.001

Strömbergsson, S., Salvi, G., & House, D. (2015). Acoustic and perceptual evaluation of category goodness of/t/and/k/in typical and misarticulated children's speech. *The Journal of the Acoustical Society of America, 137*(6), 3422–3435. https://doi.org/10.1121/1.4921033

Strömbergsson, S., Holm, K., Edlund, J., Lagerberg, T., & McAllister, A. (2020). Audience response system-based evaluation of intelligibility of children's connected speech-validity, reliability and listener differences. *Journal of Communication Disorders, 87*, 106037. https://doi.org/10.1016/j.jcomdis.2020.106037

Sturm, J. A., & Seery, C. H. (2007). Speech and articulatory rates of school-age children in conversation and narrative contexts. *Language, Speech, and Hearing Services in Schools, 38*, 47–59. https://doi.org/10.1044/0161-1461(2007/005)

Subara-Zukic, E., Cole, M. H., McGuckian, T. B., Steenbergen, B., Green, D., Smits-Engelsman, B., Wilson, P. H. (2022). Behavioral and neuroimaging research on developmental coordination disorder (DCD): A combined systematic review and meta-analysis of recent findings. *Frontiers in Psychology, 13, 2.* https://doi.org/10.3389/fpsyg.2022.809455

Sugathan, N., & Maruthy, S. (2021). Predictive factors for persistence and recovery of stuttering in children: A systematic review. *International Journal of Speech-Language Pathology, 23*(4), 359–371. https://doi.org/10.1080/17549507.2020.1812718

Sugden, E., Baker, E., Munro, N., & Williams, A. L. (2016). Involvement of parents in intervention for childhood speech sound disorders: A review of the evidence. *International Journal of Language & Communication Disorders, 51*(6), 597–625. https://doi.org/10.1111/1460-6984.12247

Sugden, E., Lloyd, S., Lam, J., & Cleland, J. (2019). Systematic review of ultrasound visual biofeedback in intervention for speech sound disorders. *International Journal of Language & Communication Disorders, 54*(5), 705–728. https://doi.org/10.1111/1460-6984.12478

Sugden, E., Baker, E., Williams, A. L., Munro, N., & Trivette, C. M. (2020). Evaluation of parent- and speech-language pathologist–delivered multiple oppositions intervention for children with phonological impairment: A multiple-baseline design study. *American Journal of Speech-Language Pathology, 29*(1), 111–126. https://doi.org/10.1044/2019_AJSLP-18-0248

Sunderajan, T., & Kanhere, S. V. (2019). Speech and language delay in children: Prevalence and risk factors. *Journal of Family Medicine and Primary Care, 8*(5), 1642. https:/. https://doi.org/10.4103/jfmpc.jfmpc_162_19

Suri, S., Tompson, B. D., & Cornfoot, L. (2010). Cranial base, maxillary and mandibular morphology in Down syndrome. *Angle Orthodontist, 80*(5), 861–869. https://doi.org/10.2319/111709-650.1

Sutherland, D., & Gillon, G. T. (2005). Assessment of phonological representations in children with speech impairment. *Language, Speech, and Hearing Services in Schools, 36*(4), 294–307. https://doi.org/10.1044/0161-1461(2005/030)

Swanson, H. L., Trainin, G., Necoechea, D. M., & Hammill, D. D. (2003). Rapid naming, phonological awareness, and reading: A meta-analysis of the correlation evidence. *Review of Educational Research, 73*(4), 407–440. https://doi.org/10.3102/003465430730044

Syrett, K., & Kawahara, S. (2014). Production and perception of listener-oriented clear speech in child language. *Journal of Child Language, 41*(6), 1373–1389. https://doi.org/10.1017/S0305000913000482

Tafiadis, D., Zarokanellou, V., Voniati, L., Prentza, A., Drosos, K., Papadopoulos, A., & Ziavra, N. (2021). Evaluation of diadochokinesis in Greek preschoolers with speech sound disorders using a diadochokinetic rates protocol. *Communication Disorders Quarterly, 43*(3), 172–181. https://doi.org/10.1177/15257401211017065

Taft, M. (1986). Lexical access codes in visual and auditory word recognition. *Language and Cognitive Processes, l*(4), 297–308.

Tager-Flusberg, H. (1981). On the nature of linguistic functioning in early infantile autism. *Journal of Autism and Developmental Disorders. 11*, 45–56.

Tallal, P. (2000). Experimental studies of language learning impairments: From research to remediation. In D. V. M. Bishop & L. B. Leonard (Eds.), *Speech and language impairments in children: Causes, characteristics, intervention and outcome* (pp. 131–155). Psychology Press.

Tamburelli, M., Sanoudaki, E., Jones, G., & Sowinska, M. (2015). Acceleration in the bilingual acquisition of phonological structure: Evidence from Polish–English bilingual children. *Bilingualism: Language and Cognition, 18*(4), 713–725. https://doi.org/10.1017/S1366728914000716

Tambyraja, S. R., Farquharson, K., & Justice, L. M. (2023). Phonological processing skills in children with speech sound disorder: A multiple case study approach. *International Journal of Language & Communication Disorders, 58*(1), 15–27. https://doi.org/10.1111/1460-6984.12764

Tanaka, H., Ishikawa, T., Lee, J., & Kakei, S. (2020). The cerebro-cerebellum as a locus of forward model: A review. *Frontiers in Systems Neuroscience, 14*, 19. https://doi.org/10.3389/fnsys.2020.00019

Tang, Y., Liu, Q., Wang, W., & Cox, T. J. (2018). A non-intrusive method for estimating binaural speech intelligibility from noise-corrupted signals captured by a pair of microphones. *Speech Communication, 96*, 116–128. https://doi.org/10.1016/j.specom.2017.12.005

Tanna, R. J., Lin, J. W., & De Jesus, O. (2022). Sensorineural hearing loss. *StatPearls* [Internet]. StatPearls Publishing.

Taruna, R. (2022). Phonological memory and phonological awareness in children: A meta-analysis. *Jurnal Keterapian Fisik, 7*(2),105–114. https://doi.org/10.37341/jkf.v0i0.380

Tate, R. L., & Perdices, M. (2019). *Single-case experimental designs for clinical research and neurorehabilitation settings: Planning, conduct, analysis and reporting*. Routledge.

Tausche, E., Luck, O., & Harzer, W. (2004). Prevalence of malocclusions in the early mixed dentition and orthodontic treatment need. *European Journal of Orthodontia*, *26*(3), 237–44. https://doi.org/10.1093/ejo/26.3.237.

Tavares, E. L. M., Brasolotto, A. G., Rodrigues, S. A., Pessin, A. B. B., & Martins, R. H. G. (2012). Maximum phonation time and s/z ratio in a large child cohort. *Journal of Voice*, *26*(5), 675.e1–4. https://doi.org/10.1016/j.jvoice.2012.03.001

Taylor, M. J., Rosenqvist, M. A., Larsson, H., Gillberg, C., D'Onofrio, B. M., Lichtenstein, P., & Lundström, S. (2020). Etiology of autism spectrum disorders and autistic traits over time. *JAMA Psychiatry*, *77*(9), 936–943. https://doi.org/10.1001/jamapsychiatry.2020.0680

Taylor, R. L. (2000). *Assessment of exceptional students: Educational and psychological procedures* (5th ed.). Allyn & Bacon.

Temperley, D. (2009). Distributional stress regularity: A corpus study. *Journal of Psycholinguistic Research*, *38*, 75–92. https://doi.org/10.1007/s10936-008-9084-0

Templin, M. C. (1957). *Certain language skills in children; Their development and interrelationships*. University of Minnesota Press.

Templin, M. C., & Darley, F. L. (1968). *The Templin-Darley Tests of Articulation*. University of Iowa Press.

Tenenbaum, E. J., Carpenter, K. L., Sabatos-DeVito, M., Hashemi, J., Vermeer, S., Sapiro, G., & Dawson, G. (2020). A six-minute measure of vocalizations in toddlers with autism spectrum disorder. *Autism Research*, *13*(8), 1373–1382. https://doi.org/10.1002/aur.2293

Terband, H., & Van Brenk, F. (2023). Modeling responses to auditory feedback perturbations in adults, children, and children with complex speech sound disorders: Evidence for impaired auditory self-monitoring? *Journal of Speech, Language, and Hearing Research*, *66*(5), 1563–1587. https://doi.org/10.1044/2023_JSLHR-22-00379

Terband, H., Maassen, B., & Maas, E. (2019). A psycholinguistic framework for diagnosis and treatment planning of developmental speech disorders. *Folia Phoniatrica et Logopaedica*, *71*(5-6), 216–227. https://doi.org/10.1159/000499426

Terband, H., Spruit, M., & Maassen, B. (2018). Speech impairment in boys with fetal alcohol spectrum disorders. *American Journal of Speech-language Pathology*, *27*(4), 1405–1425. https://doi.org/10.1044/2018_AJSLP-17-0013

Terband, H., Maassen, B., Guenther, F. H., & Brumberg, J. (2014). Auditory–motor interactions in pediatric motor speech disorders: Neurocomputational modeling of disordered development. *Journal of Communication Disorders*, *47*, 17–33. https://doi.org/10.1016/j.jcomdis.2014.01.001

Terband, H., van Brenk, F., & van Doornik-van der Zee, A. (2014). Auditory feedback perturbation in children with developmental speech sound disorders. *Journal of Communication Disorders*, *51*, 64–77. https://doi.org/10.1016/j.jcomdis.2014.06.009

Terband, H., Namasivayam, A., Maas, E., van Brenk, F., Mailend, M. L., Diepeveen, S., . . . Maassen, B. (2019). Assessment of childhood apraxia of speech: A review/tutorial of objective measurement techniques. *Journal of Speech, Language, and Hearing Research*, *62*(8S), 2999–3032. https://doi.org/10.1044/2019_JSLHR-S-CSMC7-19-0214

Tessel, C. A., & Luque, J. S. (2021). A comparison of phonological and articulation-based approaches to accent modification using small groups. *Speech, Language and Hearing*, *24*(3), 145–158. https://doi.org/10.1080/2050571X.2020.1730544

Thatcher, K. L. (2010). The development of phonological awareness with specific language-impaired and typical children. *Psychology in the Schools*, *47*(5), 467–480.

Thelen, E. (1979). Rhythmical stereotypies in normal human infants. *Animal Behaviour*, *27*(Pt. 3), 699–715. https://doi.org/10.1016/0003-3472(79)90006-X

Thelen, E. (2000). Motor development as foundation and future of developmental psychology. *International Journal of Behavioral Development*, *24*(4), 385–397. https://doi.org/10.1080/016502500750037937

Thiessen, E. D., Girard, S., & Erickson, L. C. (2016). Statistical learning and the critical period: How a continuous learning mechanism can give rise to discontinuous learning. *Wiley Interdisciplinary Reviews: Cognitive Science*, *7*(4), 276-288. https://doi.org/10.1002/wcs.1394

Thijs, Z., Bruneel, L., De Pauw, G., & Van Lierde, K. M. (2022). Oral myofunctional and articulation disorders in children with malocclusions: A systematic review. *Folia Phoniat-*

rica et Logopaedica, *74*(1), 1–16. https://doi.org/10.1159/000516414

Thomas, D. C., McCabe, P., & Ballard, K. J. (2014). Rapid syllable transitions (ReST) treatment for childhood apraxia of speech: The effect of lower dose-frequency. *Journal of Communication Disorders*, *51*, 29–42. https://doi.org/10.1016/j.jcomdis.2014.06.004

Thomas, D. C., McCabe, P., & Ballard, K. J. (2018). Combined clinician-parent delivery of rapid syllable transition (ReST) treatment for childhood apraxia of speech. *International Journal of Speech-Language Pathology*, *20*(7), 683–698. https://doi.org/10.1080/17549507.2017.1316423

Thomas, D. C., McCabe, P., Ballard, K. J., & Bricker-Katz, G. (2018). Parent experiences of variations in service delivery of Rapid Syllable Transition (ReST) treatment for childhood apraxia of speech. *Developmental Neurorehabilitation*, *21*(6), 391–401. https://doi.org/10.1080/17518423.2017.1323971

Thomas, D. C., McCabe, P., Ballard, K. J., & Lincoln, M. (2016). Telehealth delivery of Rapid Syllable Transitions (ReST) treatment for childhood apraxia of speech. *International Journal of Language & Communication Disorders*, *51*(6), 654–671. https://doi.org/10.1111/1460-6984.12238

Thomas, E. S., & Zwolan, T. A. (2019). Communication mode and speech and language outcomes of young cochlear implant recipients: A comparison of auditory-verbal, oral communication, and total communication. *Otology & Neurotology*, *40*(10), e975–e983. https://doi.org/10.1097/MAO.0000000000002405

Thomas, S., Patel, S., Gummalla, P., Tablizo, M. A., & Kier, C. (2022). You cannot hit snooze on OSA: Sequelae of pediatric obstructive sleep apnea. *Children*, *9*(2), 261. https://doi.org/10.3390/children9020261

Thomas-Stonell, N., Oddson, B., Robertson, B., & Rosenbaum, P. (2010). Development of the FOCUS (Focus on the Outcomes of Communication Under Six): A communication outcome measure for preschool children. *Developmental Medicine & Child Neurology*, *52*, 47–53. https://doi.org/10.1111/j.1469-8749.2009.03410.x

Thomas-Stonell. N., Washington, K., Oddson, B., Robertson, B, & Rosenbaum, P. (2013). Measuring communicative participation using the FOCUS©: focus on the outcomes of communication under six. *Child Care Health & Development*, *39*(4), 474–80.

Thompson, C. K. (2007). Complexity in language learning and treatment. *American Journal of Speech-Language Pathology*, *16*(1), 3–5. https://doi.org/10.1044/1058-0360(2007/002).

Thoonen, G., Maassen, B., Wit, J., Gabreels, F., & Schreuder, R. (1996). The integrated use of maximum performance tasks in differential diagnostic evaluations among children with motor speech disorders. *Clinical Linguistics & Phonetics*, *10*(4), 311–336. https://doi.org/10.3109/02699209608985178

Thurstone, L. L. (1928). The measurement of opinion. *The Journal of Abnormal and Social Psychology*, *22*, 415.

Tiemeier, H., Lenroot, R. K., Greenstein, D. K., Tran, L., Pierson, R., & Giedd, J. N. (2010). Cerebellum development during childhood and adolescence: A longitudinal morphometric MRI study. *Neuroimage*, *49*(1), 63–70. https://doi.org/10.1016/j.neuroimage.2009.08.016

Tilsen, S. (2016). Selection and coordination: The articulatory basis for the emergence of phonological structure. *Journal of Phonetics*, *55*, 53–77. https://doi.org/10.1016/j.wocn.2015.11.005

Tiwari, S., Kallianpur, D., & DeSilva, K. A. (2017). Communication impairments in children with inborn errors of metabolism: A preliminary study. *Indian Journal of Psychological Medicine*, *39*(2), 146–151. https://doi.org/10.4103/0253-=7176.203125

Tjaden, K. K., & Liss, J. M. (1995a). The role of listener familiarity in the perception of dysarthric speech. *Clinical Linguistics and Phonetics*, *9*, 139–154. https://doi.org/10.3109/02699209508985329

Tjaden, K. K., & Liss, J. M. (1995b). The influence of familiarity on judgments of treated speech. *American Journal of Speech-Language Pathology*, *4*(1), 39–47. https://doi.org/10.1044/1058-0360.0401.39

To, C. K. S., McLeod, S., Sam, K. L., & Law, T. (2022). Predicting which children will normalize without intervention for speech sound disorders. *Journal of Speech, Language, and Hearing Research*, *65*(5), 1724–1741. https://doi.org/10.1044/2022_JSLHR-21-00444

Toki, E. I., Pange, J., & Mikropoulos, T. A. (2012). An online expert system for diagnostic assessment procedures on young children's oral speech and language. *Procedia Computer*

Science, 14, 428–437. https://doi.org/10.1016/j.procs.2012.10.049

Tomasino, B., & Gremese, M. (2016). The cognitive side of M1. *Frontiers in Human Neuroscience, 10*, 298. https://doi.org/10.3389/fnhum.2016.00298

Tomes, C. S. (1872). On the developmental origin of the v-shaped contracted maxilla. *Monthly review of Dental Surgery, 1*, 2–5

Toomim, H. (2000). A report of preliminary data: QEEG, SPECT, and HEG; Targeted treatment positions for neurofeedback. *Applied Psychophysiology and Biofeedback, 25*(4), 253–254.

Torrance, G. W., Feeny, D., & Furlong, W. (2001). Visual analog scales: Do they have a role in the measurement of preferences for health states? *Medical Decision Making, 21*, 329–334.

Torres, F., Fuentes-López, E., Fuente, A., & Sevilla, F. (2020). Identification of the factors associated with the severity of the speech production problems in children with comorbid speech sound disorder and developmental language disorder. *Journal of Communication Disorders, 88*, 106054. https://doi.org/10.1016/j.jcomdis.2020.106054

Torres-Moreno, M. J., Aedo-Muñoz, E., Hernández-Wimmer, C., Brito, C. J., & Miarka, B. (2022). Fundamental contributions of neuroscience to motor learning in children: A systematic review. *Motricidade, 18*(2). https://doi.org/10.6063/motricidade.25216

Tourville, J. A., & Guenther, F. H. (2011). The DIVA model: A neural theory of speech acquisition and production. *Language and Cognitive Processes, 26*(7), 952–981. https://doi.org/10.1080/01690960903498424

Tracy, J. L. (2014). An evolutionary approach to understanding distinct emotions. *Emotion Review, 6*(4), 308–312. https://doi.org/10.1177/1754073914534478

Tremblay, S., Houle, G., & Ostry, D. J. (2008). Specificity of speech motor learning. *Journal of Neuroscience, 28*(10), 2426–2434. https://doi.org/10.1523/JNEUROSCI.4196-07.2008

Trewartha, K. M., & Phillips, N. A. (2013). Detecting self-produced speech errors before and after articulation: An ERP investigation. *Frontiers in Human Neuroscience, 7*, 763. https://doi.org/10.3389/fnhum.2013.00763

Troncone, A., & Esposito, A. (2011). On the recognition of emotional voices by typical and speech impaired children. *Neural Nets WIRN11* (pp. 228–234). IOS Press.

Trost, J. E. (1981). Articulatory additions to the classical description of the speech of persons with cleft palate. *The Cleft Palate Journal, 18*(3), 193–203.

Tsuji, S., & Cristia, A. (2014). Perceptual attunement in vowels: A meta-analysis. *Developmental Psychobiology, 56*, 179–191. https://doi.org/10.1002/dev.21179

Ttofari Eecen, K., Eadie, P., Morgan, A. T., & Reilly, S. (2019). Validation of Dodd's Model for Differential Diagnosis of childhood speech sound disorders: A longitudinal community cohort study. *Developmental Medicine & Child Neurology, 61*(6), 689–696.

Tubbs, R. S., Shoja, M. M., & Loukas, M. (2016). *Bergman's comprehensive encyclopedia of human anatomic variation*. Wiley & Sons.

Tumanova, V., Conture, E. G., Lambert, E. W., & Walden, T. A. (2014). Speech disfluencies of preschool-age children who do and do not stutter. *Journal of Communication Disorders, 49*, 25–41. https://doi.org/10.1016/j.jcomdis.2014.01.003

Turk, A., & Shattuck-Hufnagel, S. (2013). What is speech rhythm? A commentary on Arvaniti and Rodriquez, Krivokapić, and Goswami and Leong. *Laboratory Phonology, 4*(1), 93–118.

Tyler, A. A. (2008, November). What works: Evidence-based intervention for children with speech sound disorders. In *Seminars in Speech and Language 29*(4), 320–330).

Tyler, A. A., & Tolbert, L. C. (2002). Speech-language assessment in the clinical setting. *American Journal of Speech-Language Pathology, 11*, 215–220.

Tyler, A. A., & Watterson, K. H. (1991). Effects of phonological versus language intervention in preschoolers with both phonological and language impairment. *Child Language Teaching and Therapy, 7*, 141–160.

Tyler, A. A., Edwards, M. L., & Saxman, J. H. (1987). Clinical application of two phonologically based treatment procedures. *Journal of Speech and Hearing Disorders. 52*, 393–409. https://doi.org/10.1044/jshd.5204.393

Ueno, T., Saito, S., Rogers, T. T., & Ralph, M. A. L. (2011). Lichtheim 2: Synthesizing aphasia and the neural basis of language in a neurocomputational model of the dual dorsal-ventral language pathways. *Neuron, 72*(2), 385–396. https://doi.org/10.1016/j.neuron.2011.09.013

Ungerleider, L. G., & Haxby, J. V. (1994). 'What' and 'where' in the human brain. *Current Opin-*

ion in Neurobiology, *4*(2), 157–165. https://doi.org/10.1016/0959-4388(94)90066-3

Uong, E. C., McDonough, J. M., Tayag-Kier, C. E., Zhao, H., Haselgrove, J., Mahboubi, S., . . . Arens, R. (2001). Magnetic resonance imaging of the upper airway in children with Down syndrome. *American Journal of Respiratory and Critical Care Medicine*, *163*(3), 731–736. https://doi.org/10.1164/ajrccm.163.3.2004231

U. S. Food and Drug Administration, & National Institutes of Health. (2016). *BEST (Biomarkers, Endpoints, and other tools) resource*. FDA-NIH Biomarker Working Group.

U.S. Food and Drug Administration (2020). *Patient-focused drug development: Collecting comprehensive and representative input. Final guidance document.* https://www.fda.gov/media/139088/download (2020).

Vacca, R. A., Bawari, S., Valenti, D., Tewari, D., Nabavi, S. F., Shirooie, S., . . . Nabavi, S. M. (2019). Down syndrome: Neurobiological alterations and therapeutic targets. *Neuroscience & Biobehavioral Reviews*, *98*, 234–255. https://doi.org/10.1016/j.neubiorev.2019.01.001

Vallino, L.D., & Tompson, B. (1993). Perceptual characteristics of consonant errors associated with malocclusion. *Journal of Oral and Maxillofacial Surgery*, *51*, 850–856.

van Abswoude, F., Mombarg, R., de Groot, W., Spruijtenburg, G. E., & Steenbergen, B. (2021). Implicit motor learning in primary school children: A systematic review. *Journal of Sports Sciences*, *39*(22), 2577–2595. https://doi.org/10.1080/02640414.2021.1947010

van Borsel, J., & D'haeseleer, L. (2019). The Process Density Index as a measure of phonological development: Data from Dutch. *Communication Disorders Quarterly*, *40*(4), 220–227. https://doi.org/10.1177/15257401187905

van Borsel, J., Dor, O., & Rondal, J. (2008). Speech fluency in fragile X syndrome. *Clinical Linguistics & Phonetics*, *22*(1), 1–11. https://doi.org/10.1080/02699200701601997

van Bysterveldt, A. K., Gillon, G., & Foster-Cohen, S. (2010) Integrated speech and phonological awareness intervention for pre-school children with Down syndrome, *International Journal of Language & Communication Disorders*, *45*(3), 320–335, https://doi.org/10.3109/13682820903003514

Vance, M., Stackhouse, J., & Wells, B. (2005). Speech-production skills in children aged 3–7 years. *International Journal of Language & Communication Disorders*, *40*(1), 29-48. https://doi.org/10.1080/1368282041000171 6172

VandenBos, G. R. (Ed.) (2007). *APA dictionary of psychology*. American Psychological Association.

Vander Ghinst, M., Bourguignon, M., Niesen, M., Wens, V., Hassid, S., Choufani, G., . . . De Tiège, X. (2019). Cortical tracking of speech-in-noise develops from childhood to adulthood. *Journal of Neuroscience*, *39*(15), 2938–2950. https://doi.org/10.1523/JNEUROSCI.1732-18.2019

Van Der Merwe, A. (2021) New perspectives on speech motor planning and programming in the context of the four-level model and its implications for understanding the pathophysiology underlying apraxia of speech and other motor speech disorders. *Aphasiology*, *35*(4), 397–342. https://doi.org/10.1080/02687038.2020.1765306

Vander Stappen, C., & Reybroeck, M. V. (2018). Phonological awareness and rapid automatized naming are independent phonological competencies with specific impacts on word reading and spelling: An intervention study. *Frontiers in Psychology*, *9*, 320. https://doi.org/10.3389/fpsyg.2018.00320

Vanderwegen, J., Van Nuffelen, G., Elen, R., & De Bodt, M. (2019). The influence of age, sex, visual feedback, bulb position, and the order of testing on maximum anterior and posterior tongue strength in healthy Belgian children. *Dysphagia*, *34*(6), 834–851. https://doi.org/10.1007/s00455-019-09976-x

Van Engen, K. J., & Peelle, J. E. (2014). Listening effort and accented speech. *Frontiers in Human Neuroscience*, *8*, 577. https://doi.org/10.3389/fnhum.2014.00577

Vanhove, J. (2013). The critical period hypothesis in second language acquisition: A statistical critique and a reanalysis. *PLoS ONE*, *8*(7), e69172. https://doi.org/10.1371/journal.pone.0069172

Van Lieshout, P. (2004). Dynamical systems theory and its application in speech. In B. Maassen et al. (Eds.), *Speech motor control in normal and disordered speech* (pp. 51–82). Oxford University Press.

Van Lieshout, P. H., & Goldstein, L. M. (2008). Articulatory phonology and speech impairment. In M. J. Ball, M. R. Perkins, N. Müller,

& S. Howard (Eds.), *The handbook of clinical linguistics* (pp. 467–479). Blackwell.

van Mourik, M., Catsman-Berrevoets, C. E., Paquier, P. F., Yousef-Bak, E., & Van Dongen, H. R. (1997). Acquired childhood dysarthria: Review of its clinical presentation. *Pediatric Neurology, 17*(4), 299–307.

Van Riper, C. (1954, 1947, 1939). *Speech correction: Principles and methods.* Prentice-Hall.

Van Riper, C. (1978). *Speech correction: Principles and methods* (6th ed.). Prentice-Hall.

van Santen, J. P., Prud'hommeaux, E. T., & Black, L. M. (2009). Automated Assessment of Prosody Production. *Speech Communication, 51*(11), 1082–1097. https://doi.org/10.1016/j.specom.2009.04.007

van Zelst, A. L., & Earle, F. S. (2021). A case for the role of memory consolidation in speech-motor learning. *Psychonomic Bulletin & Review, 28*, 81–95. https://doi.org/10.3758/s13423-020-01793-

Vashdi, E., Avramov, A., Falatov, Š., Huang, Y. C., Jiang, P. R., & Mamina-Chiriac, P. T. (2021). The correlation between non-speech oral motor exercises (NSOME) and speech production in childhood apraxia of speech treatment. A wide clinical retrospective research. *BRAIN. Broad Research in Artificial Intelligence and Neuroscience, 11*(3Suppl.), 98–113. https://doi.org/10.18662/brain/11.3Sup1/126

Ventura, P., Kolinsky, R., Fernandes, S., Querido, L., & Morais, J. (2007). Lexical restructuring in the absence of literacy. *Cognition, 105*(2), 334–361. https://doi.org/10.1016/j.cognition.2006.10.002

Vermiglio, A. J. (2014). On the clinical entity in audiology:(Central) auditory processing and speech recognition in noise disorders. *Journal of the American Academy of Audiology, 25*(9), 904–917.

Vickie, Y. Y., Kadis, D. S., Goshulak, D., Namasivayam, A. K., Pukonen, M., Kroll, R. M., . . . Pang, E. W. (2018). Impact of motor speech intervention on neural activity in children with speech sound disorders: Use of Magnetoencephalography. *Journal of Behavioral and Brain Science, 8*(07), 415. https://doi.org/10.4236/jbbs.2018.87026

Vigliocco, G., Shi, J., Gu, Y., & Grzyb, B. (2020, June). Child directed speech: Impact of variations in speaking-rate on word learning. *Proceedings of the 42nd Annual Meeting of the Cognitive Science Society* (Vol. 42, pp. 1043–1049). Cognitive Science Society.

Vihman, M. (1993). Variable paths to early word production. *Journal of Phonetics, 21*, 61–82. https://doi.org/10.1016/S0095-4470(19)31321-X

Vihman, M. M. (2018). The development of prosodic structure: A usage-based approach. In P, Prieto & N. Esteve-Gibert (Eds.), *The development of prosody in first language acquisition* (pp. 185–206). John Benjamins.

Vihman, M. M. (2022). The developmental origins of phonological memory. *Psychological Review, 129*(6), 1495–1508. https://doi.org/10.1037/rev0000354

Vihman, M. M., DePaolis, R. A., & Davis, B. L. (1998). Is there a "trochaic bias" in early word learning? Evidence from infant production in English and French. *Child Development, 69*(4), 935–949. https://doi.org/10.1111/j.1467-8624.1998.tb06152.x

Vihman, M. M., Macken, M. A., Miller, R., Simmons, H., & Miller, J. (1985). From babbling to speech: A re-assessment of the continuity issue. *Language, 61*, 397–445. https://doi.org/10.2307/414151

Vila, P. M., & Lieu, J. E. (2015). Asymmetric and unilateral hearing loss in children. *Cell and Tissue Research, 361*, 271–278. https://doi.org/10.1007/ s00441-015-2208-6.

Vilain, A., Dole, M., Loevenbruck, H., Pascalis, O., & Schwartz, J. L. (2019). The role of production abilities in the perception of consonant category in infants. *Developmental Science, 22*(6), e12830. https://doi.org/10.1111/desc.12830

Visser-Bochane, M. I., Reijneveld, S. A., Krijnen, W. P., Van der Schans, C. P., & Luinge, M. R. (2020). Identifying milestones in language development for young children ages 1 to 6 years. *Academic Pediatrics, 20*(3), 421–429. https://doi.org/10.1016/j.acap.2019.07.003

Vissers, C. T. W., Tomas, E., & Law, J. (2020). The emergence of inner speech and its measurement in atypically developing children. *Frontiers in Psychology, 279*. https://doi.org/10.3389/fpsyg.2020.00279

Vitale, G. J. (1986). *Test of Oral Structures and Functions.* Educational Publications.

Vlach, H. A., & Sandhofer, C. M. (2012). Fast mapping across time: Memory processes support children's retention of learned words. *Frontiers in Psychology, 3*, 46. https://doi.org/10.3389/fpsyg.2012.00046

Vogler, R. C., Ii, F. W., & Pilgram, T. K. (2000). Age-specific size of the normal adenoid pad on magnetic resonance imaging. *Clinical Otolaryngology & Allied Sciences, 25*, 392–395. https://doi.org/10.1046/j.1365-2273.2000.00381.x

Vohr, B., Jodoin-Krauzyk, J., Tucker, R., Johnson, M.J., Topol. D., & Ahlgren, M. (2008). Early language outcomes of early-identified infants with permanent hearing loss at 12 to 16 months of age. *Pediatrics, 122*(3), 535–544. https://doi.org/10.1542/peds.2007-2028 PMID: 18762523.

Volkov, S. I., Ginter, O. V., Covantev, S., & Corlateanu, A. (2020). Adenoid hypertrophy, craniofacial growth and obstructive sleep apnea: A crucial triad in children. *Current Respiratory Medicine Reviews, 16*(3), 144–155.

Vorperian, H. K., & Kent, R. D. (2007). Vowel acoustic space development in children: A synthesis of acoustic and anatomic data. *Journal of Speech, Language, and Hearing Research, 50*(6), 1510–1545. https://doi.org/10.1044/1092-4388(2007/104)

Vorperian, H.K., Kent, R.K., Lee, Y. & Bolt, D.M. (2019). Corner vowels in males and females ages 4 to 20 years: Fundamental and F1-F4 formant frequencies. *The Journal of the Acoustical Society of America, 146*(5), 3255–3274. https://doi.org/10.1121/1.5131271

Vorperian, H. K., Kent, R. D., Lee, Y., & Buhr, K. A. (2023). Vowel production in children and adults With Down syndrome: Fundamental and formant frequencies of the corner vowels. *Journal of Speech, Language, and Hearing Research, 66*(4), 1208–1239.

Vorperian, H. K., Kent, R. D., Lindstrom, M. J., Kalina, C. M., Gentry, L. R., & Yandell, B. S. (2005). Development of vocal tract length during early childhood: A magnetic resonance imaging study. *Journal of the Acoustical Society of America, 117*, 338–350. https://doi.org/10.1121/1.1835958

Vorperian, H. K., Wang, S., Chung, M. K., Schimek, E. M., Durtschi, R. B., Kent, R. D., . . . Gentry, L. R. (2009). Anatomic development of the oral and pharyngeal portions of the vocal tract: An imaging study. *The Journal of the Acoustical Society of America, 125*(3), 1666–1678. https://doi.org/10.1121/1.3075589

Vouloumanos, A., & Werker, J. F. (2007). Listening to language at birth: Evidence for a bias for speech in neonates. *Developmental Science, 10*(2), 159–164. https://doi.org/10.1111/j.1467-7687.2007.00549.x

Vukovic, M., Jovanovska, M., & Rajic, L. J. (2022). Phonological awareness in children with developmental language disorder. *Archives of Public Health, 14*(1). doi.org/10.3889/aph.2022.6046

Vygotsky, L. S. (1986). *Thought and language* (A. Kozulin, Trans.). MIT Press.

Waddington, C. H. (1942). The epigenotype. *Endeavour, 1*, 18–20.

Wadsworth, S. D., Maul, C. A., & Stevens, E. J. (1998). The prevalence of orofacial myofunctional disorders among children identified with speech and language disorders in grades kindergarten through six. *International Journal of Orofacial Myology, 24*, 1–19

Wagner, M., & Watson, D. G. (2010). Experimental and theoretical advances in prosody: A review. *Language and Cognitive Processes, 25*(7-9), 905–945. https://doi.org/10.1080/01690961003589492

Waldstein, R. S., & Baum, S. R. (1991). Anticipatory coarticulation in the speech of profoundly hearing–impaired and normally hearing children. *Journal of Speech, Language, and Hearing Research, 34*(6), 1276–1285. https://doi.org/10.1044/jshr.3406.1276

Walker, J. F., & Archibald, L. M. (2006). Articulation rate in preschool children: A 3-year longitudinal study. *International Journal of Language & Communication Disorders, 41*(5), 541–565. https://doi.org/10.1080/10428190500343043

Wallace, I. F., Berkman, N. D., Watson, L. R., Coyne-Beasley, T., Wood, C. T., Cullen, K., & Lohr, K. N. (2015). Screening for speech and language delay in children 5 years old and younger: A systematic review. *Pediatrics, 136*(2), e448–e462. https://doi.org/10.1542/peds.2014-3889

Wallentin, M. (2009). Putative sex differences in verbal abilities and language cortex: A critical review. *Brain and Language, 108*(3), 175–183. https://doi.org/10.1016/j.bandl.2008.07.001

Walley, A. C., Metsala, J. L., & Garlock, V. M. (2003). Spoken vocabulary growth: Its role in the development of phoneme awareness and early reading ability. *Reading and Writing, 16*(1), 5–20.

Walsh, J., & Tunkel, D. (2017). Diagnosis and treatment of ankyloglossia in newborns and infants: a review. *JAMA Otolaryngology-Head*

& Neck Surgery, *143*(10), 1032–1039. https://https://doi.org/10.1001/jamaoto.2017.0948

Walton, J. H., & Orlikoff, R. F. (1994). Speaker race identification from acoustic cues in the vocal signal. *Journal of Speech, Language, and Hearing Research*, *37*(4), 738–745. https://doi.org/10.1044/jshr.3704.738

Wang, D., Mason, R. A., Lory, C., Kim, S. Y., David, M., & Guo, X. (2020). Vocal stereotypy and autism spectrum disorder: A systematic review of interventions. *Research in Autism Spectrum Disorders*, *78*, 101647. https://doi.org/10.1016/j.rasd.2020.101647

Wang, J., Joanisse, M. F., & Booth, J. R. (2020). Neural representations of phonology in temporal cortex scaffold longitudinal reading gains in 5-to 7-year-old children. *NeuroImage*, *207*, 116359. https://doi.org/10.1016/j.neuroimage.2019.116359

Wang, J., Yang, X., Hao, S., & Wang, Y. (2022). The effect of ankyloglossia and tongue-tie division on speech articulation: A systematic review. *International Journal of Paediatric Dentistry*, *32*(2), 144–156. https://doi.org/10.1111/ipd.12802

Wang, Y. T., Green, J. R., Nip, I. S., Kent, R. D., & Kent, J. F. (2010). Breath group analysis for reading and spontaneous speech in healthy adults. *Folia Phoniatrica et Logopaedica*, *62*(6), 297–302. https://doi.org/10.1159/000316976

Wang, Y., Chung, M. K., & Vorperian, H. K. (2016). Composite growth model applied to human oral and pharyngeal structures and identifying the contribution of growth types. *Statistical Methods in Medical Research*, *25*, 1975–1990. https://doi.org/10.1177/0962280213508849

Ward, R., Hennessey, N., Barty, E., Elliott, C., Valentine, J., & Cantle Moore, R. (2022). Clinical utilisation of the Infant Monitor of vocal Production (IMP) for early identification of communication impairment in young infants at-risk of cerebral palsy: A prospective cohort study. *Developmental Neurorehabilitation*, *25*(2), 101–114. https://doi.org/10.1080/17518423.2021.1942280

Ward, R., Leitão, S., & Strauss, G. (2014). An evaluation of the effectiveness of PROMPT therapy in improving speech production accuracy in six children with cerebral palsy. *International Journal of Speech-Language Pathology*, *16*(4), 355–371. https://doi.org/10.3109/17549507.2013.876662

Waring, R., & Knight, R. (2013). How should children with speech sound disorders be classified? A review and critical evaluation of current classification systems. *International Journal of Language & Communication Disorders*, *48*(1), 25–40. https://doi.org/10.1111/j.1460-6984.2012.00195.x

Waring, R., Rickard Liow, S., Dodd, B., & Eadie, P. (2022). Differentiating phonological delay from phonological disorder: Executive function performance in preschoolers. *International Journal of Language and Communication Disorders*, *57*(2), 288–302. https://doi.org/10.1111/1460-6984.

Warner-Czyz, A. D., Roland Jr, J. T., Thomas, D., Uhler, K., & Zombek, L. (2022). American Cochlear Implant Alliance Task Force guidelines for determining cochlear implant candidacy in children. *Ear and Hearing*, *43*(2), 268. https://doi.org/10.1097/AUD.0000000000001087

Washington, J. A., & Craig, H. K. (1998). Socioeconomic status and gender influences on children's dialectal variations. *Journal of Speech, Language, and Hearing Research*, *41*(3), 618626. https://doi.org/10.1044/jslhr.4103.618

Wasserman, T., Wasserman, L.D. (2023). Apraxia, dyspraxia, and motor coordination disorders: Definitions and confounds. In T. Wasserman (Ed.), *Apraxia: The neural network model. Neural network model: Applications and implications*. Springer. https://doi.org/10.1007/978-3-031-24105-5_1

Watts, E., & Rose, Y. (2020). Markedness and implicational relationships in phonological development: A cross-linguistic investigation. *International Journal of Speech-Language Pathology*, *22*(6), 669–682. https://doi.org/10.1080/17549507.2020.1842906

Webb, A. N., Hao, W., & Hong, P. (2013). The effect of tongue-tie division on breastfeeding and speech articulation: A systematic review. *International Journal of Pediatric Otorhinolaryngology*, *77*(5), 635–646. https://doi.org/10.1016/j.ijporl.2013.03.008

Weinberg, S. M., Raffensperger, Z. D., Kesterke, M. J., Heike, C. L., Cunningham, M. L., Hecht, J. T., . . . Marazita, M. L. (2016). The 3D Facial Norms Database: Part 1. A web-based craniofacial anthropometric and image repository for the clinical and research community. *The Cleft Palate-Craniofacial Journal*, *53*, 185–197. https://doi.org/10.1597/15-199

Weinrich, B., Brehm, S. B., Knudsen, C., McBride, S., & Hughes, M. (2013). Pediatric normative data for the KayPENTAX phonatory aerodynamic system model 6600. *Journal of Voice, 27*(1), 46–56. https://doi.org/10.1016/j.jvoice.2012.09.001

Weiss, C. A. (1982). *Weiss Intelligibility Test.* CC Publications.

Wells, B., & Peppé, S. (2003). Intonation abilities of children with speech and language impairments. *Journal of Speech, Language, and Hearing Research, 46*(1) 5–20. https://doi.org/10.1044/1092-4388(2003/001)

Wells, B., Peppé, S., & Goulandris, N. (2004). Intonation development from five to thirteen. Journal of *Child Language, 31*(4), 749–778. https://doi.org/10.1017/S030500090400652X

Werker, J. F., & Curtin, S. (2005). PRIMIR: A developmental framework of infant speech processing. *Language Learning and Development, 1*(2), 197–234. https://doi.org/10.1080/15475441.2005.9684216

Werker, J. F., & Hensch, T. K. (2015). Critical periods in speech perception: New directions. *Annual Review of Psychology, 66*(1), 173–196. https://doi.org/10.1146/annurev-psych-010814-015104

Werker, J. F., & McLeod, P. J. (1989). Infant preference for both male and female infant-directed talk: A developmental study of attentional and affective responsiveness. *Canadian Journal of Psychology, 43*, 230–246.

Werker, J. F., & Tees, R. C. (1984). Cross-language speech perception: Evidence for perceptual reorganization during the first year of life. *Infant Behavior and Development*, 7(1), 49–63. https://doi.org/10.1016/S0163-6383(84)80022-3

Werker, J. F., & Tees, R. C. (1992). The organization and reorganization of human speech perception. *Annual Review of Neuroscience, 15*(1), 377–402.

Werker, J. F., & Tees, R. C. (2005). Speech perception as a window for understanding plasticity and commitment in language systems of the brain. *Developmental Psychobiology: The Journal of the International Society for Developmental Psychobiology, 46*(3), 233–251. https://doi.org/10.1002/dev.20060

Werker, J. F., & Yeung, H. H. (2005). Infant speech perception bootstraps word learning. *Trends in Cognitive Sciences, 9*(11), 519–527. https://doi.org/10.1016/j.tics.2005.09.003

Werner, L. (2007). What do children hear? How auditory maturation affects speech perception. *The ASHA Leader, 12*(4), 6–33. https://doi.org/10.1044/leader.FTR1.12042007.6

Wertzner, H. F., Amaro, L., & Galea, D. E. D. S. (2007). Phonological performance measured by speech severity indices compared with correlated factors. *São Paulo Medical Journal, 125*, 309–314.

Wertzner, H. F., Neves, L. P., & Jesus, L. M. T. (2022). Oral and laryngeal articulation control of voicing in children with and without speech sound disorders. *Children, 9*, 649. https://doi.org/10.3390/children9050649

Werwach, A., Mürbe, D., Schaadt, G., & Männel, C. (2021). Infants' vocalizations at 6 months predict their productive vocabulary at one year. *Infant Behavior and Development, 64*, 101588. https://doi.org/10.1016/j.infbeh.2021.101588

West, K. L., & Iverson, J. M. (2021). Communication changes when infants begin to walk. *Developmental Science, 24*(5), e13102. https://doi.org/10.1111/desc.13102

Westbury, J. R., & Dembowski, J. (1993). Articulatory kinematics of normal diadochokinetic performance. *Annual Bulletin of the Research Institute of Logopedics and Phoniatrics, 27*, 13–36.

Westbury, J. R., Hashi, M., & Lindstrom, M. J. (1998). Differences among speakers in lingual articulation for American English /ɹ/. *Speech Communication, 26*(3), 203–226. https://doi.org/10.1016/S0167-6393(98)00058-2

Weston, A. D., & Shriberg, L. D. (1992). Contextual and linguistic correlates of intelligibility in children with developmental phonological disorders. *Journal of Speech, Language, and Hearing Research, 35*(6), 1316–1332. https://doi.org/10.1044/jshr.3506.1316

Whalen, D. H., Levitt, A. G., & Wang, Q. (1991). Intonational differences between the reduplicative babbling of French- and English learning infants. *Journal of Child Language, 18*, 501–516. https://doi.org/10.1017/S0305000900011223

Whalley, K., & Hansen, J. (2006). The role of prosodic sensitivity in children's reading development. *Journal of Research in Reading, 29*(3), 288–303. https://doi.org/10.1111/j.1467-9817.2006.00309.x

What Works Clearinghouse (WWC). (2012). *Early childhood education interventions for children with disabilities*. Institute of Education Sciences. U. S. Department of Education. https://ies.ed.gov/ncee/wwc/Docs/InterventionReports/wwc_pat_060512.pdf

Whelan, B. M., Theodoros, D., Mcmahon, K. L., Copland, D., Aldridge, D., & Campbell, J. (2021). Substrates of speech treatment-induced neuroplasticity in adults and children with motor speech disorders: A systematic scoping review of neuroimaging evidence. *International Journal of Speech-Language Pathology*, *23*(6), 579–592. https://doi.org/10.1080/17549507.2021.1908425

Whitall, J., Bardid, F., Getchell, N., Pangelinan, M. M., Robinson, L. E., Schott, N., & Clark, J. E. (2020). Motor development research: II. The first two decades of the 21st century shaping our future. *Journal of Motor Learning and Development*, *8*(2), 363–390. https://doi.org/10.1123/jmld.2020-0007

White, A. N., Chevette, M., Hillerstrom, H., & Esbensen, A. (2022). Parental perspectives on research for Down syndrome. *Journal of Applied Research in Intellectual Disabilities*, *35*(1), 179–187. https://doi.org/10.1111/jar.12937

Whitehill, T. L., & Wong, C. C-Y. (2006). Contributing factors to listener effort for dysarthric speech. *Journal of Medical Speech-Language Pathology*, *14*, 335–341.

Whitehill, T. L., Lee, A. S., & Chun, J. C. (2002). Direct magnitude estimation and interval scaling of hypernasality. *Journal of Speech, Language, and Hearing Research*, *45*, 80–88.

Whitelaw, G. M., & Yuskow, K. (2006). Neuromaturation and neuroplasticity of the central auditory system. In T. K. Parthasarathy (Ed.), *An introduction to auditory processing disorders in children* (pp. 21–38). Lawrence Erlbaum Associates.

Whiteside, S. P., Dobbin, R., & Henry, L. (2003). Patterns of variability in voice onset time: A developmental study of motor speech skills in humans. *Neuroscience Letters*, *347*(1), 29–32. https://doi.org/10.1016/S0304-3940(03)00598-6

Whitford, T. J., Jack, B. N., Pearson, D., Griffiths, O., Luque, D., Harris, A. W., . . . Le Pelley, M. E. (2017). Neurophysiological evidence of efference copies to inner speech. *Elife*, *6*, e28197. 97. https://doi.org/10.7554/eLife.28197

Wieling, M., & Tiede, M. (2017). Quantitative identification of dialect-specific articulatory settings. *The Journal of the Acoustical Society of America*, *142*(1), 389–394. https://doi.org/10.1121/1.4990951

Wightman, D. C., & Lintern, G. (2017). *Part-task training for tracking and manual control* (pp. 227–243). Routledge.

Wild, A., Vorperian, H. K., Kent, R. D., Bolt, D. M., & Austin, D. (2018). Single-word speech intelligibility in children and adults with Down syndrome. *American Journal of Speech-Language Pathology*, *27*(1), 222–236. https://doi.org/10.1044/2017_AJSLP-17-0002

Williams, A. L. (2000a). Multiple oppositions: Theoretical foundations for an alternative contrastive intervention approach. *American Journal of Speech-Language Pathology*, *9*(4), 282–288. https://doi.org/10.1044/1058-0360.0904.282

Williams, A. L. (2000b). Multiple oppositions: Case studies of variables in phonological intervention. *American Journal of Speech-Language Pathology*, *9*(4), 289–299. https://doi.org/10.1044/1058-0360.0904.289

Williams, A. L., McLeod, S., McCauley, R. J. (Eds.). (2010). *Interventions for speech sound disorders in children*. Brookes Publishing.

Williams, J. H., Whiten, A., Suddendorf, T., & Perrett, D. I. (2001). Imitation, mirror neurons and autism. *Neuroscience & Biobehavioral Reviews*, *25*(4), 287–295. https://doi.org/10.1016/S0149-7634(01)00014-8

Williams, P., & Stackhouse, J. (2000). Rate, accuracy and consistency: Diadochokinetic performance of young, normally developing children. *Clinical Linguistics & Phonetics*, *14*(4), 267–293. https://doi.org/10.1080/02699200050023985

Williams, P., & Stephens, H. (2004). *Nuffield Dyspraxia Programme* (3rd ed.). The Miracle Factory.

Wilson, C., Page, A. D., & Adams, S. G. (2020). Listener ratings of effort, speech intelligibility, and loudness of individuals with Parkinson's disease and hypophonia. *Canadian Journal of Speech-Language Pathology & Audiology*, *44*(2).

Wilson, E. M., Abbeduto, L., Camarata, S. M., & Shriberg, L. D. (2019). Estimates of the prevalence of speech and motor speech disorders in adolescents with Down syndrome. *Clinical Linguistics & Phonetics*, *33*(8), 772–789. https://doi.org/10.1080/02699206.2019.1595735

Wilson, E. M., Green, J. R., Yunusova, Y., & Moore, C. A. (2008). Task specificity in early oral motor development. *Seminars in speech and language*, *29*(4), 257–266.

Wilson, I., & Gick, B. (2014). Bilinguals use language-specific articulatory settings. *Journal of Speech, Language, and Hearing Research*, *57*(2), 361–373. https://doi.org/10.1044/2013_JSLHR-S-12-0345

Wilson, R. (2013, December 22). What dialect do you speak? A map of American English. *The Washington Post*. https://www.washingtonpost.com/blogs/govbeat/wp/2013/12/02/what-dialect-to-do-you-speak-a-map-of-american-english/

Wiltshire, C. E., Chiew, M., Chesters, J., Healy, M. P., & Watkins, K. E. (2021). Speech movement variability in people who stutter: A vocal tract magnetic resonance imaging study. *Journal of Speech, Language, and Hearing Research*, *64*(7), 2438–2452. https://doi.org/10.1044/2021_JSLHR-20-00507

Winsler, A., Carlton, M. P., & Barry, M. J. (2000). Age-related changes in preschool children's systematic use of private speech in a natural setting. *Journal of Child Language*, *27*(3), 665A687. https://doi.org/10.1017/S0305000900004402

Witzel, M. A., Rich, R. H., Margar-Bacal, F., & Cox, C. (1986). Velopharyngeal insufficiency after adenoidectomy: An 8-year review. *International Journal of Pediatric Otorhinolaryngology*, *11*(1), 15–20. https://doi.org/10.1016/s0165-5876(86)80023-4

Wolf, M., Primov-Fever, A., Amir, O., & Jedwab, D. (2005). The feasibility of rigid stroboscopy in children. *International Journal of Pediatric Otorhinolaryngology*, *69*(8), 1077–1079. https://doi.org/10.1016/j.ijporl.2005.03.004

Wolfram, W., Carter, P., & Moriello, B. (2004). Emerging Hispanic English: New dialect formation in the American South. *Journal of Sociolinguistics*, *8*(3), 339–358. https://doi.org/10.1111/J.1467-9841.2004.00264.X

Wolk, L., & Brennan, C. (2013). Phonological investigation of speech sound errors in children with autism spectrum disorders, *Speech, Language and Hearing*, *16*(4) 239–246. https://doi.org/10.1179/2050572813Y.0000000020

Wolk, L., Abdelli-Beruh, N. B., & Slavin, D. (2012). Habitual use of vocal fry in young adult female speakers. *Journal of Voice*, *26*(3), e111–e116. https://doi.org/10.1016/j.jvoice.2011.04.007

Wolpert, D. M., Ghahramani, Z., & Jordan, M. I. (1995). An internal model for sensorimotor integration. *Science*, *269*(5232), 1880–1882. https://doi.org/10.1126/science.7569931

Wood, S. E., Timmins, C., Wishart, J., Hardcastle, W. J., & Cleland, J. (2019). Use of electropalatography in the treatment of speech disorders in children with Down syndrome: A randomized controlled trial. *International Journal of Language & Communication Disorders*, *54*(2), 234–248. https://doi.org/10.1111/1460-6984.12407

Woolnough, O., Forseth, K. J., Rollo, P. S., & Tandon, N. (2019). Uncovering the functional anatomy of the human insula during speech. *elife*, *8*, e53086. https://doi.org/10.7554/eLife.53086

World Health Organization (1988). *Health promotion glossary*.

World Health Organization (2001). *International Classification of Functioning, Disability and Health (ICF)* (1st ed.).

World Health Organization (2001). *The world health report 2001: Mental health: New understanding, new hope*. World Health Organization.

World Health Organization (2007), *International classification of functioning, disability, and health: Children and youth version* (ICF-CY). https://healthengine.com.au/info/parentg-socialenvironment-and-its-effects-onchild-development

World Health Organization. (2016). *International statistical classification of diseases and related health problems* (10th ed.). https://icd.who.int/browse10/2016/en

Wöstmann, M., Herrmann, B., Maess, B., & Obleser, J. (2016). Spatiotemporal dynamics of auditory attention synchronize with speech. *Proceedings of the National Academy of Sciences*, *113*(14), 3873–3878. https://doi.org/10.1073/pnas.1523357113

Wrembel, M., Marecka, M., & Kopečková, R. (2019). Extending perceptual assimilation model to L3 phonological acquisition. *International Journal of Multilingualism*, *16*(4), 513–533. https://doi.org/10.1080/14790718.2019.1583233

Wren, Y. E., Roulstone, S. E., & Miller, L. L. (2012). Distinguishing groups of children with persistent speech disorder: Findings from a prospective population study. *Logopedics Phoniatrics Vocology*, *37*(1), 1–10. https://doi.org/10.3109/14015439.2011.625973

Wren, Y., Titterington, J., & White, P. (2021). How many words make a sample? Determining the minimum number of word tokens needed in connected speech samples for child speech assessment. *Clinical Linguistics & Phonetics, 35*(8), 761–778. https://doi.org/10.1080/02699206.2020.1827458

Wren, Y., Harding, S., Goldbart, J., & Roulstone, S. (2018). A systematic review and classification of interventions for speech-sound disorder in preschool children. *International Journal of Language & Communication Disorders, 53*(3), 446–467. https://doi.org/10.1111/1460-6984.12371

Wu, H., & Leung, S.-O. (2017) Can Likert scales be treated as interval scales?—A simulation study. *Journal of Social Service Research, 43*(4), 527–532. https://doi.org/10.1080/01488376.2017.1329775

Wu, Y., Muentener, P., & Schulz, L. E. (2017). One-to four-year-olds connect diverse positive emotional vocalizations to their probable causes. *Proceedings of the National Academy of Sciences, 114*(45), 11896–11901. https://doi.org/10.1073/pnas.1707715114

Wulf, G. (2007). Self-controlled practice enhances motor learning: Implications for physiotherapy. *Physiotherapy, 93*(2), 96–101. https://doi.org/10.1016/j.physio.2006.08.005

Wulf, G., & Lewthwaite, R. (2016). Optimizing performance through intrinsic motivation and attention for learning: The OPTIMAL theory of motor learning. *Psychonomic Bulletin Reviews, 23*, 1382–1414.

Wulf, G., Shea, C., & Lewthwaite, R. (2010). Motor skill learning and performance: A review of influential factors. *Medical Education, 44*(1), 75–84. https://doi.org/10.1111/j.1365-2923.2009.03421.x

Wuyts, F., Heylen, L., Mertens, F., De Bodt, M., & Van de Heyning, P. (2002). Normative voice range profiles of untrained boys and girls. *Journal of Voice, 16*(4), 460–465.

Wysocka, M. (2019). The possibilities of applying music in logopedic therapy. A survey of research. *Logopedia, 48*(1), 5–18.

Xi, X., Li, P., Baills, F., & Prieto, P. (2020). Hand gestures facilitate the acquisition of novel phonemic contrasts when they appropriately mimic target phonetic features. *Journal of Speech, Language, and Hearing Research, 63*(11), 3571–3585. https://doi.org/10.1044/2020_JSLHR-20-00084

Xu, F., Xu, J., Zhou, D., Xie, H., & Liu, X. (2022). A bibliometric and visualization analysis of motor learning in preschoolers and children over the last 15 years. *Healthcare, 10*(8), 1415. https://doi.org/10.3390/healthcare10081415

Xu, Y. (2011). Speech prosody: A methodological review. *Journal of Speech Sciences, 1*, 85–115.

Xue, S. A. & Hao, J. G. (2006). Normative standards for vocal tract dimensions by race as measured by acoustic pharyngometry. *Journal of Voice, 20*, 391–400. https://doi.org/10.1016/j.jvoice.2005.05.001

Xue, W., van Hout, R., Cucchiarini, C., & Strik, H. (2021). Assessing speech intelligibility of pathological speech: test types, ratings and transcription measures. *Clinical Linguistics & Phonetics*, 37(1), 1–25. https://doi.org/10.1080/02699206.2021.2009918

Yairi, E. (1981). Disfluencies of normally speaking two-year-old children. *Journal of Speech, Language, and Hearing Research, 24*(4), 490–495. https://doi.org/10.1044/jshr.2404.490

Yairi, E., & Ambrose, N. (2013). Epidemiology of stuttering: 21st century advances. *Journal of Fluency Disorders, 38*(2), 66–87. https://doi.org/10.1016/j.jfludis.2012.11.002

Yankowitz, L. D., Schultz, R. T., & Parish-Morris, J. (2019). Pre-and paralinguistic vocal production in ASD: Birth through school age. *Current Psychiatry Reports, 21*(12), 1–22. https://doi.org/10.1007/s11920-019-1113-1

Yankowitz, L. D., Petrulla, V., & Plate, S. (2022). Infants later diagnosed with autism have lower canonical babbling ratios in the first year of life. *Molecular Autism, 13*(1), 28. https://doi.org/10.1186/s13229-022-00503-8

Yaruss, J. S. (1998). Real-time analysis of speech fluency procedures and reliability training. *American Journal of Speech-Language Pathology, 7*(2), 25–37. https://doi.org/10.1044/1058-0360.0702.25

Yaruss, J. S., & Logan, K. J. (2002). Evaluating rate, accuracy, and fluency of young children's diadochokinetic productions: A preliminary investigation. *Journal of Fluency Disorders, 27*(1), 65–86. https://doi.org/10.1016/S0094-730X(02)00112-2

Yaruss, J. S., & Pelczarski, K. (2007). Evidence-based practice for school-age stuttering: Balancing existing research with clinical practice. *EBP Briefs, 2*(4), 1–8.

Yaruss, J. S., & Quesal, R. W. (2006). Overall Assessment of the Speaker's Experience of

Stuttering (OASES): Documenting multiple outcomes in stuttering treatment. *Journal of Fluency Disorders, 31*(2), 90–115. https://doi.org/10.1016/j.jfludis.2006.02.002

Yaruss, J. S., Newman, R. M., & Flora, T. (1999). Language and disfluency in nonstuttering children's conversational speech. *Journal of Fluency Disorders, 24*(3), 185–207. https://doi.org/10.1016/S0094-730X(99)00009-1

Yathiraj, A., & Vanaja, C. S. (2015). Age related changes in auditory processes in children aged 6 to 10 years. *International Journal of Pediatric Otorhinolaryngology, 79*(8), 1224–1234. https://doi.org/10.1016/j.ijporl.2015.05.018

Yi, H., Pingsterhaus, A., & Song, W. (2021). Effects of wearing face masks while using different speaking styles in noise on speech intelligibility during the COVID-19 pandemic. *Frontiers in Psychology, 28*. https://doi.org/10.3389/fpsyg.2021.682677

Yip, M. (2002). *Tone*. Cambridge University Press. https://doi.org/10.1017/CBO9781139164559

Yoder, P. J., Woynaroski, T., & Camarata, S. (2016). Measuring speech comprehensibility in students with Down syndrome. *Journal of Speech, Language, and Hearing Research, 59*(3), 460–467. https://doi.org/10.1044/2015_JSLHR-S-15-0149

Yorkston, K. M., Strand, E. A., & Kennedy, M. R. (1996). Comprehensibility of dysarthric speech: Implications for assessment and treatment planning. *American Journal of Speech-Language Pathology, 5*(1), 55–66. https://doi.org/10.1044/1058-0360.0501.55

Yorkston, K. M., Beukelman, D. R., Strand, E. A., & Bell, K. R. (1999). *Management of motor speech disorders in children and adults* (2nd ed.). Pro-Ed.

Yorkston, K. M., Hakel, M., Beukelman, D. R., & Fager, S. (2007). Evidence for effectiveness of treatment of loudness, rate, or prosody in dysarthria: A systematic review. *Journal of Medical Speech-Language Pathology, 15*(2), xi–xi.

Yoshizawa, S., Ohtsuka, M., Kaneko, T., & Iida, J. (2018). Assessment of hypoxic lip training for lip incompetence by electromyographic analysis of the orbicularis oris muscle. American *Journal of Orthodontics and Dentofacial Orthopedics, 154*(6), 797–802.

Yoss, K. A., & Darley, F. L. (1974). Developmental apraxia of speech in children with defective articulation. *Journal of Speech and Hearing Research, 17*(3), 399–416. https://doi.org/10.1044/jshr.1703.399

Young, E. H. & Hawk, S. S. (1955). *Moto-kinesthetic speech training*. Stanford University Press.

Yu, B., Nair, V. K., Brea, M. R., Soto-Boykin, X., Privette, C., Sun, L., . . . Hyter, Y. D. (2022). Gaps in framing and naming: Commentary to "A Viewpoint on Accent Services," *American Journal of Speech-Language Pathology*, 1–6. https://doi.org/10.1044/2022_AJSLP-22-00060

Yuskaitis, C. J., Parviz, M., Loui, P., Wan. C. Y., & Pearl, P. L. (2015). Neural mechanisms underlying musical pitch perception and clinical applications including developmental dyslexia. *Current Neurology and Neuroscience Reports, 15*(8), 51. https://doi.org/10.1007/s11910-015-0574-9.

Zajac, D. J. (2015). The nature of nasal fricatives: Articulatory-perceptual characteristics and etiologic considerations. *Perspectives on Speech Science and Orofacial Disorders, 25*, 17–28. https://doi.org/10.1044/ssod25.1.17

Zajac, D., Plante, C., Lloyd, A., & Haley, K. (2010). Reliability and validity of a computer mediated single-word intelligibility test: Preliminary findings for children with repaired cleft lip and palate. *Cleft Palate-Craniofacial Journal. 48*(5), 538–548. https://doi.org/10.1597/09-166

Zanon, A., Sorrentino, F., Franz, L., & Brotto, D. (2019) Gender-related hearing, balance and speech disorders: A review. *Hearing, Balance and Communication, 17*(3), 203–212. https://doi.org/10.1080/21695717.2019.1615812

Zarzo-Benlloch, M., Cervera-Mérida, J. F., & Ygual-Fernández, A. (2017). Variables that influence articulation accuracy in children with Down syndrome and specific language disorder: Similarities and differences. In *Advances in speech-language pathology*. IntechOpen. https://doi.org/10.5772/intechopen.69933

Zecker, S. G. (2004). Attention-Deficit/Hyperactivity Disorder: Information for school-based practitioners. *Perspectives on Neurophysiology and Neurogenic Speech and Language Disorders, 14*(3), 8–13. https://doi.org/10.1044/nnsld14.3.8

Zeigler, K., & Camarota, S. A. (2019). *67.3 million in the United States spoke a foreign language at home in 2018*. Center for Immigration Studies. https://cis.org/sites/default/files/2019-10/camarota-language-19_0.pdf

Zhang, S., Zhao, J., Guo, Z., Jones, J. A., Liu, P., & Liu, H. (2018). The association between genetic variation in FOXP2 and sensorimotor control of speech production. *Frontiers in Neuroscience, 12*, 666. https://doi.org/10.3389/fnins.2018.00666

Zhao, H., He, X., & Wang, J. (2022). Efficacy of infant's release of ankyloglossia on speech articulation: A randomized trial. *Ear, Nose & Throat Journal*. https://doi.org/10.1177/01455613221087946

Zicari, A. M., Albani, F., Ntrekou, P., Rugiano, A., Duse, M., Mattei, A., & Marzo, G. (2009). Oral breathing and dental malocclusions. *European Journal of Paediatric Dentistry, 10*(2), 59–64.

Ziegler, J. C., & Goswami, U. (2005). Reading acquisition, developmental dyslexia, and skilled reading across languages: A psycholinguistic grain size theory. *Psychological Bulletin, 131* (1), 3–29.

Žigman, T., Petković Ramadža, D., Šimić, G., & Barić, I. (2021). Inborn errors of metabolism associated with autism spectrum disorders: Approaches to intervention. *Frontiers in Neuroscience, 15*, 673600. https://doi.org/10.3389/fnins.2021.673600

Zraick, R. I., & Liss, J. M. (2000). A comparison of equal-appearing interval scaling and direct magnitude estimation of nasal voice quality. *Journal of Speech, Language, and Hearing Research, 43*, 979–988.

Zumbansen, A., Peretz, I., & Hébert, S. (2014). Melodic intonation therapy: Back to basics for future research. *Frontiers in Neurology, 5*, 7. https://doi.org/10.3389/fneur.2014.00007

Zur, K. B., Cotton, S., Kelchner, L., Baker, S., Weinrich, B., & Lee, L. (2007). Pediatric Voice Handicap Index (pVHI): A new tool for evaluating pediatric dysphonia. *International Journal of Pediatric Otorhinolaryngology, 71*(1), 77–82. https://doi.org/10.1017/S0305000900011223

Zwicker, J. G., & Harris, S. R. (2009). A reflection on motor learning theory in pediatric occupational therapy practice. *Canadian Journal of Occupational Therapy, 76*(1), 29–37. https://doi.org/10.1177/000841740907600108

INDEX

Note: Page numbers in **bold** reference non-text material.

A

AAE (African American English), 271
  dialect shifting, 273
AAPS-3 (*Arizona Articulation Proficiency Scale, 3rd ed.)*, 131
AAVE (African American Vernacular English), 271
ABI (Acquired brain injury), dysarthria and, 305
ABR (Auditory brainstem response), 42
Academics, OSAS and, 30
Acceleration, in bilingual phonological development, 266
Accent
  addition, 273–274
  coaching, 273–274
  defined, 269
  elimination, 273–274
  expansion, 273–274
  modification, 273–274
  reduction, 273–274
Accentedness
  assessing, 234
  defined, 221
Accessibility account, 61
Accuracy
  assessing, comprehensibility, 232
  defined, 146
  speech, defined, 219–220
Acoustic
  measures, pitch perturbation quotient (PPQ), 164
  parameters, 163–164
    age and, 163
  phonology and, 198–199
Acoustic analysis of, 147–148
  fricatives, 148
    calculation of spectral moments, 106–107
  stops, 147
  vowels, 147–148
Acoustic studies
  of speech development, 104–108
    instrumental methods, 108
    spectral moments, 106–107
    speech banana, 104–105
    temporal patterns, 107–108
    voice, 106
    vowel formant frequencies, 105–106
  voice disorders, children with, 163–164
Acquired brain injury (ABI), dysarthria and, 305
Acquisition
  asymmetric, 262
  described, 245
  guided, 262
  of language, critical period for, 259–262
  natural, 262
  simultaneous, of languages, 262
  of speech sounds, 79
  successive, of languages, 262
  symmetric, 262
Active tone, 145
Acute otitis media (AOM), 313
Adaptive
  movements, 253
  bilingualism, 262
Adenoid, 29
  adenotonsillar hypertrophy of, 290
  faces, 316–317
  hypertrophy, 30, 46
Adenotonsillar hypertrophy, 290–291

ADHD (Attention deficit hyperactivity disorder), 293
behavioral intervention, 293
cerebellum and, 77
craniofacial anomalies and, 50
emotions and, 55
fragile X syndrome, 312
HEG (Hemoencephalography) and, 330
medications for, 293
ADSV™ (Analysis of Dysphonia in Speech and Voice), 163
Adult acquired dysarthria, 140–141
Adults, alveoli and, 23
Aerodynamic
properties, in speech, 151
studies, voice and, 164–165
Aerodynamics, of speech production, 331
AERP (Auditory event-related potential), 42
components of, **42**
cortical
"late," 42
"slow," 42
Affect, prosody and, 174
African American English (AAE), 271
dialect shifting, 273
African American Vernacular English (AAVE), 271
Age
of parents, ASD (Autism spectrum disorder) and, 294
positive transfer and, 266
Aggression, fragile X syndrome, 312
Ahhs, 54
AI (Artificial intelligence), components of, 15
Air
conducted feedback, 70
pressure
intraoral, 151
subglottal, 151
Airway functions, Down syndrome and, 308
Alcohol related
birth defects (ARBD), 309
neurodevelopmental disorder (ARND), 309
Alternating Motion Rate (AMR), 126–128
Alveolar fricatives /z/ and /s/, **103**
Alveoli, increase of, 23
Alzheimer's disease, Down syndrome and, 307
American English, voiceless stops in, 193
American Sign Language (ASL), 254, 268
American Speech-Language Association (ASHA), 7, 118, 258, 276
CAS (Childhood apraxia of speech), described by, 301
early intervention, defined, 154
fluency defined by, 220–221
Practice Portal, **122**
American Speech-Language-Hearing Association, on speech sound disorders, 279
Amortized control, motor control and, 241
Amphetamines, ADHD (Attention deficit hyperactivity disorder) and, 293
Amplification, 247
AMR (Alternating Motion Rate), 126–128
Amusement, 54
Amygdala, 75
Analysis of Dysphonia in Speech and Voice (ADSV™), 163
Analytical validation, described, 285
Anatomic development, 21–22
Ancestry, genetic, 275
Anger, 54
Angle's classes of occlusion, **36**
Ankyloglossia, 28, 291–292
prevalence of, 291–292
Anterior tongue, fibers of, 27
Anticipatory coarticulation, 65
AOM (Acute otitis media), 313
APA Dictionary of Psychology, 63, **136**
APD (Articulation/phonological disorders), 285
Apert syndrome, 50
Apraxia of speech, 47, 67
childhood, 5, 207
diagnosing, childhood, 140
organic disorders and, 281
see also Childhood apraxia of speech
Apraxia Profile: A Descriptive Assessment Tool for Children, 143
ARBD (Alcohol related birth defects), 309
Arizona Articulation Proficiency Scale, 3rd ed. (AAPS-3), 131
ARND (Alcohol-related neurodevelopmental disorder), 309

Arteriovenous malformation, congenital, CMD (Cerebellar mutism) and, 297
Articulate Instruments, 148
Articulation, 65–67, 100
atypical, 297
based disorder, 288
compensatory, 253
defined, 65
disorders, 4
Down syndrome and, 307
lingual-labial, 34
oral, phonation accompanied by, 81
of /ɹ/, 99
rate, defined, 175
reduced, CP (Cerebral palsy) and, 299
of /s/ and /z/, 104
supralaryngeal structures and, 65
tests, 130–132
vowels and, 93
Articulation/phonological disorders (APD), 6, 285
Articulatory
goodness, 96
imagery, 73
phonology, 98–99
approach, 287
Artificial intelligence (AI), components of, 15
ASD (Autism spectrum disorder), 293–297
atypical articulation and, 297
cerebellum and, 77
craniofacial anomalies and, 50
emotions and, 55
fragile X syndrome, 312
gene disorders, 282
hypotonia and, 314, 315
manual signs and, 268
MPAs and, 50
primitive reflexes and, **40**
speech characteristics of, 294
ASHA (American Speech-Language-Hearing Association), 118, 258, 276
CAS (Childhood apraxia of speech), described by, 301
early intervention, defined, 154
fluency defined by, 220–221
NOMS, 328
Practice Portal, **122**
on speech sound disorders, 279
ASL (American Sign Language), 254, 268
ASP (Automatic Selective Perception) model, 264
Asperger's syndrome, 294
Aspirated stops, in syllable initial position, 108
Assimilation processes, 94
Asymmetric acquisition, 262
Ataxia
cerebellar, CMD (Cerebellar mutism) and, 298
CP (Cerebral palsy) and, 298, 299
Atomoxetine, ADHD (Attention deficit hyperactivity disorder) and, 293
Attention-deficit disorder
OSAS and, 30
primitive reflexes and, **40**
Attention deficit hyperactivity disorder (ADHD), 293
behavioral intervention, 293
cerebellum and, 77
craniofacial anomalies and, 50
emotions and, 55
fragile X syndrome, 312
HEG (Hemoencephalography) and, 330
medications for, 293
Attention, focus of, 248, 251
Attunement, perceptual, 43
Atypical prosody, 184
Atypical Rhythm Risk Hypothesis, 171
Atypical rhythm/stress pattern, CP (Cerebral palsy) and, 299
Auditory
brainstem response (ABR), 42
discrimination, 247
FASD (Fetal alcohol spectrum disorders) and, 309
event-related potential (AERP), 42
components of, **42**
"late" cortical, 42
"slow" cortical, 42
feedback, 70, 97
speech development and, 70
filtering, FASD (Fetal alcohol spectrum disorders) and, 310
pathway, maturation of, 211
perceptual
methods, 295
ratings, 163

Auditory *(continued)*
processing, OM (Otitis media) and, 314
rating scales, objective voice measures and, 164
stream formation, described, 210
streaming, **212**
system, 40–47
diagram of nervous, **41**
verbal
imagery, 73
therapy, cochlear implant and, 269
word images, linked to motor word images, 74–75
Autism and Developmental Disabilities Monitoring Network, 293–294
Autism spectrum disorder (ASD), 8, 293–297
ASD (Autism spectrum disorder), 294
cerebellum and, 77
craniofacial anomalies and, 50
emotions and, 55
fragile X syndrome, 312
gene disorders, 282
hypotonia and, 314, 315
manual signs and, 268
MPAs and, 50
primitive reflexes and, **40**
Automatic Selective Perception (ASP) model, 264
Autonomy, partial, of subsystems, 240–241
Autosegmental phonology, 195–196
Autosomal patterns
dominant, 49
recessive, 49
Autosomes, 47
Awe, 54

B

B cells, 30
Babble
reiterated, 84
repetitive, vocal development and, 82, 84
variegated, 84
Babbling, 82
fragile X syndrome, 312
goal, 86–87
jaw movement and, **33**
mean level of, 87
prosodic patterns in, 174
speech disorders and, **88**
Backward
coarticulation, 65
masking, 211
Bacterial infections, hearing loss and, 313
Bankson–Bernthal Test of Phonology (BBTOP), 131
BBTOP (*Bankson–Bernthal Test of Phonology*), 131
Behavior
cerebellum and, 77
problems, OSAS and, 30
stage-like, 80
Bilabials, consonants and, 86
Bilateral
cleft palate, 305
superior temporal gyrus, phonological memory and, 202
advantage, 267–268
Bilingual Processing Rich Information from Multidimensional Interactive Representations (PRIMIR), 264
Bilingualism, 262–269
bimodal
described, 269
sign languages and, 268–269
children with, phonological development in, 266
models of, 263–264
nonlinguistic cognition and, 268
Bimodal bilingualism
described, 269
sign language and, 268–269
Biofeedback, 329–331
Down syndrome and, 309
studies of, **332–333**
Biological factors, speakers characteristics and, 111
Biomarkers
for children, 285
defined, 284
speech, 284–285
Biopsychosocial model, speech disorders and, 9
Bipedalism, 82
Birth weight, hearing loss and, 313
Bite, **39**

Black English, 271
Bleeding, CMD (Cerebellar mutism) and, 297
Blocked practice, 250
Blow-smile sequence, 129
Body movements, 56
BoDySKiD (Bogenhausen Dysarthria Scales for Childhood Dysarthria), 141, 143, 187
Bogenhausen Dysarthria Scales for Childhood Dysarthria (BoDySKiD), 141, 143, 187
Bone-conducted feedback, 70
BoNT-A injection, CP (Cerebral palsy) and, 300
Bootstrapping, prosodic, 174
Botulinum toxin, CP (Cerebral palsy) and, 300
Boundary
  phrase, 185
  prosody and, 174
Box scales, 138
Bracing
  lateral, 99
  tongue, 99
Brain
  cerebrum, 77
  changes in, second language and, 261
Brainstem
  auditory pathway and, 43
  behavioral responses and, 43
  cerebellum, 77–78
Brazilian Portuguese, syllable-timed language, 166
Breastbone, 22
Breastfeeding, ankyloglossia and, 291
Breathiness, 162
Breathing
  mouth, 30–31, 316
    craniofacial/oral features associated with, **318**
    treating, 31
  sleep-disordered, 31
  speech, 23
Breathy voice, 162
Broad
  focus, 175
  transcriptions, 132
Broca, Paul, 75
Broca's area, 348
  described, 75
  word images, linked to Wernicke's area, 74–75
Browman, Catherine P., 98
Buccal cusp tips, 35
Bucket handle mechanical action, 22–23
  adult ribs and, 22–23

C

CAAP (*Clinical Assessment of Articulation and Phonology*), 131
Canonical
  babbling (CB), 81–82, 84, 155
    delayed, CP (Cerebral palsy) and, 299
    fragile X syndrome, 312
    ratio (CBR), 81–82
  syllable, defined, 81
Cantonese, syllable-timed language, 166
CAPE-V (Consensus Auditory-Perceptual Evaluation of Voice), 162
  GRBAS (Grade, Roughness, Breathiness, Asthenia, and Strain scale) and, 164
Cardiopulmonary disease, OSAS and, 30
Cartilage, thyroid, in newborn, 37
CAS (Childhood apraxia of speech), 5, 207
  atypical DDK and, 129
  coarticulatory transitions, lengthened/disrupted, 302–303
  described by ASHA, 301
  diagnosing, 140
  Down syndrome and, 308
  errors, inconsistent, 303–304
  gene disorders and, 282
  integrated view of, 304
  prosody, inappropriate, 302
Cascade
  defined, 114
  speech development and, 113–114
Case history, detailed, phonology, 213
Category goodness ratings, 96
The Caterpillar Passage, 180
CB (Canonical babbling), 81–82, 84, 155
  fragile X syndrome, 312
CBR (Canonical babbling ratio), 81–82
CCD (Common clinical distortions only), 128

CDC (Centers for Disease Control)
autism, prevalence of, 293
on hearing loss, 46–47
CDS (Child directed speech), 173
Centers for Disease Control (CDC)
autism, prevalence of, 293
on hearing loss, 46–47
Central
hypotonia, 314
incisors, 34
nervous system (CNS)
defined, 237
IMD (Inherited metabolic disorders) and, 315
neuroplasticity and, 243
Cerebellar
ataxia, CMD (Cerebellar mutism) and, 298
cerebellar mutism (CM), 297–298
with dysarthria (CMD), 297–298
mutism (CM), 298
hypotonia and, 314
peduncle invasion, superior, CMD
speech, CMD (Cerebellar mutism) and, 298
tumors, 297
Cerebellitis, CMD (Cerebellar mutism) and, 297
Cerebello-thalamo-cortical pathway, 77
Cerebellum, 77–78
neural connections and, 1
primary role of, 77
Cerebral cortex, neural connections and, 1
Cerebral palsy (CP), 298–301
craniofacial anomalies and, 50
described, 298
double nonspeech movements and, 129
hypotonia and, 314, 315
pervasive effects of, 299
primitive reflexes and, **40**
respiratory abilities and, 23
studies on dysarthria and, 305
VSA (Vowel Space Area) and, 230
Cerebro-cerebellar circuits, 240
Cerebrum, 77
CFCS Communication Function Classification System, CP (Cerebral palsy) and, 299
CGG triplet, fluency disorders and, 311
Chemical, exposure, ASD (Autism spectrum disorder) and, 294
Chicano English, 271
Child directed speech (CDS), 173
Childhood apraxia of speech (CAS), 5, 301–304
atypical DDK and, 129
coarticulatory transitions, lengthened/disrupted, 302–303
diagnosing, 140
Down syndrome and, 308
errors, inconsistent, 303–304
disintegrative disorder, 294
dysarthria, 5, 140
gene disorders and, 282
integrated view of, 304
prosody, inappropriate, 302
see also Apraxia of speech
Children
assessing speech production in, 96
bilingual, phonological development in, 266
cerebellar tumors and, 297
feral, 260
ICF and, 118
lung volume of, 23
onset disorders, cerebellum and, 77
phonological processing in, model of, 209–213
prosody assessment of, **186**
with R-SSDs, 99
speaking rate, 107
speech, phonological production, 205–206
speech disorders
adenoid faces, 316–317
adenotonsillar hypertrophy, 290–291
ADHD (Attention deficit hyperactivity disorder), 293
ankyloglossia, 291–292
ASD (Autism spectrum disorder), 293–297
CAS (Childhood apraxia of speech), 301–304
cleft palate, 305–306
clinical considerations for, 254–256
CM (Cerebellar mutism), 297–298
CMD (Cerebellar mutism with dysarthria), 297–298

CP (cerebral palsy), 298–301
DCD (Developmental coordination disorder), 306–307
dentofacial disharmonies, 315–316
Down syndrome, 307–309
dysarthria, 304–305
FASD (Fetal alcohol spectrum disorders), 309–310
fluency disorders, 310–311
fragile X syndrome, 311–312
hearing disorders, 312–314
hypotonia, 314–315
IMD (Inherited metabolic disorders), 315
long-face syndrome, 316–317
malocclusion, 315–316
mouth breathing, 316–317
OMDs (Orofacial myofunctional disorders), 317, 319
OPD (Oral placement disorder), 317
SSD (Speech sound disorder), 285–290
risk factors, 282–284
speech
repairs, self-initiated, 69
sequencing errors by, 69
sound acquisition, 3 years and older, 92–94
voice disorders in, 162–165
prevalence of, 163
risk factors, **163**
Children's Test of Nonword Repetition (CNRep), 207
Chinese, tonal language, 166
Chromogranin A, comprehensibility assessment and, 232
Chromosomal anomalies, 281
Chromosome, **48**
described, 47
Chronic
nasal airway obstruction, 316
serous otitis media, FASD (Fetal alcohol spectrum disorders) and, 310
suppurative otitis media (CSOM), 313
Chunking, prosody and, 174–175
CIMT (Constraint induced movement therapy), CP (Cerebral palsy) and, 301
Cingulate gyrus, 75
Clear speech, 179–180, 247
Cleft lip, 6
associated problems, 305
Cleft palate, 6, 305–306
associated problems, 305
Clefting, 50
Clinical
considerations, for speech disorders in children, 254–256
phonetics, 132
phonology, 192
Clinical Assessment of Articulation and Phonology (CAAP), 131
Clinical Linguistics & Phonetics, 109
Clonidine, extended-release, ADHD (Attention deficit hyperactivity disorder) and, 293
CM (Cerebellar mutism), 297–298
hypotonia and, 314
CMD (Cerebellar mutism with dysarthria), 297–298
CNRep (Children's Test of Nonword Repetition), 207
CNS (Central nervous system)
defined, 237
IMD (Inherited metabolic disorders) and, 315
neuroplasticity and, 243
Coarticulation, 65
described, 65–66
resistance, 66
Coarticulatory aggressiveness, 66
Cochlear implant, 268–269
Cochlear Implant Alliance Task Force, 269
Cocktail party problem, 210
Code
meshing, 274
switching, 274–275
Cognition
CMD (Cerebellar mutism) and, 298
fragile X syndrome, 312
nonlinguistic, bilingualism and, 268
Cognitive operations, cerebellum and, 77
Cohort theory, 203
Colonial heritage language, 263
Commissioning Support Programme, 327, 328
Common clinical distortions only (CCD), 128

Communication
  development, red flags, **156–157**
  disorders, 279
    gender differences in, 110
    sex as risk factor, 111
  Down syndrome, 307
  efficiency, defined, 220
  functional, diagram of, **218**
  gestures and, 111
  infants, vocalizations, 79–88
  nonverbal, 55–56
  process, early stages, 59–60
  tadoma, 199
  verbal, 55–56
Communication Function Classification System (CFCS), CP (Cerebral palsy) and, 299
Communicative efficiency, assessing, 232–233
Compensatory
  articulations, 253
  movement, 253
Complexity
  assumption of, 334
  diagram of, **334**
  as intervention, 334–335
  speech/language and, 331, 334–335
Compound acquisition, of languages, 262
Comprehensibility
  assessing, 231–234
    accuracy, 232
    communicative efficiency, 232–233
    fluency, 233
    global ratings, 231
    listening effort, 232
    naturalness, 233–234
    orthography-based measures, 231–232
  defined, 218–219
  of speech, **219**
Comprehension-based model WEAVER++ (Word Encoding by Activation and VERification), self-monitoring and, 70
Computational models, 14–15
Computer
  aided therapy, 335
  based, expert systems, 15
Conceptual Act Theory, 55
Conceptual representation, 59–60
Condensed inner speech, 74
Conductive hearing loss, FASD (Fetal alcohol spectrum disorders) and, 310
Congenital
  anomaly
    organic disorders and, 281
    as speech order risk factor, 284
  arteriovenous malformation, CMD (Cerebellar mutism) and, 297
  blindness, hypotonia and, 314
  hearing loss, 312
    sensorineural, 312
Connected speech, analysis of, 134
Connected Speech Transcription Protocol (CoST P), 134
Connectionist models, language comprehension/production and, 67
Consanguinity, as speech order risk factor, 284
Consensus Auditory-Perceptual Evaluation of Voice (CAPE-V), 162
Consistency
  sound, 220
  of speech production, 94–96
Consolidation, memory, 253–254
Consonants, **93**
  devoicing, 289
  final deletion of, 94
  front oral, cleft palate and, 306
  inventories, initial-position, **135**
  lateral, /l/, 101
  rhotic /ɹ/, 99
Constant practice, 250
Constraint induced movement therapy (CIMT), CP (Cerebral palsy) and, 301
Constraints, 289
  OT (Optimality theory), 196–197
Contempt, 54
Content words, 176–177
Contentment, 54
Context bias, VAS (Visual Analog Scale), 139
Contextual Probes of Articulation Competence–Spanish, 272
Contralateral
  cerebellar cortex, corticoponto-cerebellar pathway and, 77
  thalamus, 77

Contrast Therapy, 335–336
Contrastive analysis
  hypothesis, 267
  pair of languages and, 266–267
Contrasts, covert, 108–109
  defined, 109
Conversation, turn-taking, 167
Conversational speech, adult, 123
Coordinate bilingualism, 262
Coordination, multi-joint, motor control and, 241
Copy, efference, 14
Core vocabulary therapy (CVT), 336
Coronals, consonants and, 86
Cortex, auditory pathway and, 43
Corticoponto-cerebellar pathway, 77
Corticospinal damage, CMD (Cerebellar mutism) and, 298
Cortisol levels, comprehensibility assessment and, 232
Costal cartilage, 22
Cover-body theory, 37
Covert
  contrasts, 108–109
    defined, 109
  speech, 57, 73
    development of, 112–113
CP (Cerebral palsy), 298–301
  craniofacial anomalies and, 50
  described, 298
  double nonspeech movements and, 129
  hypotonia and, 314, 315
  pervasive effects of, 299
  primitive reflexes and, **40**
  respiratory abilities and, 23
  studies on dysarthria and, 305
  VSA (Vowel Space Area) and, 230
CPH (Critical period hypothesis), 259
Cranial
  neuropathies, CMD (Cerebellar mutism) and, 298
  nerve examination, 146
Craniofacial
  anatomy, FASD (Fetal alcohol spectrum disorders) and, 309
  anomalies, 50
    Down syndrome and, 308
  dysmorphology, Down syndrome and, 309
  measurements, reference points, **51**
  structures, growth trajectories of, **41**
  system
    genes and, 47
    modular growth of, 40
Creaky voice quality, 162, 270
Cri du chat syndrome, 50
Cricothyroid muscle, voice pitch and, muscles, 296
Critical period
  defined, 259
  of language acquisition, 259–262
  hypothesis (CPH), 259
Croak, voice, 270
Crossbite, defined, **37**
Crosslinguistic Nonword Repetition framework, 207
Cross
  linguistic transfer, 266
  speaker switching, 274
Crouzon syndrome, 50
Crowding, defined, **37**
CSOM (Chronic suppurative otitis media), 313
Cueing techniques, 346
Cues
  nonverbal, 56
  vocal emotions, 56
Cul-de-sac resonance, 150
Cultural diversity, 276
Curvilinear analogue scales, 138
CV syllables, 202
CVCV syllables, 202
CVT (Core vocabulary therapy), 336
Cycles approach, 336–337
Cytomegalovirus, hearing loss and, 313

D

Darwin, Charles, *Expressions of the Emotions in Man and Animals*, 54
DCD (Developmental coordination disorder), 306–307
  prevalence of, 307
  speech gestures and, 307
DDK (Diadochokinesis), 126–128, 146, 350
  atypical, 129
  consonants and, **153**

DDK (Diadochokinesis) *(continued)*
defined, 126
mean rates, **127**
rate, as index of movement limitations, 130
regularity, as index of ability to maintain uniform temporal pattern, 130
scale to rate, 127–128
task, 130, 300
Deaffrication, 94
DEAP (*Diagnostic Evaluation of Articulation and Phonology: Articulation Assessment*), 131
Deceleration, in bilingual phonological development, 266
Deciduous dentition, 34
Declarative sentence, 178
Declaratives, HRT (High rising terminal) on, 270
Decomposition, task, 249
Deep bite, defined, **37**
Degenerative disease, CMD (Cerebellar mutism) and, 297
Deictic gestures, 111
Delay
defined, 257
speech, 257–258
Delayed auditory maturation, FASD (Fetal alcohol spectrum disorders) and, 310
Delphi study, 29
Demographic variability, described, 285
DEMSS (Dynamic Evaluation of Motor Speech Skill), 143, 187
Dental
anomalies, cleft palate and, 305
disharmonies, 315
emergence, 34
malocclusion, Down syndrome and, 308
occlusion, 35
Dentofacial disharmonies, 315–316
Department of Education, 343
Depression, HEG (Hemoencephalography) and, 330
Desire, 54
Development
coordination disorders, 8
language disorder, 8
socio-emotional, 53
Developmental
apraxia of speech, 301
coordination disorder (DCD), 306–307
prevalence of, 307
delay, defined, **136**
dentofacial deformities, 315
disorders, 8, 294
dyspraxia, CP (Cerebral palsy) and, 299
fluency disorder, 207–208
Developmental Functional Modules (DFMs)
defined, 84–85
infant vocalizations and, 84–85
Developmental language disorder (DLD), 208, 279
SSD (Speech sound disorder) and, 208
Developmental neuroscience, speech disorders and, 349–350
reference data, measuring intelligibility, 227
speech gestures and, 307
stuttering
cerebellum and, 77
emotions and, 55
Deviated septum, nasal obstruction and, 316
Devoicing, Prevocalic, 94
DFMs (Developmental Functional Modules)
defined, 84–85
infant vocalizations and, 84–85
Diabetes, ASD (Autism spectrum disorder) and, 294
Diacritic marks, 132
Diadochokinesia, defined, 126
Diadochokinesis (DDK), 126–128, 130, 146, 300
atypical, 129
consonants and, **153**
defined, 126
mean rates, **127**
rate, 350
as index of movement limitations, 130
regularity, as index of ability to maintain uniform temporal pattern, 130
scale to rate, 127–128

Diagnostic and Statistical Manual of Mental Disorders 5th ed. (*DSM–5)*, 286
Diagnostic Evaluation of Articulation and Phonology: Articulation Assessment (DEAP), 131
Dialect
  commonly encountered, 271
  defined, 269–270
  gender and, 270
  vs. language, 273
  representation, 271
  shifting, 273
Diaphragm, described, 22
Diastema, defined, **37**
Difference
  defined, 258
  speech, 257
Digital
  biomarker, defined, 284
  therapy, game based, 293
Diglossia, 274–275
Dimorphism, sexual, 25
Diplegia, CP (Cerebral palsy) and, 299
Direct Magnitude Estimation (DME), 137
  intelligibility and, 224
Directions Into Velocities of Articulators (DIVA) model, 14
Discourse, turn-taking, 167
Discrimination
  auditory, 247
  tests, two-pint, 121
Disfluency, 4
Disgust, 54, 55
Disorder
  defined, 258
  X, 5, 6
Distributed practice, 250
DIVA (Directions Into Velocities of Articulators) model, 14, 199
DLD (Developmental language disorder), 208, 279
  SSD (Speech sound disorder) and, 208
DME (Direct Magnitude Estimation), 137
  intelligibility and, 224
DNA, 47
Dodd's Model for Differential Diagnosis (MDD), 286
Dorsal
  consonants, 86
  pathways
    disruption of, speech/language disorders and, 77
    language and, 75–77
    upper, 76
  rhizotomy, CP (Cerebral palsy) and, 300
Down syndrome (DS), 6, 8, 50, 307–309
  emotions and, 55
  hypotonia and, 314, 315
  life expectancy, 307
  manual signs and, 268
  primitive reflexes and, **40**
  speech disorders and, 141
  VSA (Vowel Space Area) and, 230
Drift, described, 148
Driving simulators, comprehensibility assessment and, 232
DS (Down syndrome), 6, 8, 50, 307–309
  emotions and, 55
  hypotonia and, 314, 315
  life expectancy, 307
  manual signs and, 268
  primitive reflexes and, **40**
  speech disorders and, 141
  VSA (Vowel Space Area) and, 230
DSM–5 (Diagnostic and Statistical Manual of Mental Disorders 5th ed.*)*, 286
  DCD (Developmental coordination disorder), diagnosing, 306
DST (Dynamic systems theory), 11–12, 289
DTTC (Dynamic Temporal and Tactile Cueing), 337, 340
  MSTP (Motor speech treatment protocol) and, 339
Dual-pathway model, 73
Dynamic Evaluation of Motor Speech Skill (DEMSS), 143, 187
Dynamic systems theory (DST), 11–12, 289
Dynamic Temporal and Tactile Cueing (DTTC), 337, 340
  MSTP (Motor speech treatment protocol) and, 339
Dysarthria, 5
  adult acquired, 140–141
  atypical movements and, 288

Dysarthria *(continued)*
cerebellar mutism with, 297–298
childhood, 5, 140
CMD (Cerebellar mutism) and, 297
CP (Cerebral palsy) and, 299, 300
diagnosis of, 140, 146–147
differential diagnosis of, 129
Down syndrome and, 308, 309
hypotonia and, 314
mutism and, 298
organic disorders and, 281
Dyskinetic, CP (Cerebral palsy), 298
movements, 299
Dysmorphic, facial skeletal, FASD (Fetal alcohol spectrum disorders), 309
Dysphagia, CMD (Cerebellar mutism) and, 297
Dysphonia, muscle tension, 162
Dyspraxia
differential diagnosis of, 129
orofacial, 281

E

EAIS (Equal Appearing Interval Scale), 136–137
Ear, 40
advantage,181
fragile X syndrome, 312
infections, cleft palate and, 305
misplaced, 310
EAR (Electronically Activated Recorder), 72
Early Hearing Detection and Intervention (EHDI) programs, 47
Early intervention (EI), defined, 154
Ebonics, 271
EBP (Evidence-based practice), 321–324
implementation science and, 324
LoE (Levels of evidence), 322–324
pillars of, **321**
SSDS (Single-subject design study), 323–324
Education, as speech order risk factor, 284
EEG (Electroencephalography), 75, 330
spikes, comprehensibility assessment and, 232
Efference copy, 14
Efficiency, Communication, defined, 220
Ego centric speech, 112
EHR (Electronic health records), 282
EI (Early intervention), defined, 154
Ekman, Paul, 54
on emotions, 54
Electroencephalography (EEG), 75, 330
Electromyography (EMG), 330–331
Electronic health records (EHR), 282
Electronically Activated Recorder (EAR), 72
Electropalatography (EPG), 148–149, 330–331
Embarrassment, 55
Embedding, discussed, 241–242
Embodiment, discussed, 241
Embolism, CMD (Cerebellar mutism) and, 297
Emergence, dental, 34
Emergent account, 61
EMG (Electromyography), 330–331
Emotional
prosody, 182
speech expressions, 72
word knowledge, 72
Emotions
cerebellum and, 77
defined, 53
developmental interactions, 55
facial expression of, 53–54
negative, 54–55
neural circuits of, 54
positive, 54
speech and, 176–177
vocal
behavior and, 83
expressions and, 54–55
Empty Set Therapy, 335, 337–338
Enabling, discussed, 242
Encoding
phonetic, 63
phonological, 61
Enculturation, discussed, 242
End aversion bias, VAS (Visual Analog Scale), 139
Endoscopy, voice and, 165
English, non-tonal language, 166–167
English-Spanish Assessment, 272
Enuresis, OSAS and, 30

Envelope, motor functions, 122–123
Environmental factors, ASD (Autism spectrum disorder) and, 294
EPG (Electropalatography), 148–149, 330–331
Epidemiology, defined, 5
Epigenetics, 47
  defined, 51–52
  genetics and, relationship between, **52**
  speech anatomy and, 50–53
Epiglottis, of neonates, 24
Epilepsy, gene disorders, 282
Equal Appearing Interval Scale (EAIS), 136–137
Errors
  detection of, 70–71
  inconsistency, 303
  phonological, 69
  self-monitoring and
    correction of, 70
    detection of, 70
  sequencing, speech, 67
  speech sequencing, by children, 69
Estes, Graf, 208
Estradiol, minipuberty and, 110
ET (Eustachian tube), 46
  orientation of, **46**
Etiologies, classes of, 279–281
Etiology, defined, 4–5
Eustachian tube (ET), 46, **46**
  cleft palate and, 306
Evidence Maps, 324
Evidence-based practice (EBP), 321–324
  implementation science and, 324
  LoE (Levels of evidence), 322–324
  pillars of, **321**
  SSDS (Single-subject design study), 323–324
Evoked brainstem response, 43
Examination
  oral
    mechanisms, 118–121
    peripheral, 118–121
  orofacial, **120**
Executive function, FASD (Fetal alcohol spectrum disorders) and, 309
Expanded inner speech, 73–74
Expert systems, 15
Expertise, described, 15
Explicit motor learning, vs. implicit motor learning, 244–245
Expressions of the Emotions in Man and Animals, 54
An expressive word: A study and guide in speech mechanics, psychology, philosophy, and aesthetics in life and on the stage, **93**
Extended mapping, 203
Extensions to the International Phonetic Alphabet for Disordered Speech (extIPA), 162
External
  Ear, 40
  feedback, self-monitoring and, 70
  focus, 248
    of attention, 251
extIPA (Extensions to the International Phonetic Alphabet for Disordered Speech), 162
Extrinsic
  feedback, 251
  muscles, tongue and, 26, **27**
Eyes, fragile X syndrome, 312

F

Face, fragile X syndrome, 312
Facial
  expression of emotions, 53–54
  expressions of emotions, 56
  skeleton, 40
    hyperdivergent, 316
Factorization, information, motor control and, 240
Failure to thrive, OSAS and, 30
Faithfulness constraints, OT (Optimality theory), 197
Family history, as speech order risk factor, 284
Fasciculi, longitudinal, 76
Fasciculus
  fronto-occipital, 76
  inferior, 76
FASD (Fetal alcohol spectrum disorders), 8, 50, 309–310
  boys speech impairment, 309
  hypotonia and, 315
  speech disorders and, 141

Fast
  mapping, phonological memory and, 203
  twitch fibers, 27
Fatigue scale, comprehensibility assessment and, 232
FDA (Food and Drug Administration)
  ADHD (Attention deficit hyperactivity disorder) and, game based digital therapy, 293
  ADHD medications and, 293
FDA-2 (Frenchay Dysarthria Assessment-2nd edition), 119
Fear, 54, 55
Feedback
  air-conducted, 70
  auditory, 70, 97
  bone-conducted, 70
  cleft palate and, 305
  control, internal models and, 66
  defined, 250–251
  extrinsic, 251
  frequency/timing of, 252
  intrinsic, 251
  somatosensory, 70
  speech production and, 67
Feedforward-feedback model, of speech production, **14**
Feral children, 260
Fetal alcohol spectrum disorders (FASD), 8, 50, 309–310
  hypotonia and, 315
  speech disorders and, 141
Fetus, teratogenic to, 309
Fibers, of tongue, 27
Filters, 289
Final consonant deletion, 94
First language, 267
Fisher–Logemann Test of Articulation (FLTA), 131
Fitts and Posner stage model
  features of, **238**
  motor learning, 238–239
Fitts' Law, 64
"Five-for-five rule," 125
Flesch–Kincaid, grade level, 180
Fletcher, S.G., 126
Floppy infant syndrome, 314
FLTA (*Fisher–Logemann Test of Articulation*), 131
Fluency
  assessing, 233
  defined, 220–221
  disorders, 310–311
FM devices, 269
FMR1 gene, fluency disorders and, 312
fMRI (Functional magnetic resonance imaging), 75
FND (Functional neurological disorder), 280
fNIRS (Functional near-infrared spectroscopy), 75
Focus
  of attention, 248
  attentional, 251
  broad, 175
  external, 248
  internal, 248
  prosody and, 175
FOCUS (Focus on the Outcomes of Communication Under Six), 118, 328
Focus on the Outcomes of Communication Under Six (FOCUS), 118, 328
Follicle-stimulating hormone (FSH), minipuberty and, 110
Food and Drug Administration (FDA)
  ADHD (Attention deficit hyperactivity disorder),
    game based digital therapy, 293
    medications and, 293
Foreign accent, 273–274
Formant frequencies, 25
  vowel, 105–106, **230**
Fortitions, 195
Forward coarticulation, 65
Fourth ventricle invasion, CMD (Cerebellar mutism) and, 298
FOXP2 gene, 281, 282
Fragile X syndrome, 8, 50, 311–312
  hypotonia and, 314
  protein and, 312
French, syllable-timed language, 166
Frenchay Dysarthria Assessment-2nd edition (FDA-2), 119
Frenotomy, 292
Frenulum, defined, 28

Frenum, defined, 28
Fricatives
/ʃ/, 101
/s/, 101
acoustic analysis of, 148
calculation of spectral moments, 106–107
alveolar /z/ and /s/, **103**
interdental, 101
interdental /d/ and /θ/, **103**
maximum prolongation duration of, /s/ and /z/, 125–126
Front oral consonants, cleft palate and, 306
Frontal gyrus, inferior, 75
Fronting, 94
FSH (Follicle-stimulating hormone), minipuberty and, 110
Fujiki, R.B., 164
Function words, 176–177
Functional
assessment, 119
etiology, 279–281
flexibility
observation of, 83
vocal development and, 82
sound disorders, 279
magnetic resonance imaging (fMRI), 75
matrix hypothesis, **52**
integrated, **52**
MRIs, comprehensibility assessment and, 232
near-infrared spectroscopy (fNIRS), 75
neurological disorder (FND), 280
frequency, vocal, 25
speech disorders
defined, 280
of oropharynx, 30

G

Gag reflex, **39**
Game based digital therapy, 293
Gender, 47–49
code, 111
dialects and, 270
differences in language development, 109–111
muscle tension dysphonia and, 162
speech differences in, 110
voice disorders, puberty and, 162, **163**
Gene disorders
CAS (Childhood apraxia of speech), 282
epilepsy, 282
General growth, 40
Generalized motor program (GMP), 12–13
Generative phonology, 193–194, **194**
rewrite rule, **194**
Genes, **48**
craniofacial system and, 47
Genetics, 47
ancestry, 275
ASD (Autism spectrum disorder) and, 294
speech
anatomy and, 50–53
language disorders and, 281–282
Genomics, speech/language disorders and, 281–282
Genotype, 47
Gestural phonology, 198
Gestures
communicative, 111
undifferentiated, 148
walking and, 82
GFTA-2 (*Goldman–Fristoe Test of Articulation, 2nd ed.*), 131
Given information, defined, 172
Givenness, defined, 172
Gliding, 94
Global, factors involved, speech intelligibility, 231
Glottals
consonants and, 86
fry, 270
rattle, 270
scrape, 270
GM (Gray matter), changes in, second language and, 261
GMFCS (Gross Motor Function Classification System), CP (Cerebral palsy) and, 299
GMP (Generalized motor program), 12–13
Goal babbling, 86–87
Goldman–Fristoe Test of Articulation, 2nd ed. (GFTA-2), 131

Goldstein, Louis, 98
Gonadotropic hormones, minipuberty and, 110
Goodness, articulatory, 96
Grade, Roughness, Breathiness, Asthenia, and Strain scale (GRBAS), 162
Grating orientation test, 122
Gray matter (GM), changes in, second language and, 261
GRBAS (Grade, Roughness, Breathiness, Asthenia, and Strain scale), 162
  CAPE-V (Consensus Auditory-Perceptual Evaluation of Voice) and, 164
Gross Motor Function Classification System (GMFCS), CP (Cerebral palsy) and, 299
Growls, 54
Guanfacine, ADHD (Attention deficit hyperactivity disorder) and, 293
Guided acquisition, 262
Gyri, 75
Gyrus
  bilateral superior temporal, phonological memory and, 202
  inferior frontal, 76
    phonological memory and, 202
  superior temporal, 76

H

Habitual mouth breathing, 30–31
  treating, 31
Handicap, voice, 165
HAPP-3 (*Hodson Assessment of Phonological Patterns, 3rd ed.*), 131
Happiness, 54
Harsh, whispery, CMD (Cerebellar mutism) and, 297
Head, modular growth of, 40
Health
  approach, development of, 239
  promotion of, 326
  related models, speech disorders and, 8–10
Hearing
  aids, 269
  defined, 1
  disorders, 312–314
  FASD (Fetal alcohol spectrum disorders) and, 309
  impairment, cleft palate and, 305
  loss
    CDC on, **46**
    classification of, **313**
    congenital, 312
    Down syndrome and, 308
    environmental causes of, 313
    FASD (Fetal alcohol spectrum disorders) and, 310
    speech disorders and, 281
    as speech order risk factor, 284
HEG (Hemoencephalography), 330
Heightened palate, FASD (Fetal alcohol spectrum disorders) and, 309
Hemiplegia, CP (Cerebral palsy) and, 299
Hemoencephalography (HEG), 330
Hemorrhage, CMD (Cerebellar mutism) and, 297
Hereditary metabolic disorders, 315
Heritage language, 262
  colonial, 263
  immigrant, 263
  indigenous, 263
Heterogeneity, SSD (Speech sound disorder) and, 290
Hierarchy motor control, principles of, 240–241
High
  frequency syllables, 202
  rising terminal (HRT), 270
Hispanic English, 271
Hoarse voice, CMD (Cerebellar mutism) and, 297
Hodson Assessment of Phonological Patterns, 3rd ed. (HAPP-3), 131
Homo
  loquens, 311
  sapiens, 1
Horizontal visual analog scale (HVAS), 138
Hormonal activity, sex differences and, 110
HRT (High rising terminal), 270
Human motor skills, compared to speech motor control, 254
Hunter, E.J., 161, 162
HVAS (Horizontal visual analog scale), 138
Hyoid bone, thyroid cartilage and, 37

Hyperbilirubinemia, hearing loss and, 313
Hyperdivergent, 316
facial skeletal, 316
Hyperfunction, laryngeal, 296
Hypernasal, speech, cleft palate and, 306
Hypernasality, 150
CP (Cerebral palsy) and, 299
Hypertonicity, CP (Cerebral palsy) and, 299
Hypertrophic turbinates, 316
Hypertrophy
adenoid, 30, 46
obstructive, 46
Hyponasality, 150
Hypothesis, contrastive analysis, 267
Hypotonia, 145
Down syndrome and, 308
Hypotonicity, Down syndrome and, 308
Hypoxia, hearing loss and, 313

I

Iambs, 174
Iatrogeny, defined, 325
ICD (International Classification of Diseases), 282
ICD-10 (International Statistical Classification of Diseases and Related Health Problems 10th ed.*)*, 306
ICF (International Classification of Functioning, Disability and Health), 117–118
for children/youth, 118
ICF-CY (International Classification of Functioning, Disability and Health: Children & Youth Version), 118, 234
purpose of, 9–10
ICF-CY levels, CP (Cerebral palsy) and, 301
ICS (Intelligibility in Context Scale), 223–224
Ideative gestures, 111
Idiolect, 270–271
Idiopathic, defined, 5
IDS (Infant-directed speech), 173
II-1.25 (Intelligibility Index–1.25), 226
IIAN (Intelligibility Index–Age Normalized), 226
II-AS (Intelligibility Index–All Syllables), 226
II-O (Intelligibility Index–Original), 226
II-PS (Intelligibility Index–PS), 226
ILS (incompetent lip seal), 31–32
Imagery
articulatory, 73
motor, 246
speech, 73
voice, 73
IMD (Inherited metabolic disorders), 315
Imitation, 247–248
Immigrant heritage language, 263
Immune, activation, ASD (Autism spectrum disorder) and, 294
IMP (Infant Monitor of Vocal Production), 154
CP (Cerebral palsy) and, 299
Implementation science, 324
Implicational relationship, 197
Implicit motor learning, vs. explicit motor learning, 244–245
Inborn errors of metabolism, 315
Incisors, central, 34
Incompetent lip seal (ILS), 31–32
Incomplete cleft palate, 305
Inconsistency
assessed, 303
described, 303
of speech production, 95
Independent analysis, 135
Indigenous heritage language, 263
Infant Monitor of Vocal Production (IMP), 154
CP (Cerebral palsy) and, 299
Infant-directed speech (IDS), 173
Infants
defined, 1
emotional expressions and, 55
lung volume of, 23
phonetic development in, metrics of, 87–88
reflexes, 38–40
respiratory system of, 22
skull, **33**
speech development and, milestones of, 88, **89–91**

Infants *(continued)*
vocal tract of, 24, **25**
vocalizations, 79–88
capabilities/processes of, 82–84
developmental functional modules, 84–86
goal babbling, 86
metrics of phonetic development, 87–88
stage models of, 79–82
word boundaries and, 43
Infections, hearing loss and, 313
Inferior
frontal gyrus, 75, 76
parietal lobule, 75
phonological memory and, 202
Inflammation, CMD (Cerebellar mutism) and, 297
Information factorization, motor control and, 240
Infra-red spectroscopy, comprehensibility assessment and, 232
Inheritance, patterns of, 49
Inherited metabolic disorders (IMD), 315
Inner
ear, 40
auditory pathway and, 43
monologue, 73
speech, 57, 73–74
condensed, 74
development of, 112–113
expanded, 73–74
voice, 73
Instrumental methods, 108, 147–151
Integrated
functional matrix hypothesis, **52**
therapy or integrated stimulation therapy, 340
Integrated Psycholinguistic Model of Language Processing (IPMSP), 344
Intelligence, hypotonia and, 314
Intelligibility
assessing, 222–231
choices in, **224**
developmental reference data, 227
factors involved in speech, 227–231
item identification, 225–227
judgement of, 224
parental report, 223–224
questions, 223
rating scale, 224–225
defined, 217–218
Down syndrome, 307
item identification, 224–227
spontaneous speech, 225–226
judging, 224
rating scale, 224–225
reduced, 281
scores, children, **229**
of speech, production of fluent, 217
tests, features of, **228**
Intelligibility in Context Scale (ICS), 223
Intelligibility Index
1.25 (II-1.25), 226
Age Normalized (IIAN), 226
All Syllables (II-AS), 226
Original (II-O), 226
PS (II-PS), 226
Intensity of practice, 249
Interaction, prosody and, 174
Interdental fricatives, 101
Interdental fricatives /d/ and /θ/, **103**
Interest, 54
Interlanguage, 267
Internal
bleeding, CMD (Cerebellar mutism) and, 297
feedback, self-monitoring and, 70
focus, 248
of attention, 251
models, 14
feedback control and, 66
motor overflow and, 66–67
International Classification of Diseases (ICD), 282
International Classification of Functioning, Disability, and Health (ICF-CY), 117–118, 234
strength, defined, 144
purpose of, 9–10
Interrogative sentence, 178
Intervention, complexity as, 334–335
Intonation, described, 159
Intonation contour, 159
Intonational
phrase, 168
defined, 167
Intraoral air pressure, 151
Intrasentential code-switching, 274

Intrinsic
feedback, 251
muscles, tongue and, 26, **27**
Intrusive approaches, intelligibility, 223
IOPI (Iowa Oral Performance Instrument), 144
Iowa Oral Performance Instrument (IOPI), 144
IPMSP (Integrated Psycholinguistic Model of Language Processing), 344
Italian, syllable-timed language, 166

J

Jaw
disharmonies, 315
motor control of, **33**
movements
babbling and, **33**
dependent, 32
independent, 32
Journal of Phonetics, 3
on phonetic and phonological domains, 261

K

Kaufman Speech Praxis Test for Children (KSPT), 141
Keating, P., 171
Khan–Lewis Phonological Analysis, 2nd ed. (KLPA–2), 131
Kidd, G.R., 264
KLPA–2 (*Khan–Lewis Phonological Analysis, 2nd ed.*), 131
Knowledge of Performance (KP), 251–252
Knowledge of Results (KR), 251
KP (Knowledge of Performance), 251
KR (Knowledge of Results), 251
KSPT (Kaufman Speech Praxis Test for Children), 141

L

L2 learning
factors that affect, **265**
individual differences in, 264–266
L8NRT (Late-8 Non-word Repetition Task), 207
Labial Complex DFM, 85, 86
In the labyrinths of language, **93**
Lamina propria, 37
Language
acquisition of
critical period for, 259–262
device, 259
cerebellum and, 77–78
connectionist models and
comprehension, 67
production, 67
development, described, 79
developmental interactions, 55
dialect vs., 273
disorders, dorsal pathway disruption and, 77
fragile X syndrome, 312
gene, 281
heritage, 263
colonial, 263
immigrant, 263
indigenous, 263
impairment, preoperative as risk factor, 298
learning, second, 2–3
pathways of, dorsal/ventral, 75–77
processing, streams/systems, **76**
spoken
at home in U.S., 263
neural networks of, 74–78
processing, 43
production model of, **59**
spontaneous MLU decreased, 298
stress-times, 166
syllable-timed, 166
universal receptors, 43
Laryngeal
anomalies, Down syndrome and, 308
DFM, 84
diadochokinesis (LDDK), 126
dysmorphologies, Down syndrome and, 308
hyperfunction, 296
motor area, 296
muscle
voice pitch and, 296
resistance (RL), defined, 164
system, 21, 37–38
Laryngealization, 270

Laryngomalacia, Down syndrome and, 308
Larynx, 37
Latch, ankyloglossia and, 291
Late acquired
  sounds, 99–104
    story of /ð/ and /θ/, 100–102
    story of /l/, 100
    story of /ɹ/, 99–100
  "late" cortical AERP, 42
Late-8 Non-word Repetition Task (L8NRT), 207
Lateral
  bracing, 99
  consonant /l/, 101
Laughs, 54
LDDK (Laryngeal diadochokinesis), 126
Learning
  basis, gender differences and, 110
  implicit vs. explicit, 244–245
Lee Silverman Voice Treatment (LSVT®), 338
  CP (Cerebral palsy) and, 300
Left
  ear advantage, 181
  handedness, CMD (Cerebellar mutism) and, 298
Lemma, defined, 10, 60
Lenitions, 195
Lethologica, defined, 60
Levels of evidence (LoE), 322–324
Levelt, Willem J. M., *Speaking: From Intention to Articulation*, 57
Levelt's theory of language production, 58–59
Lexical
  selection, 60
  storage, memory access to, 200, 203
Lexicon, mental, 60
LH (Luteinising hormone), minipuberty and, 110
Lichtheim, Ludwig, dual-pathway model, 74
Lichtheim's house, 75
Life-long plasticity, 3
Likert scale, 138, 165, 224, 225
Lingual
  frenulum, described, 28–29
  gnosis, 139
  labial articulation, 34
  praxis, 139
Lingual Complex DFM, 85
Linguistic
  diversity, 276
  factors involved
    speech intelligibility, 229–231
    speech intelligibility and, 227, 229
  focus, defined, 185
  level, 58–63
    conceptual representation, 59–60
    lemma/lexeme, 60
    phonetic encoding, 63
    phonological encoding, 61–63
  processing, bilingualism and, 268
  symbolic planning, 64
  utterance, producing, 71–73
Lip-jaw coordination, 32–33
Lips, 31–32
  incomplete seal of, 31–32
  reading, 231
  strength, Down syndrome and, 308
Liquids /ɹ/ and /l/, 99
Listener effect
  assessing, comprehensibility, 232
  defined, 220
Literacy domains, fragile X syndrome, 312
LoE (Levels of evidence), 322–324
Long-face syndrome, 50, 53, 316–317
  fragile X syndrome, 312
Longitudinal, fasciculi, middle/inferior, 76
Long-term memory, 201
  short-term memory and, 266
Loudness, described, 161
Lower, ventral pathway, 76
LSVT® (Lee Silverman Voice Therapy), CP (Cerebral palsy) and, 300, 338
LSVT BIG, 338
LSVT LOUD, 338
  CP (Cerebral palsy) and, 301
  Down syndrome and, 309
Lungs, volume, infants, 23
Luteinising hormone (LH), minipuberty and, 110
Lymph, defined, 30
Lymphoid hypertrophy, 291

M

M cells, 30
Macroglossia, Down syndrome and, 308

Macro-orchidism, fragile X syndrome, 312
MACS (Manual Ability Classification System), CP (Cerebral palsy) and, 299
Magnetoencephalography (MEG), 75
Mainstream American English, 273
Mainstream dialect, 270
Male sex, as speech order risk factor, 284
Malocclusion, **36**, 315–316
  described, 35
  terminology, **37**
MAMS (Movement, Articulation, Mandibular and Sensory awareness) assessment, 122
Mandarin Chinese, syllable-timed language, 166
Mandible, 32–33
Mandibular
  DFM, 85
  hypoplasia, Down syndrome and, 308
  musculature, 32
Manual Ability Classification System (MACS), CP (Cerebral palsy) and, 299
Mapping
  extended, 203
  fast, 203
Markedness
  constraints, OT (Optimality theory), 197
  defined, 197
Masking, backward, 211
Mass practice, 250
Mastitis, ankyloglossia and, 291
Maternal diabetes, ASD (Autism spectrum disorder) and, 294
Matryoshka dolls, 331
Maxillary
  gingiva, 292
  hypoplasia, Down syndrome and, 308
  labial frenulum, 292
Maximal opposition approach, 335–336
Maximum performance tasks, 122–130
  AMR (Alternating Motion Rate), 126–128
  Maximum Phonation Time (MPT), 123–126, 146
  MPD (Maximum Phonation Duration), 123–126
  SMR (Sequential Motion Rate), 126–128
Maximum Phonation Duration (MPD), 123–126
Maximum Phonation Time (MPT), 123–126, 146
Maximum Prolongation Time (MPT), 123–126
Maximum Repetition Rate (MRR), 129
Maximum Repetition Rate of Trisyllables (MRR-Tri), 303
MBCT (Melodic Based Communication Therapy), 339
MBL (Mean babbling level), 147
MBOPP (Multi-Dimensional Battery of Prosody Perception), 185
MCP (Measure for Cluster Proximity), 134
MD (Myofunctional devices), 342
MDD (Dodd's Model for Differential Diagnosis), 286
MDVP™ (Multidimensional Voice Program), 163
Mean babbling level (MBL), 87, 147
  length of utterance (MLU), 125
    decreased, CMD (Cerebellar mutism) and, 298
Measure for Cluster Proximity (MCP), 134
Medical models, speech disorders and, 8–10
Medications, hearing loss and, 313
Medulloblastoma, CMD (Cerebellar mutism) and, 298
MEG (Magnetoencephalography), 75
Melodic Based Communication Therapy (MBCT), 339
Melodic intonation therapy (MIT), 182, 338–339
Memory
  access to lexical storage, 200
  consolidation, 253–254
  long-term, 201
  phonological, 200, 201–203
    fast mapping and, 203
  working, model of, **201**
Mental
  health, positive, 326
  lexicon, 60
  practice, 246
  rehearsal, 246
Message content, questions regarding, 232
Mesulam's theory, 75

Metabolism, inborn errors of, 315
Metaphon therapy, 338
Metathetic attributes, 137
Meter-shaped scales, 138
Methodology approaches to speech disorders, 8–15
Methylphenidate, ADHD (Attention deficit hyperactivity disorder) and, 293
Metrics, of phonetic development, in infants, 87–88
Mexican-American English, 271
Middle ear, 40
Middle latency response (MLR), 42
Midface skeleton, Down syndrome and, 308
Midline shift, defined, **37**
Mild hearing loss, 313
Milk dentition, 34
Miller, G.A., 137
Mimetic muscles, 53
Minimal pair approach, 335
Minipuberty, 110
Minor physical anomalies (MPAs), 50
Mirror neurons, 247–248
Misplaced ear, 310
MIT (Melodic intonation therapy), 182, 338–339
MLB (Mean level of babbling), 87
MLR (Middle latency response), 42
MLU (Mean length of utterance), 125
  decreased, CMD (Cerebellar mutism) and, 298
Modal voice quality, 162
Modular objectives, motor control and, 241
Modules
  developmental functional, 84
    infant vocalizations and, 84–85
Monitoring
  speech production, 67
  techniques, 346
Monologue, inner, 73
Monosyllabic utterances, CP (Cerebral palsy) and, 299
Monotone, voice, 297
Mora-timed rhythms, rhythms, 183
Morphosyntax, closure of, 3
Motherese, 296
Moto-kinesthetic method, 340
Motor
  action, absent, 288
  behavior
    defined, 237
    modeling of, 246–247
  control
    cerebro-cerebellar circuits, 240
    CP (Cerebral palsy) and, 299
    defined, 237
    hierarchy/modules of, 240–241
    internal models of, 66
    jaw, **33**
    modular objectives and, 241
    multi-joint coordination and, 241
    neural systems for, 239–241
    of skilled movements, 242–243
    of speech, 64
    speech, 254
    temporal abstraction and, 241
    variability of movements, 240
    voluntary, 237
  coordination, cerebellum and, 77
  cortex, 296
  development of
    contemporary research, 239
    study of, 289
  disorders, 141
    CMD (Cerebellar mutism) and, 298
    difficulty of term, 290
  factors, 288
  function, developmental disorder defined, 306
  functions envelope, 122–123
  generalization, 244
  imagery, 246
  learning, 238
    Fitts and Posner stage model, 238–239
    hypothetical example of, **246**
    implicit vs. explicit, 244–245
    motor performance and, 243
    neuroplasticity and, 243
    phases of, 245
    of speech, 97–99
    stages of, 238–239
  neuroscience of, development, 239
  overflow, internal models and, 66–67
  patterns of, of speech, 79
  performance, motor learning and, 243
  phonetic, 213

planner, 64
planning, 63
programming disorder, 288
program
defined, 63
generator, 64
programming, 63
Down syndrome and, 309
skill
acquisition of, 97
human, 254
leaning of, 97
speech
assessing speech motor skills, 141
four tests, **142**
control, 97
delay (MSD), 5
disorder (MSD
hierarchy (MSH), 187
pediatric disorder, 140
treatment protocol (MSTP), 339
word images, linked to auditory word images, 74–75
Mouth
breathing, 30–31, 316–317
craniofacial/oral features associated with, **318**
treating, 31
Movement, Articulation, Mandibular and Sensory awareness (MAMS) assessment, 122
Movement
error, revealed by, 95–96
specification, 64
Movements
atypical, dysarthria and, 288
compensatory/adaptive movements, 253
context of, 248–249
skilled, motor control of, 242–243
variability of, motor control and, 240
MPAs (Minor physical anomalies), 50
MPD (Maximum Phonation Duration), 123–126
MPT (Maximum Phonation Time), 123–126
MPT (Maximum Prolongation Time), 123–126
MRR (Maximum Repetition Rate), 129
MRR-Tri (Maximum Repetition Rate of Trisyllables), 303
MSD (Motor speech disorder), 5
MSH (Motor Speech Hierarchy), 141, 187
assessing speech motor skills, 141
MSTP (Motor speech treatment protocol), 339
Multi-Dimensional Battery of Prosody Perception (MBOPP), 185
Multidimensional Voice Program (MDVP™), 163
Multifactorial, etiology, 5, 279–281
Multi-joint coordination, motor control and, 241
Multilingualism, defined, 262
Multimodal therapy, 340
Multiple oppositions therapy, 340
Multiple sclerosis, 280
Multiword utterances, children and, 69–70
Muscle power function, defined, 144
Muscle tension dysphonia, 162
Muscle tone
CMD (Cerebellar mutism) and, 297
defined, 145
Muscular
hydrostat, 26, 31
hypotonia, CMD (Cerebellar mutism) and, 297
Musculoskeletal system, disorders of, 30
Mutism, dysarthria and, 298
Myofunctional devices (MD), 342
Myoton-3, 146
Myotonometer™, 146

N

Narrow
focus, 175
transcriptions, 132
Nasal
airway obstruction, chronic, 316
cavity, 24
deformity, exterior, 316
Nasalance
defined, 150
used measure of, 150
Nasality, defined, 150
Nasalization, defined, 150
Nasally radiated sound energy, 150
Nasoendoscope, 165

Nasometer, velopharyngeal opening and, 150
Nasometry, 150–151, **150**
  cleft palate and, 306
Nasopharyngoscopy, cleft palate and, 306
National Library of Medicine, speech disorder, defined, 4
Native language magnet/neural commitment theory, 44
Native speech, fluent, 242
Natural
  acquisition, 262
  history, 5
  phonology, 194–195
    basic model of, **195**
  processes, phonological rules and, 195
  reference vowel framework, 86
Naturalness
  assessing, 233–234
  defined, 221
NDP (Nuffield dyspraxia program), 341
ND-PAE (Neurobehavioral disorder associated with prenatal alcohol exposure), 309
Negative transfer, 266
Neonatal, reflexes, 38–40
Neonate
  alveoli and, 23
  thorax, 22
  vocal tract of, 23–24
Nesting dolls, 331
Neural
  circuits of emotions, 54
  connections, 1
  growth, 40
  networks, spoken language and, 74–78
  plasticity, adults and, 260
  systems, for motor control, 239–241
Neurobehavioral disorder associated with prenatal alcohol exposure (ND-PAE), 309
Neurocomputational models, 199
Neurocranium, 40
Neurodevelopmental disorders
  hypotonia and, 315
  manual signs and, 268
Neurofeedback, 330
Neurofibromatosis, hypotonia and, 314
Neurology
  overshooting, 146
  undershooting, 146
Neurons, mirror, 247–248
Neuroplasticity
  central nervous system (CNS) and, 243
  motor learning and, 243
  shaped by, 260–262
Neuropsychiatric
  CMD (Cerebellar mutism) and, 298
  disorders, 280
New information, 172
Newborn, reflexes, 38–40
Node structure theory, self-monitoring and, 70–71
Nodes, prolonged activation of uncommitted, 71
Nominal gestures, 111
"The Non-Anomalous Nature of Anomalous Utterances," 68
Non persistent speech disorder (non-PSD), 128
Nonintrusive approaches, intelligibility, 223
Nonlinguistic cognition, bilingualism and, 268
Nonmainstream dialect, 270
Nonmaleficence, defined, 325
Nonspeech oral movements (NSOMs), 128, 130, 341
Nonstandard dialect, 270
Nonstimulants, ADHD (Attention deficit hyperactivity disorder) and, 293
Nonsyndromic clefting, 50
Non-tonal languages, 166
Nonverbal
  communication, 55–56
  vocalizations, emotional expressions and, 55
Nonword repetition (NWR), 207
Nonword repetition test (NWRT), 207
  DLD (Developmental language disorder) and, 208
Nonwords
  producing, 71–73
    affect, 72–73
Noonan syndrome, 50
Nouns, published inventories and, 336

NSOMs (Nonspeech oral movements), 128, 130, 341
NWR (Nonword repetition), 207
NWRT (Nonword repetition test), 207
  DLD (Developmental language disorder) and, 208

O

Objective
  intelligibility measures (OIMs), 222–223
  quantitative assessment, 144
  voice measures, auditory-perceptual rating scales and, 164
Obstructive
  hypertrophy, 46
  sleep apnea syndrome (OSAS), 30
Occlusion
  Angle's classes of, **36**
  dental, 35
Occult cleft palate, cleft palate and, 305
OIMs (Objective intelligibility measures), 222–223
OM (Otitis media), 313
  chronic serous, FASD (Fetal alcohol spectrum disorders) and, 310
  with effusion, 313
OMDs (Orofacial myofunctional disorders), 317, 319
OMT (Orofacial myofunctional therapy), 342
Onset-rime, 205
Oohs, 54
OOM (Orbicularis oris muscle), 31
OPD (Oral placement disorder), 317
Open bite, defined, **37**
Opposition therapy, 335–336
  multiple, 340
OPTIMAL (Optimizing Performance through Intrinsic Motivation and Attention for Learning), 252
Optimality theory (OT), 196–197
  diagram of, **196**
Optimizing Performance through Intrinsic Motivation and Attention for Learning (OPTIMAL), 252
Oral
  anatomy, tongue-tie, 28
  articulation, phonation accompanied by, 81
  cavity, 24
  habits, as speech order risk factor, 284
  mechanisms examination, 118–121, 146
  motor control, FASD (Fetal alcohol spectrum disorders) and, 309
  peripheral examination, 118–121
  placement disorder (OPD), 317
  stereognosis, 121–122
Orally radiated sound energy, 150
Orbicularis oris muscle (OOM), 31
Organic
  disorders, 280
    ethologic categories of, 281
  etiology, 279–281
  sound disorders, 279
Organization, segmental type of, 66
Orientation test, grating, 122
Orofacial
  dyspraxia, 281
  examination, **120**
  myofunctional
    disorders (OMDs), 317, 319
    therapy (OMT), 342
  praxis, 139, 140
  reflexes, 38–40
  strength, 144, 146
  system, sensory function assessing, 121–122
  tone of, 146
Oropharynx, functional disorders of, 30
Orthographic transcription, measuring intelligibility, 225
OSAS (Obstructive sleep apnea syndrome), 30
OT (Optimality theory), 196–197
  diagram of, **196**
Otitis media (OM), 313
  chronic serous, FASD (Fetal alcohol spectrum disorders) and, 310
Otolaryngology, adenoid hypertrophy and, 30
Ototoxic medications, hearing loss and, 313
Outcome, measures, 327–329
Overjet, defined, **37**
Overshooting, neurology, 146
Overt speech, 57

P

P arm, **48**
PA (Phonological awareness), 200, 203–205, 342–343
PAD (Phonological/articulatory disorders), 285
Pain, 55
Palatine tonsils
  adenotonsillar hypertrophy of, 290
  inflammation of, 30
PAM (The perceptual assimilation model), 263–264
Parental report, intelligibility assessment and, 223–224
Parentese, 296
Parent-infant interactions, vagus nerve and, 83
Parietal lobule, inferior, 75
Partial, cleft palate, 305
Partial
  autonomy, of subsystems, 240–241
  fetal alcohol syndrome (pFAS), 309
Passive tone, 145
PAT–3 (*Photo-Articulation Test, 3rd ed.*), 131
Pathogenesis, defined, 5
Patient-reported outcomes, 329
PCC (Percent consonants correct), 133, 147, 226
PCC-R (Percent Consonants Correct-Revised), 133
pCMS (Post-operative cerebellar mutism syndrome), 297
PDI (Phonological Density Index), 206
Peabody Picture Vocabulary Test (PPVT-4), 272–273
Pediatric
  adenoid hypertrophy and, 30
  motor speech disorder, diagnostic categories of, 140
  speech, disorders/variations, 3–8
Pediatric Voice Handicap Index (pVHI), 165
Pediatric Voice Outcome Survey (PVOS), 165
Pediatric Voice-Related Quality-of-Life Survey (PVRQOL), 165
Pedigree, 47
  chart, 47, **48**
Pentax Medical, 163
PEPPER (Phonetic and phonologic evaluation records), 187
PEPS-C (Profiling Elements of Prosody in Speech-Communication), 185
Percent
  consonants correct (PCC), 133, 147
    Revised (PCC-R), 133
  vowels correct (PVC), 133
Percentage of Consonants Correct (PCC), 226
Percentage of Intelligible Correct Syllables (PICS), 133
The Percentage of Intelligible Correct Syllables (PICS), 226
Percentage of Intelligible Syllables (PINTS), 134
Perception
  based theory, self-monitoring and, 70
  components of, 71–72
  described, 209
  phonological processing in, children, 209, 211
Perceptual
  assimilation model (PAM), 263–264
  attunement, 43
  magnetic effect, **45**
  methods, of speech production, 117
Permanent dentition, 34
Persistent speech disorder (PSD), 128
Pervasive development disorders, 294
Peterson, G.E., 105
pFAS (Partial fetal alcohol syndrome), 309
Pharyngeal
  arches, palatine tonsil and, 30
  cavity, 24
  reflex, **39**
  tonsil, 29
    adenotonsillar hypertrophy of, 290
Pharyngolaryngeal, DFM, 85
Pharynx
  adenotonsillar hypertrophy of, 290
  of neonates, 24
Phecodes, 282
Phenomenology, defined, 4
Phenotype, 47
Phonation
  articulation accompanied by, 81

defined, 159
Down syndrome and, 307
pulse, 270
simple, 81
Phoneme, 79
collapse, 336
mastery of production of, 92
prototypes, 44
specific nasal air emission, 150
Phonemic transcriptions, 95, 132
Phonetic
development, in infants, metrics of, 87–88
domains, malleability of, 261
drift, 3
encoding, 63
inventory, 134–136
defined, 134–135
motor, 213
described, 209
pattern, perceiving/producing, **71**
placement method, 340
restricted repertoires, CP (Cerebral palsy) and, 299
settings, 3
transcriptions, 68, 95, 132
Phonetic and phonologic evaluation records (PEPPER), 187
Phonetics, described, 191
Phonetogram, 128
Phonological
access to lexical storage, 203
awareness (PA), 200, 203–205
development
in bilingual children, 266
delayed, 295
disorders, 4, 6
encoding, 61–63
errors in, 67–68, 69
factors involved, speech intelligibility and, 227, 229
long-term memory (pLTM), 201–202
loop, 202
mean length of utterance (pMLU), 134, 147, 272
memory, 200, 201–203
fast mapping and, 203
neighborhood
defined, 62
density, 62
patterns, 147
phrase, 168
process
analysis, 147
defined, 94
processes
atypical, 295
development of speech and, 79, 94, 147
processing, 200
in children, model of, 209–213
suppression of, 94, **95**
production, 200, 205–209
children's speech, 205–206
representation (PR), 61, 202
rhythm, prosodic phrasing and, 166
short-term (pSTM), 201–202
Phonological awareness (PA), 342–343
Phonological Density Index (PDI), 206
Phonological mean length of utterance (pMLU),134, 147, 272
Phonological/articulatory disorders (PAD), 285
Phonology
acoustics and, 198–199
articulatory, 98–99
autosegmental, 195–196
clinical assessment guidelines, 213–214
defined, 191, 198–199
generative, 193–194
gestural, 198
natural, 194–195
primary concern of, 191–192
speech sample, 213–214
structure of, diagram of, **192**
theories of, 192–198
PhonoSens, 344
Phonotrauma, 163
Photo-Articulation Test, 3rd ed. (PAT-3), 131
Phrase
boundaries, defined, 185
final lengthening, 178–179
defined, 172
Phrasing, defined, 172
Physical and Rehabilitation Medicine (PRM), VAS (Visual Analog Scale), 139

Physiologic development, 21–22
Physiological level
  speech production, 63–67
    planning/programming, 63–64
PICS (Percentage of Intelligible Correct Syllables), 133, 226
Pierre Robin syndrome, 50
PINTS (Percentage of Intelligible Syllables), 134
Pitch
  contour, 159
  laryngeal hyperfunction and, 296
  pattern, 159
  perturbation quotient (PPQ), acoustic measures of, 164
  as prosodic feature, 295–296
Plasticity
  described, 243
  learning, 2–3
  life-long, 3
  neural, adults and, 260
Playground problem, 209, 211
PLM (Principles of Motor Learning), 243–254
  framework/clinical applications, 246–254
    amount of practice, 249
    compensatory/adaptive movements, 253
    feedback frequency/timing, 252
    feedback type, 250–252
    focus of attention, 248
    imitation, 247–248
    memory consolidation, 253–254
    motor behavior modeling, 246–247
    motor imagery, 246
    movement context, 248–249
    practice schedule, 250
    practice variability, 250
    stimulability, 252–253
    task decomposition, 249
    type of practice, 250
  MSTP (Motor speech treatment protocol) and, 339
pLTM (Phonological long-term memory), 201–202
PML (Principles of motor learning), 339
pMLU (Phonological Mean Length of Utterance), 134, 147, 272
  neumotachograph, 151
Point vowels, 87
Polyvagal theory, vocal development and, 83
Pons, corticoponto-cerebellar pathway and, 77
Popcorning, 270
Positive transfer, 266
Postbite, defined, **37**
Posterior, tongue, fibers of, 27
Posterior cranial fossa, CMD (Cerebellar mutism) and, 298
Postoperative
  cerebellar mutism syndrome (pCMS), 297
  speech, language deficits and, 298
Post-surgery, intelligibility, cleft palate and, 306
PPQ (Pitch perturbation quotient), acoustic measures of, 164
PPVT-4 (Peabody Picture Vocabulary Test), 272–273
PR (Phonological representation), 61, 202
Practice
  amount of, 249
  constant vs. variable, 250
  hypothesis, variability of, 244
  patterns, 348–349
  schedule, 250
  type of, 250
The Practice Portal, **122**, 324
Prader-Willi syndrome, hypotonia and, 314
Praxis
  defined, 139
  orofacial, 139, 140
  in speech production, 141
Praxis and Speech Motor Control, 130
p-RDA (Radboud Dysarthria Assessment), 146
Pre-Kindergarten National Outcome Measure System (Pre-K NOMS), Therapy Outcome Measures (TOM), 118
Prelexical vocalizations, 87
Preston, J.L., 128
Prevention
  defined, 5
  resources on, 325–326

types of, 325
Prevocalic
devoicing, 94
prevoicing, 94
Prevoicing, Prevocalic, 94
Primary
dentition, 34
prevention, 325
PRIMIR (Bilingual Processing Rich Information from Multidimensional Interactive Representations), 264
Primitive reflexes, 38–40
persistence of, **40**
Primordial prevention, 325
Principles of Motor Learning (PLM), 243–254, 339
framework/clinical applications, 246–254
amount of practice, 249
compensatory/adaptive movements, 253
feedback frequency/timing, 252
feedback type, 250–252
focus of attention, 248
imitation, 247–248
memory consolidation, 253–254
motor behavior modeling, 246–247
motor imagery, 246
movement context, 248–249
practice schedule, 250
practice variability, 250
stimulability, 252–253
task decomposition, 249
type of practice, 250
MSTP (Motor speech treatment protocol) and, 339
Private speech, 73–74
development of, 112–113
PRM (Physical and Rehabilitation Medicine), VAS (Visual Analog Scale), 139
ProCAD (Profile of Childhood Apraxia of Speech and Dysarthria), 143
Process analysis, 290
oriented profiling, 287–288
of prosody, 183–184
Processing rich information from multidimensional interactive representations (PRIMIR), 44
Production
based theory, self-monitoring and, 70–71
of a word, 95
Profile of Childhood Apraxia of Speech and Dysarthria (ProCAD), 143
Profiling Elements of Prosody in Speech-Communication (PEPS-C), 185
Prominence, defined, 172
PROMPT (Prompts for Restructuring Oral Muscular Phonetic Targets), 141, 340, 344
MSTP (Motor speech treatment protocol) and, 339
Prompts for Restructuring Oral Muscular Phonetic Targets (PROMPT), 141, 340, 344
MSTP (Motor speech treatment protocol) and, 339
Pronunciation instruction, 273–274
PROP (Prosody Profile), 187
Proportion of whole-word proximity (PWP), 147, 272
Prosodic
entrainment, 167, 188
word, 168
Prosody, 159, 165–170
analysis of, automatic acoustic, 188–189
assessment of
in children, **186**
as other tests component, 187–188
atypical, 295
bootstrapping, 174
clinical
applications of, 184–185
tests of, 185–187
conversational, 188
cube, 185
development of, 175–180, **181**
affect, 176–177
boundary effects, 178–179
content/function words, 177–178
declarative vs. interrogative contrast, 178
general patterns, 173–175
phonological processes, 175–176
register/speaking style, 179–180
speaking/articulation rate, 175–176
specific features, 175–180

Prosody *(continued)*
Down syndrome and, 307
hemispheric processing of linguistic, **182**
hierarchy of, 167, **168**
information flow, in English, **183**
interventions, 344–345
neural mechanisms of, 180–183
phonetic effects of, 171–172
process analysis of, 183–184
reading, 180
schematic representation of, **169**
study of, prospects of detailed, 188–189
S-W words, 178
voice profile, 296
Prosody Profile (PROP), 187
Prosody-Voice Screening Pro file (PVSP), 187
Protective factor, defined, 284
Prothetic attributes, 137
Protophones
defined, 83–84
vocal development and, 82
PSD (Persistent speech disorder), 128
pSTM (Phonological short-term), 201–202
Psycholinguistic models, speech disorders and, 10
Psychosocial, stress testing, 55
Puberty, voice disorders, 162, **163**
Puerto Rican dialect of Spanish, 272
Pulsatile, 270
Pulse phonation, 270
Pupil diameter, comprehensibility assessment and, 232
PVC (Percent vowels correct), 133
pVHI (Pediatric Voice Handicap Index), 165
PVOS (Pediatric Voice Outcome Survey), 165
PVRQOL (Pediatric Voice-Related Quality-of-Life Survey), 165
PVSP (Prosody-Voice Screening Pro file), 187
PWP (Proportion of whole-word proximity), 147, 272

Q

Q arm, **48**
qEEG (Quantitative Electroencephalography), 330
QPR (Quality of Phonological Representations), 61
QPR (Quality of representation) task, 202–203
Quadriplegia, CP (Cerebral palsy) and, 299
Quadrupedal locomotion, 82
Quality-of-life, voice, 165
Quality of Phonological Representations (QPR), 61
Quality of representation (QPR) task, 202–203
Quantitative assessment, objective, 144
Quantitative Electroencephalography (qEEG), 330
Quaternary prevention, 325
Questionnaires, comprehensibility assessment and, 232

R

Radboud Dysarthria Assessment (p-RDA), 146
Railroad track ear, 310
RAN (Rapid automatized naming), 206
Random practice, 250
Range of motion (ROM), 130, 145
rAOM (Recurrent AOM), 313
Rapid
automatized naming (RAN), 206
serial naming, 206
syllable transition treatment (ReST), 339, 345
Rate
constraint processing theory, 45
reduction therapy, 345–346
Rating scales, 136–139
defined, 136
hybrid, 138
intelligibility, 224–225
Ratings of intelligibility along with PCC, 328
RCSLT (Royal College of Speech and Language Therapists), define speech sound disorders, 286, 327
Reaction times, comprehensibility assessment and, 232
Reading
fluency, defined, 180
prosody and, 180

rates, 176
Recall schema, 13
Receptors, sensory, tongue, 27
Recognition schema, 13
Recurrent AOM (rAOM), 313
Red flags, described, 155
Reference data, developmental, measuring intelligibility, 227
Reflexes, orofacial, 38–40
Register, speaking style, 179–180
Rehabilitation, principles of, 243
Reinke's space, ss
Reiterated babble, 84
Relational analysis/assessment, 135, 147
Relationship, implicational, 197
Relief, 54
Repetitive
babble, vocal development and, 82, 84
Representation
described, 209
phonological, 212
Representational gesture, 111
Residual speech sound dis order (R-SSD), sounds, story of /s/ and /z/, 99
Resonance
disorders, 4
Down syndrome and, 307
Respiration, Down syndrome and, 307
Respiratory
DFM, 84
rate, birth to adolescence, 23
system, 21, 22–23
described, 22
growth of, 23
times, comprehensibility assessment and, 232
ReST (Rapid syllable transition treatment), 339, 345
Resting tone, 145
Retention, described, 245
Rhotic consonant /ɹ/, 99
Rhyme, 205
Rhythm, speech, described, 170–171
Rhythmic stereotypes, 84
Rib cage, described, 22
Ribs
adult, 22–23
breathing and, 22
cartilage connections, 22
Right ear advantage, 181
Right-to-left coarticulation, 65
Rigidity, of muscle, 145
Risk factors
defined, 282–283
speech disorders, in children, 282–284
R_L (Laryngeal resistance), 164
Roberts syndrome, 50
ROM (Range of motion), 130, 145
Rooting reflex, **39**
Royal College of Speech and Language Therapists (RCSLT), define speech sound disorders, 286, 327
R-SSD (Residual speech sound dis order), 99

S

Sadness, 54, 55
Saethre-Chotzen syndrome, 50
Sagittal malocclusions, 35, **36**
Schema theory, 12–13
Schizophrenia, MPAs and, 50–51
Screen ing Test for Developmental Apraxia of Speech — Second Edition (STDAS-2), 143
SCU (Syllables correctly understood), 226
SDCS (Speech Disorders Classification System), 5, 286–287, **287**
Second language, brain changes and, 261
Second language learning (SLA), 266–267
Secondary
dentition, 34
prevention, 325
Segmental errors, 95
Segmentation, described, 249
Self-controlled practice, 250
Self-cueing, 346
Self-directed speech, 73–74
development of, 112–113
Self-monitoring, 70–71, 346
children and, 69–70
defined, 70
theories on, 70–71
verbal, 70
Self-talk, 73–74
Semantic
neighborhoods, 60
density, 60, 62

Semantic *(continued)*
processing, 75
relations, prosodic phrasing and, 166
Sensitivity, tongue and, 27–28
Sensorimotor, defined, 1
Sensorineural hearing loss, 312
FASD (Fetal alcohol spectrum disorders) and, 310
Sensory
disorders, fragile X syndrome, 312
receptors, tongue, 27
Sequencing error, speech, 67
Sequential Motion Rate (SMR), 126–128
Serotonin reuptake inhibitors, ASD (Autism spectrum disorder) and, 294
Sex, 47–49
differences
hormonal activity and, 110
in language development, 109–111
as risk factor, of communication disorders, 111
steroids, minipuberty and, 110
Sexual dimorphism, 25
cerebellum and, 77
SGD (Speech generating device), 7
SHAPE (*Smit–Hand Articulation and Phonology Evaluation*), 131
Shedding, teeth, 34
Short-term memory/categorization
7 points of gradation, 137
information in, 266
Shrieks, 54
SIE (Spanish-Influenced English), 271
Sighs, 54
Sign language, **64**
American, 254
bimodal bilingualism and, 268–269
Silent speech, 73
Simplification, described, 249
Simultaneous acquisition, of languages, 262
Single-subject design study (SSDS), 323–324
LoE (Levels of evidence), 324
SIT (Speech Intelligibility Treatment), CP (Cerebral palsy) and, 300
Sketchpad, visuo-spatial, 201
Skin
conductance, comprehensibility assessment and, 232
fragile X syndrome, 312
Skull
infant, **33**
modular growth of, 40
SLA (Second language learning), 266–267
Sleep
apnea, Down syndrome and, 308
disordered breathing, 31
SLM (Speech learning model), 263
SLM-r (Speech learning model-revised), 263
"Slow" cortical AERP, 42
Slow-twitch fibers, 27
Smart-Palate, 148
SMC (Speech motor chaining), 339, 346–347
Smit–Hand Articulation and Phonology Evaluation (SHAPE), 131
SMOG Index, 180
SMR (Sequential Motion Rate), 126–128
SMSD (Speech motor skill development), 241–242
Social anxiety, fragile X syndrome, 312
Social Cognitive Theory, 247
Social living, grammar of, 53
Social-behavioral issues, FASD (Fetal alcohol spectrum disorders) and, 309
Socialization, developmental interactions, 55
Sociocultural
basis, gender differences and, 110
factors, speakers characteristics and, 111
Socio-emotional development, 53
Sociolect, 270–271
SODA (Substitutions, omissions, distortions, and additions), 131, 134, 303
Soft palate, of neonates, 24
Soft skin, fragile X syndrome, 312
Somatic growth, 40
Somatosensory feedback, 70
Sonography, 149
Sound
consistency, 220

  defined, 199
  energy, orally/nasally, 150
Sound Patterns of English, 193
Sounds
  late acquired, 99–104
    story of /ð/ and /θ/, 100–102
    story of /l/, 100
    story of /ɹ/, 99–100
    story of /s/ and /z/, 102–104
Source-filter theory, 159
Spanglish, 271
Spanish
  influenced English, 271–273
  Puerto Rican dialect of, 272
  syllable-timed language, 166
Spastic, CP (Cerebral palsy), 298
Spasticity, of muscle, 145
Spatial resolution, tongue and, 27–28
SPAT–II (*Structured Photographic Articulation Test, 2nd ed.*), 131
Spatiotemporal
  goals, speech and, 97
  index (STI), 107
    CP (Cerebral palsy) and, 300
Speaking
  louder, 161
  rate, 176
    of children, 107
    defined, 175
Speaking: From Intention to Articulation, 57
Special
  delivery, forms of, 327
  moments, 106–107
Speech, 93–94
  accuracy, 133
    defined, 219–220
  acoustic output of, 331
  acts, defined, 172, **173**
  aerodynamic properties in, 151
  anatomy
    epigenetics and, 50–53
    genetics and, 50–53
  apraxia of, 47, 67
    childhood, 5, 207
    diagnosing, childhood, 140
    organic disorders and, 281
  assessment, birth to three, 154–155
  atypical features of, 295
  banana, for children, 104–105
  biomarkers, 284–285
  breathing, 23
  cerebellum and, 77–78
  children, phonological production, 205–206
  clear, 179–180, 247
  connected, analysis of, 134
  conversational, adult, 123
  covert, 57, 73
  delay, 257–258
  described, **2**, 57–58
  development, 2–3
    acoustic studies of, 104–108
    auditory feedback and, 70
    babbling and, **88**
    cascades/systems views of, 113–114
    defined, 2
    milestones of, 88, **89–91**
    motor perspectives on, 241–242
    sex/gender differences, 109–111
  deviations in, 257
  difference, 257
    defined, 4, 258
  Down syndrome and, 308
  ego-centric, 112
  expanded inner, 73–74
  expressions, emotional, 72
  as external thought, **74**
  fragile X syndrome, 312
  gestures, DCD (Developmental coordination disorder), 307
  imagery, 73
  inconsistency, CAS (Childhood apraxia of speech), 303
  infant-directed, 296
  inner, 73–74
    condensed, 74
    development of, 112–113
  language therapy, cleft palate and, 306
  linguistic level, 58–63
    conceptual representation, 59–60
    lemma/lexeme, 60
    phonetic encoding, 63
    phonological encoding, 61
    speech planning/programming, 63–64
  mechanism examination, 118–121

Speech *(continued)*
motor
control, 64, 97, 254
learning, 97–99
patterns of, 79
planning/programming, FASD (Fetal alcohol spectrum disorders) and, 309
musculature of, 254
neuroscience of, developmental, 77–78
overt/covert, 57
private, 73–74
development of, 112–113
production
aerodynamics of, 331
assessed, 117
assessing in children, 96
assessment methods, 152–154
consistency/variability of, 94
Down syndrome, 307
errors in, 67–70
four-level model of, 63–64
monitoring/feedback in, 67
physiological level of, 63–67
praxis in, 141
systems of, 152–154
prosody and, 166
rate, slow, 297
reading, 231
repairs, self-initiated, 69
rhythm, described, 170–171
self-directed, 73–74
sequencing errors, 67
by children, 69
sex-specific features of, 110
silent, 73
sound acquisition, 7, 79, 241–242
children, 3 years and older, 92–94
defined, 7
discussed, 6
disorders, 7, 279
sequences, 7
disorder (SSD), 285
children with, 163, 285–290
clinical populations presenting, Venn diagram, **259**
criteria for, 286
defined, 6
DLD (Developmental language disorder) and, 208
heterogeneity and, 290
sounds
mastery, profile of, **92**
positional targets and, 97
vowels and, 93–94
spontaneous, measuring intelligibility, 225–226
suprasegmental aspects of, CMD (Cerebellar mutism) and, 297
system framework, **152**
traditional therapy, 347–348
uniqueness of, 1
The Speech Chain, 58
Speech disorders, 257
approaches to, 8–15
health-related models, 8–10
medical models, 8–10
biopsychosocial model and, 9
clinical considerations for children with, 254–256
defined,4, 258
developmental neuroscience and, 349–350
dorsal pathway disruption and, 77
Down syndrome and, 308
health-related models and, 8–10
indications of, 299
medical models and, 8–10
non persistent speech disorder (non-PSD), 128
practice patterns, 348–349
production, 2
feedforward-feedback model of, **14**
individual units of, 6
models, 10
psycholinguistic models and, 10
risk factors, 282–284
segments, 7
treatment, 326–329
adaptive cueing, 346
biofeedback, 329–331
complexity of, 331, 334–335
computer-aided therapy, 335
contrast/opposition therapy, 335–336
core vocabulary therapy, 336
cycles, 336–337

DTTC, 337
empty set therapy, 337–338
forms of special delivery, 327
goals/target of, 326
LSVT® (Lee Silverman Voice Therapy), 338
MD (Myofunctional devices), 342
method of, 326–327
MIT (Melodic intonation therapy), 338–339
motor learning, 339
MSTP (Motor speech treatment protocol), 339–340
multimodal therapy, 340
multiple oppositions, 340
NDP (Nuffield dyspraxia program), 341
NSOMs (Nonspeech oral movements), 341
OMT (Orofacial myofunctional therapy), 342
outcome measures, 327–329
PA (Phonological awareness), 342–344
PhonoSens, 344
PROMPT (Prompts for Restructuring Oral Muscular Phonetic Targets), 344
prosody interventions, 344–345
rate reduction therapy, 345–346
ReST (Rapid syllable transition treatment), 345
self-cueing, 346
SMC (Speech motor chaining), 346–347
SSIT (Speech Systems Intelligibility Treatment), 347
support, 327
systems approach, 347
tDCS (Transcranial Direct Current Stimulation), 348
traditional speech therapy, 347–348
Speech Disorders Classification System (SDCS), 5, 286–287, **287**
Speech generating device (SGD), 7
Speech intelligibility
factors involved in, 227–231
acoustic factors, 229–231
global ratings, 231
phonological/linguistic factors, 227, 229
visual factors, 231
Speech Intelligibility Treatment (SIT), CP (Cerebral palsy) and, 300
Speech motor chaining (SMC), 339, 346–347
Speech motor skill development (SMSD), 241
Speech range profile (SRP), 128
Speech Systems Approach, CP (Cerebral palsy) and, 300
Speech Systems Intelligibility Treatment (SSIT), 347
Speech-language, pathology, adenoid hypertrophy and, 30
Speed
speech production and, 144–147
Spoken language
neural networks of, 74–78
processing, 43
production model of, **59**
Spontaneous speech
measuring intelligibility, 225–226
word/sentence lists, 226–227
Spoonerisms, 67–68
Spreading activation, 67
SRT (Syllable Repetition Task), 303
SSD (Speech sound disorder), 285
children with, 163, 285–290
clinical populations presenting, Venn diagram, **259**
criteria for, 286
defined, 6
DLD (Developmental language disorder) and, 208
heterogeneity and, 290
theoretical accounts/clinical management of, pediatric, **7**
SSDS (Single-subject design study), 323–324
LoE (Levels of evidence), 324
SSIT (Speech Systems Intelligibility Treatment), 347
SSL (Syllable structure level), 147
values of, 87–88
Stackhouse and Wells, psycholinguistic framework of, 286

Stacking dolls, 331
Stage
  fright, 73
  like behaviors, 80
  models, vocalizations and, 80–81
Stampe's theory of natural phonology, 289
Standard dialect, 270
STDAS-2 (Screen ing Test for Developmental Apraxia of Speech — Second Edition), 143
Steadiness, defined, 145
Stereognosis, oral, 121–122
Stereotypes, rhythmic, 84
Sternum, 22
Steroidogenic activity, ASD (Autism spectrum disorder) and, 294
STI (Spatiotemporal index), 107
Stimulability, described, 252–253
Stimulants, ADHD (Attention deficit hyperactivity disorder) and, 293
Stimulation, as speech order risk factor, 284
Stops, acoustic analysis of, 147
Strained-strangled voice, CP (Cerebral palsy) and, 299
Streaming
  auditory, **212**
  described, 210
Strength, defined, 144
Stress-timed language, 166
  rhythms, 183
Strohbass glottal fry, 270
Stroke, 280
Structural
  constraints, OT (Optimality theory), 197
  observations, 119
Structured Photographic Articulation Test, 2nd ed. (SPAT–II), 131
Stuttering
  cerebellum and, 77
  emotions and, 55
Subglottal air pressure, 151
Submucous cleft palate, cleft palate and, 305
Subordinate bilingualism, 262
Subphonemic difference, in sound production, 109
Substitution processes, 94
Substitutions, omissions, distortions, and additions (SODA), 131, 134, 303
Subsystems, partial autonomy of, 240–241
Subtotal cleft palate, 305
Subtractive bilingualism, 262
Successive acquisition, of languages, 262
Suck swallow- breathe pattern, 37
Sucking reflex, **39**
Superior
  cerebellar peduncle invasion, CMD (Cerebellar mutism) and, 298
  labial frenulum, 292
  temporal gyrus, 76
Support, described, 327
Suppression, of phonological processes, 94, **95**
Supralaryngeal
  articulation, 81
  implementation of prominence, 172
  structures, 64, 172
    articulation and, 65
  system, 21, 23–40
    lips, 31–32
    mandible, 32–33
    teeth, 34–37
    tongue, 26–29
    velopharynx, 29–31
  vocal tract, 25
Suprasegmental. *See* Prosody
Surgery, cleft palate and, 306
Surprisal, defined, 172
Surprise, 54
S-W words, 178
Swallowing
  CMD (Cerebellar mutism) and, 297
  Down syndrome and, 308
  reflex, **39**
Sydenham-Guttentag criteria, 6
Syllabary, 62
  core syllables in, 202
  phonological memory and, 202
Syllabification, 62
Syllable Repetition Task (SRT), 303
Syllable structure level (SSL), 147
  values of, 87–88
Syllables, 43
  blending, 205
  canonical, 81
  correctly understood (SCU), 226

deletion, 205
described, 61–62, 167
phonological structure of, **68**
reduction, 94
segmentation:, 205
structure of, **167**
structure processes, 94
in syllabary, 202
timed language, rhythms, 183
Sylvian fissures, 75
Symmetric acquisition, 262
Syndromic clefting, 50
Syntactic
constituent structure, prosodic phrasing and, 166
Synthetic microfibers, von Frey fibers and, 121
System control theory, defined, 10
Systems approach, 347
research, motor development, 239

T

T cells, 30
Tactile sensitivity, tongue and, 28
Tadoma, 199
Target language, 267
Tasks
decomposition, 249
potency of, 244
specificity of, 244
tDCS (Transcranial Direct Current Stimulation), 348
TDTA (*Templin–Darley Tests of Articulation*), 131
Teeth, 34–37
Templin–Darley Tests of Articulation (TDTA), 131
Temporal
abstraction, described, 241
patterns, 107–108
Teratogenic, to fetus, 309
Tertiary prevention, 325
Testicles, fragile X syndrome, 312
Testosterone
gender differences and, 110
minipuberty and, 110
Tetraplegia, CP (Cerebral palsy) and, 299
Thalamus, contralateral, 77
Theoretical approaches to speech disorders, 8–15
models
computational models, 13–15
dynamic systems theory, 11–12
health-related, 8–10
medical, 8–10
psycholinguistic, 10
schema theory, 12–13
speech production, 10–11
Therapy Outcome Measure (TOM), 328, 329
Thinking, verbal, 73
Thorax, neonatal, 22
Thought, as internal speech, **74**
Thurstone, L.L., 136
Thyroid cartilage, in newborn, 37
Time-by-count method, 126–127
Tip-of-the-tongue (TOT) phenomenon, defined, 60
ToBI (Tones and Break Indices), 188
Toddlers
speech development and, milestones of, 88, **89–91**
TOM (Therapy Outcome Measure), 328, 329
Tonal languages, 166
Tone
unit, 167
of voice, 72
Tones and Break Indices (ToBI), 188
Tongue, 26–29
anterior, fibers of, 27
bracing, 99
jaw coordination, 32–33
movements of, analyzed, 32
posterior, fibers of, 27
size of, 24
strength, Down syndrome and, 308
thrust/extrusion, **39**
tie, 28, 291–292
division, 292
Tonsil
palatine, inflammation of, 30
pharyngeal, 29
Tonsillectomy, 291
Tonsillitis, described, 30
Tonsilltomy, 291
Tonsils, adenotonsillar hypertrophy of, 290

TOT (Tip-of-the-tongue) phenomenon, defined, 60
Tracheal stenosis, Down syndrome and, 308
Training, principles of, 243
Transcranial Direct Current Stimulation (tDCS), 348
Transcriptions, 188
  conversational samples, 133
  defined, 132
  orthographic, measuring intelligibility, 225
  phonetic/phonemic, 95
  uses of, 132
Transfer
  in bilingual phonological development, 266
  cross-linguistic, 266
  described, 245
  negative, 266
  positive, 266
Translanguaging, 274
Transverse
  malocclusions, 35, **36**
  tongue, **39**
Trauma
  CMD (Cerebellar mutism) and, 297
  organic disorders and, 281
Treacher Colling syndrome, 50
Treatment
  defined, 5
  of the empty set, 337–338
Triplegia, CP (Cerebral palsy) and, 299
Trisomy 21. *See* Down syndrome
Triumph, 54
Trochees, 174
Trophoblast, gender differences and, 110

U

UHL (Unilateral hearing loss), 313
Ultrasound (US), 149, 330–331
  Down syndrome and, 309
Uncinate fasciculus, 76
Uncommitted nodes, prolonged activation of, 71
Undershooting, neurology, 146
Undifferentiated gestures, 148
Unilateral
  cleft palate, 305
  hearing loss (UHL), 313
Universal
  discrimination ability, 43
  language receptors, 43
Upper, dorsal pathway, 76
Uptalk, 270
US (Ultrasound), 149
U.S. census, language spoken in home, 263
U.S. National Survey of Children's Health, 268
Utterances
  described, 167–168
  SSL (Syllable structure level) and, 88

V

V3 framework, 284–285
Vagus nerve
  functions served by, 83
  parent-infant interactions and, 83
Valproate intake, ASD (Autism spectrum disorder) and, 294
Variability
  assessed, 303
  defined, 95, 303
  of practice hypothesis, 244
  revealed by, 95–96
  of speech production, 94–96
Variable practice, 250
Variegated babble, 84
VAS (Visual Analog Scale), 138
  biases, 138–139
VDLI (Vocal Development Landmarks Interview), 154
Velicepiglottic engagement, 24
Velocardiofacial syndrome, 50
Velopharyngeal
  anatomy, changes in, 291
  DFMs (Developmental Functional Modules), 85
  valving, 291
Velopharynx, 29–31
  major forms of, **29**
Ventral pathways
  language and, 75–77

lower, 76
Ventricle invasion, CMD (Cerebellar mutism) and, 298
Verbal
communication, 55–56
dyspraxia profile, 143
mediation, 73
reduced output of, 295
self-monitoring, 70
thinking, 73
Verbal Motor Assessment of Children (VMPAC), 143
Verbal Motor Production Assessment for Children, Revised (VMPAC-R), 141
Verification, described, 285
Vermis incision, CMD (Cerebellar mutism) and, 298
Vernacular dialect, 270
Vertical
analog visual scale (VVAS), 138
malocclusions, 35, **36**
VHI (Voice Handicap Index), 165
VHI-10 (Voice Handicap Index-10), 165
Vibration, sound by, 159
Video games, ADHD (Attention deficit hyperactivity disorder) and, 293
Viral infections, hearing loss and, 313
Viscerocranium, 40
Visual, factors involved, speech intelligibility, 231
Visual Analog Scale (VAS), 138
biases, 138–139
Visually impaired, visual-to-tactile substitution and, 28
Visual-to-tactile substitution, visually impaired and, 28
Visuo-spatial sketchpad, 201–203
Vital capacity, defined, 123
VMPAC (Verbal Motor Assessment of Children), 143
Focal Oromotor Function subtest, 310
VMPAC-R (Verbal Motor Production Assessment for Children, Revised), 141
VMS (Vocal motor schemes), 136
VOCA (Voice output communication aid), 7
Vocal
behavior, 217
demand, 162
response, 162
effect, 161–162
expressions of emotions, 54–55
folds, 37
structure of, **38**
fry, 270–271
function, variations in, 163
fundamental frequency, 25
organs, neural connections and, 1
pitch, 296
roll, 270
tract
1-year-old girl and 18-year-old woman, **26**
cavities of, 24
growth of, 24–25
of infants, **25**
of neonates, 23–24
Vocal Development Landmarks Interview (VDLI), 154
Vocal motor schemes (VMS), 136
Vocal range profile (VRP), 128
Vocalizations
infants, 79–88
capabilities/processes of, 82–84
developmental functional modules, 84–86
goal babbling, 86
metrics of phonetic development, 87–88
stage models of, 79–82
Voice, 160–165
defined, 159, 162
disorders, 4
in children, 162–165
defined, 280
gender, 110
handicap, 165
imagery, 73
inner, 73
loudness, 161–162
monotone, 297
pitch, f_0, 160–161
prosody profile, 296
quality, 159, 162
prosody and, 173
quality-of-life, 165

Voice *(continued)*
strained-strangled, CP (Cerebral palsy) and, 299
tone of, 72
tremor, 297
vocal effect, 161–162
The Voice Handicap Index (VHI), 165
Voice Handicap Index (VHI), 165
Voice Handicap Index-10 (VHI-10), 165
Voice onset time (VOT), 107, **108**
Voice output communication aid (VOCA), 7
Voiceless
/θ/, 102
stops
in American English, 193
in syllable initial position, 108
Volubility
fragile X syndrome, 312
vocal development and, 82, 83
Voluntary motor control, 237
von Frey fibers, 121
VoQS, 162
VOT (Voice onset time), **108**
Vowel formant frequency, **230**
Vowel space area (VSA), 105–106, 230–231
Vowels
acoustic analysis of, 147–148
distorted, 297
formant frequencies, 105–106
point, 87
quadrilaterals, **106**
speech sounds and, 93–94
VRP (Vocal range profile), 128
VRQOL instrument, 165
VSA (Vowel space area), 105–106
VSA (Vowel Space Area), 231
VVAS (Vertical visual analog scale), 138

W

Waldeyer's Ring, 29, 30
Walking, gestures and, 82
WCM (Word complexity measure), 147
Weakness, CP (Cerebral palsy) and, 299
Weaning, ankyloglossia and, 291
Weight
ankyloglossia and, 291
hearing loss and, 313
WEIRD (Western, Educated, Industrialized, Rich, and Democratic), 54
Well-being
defined, 326
promotion of, 326
Well-Formedness Condition, 196
OT (Optimality theory), 197
Wernicke, Carl, dual-pathway model, 74
Wernicke's area
described, 75
word images, linked to Broca's area, 74–75
Western, Educated, Industrialized, Rich, and Democratic (WEIRD), 54
Wheel of Emotion, 54
White matter (WM), changes in, second language and, 261
WHO (World Health Organization)
on health promotion, 326
outcome measure defined by, 327
on sex and gender, 48
Williams syndrome, 50
WM (White matter), changes in, second language and, 261
Word
boundaries, 43
awareness, 205
complexity measure (WCM), 147
Word Encoding by Activation and VERification (Comprehension-based model WEAVER++), 70
Words
core vocabulary, 336
knowledge, emotional, 72
producing, 71–73
affect, 72–73
production of, 95
Wordsworth, William, 79
Work Group on Neuroimaging Markers of Psychiatric Disorders, described, 285
Working memory, model of, **201**
World Health Assembly, ICF and, 118
World Health Organization (WHO)
on health promotion, 326
outcome measure defined by, 327
on sex and gender, 48

X

X chromosome, 47
  fragile X syndrome, 312
X-linked
  inheritance, 49
    dominant, 49
    recessive, 50
XX chromosome, 47

Y

Y chromosome, 47
Youth. *See* Children

Z

Zinc-copper cycles, ASD (Autism spectrum disorder) and, 294